Ibuprofen

Ibuprofen

A critical bibliographic review

Edited by

K D Rainsford

Sheffield Hallam University, Sheffield, UK

TAYLOR AND FRANCIS LIMITED

UK	Taylor & Francis, 11 New Fetter Lane, London EC4P 4EE
USA	Taylor & Francis Inc., 325 Chestnut Street, Philadelphia PA 19106

Taylor & Francis is an imprint of the Taylor & Francis Group

British Library Cataloguing in Publication Data

A catalogue record for this book is available from the British Library.
ISBN 0-7484-0694-8 (cased)

Library of Congress Cataloguing in Publication Data are available

Cover design by Hyberts, Wattham St Lawrence, Berkshire
Typeset in 10/14 Stone Serif by Graphicraft Ltd, Hong Kong
Printed and bound by T.J. International Ltd, Padstow, Cornwall

Ibuprofen

A critical bibliographic review

Preface

Ibuprofen is one of the safest drugs employed today for the treatment of pain, inflammation and fever. The development and extensive clinical use of this drug is one of the success stories of the pharmaceutical industry. In this day and age such successes are few since we tend to hear more of the negative or unsafe aspects attributed to the actions of many drugs. In respect of relative safety, this is really the success for ibuprofen since it has a wide range of tolerance while at the same time being often more effective on a dose-for-weight basis than aspirin and paracetamol in the treatment of many painful conditions.

In rheumatic diseases it is probably the drug of first choice in many countries. Although it is certainly not the most potent among the NSAIDs, what is clear is that it represents a good balance of efficacy over a wide dosage range compared with safety.

As the confidence over the safety of this drug developed following its introduction as one of the first of the newer NSAIDs introduced in the late 1960s, so the case developed for its switch from being a prescription-only drug to non-prescription (over-the-counter, or OTC) status worldwide. Now it is well recognized as probably being among the safer of the OTC analgesics available today. While not being without side-effects as noted in several chapters in this book, the worldwide incidence of reported adverse reactions, especially those in the gastrointestinal system, is relatively low at prescription and OTC dosages compared with others of its class.

Ibuprofen has been studied extensively not only for its mechanisms and clinical application, but also with others of its class. In this respect, like aspirin, paracetamol or indomethacin, it has become a universal standard for comparison in many clinical conditions and experimental models.

Bringing together the large amount of literature available on ibuprofen in what is the first published monograph has presented a major challenge. I am most indebted to the experts who assisted me in the preparation of chapters in this book, where we have attempted to give a balanced and comprehensive coverage of the extensive literature on the clinical studies and applications of ibuprofen; the historical aspects of its development, chemistry and pharmaceutical properties, pharmacological activity and toxicity; as well as its novel applications for treating non-pain states where ibuprofen has been of particular interest (e.g. in the prevention of colon, mammary or other cancers, Alzheimer's disease, diabetic retinopathy, treatment of lung inflammation in cystic fibrosis, to name a few). As we discover more about the molecular and cellular modes of action in relation to the actions as an anti-inflammatory agent, so insight will come regarding how this drug works in pain and inflammation but also in the above mentioned novel non-pain states where knowledge of its mechanism(s) of action(s) is particularly puzzling.

This book is dedicated to the original discoverers of ibuprofen — Dr Stewart Adams, the late Dr John Nicholson, and their colleagues at the Boots Pure Drug Company in

Nottingham (UK); and to the immense number of scientists and physicians worldwide who have undertaken investigations on this drug and without whose work we would not have so much knowledge as is available now in the public domain on this drug's actions and uses. I would also like to pay special tribute to the many colleagues who have helped in my understanding of this drug, and who encouraged me to put together this monograph. I am mindful of the fact that there are probably some points which could or should have been included; it is difficult to be exhaustive in coverage of the literature.

My special thanks go to Mrs Veronica Rainsford-Koechli and Mrs Marguerite Lyons who provided an immense amount of secretarial support in the preparation of this book.

K D Rainsford
Sheffield Hallam University
Sheffield, UK

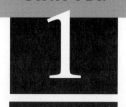

History and Development of Ibuprofen

K D RAINSFORD

Division of Biomedical Sciences and Biomedical Research Centre,
Sheffield Hallam University, Pond Street, Sheffield S1 1WB, UK

Contents

1.1 INTRODUCTION

The history of ibuprofen began over 40 years ago and is inextricably linked to understanding of the concepts of the pathogenesis of inflammatory diseases and the actions of therapeutic agents used at that time. The principal initiator of this research leading to the discovery of ibuprofen was Dr Stewart Adams (Figure 1.1), a pharmacologist in the Research Department of The Boots Pure Drug Company Ltd at Nottingham, UK. His aim was to find analgesic drugs with improved efficacy over aspirin. As with all major discoveries, there is an important personal element and what has been attempted here is to bring together information to show what were the most significant events and thoughts that were important for the discovery process. I am most indebted to Stewart Adams for a considerable amount of information and historical detail that enabled me to write this important chapter. I am also especially grateful to him for discussing what have been most interesting historical details and for giving me an insight into those earlier years and the thinking behind the discovery of ibuprofen.

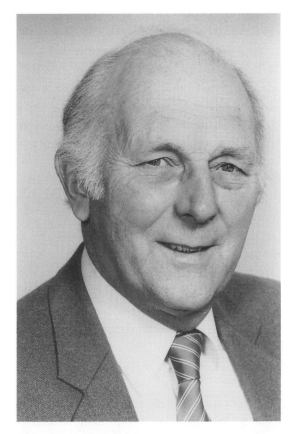

Figure 1.1: A photograph of Dr Stewart Adams taken in 1987.

Stewart Adams has written a detailed account of the pharmacological aspects of the discovery of the propionic acids (Adams, 1992). The late Dr John Nicholson, who first synthesized ibuprofen, reviewed in depth the medicinal chemistry of the propionic acids and the chemical discovery process underlying the development of ibuprofen (Nicholson, 1982). It is not proposed to give a total account of what these expert authors have already reviewed in depth. I hope more to emphasize the main thinking at the time and key events involved in the discovery of what has been one of the most successful NSAIDs developed since aspirin.

The standard drugs for treating rheumatoid arthritis and other painful arthritic diseases at the time when Stewart Adams started his research were aspirin and cortisone. The pioneering studies supported by the Empire Rheumatism Council (later to become the Arthritis and Rheumatism Council) and the Medical Research Council in the United Kingdom had established the efficacy of cortisone and aspirin in the relief of pain and soft-tissue swelling in rheumatoid arthritis. However, the shortcoming of both drugs were becoming strikingly evident even at the time of these reports.

In the 1950s when Boots were beginning this research, only a few other companies had begun research programmes into aspirin-type drugs, notably Dr T Y Shen at Merck and Co. (Rahway, NJ, USA) and Dr Steve Winder at Parke Davis (Ann Arbor, MI, USA). Before this Dr G Wilhelmi at J R Geigy AG (Basel, Switzerland) had worked on derivatives of amidopyrine and other pyrazoles. In 1958 Winder and his colleagues published an important paper indicating their thinking about the use of the ultraviolet (UV) erythema technique for determining the anti-inflammatory activity of novel compounds. This assay was similar to that in use at Boots and they had, moreover, obtained similar results with standard drugs (e.g. aspirin). The Parke Davis group eventually produced mefenamic acid, flufenamic acid and other fenamates as a result of the initial testing of compounds in this assay.

Boots, however, started with a distinct disadvantage with their meagre resources as their Pharmacology Department was housed in a group of old rambling buildings attached to a Victorian house located in the outskirts of Nottingham (Figures 1.2–1.5). It was moved there at the beginning of the Second World War from the centre of Nottingham as a precaution against bombing — a wise move since part of the Research Department was destroyed in an air raid in 1941. The first six years of the research on new aspirin-type drugs was thus carried out under most unsatisfactory conditions. Adams' laboratory (Figure 1.2) was in one of the 'front rooms' of the house and later he was able to acquire the kitchen and larder (Figure 1.4) as additional accommodation.

1.2   HISTORICAL BACKGROUND

It has been said that the road to drug development is a minefield, the path through which is both tortuous and dangerous. One of the leading medicinal chemists in the field of inflammatory drug research, T Y Shen, who developed the NSAIDs indomethacin, sulindac

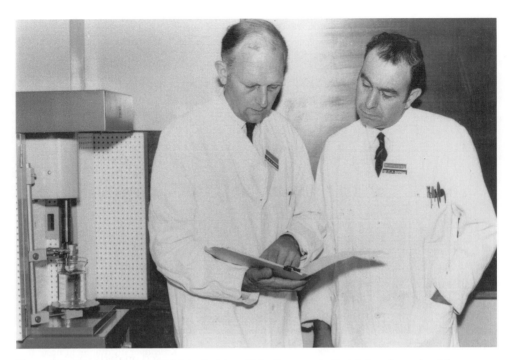

Figure 1.2: Stewart Adams with his technician, Colin Burrows, in their laboratory, about the mid-1960s.

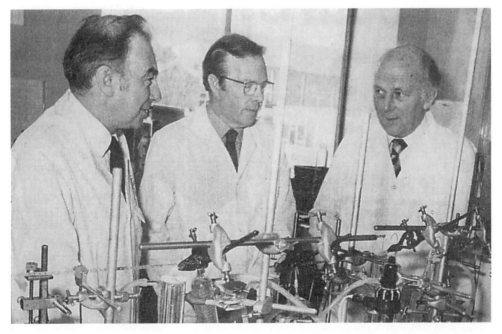

Figure 1.3: Stewart Adams (right) with Colin Burrows (left) and John Nicholson in the mid-1960s.

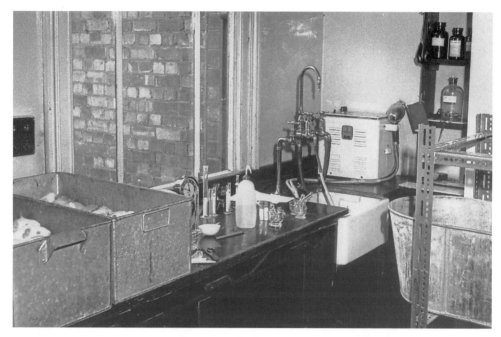

Figure 1.4: Part of the laboratory ('kitchen') in 1957 showing the Kromayer ultraviolet lamp in the background and guinea-pig holding cages on either side.

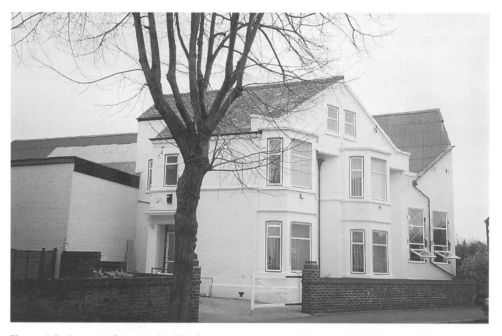

Figure 1.5: A recent photograph of the house where Stewart Adams had his laboratory in Rutland Road, West Bridgford, Nottingham and where the early pharmacological studies leading to the discovery of ibuprofen were performed.

and diflunisal at Merck and Co. (USA), described the period, 1955–1970, during which the earlier NSAIDs such as ibuprofen and indomethacin were developed as the 'golden era' of Edisonian empiricism (Shen, 1984). Without doubt this era set the stage for the later proliferation of NSAIDs in the 1970s and 1980s, many of which were discovered serendipitously (Shen, 1984) and are considered by some to represent little advance over those drugs developed previously. The mechanisms underlying the development of the rheumatic diseases for which these drugs were intended were little understood. The drugs available for treating pain and inflammation in rheumatic diseases in the 1950s to 1960s included aspirin, the other salicylates, aminophenols (phenacetin) and pyrazolones, which dated from the beginning of the century; phenylbutazone (which was originally used to solubilize aminopyrine and accidently discovered as an effective anti-inflammatory drug); and the corticosteroids discovered in the 1950s (Shen, 1984). Gold salts had also been found in the 1930s to have disease-modifying activity in rheumatoid and related arthropathies, though in the 1950s they were regarded as very toxic.

Thus, with the current remedies for rheumatic diseases being aspirin, corticosteroids, phenylbutazone and, to a lesser extent gold salts, the need was readily identified in the 1950s for a more potent drug than aspirin, one that would not produce the potentially fatal side-effect of agranulocytosis seen with phenylbutazone or the serious side-effects with corticosteroids. Indeed a report (No. 848 from the Pharmacology and Physiology Division of the Research Department at the Boots Pure Drug Company) dated 5 March 1956 and prepared by Dr Adams noted:

> *Apart from cortisone and related steroids, aspirin and phenylbutazone are the only two drugs which are universally used to bring about relief of pain and increased mobility in rheumatoid arthritis. Aspirin, because it is a very safe drug, is usually preferred.*

Also,

> *From discussions with Dr Duthie [a leading rheumatologist of the time] at Edinburgh [Northern General Hospital], Dr Bywaters [also a leading rheumatologist] at Taplow and Dr Hill at Stoke Mandeville, it is obvious that aspirin and phenylbutazone are the only established non-hormonal compounds in the treatment of rheumatoid arthritis, while aspirin and sodium salicylate are very effective in the treatment of rheumatic fever.*

Furthermore,

> *We believe that virtually no attempt has been made to investigate thoroughly the anti-inflammatory properties of salicylate-type anti-rheumatics. In view of the widespread use of aspirin and sodium salicylate over the past 50 years this seems to be an amazing omission.*

CHAPTER 1

The key to the need to develop a drug that would be superior to aspirin, less toxic than phenylbutazone and without the hormonal associations and side-effects associated with cortisone derives from the following quotes in Dr Adams' report:

> *We recently discussed our results [from guinea-pig UV erythema assays with benzoic/salicylic acids and related compounds], with Dr Duthie of the Rheumatism Research Unit, Edinburgh, and he was strongly in favour of the type of investigation [involving the development of a drug to replace existing agents] which is envisaged here. Dr Duthie who is a staunch supporter of aspirin and opposed to cortisone, believes that a 'super' aspirin or non-toxic phenylbutazone would have an immense market.*

Moreover:

> *The main disadvantage of the compounds of this type [pyrazoles] which have been used clinically e.g. phenazone, amidopyrine, and phenylbutazone, is that prolonged administration of therapeutic doses may give rise to toxic side-effects including agranulocytosis. This we believe is the main objection to the further investigation of compounds of this nature.*

It is important to note that at this stage Adams believed that the analgesic action of aspirin could be explained entirely on its anti-inflammatory properties — a hypothesis that despite some subsequent qualification has proved at least partly valid.

This report by Dr Adams is interesting from the insight that it gives to the thinking about anti-rheumatic therapies at the time and the potential for commercial developments. An interesting aspect concerning the use of aspirin and ideas about developing a 'super' aspirin is that no mention was made in the report of the gastrointestinal side-effects of aspirin that were discussed in the literature at the time. The gastrointestinal side-effects of aspirin were recognized by many rheumatologists at that time. Although not mentioned in report No. 848, it was an aim of Adams' group to produce a compound that would be 'well tolerated by the gastrointestinal tract'. Extensive studies were carried out to find those compounds with the best potential in this respect. Over the years this was always a major target in the studies by the group and it is not entirely good luck that ibuprofen is now considered to be the safest of the NSAIDs.

1.3 INITIAL STAGES

This report by Dr Adams in 1956 was making the case for development of a programme for 'non-hormonal' anti-rheumatic compounds; at this time the 'project' team was merely Adams and one technician. Adams and Colin Burrows had already modified the UV erythema assay in guinea-pigs first described by Wilhelmi (1949), who had used this to identify

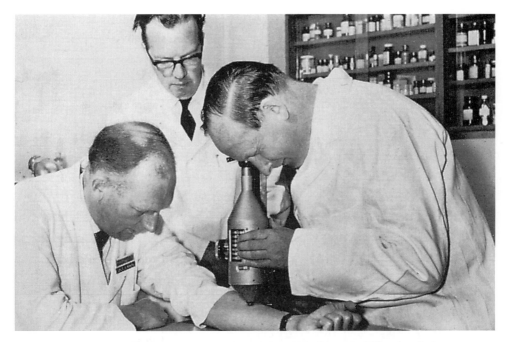

Figure 1.6: Trafuryl erythema assay on the volar surface of the forearm: Adams, Nicholson and Cobb.

the anti-inflammatory activity of phenylbutazone (Adams and Cobb, 1958). Adams and Burrows later developed a more sophisticated technique requiring only a 20-second exposure to UV without the need to anaesthetize the animal, a feature that not only removed the confounding effects of anaesthesia but also enabled them to test appreciably more compounds each day. Their technique (personal communication, Dr S S Adams, 1998) was as follows:

> *Shaved albino guinea-pigs were dosed orally with aspirin or test compound 30 min before a 20-second exposure to ultraviolet light from a Kromayer lamp. Two hours later the degree of erythema was estimated visually on a scale of 0–4 (maximum = 4) by an observer who was unaware of the dosage schedules. The 2 hr erythema could be completely suppressed by oral doses of 160 mg/kg aspirin and this drug was employed as a positive standard in each day's experiments. In fact there was only suppression of the erythema at 2 hr since it became fully developed after 24 hr.*

Adams and Cobb, 1963

One of the factors that was important in the decision to proceed with the use of this technique was the fact that corticosteroids were inactive. Thus the actions of

DATE 19.12.6 BATH NO. 271 DOSED 11.30 EXPOSED 12.20 EXAMINED 2.20 F, 2229

Animal.	Wt.	Vol	RD number	mg/kg	Result		Animal	Wt.	Vol	RD number	mg/kg	Result	
RH	780	3.12	RB1448	160	2	1	25. YHTB	720	1.44	RP1	80	1	O
2. RHT	770	3.08		160	O	2	26. YHGB	650	260	RP1	160	1	1
3. RHBT	710	0.71	Aspirin	40	1	3	27. GH	650	260		160	O	O
4. RHYT	750	50	RB1472	10	O	O	28. GHT	640	268	Aspirin	160	O	O
5. RHGT	570	114		10	O	O	29. GHRT	710	284	RB1461	20	3	3
6. RHB	690	276	RB1472	20	O	O	30. GHBT	700	140	RB1461	10	4	4
7. RHHB	690	276		20	O	O	31. GHYT	720	265	RB1461	acid 10	4	4
8. RHHB	620	248	Aspirin	160	2	3	32. GHB	630	252	RB1461	20	4	4
9. BH	760	152	Aspirin	80	1	3	33. GHTB	670	134	RB1461	40	3	4
10. BHT	680	1.36	RB1472 13599	40	1	1	34. GHRYB	660	132		40	1	3
11. BHRT	620	124		40	O	O	35. GHBTB	690	1.96	RB1461	80	1	1
12. BHYT	790	3.16	RB1472	80	2	1	36. RT	720	288		80	2	2
13. BHGT	760	284		80	1	O	37. BT	720	0.72	RB1464	20	2	4
14. BHB	760	076	Aspirin	40	2	4	38. YT	740	0.74		20	1	2
15. BHTB	830	332	S20	240	3	4	39. GT	820	164	RB1464	40	2	3
16. BHYTB	800	320	S21	240	4	4	40. RB	750	150		40	O	1
17. BHYTRB	630	252	13599	80	4	4	41. BB	630	252	RB1464	80	O	2
18. BHGTB3	700	280		80	4	4	42. YB	660	264		80	1	O
19. YH	650	260	S22	240	4	4	43. GB	710	284	13103	80	4	4
20. YHT	780	3.12	S23	240	3	4	44. RTB	740	308	13088	80	3	4
21. YHRT	580	116	Aspirin	80	O	3	45. BTB	580	232	13122	40	4	4
22. YHBT	700	0.70	RP1	40	O	O	46. YTB	700	280	S11	240	4	4
23. YHGT	750	0.75		40	O	1	47. GTB	680	272	S13	240	3	4
24. YHB	630	1.26	RP1	80	O	O	48. RTBB	600	240	S14	240	4	4
							BTRB	690	276	S15	240	4	4
							BTYB	530	252	S16	240	3	4

Figure 1.7: Extracts from the files showing the first testing of ibuprofen on 19 December 1961. Each figure is the degree of redness (on an increasing scale of 0 to 4) for each individual guinea-pig. Ibuprofen was RB 1472, an early temporary number. The two sets of readings represent observations before and after light 'stroking' of the skin in the erythematous area; the 'stroking' appeared to enhance the sensitivity of detection.

aspirin-type drugs in this assay could be regarded as specific to this class of compounds. Later pioneering studies both of Collier (1963) on the 'antagonism' of kinins by aspirin, phenylbutazone, mefenamic acid and other compounds, and of Vane (1971) showing that the anti-inflammatory, analgesic and antipyretic effects of aspirin and related

PATENT SPECIFICATION

NO DRAWINGS

971,700

Inventors: JOHN STUART NICHOLSON
and STEWART SANDERS ADAMS

Date of filing Complete Specification: Jan. 12, 1962.

Application Date: Feb. 2, 1961.   *No. 3999/61.*

Complete Specification Published: Sept. 30, 1964.

© *Crown Copyright 1964.*

Index at acceptance:—C2 C(2A2, 2A14, 2R15, 2T16, 3A8A2, 3A8B2, 3A8C3, 3A8K, 3A10A4E, 3A10A4F, 3A10A5A1, 3A10A5A2, 3A10A5E, 3A10A5F, 3A10A5G2, 3A10A5K, 3A10B2C, 3A10B5E, 3A10E3C1, 3A10E4A3, 3A10E5D, 3A10E5E, 3A10E5F1A, 3A10E5F1E, 3A10E5F2A, 3A10E5F3A, 3A10E5F3D, 3A13A3A2, 3A13A3A3, 3A13A3B1, 3A13A3F3); A5 B(1S, 2S)

International Classification:—C 07 c (A 61 k)

COMPLETE SPECIFICATION

Anti-Inflammatory Agents

We, BOOTS PURE DRUG COMPANY LIMITED, a British Company, of Station Street, Nottingham, England, do hereby declare the invention, for which we pray that a patent may be granted to us, and the method by which it is to be performed, to be particularly described in and by the following statement: —

This invention relates to phenylalkane derivatives. More particularly it relates to novel pharmaceutical and veterinary compositions which comprise as the active ingredient one or more members of a specified group of derivatives of toluene. The invention also relates to the provision of novel members of this specified group of compounds.

It is an object of the invention to provide therapeutic compositions for the relief of pain, fever and inflammation in man and animals which do not suffer from the disadvantages of similar therapeutic compositions based on aspirin, phenylbutazone or adrenocorticosteroids.

We have now discovered that compounds of the general formula I

$$R^1 \text{—}\!\!\left\langle\!\!\!\bigcirc\!\!\!\right\rangle\!\!\text{—} \overset{\displaystyle CH-X}{\underset{\displaystyle R^2}{|}}$$

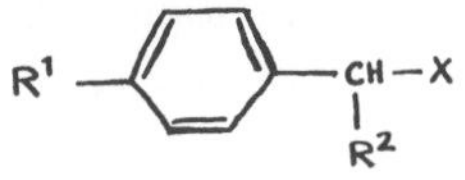

I

wherein R^1 represents ethyl, propyl, butyl, alkenyl (C_2—C_4), pentyl (except n-pentyl), alkoxy (C_2—C_3), allyloxy, phenoxy, phenylthio or cycloalkyl (C_5—C_7) optionally substituted by methyl or ethyl in the 1-position, R^2 represents hydrogen or methyl and X represents the radical COOH, COOR³ wherein R^3 represents alkyl (C_1—C_8) or optionally N-alkylated aminoalkyl (C_2—C_8), COOM wherein M represents the ammonium ion or a single

equivalent of a non-toxic metallic cation, COOH.B wherein B represents a non-toxic organic base, $CONH_2$, CH_2NH_2 or the group CH_2OR^4 where R^4 represents hydrogen or lower alkanoyl (C_1—C_3) have valuable anti-inflammatory, analgesic and antipyretic properties.

Furthermore in general the compounds exhibit low toxicity and low irritancy to the gastric mucosa, they do not have other undesirable pharmacological activities which might give rise to unwanted side effects and they are stable in the presence of water.

According to the present invention there are provided therapeutic compositions comprising as active ingredient one or more compounds of the general formula I in association with a pharmaceutically acceptable diluent or carrier.

The following compounds are typical of the active compounds of the general formula I, but do not limit the invention in any way: —

4-*n*-Propylphenylacetic acid
4-Ethoxyphenylacetic acid
4-Isopropylphenylacetic acid
4-propoxyphenylacetic acid
4-Isopropoxyphenylacetic acid
4-*s*-Butylphenylacetic acid
4-Allyloxyphenylacetic acid
4-*t*-Butylphenylacetic acid
4-Cyclopentylphenylacetic acid
4-*iso*butylphenylacetic acid
4-Cycloheptylphenylacetic acid
4-Cyclohexylphenylacetic acid
4-(1-Ethylpropyl)phenylacetic acid
4-Phenoxyphenylacetic acid
4-(1,2-dimethylpropyl)phenylacetic acid
4-Phenylthiophenylacetic acid
α-(4-Cyclohexylphenyl)propionic acid

[*Price 4s. 6d.*]

Figure 1.8: The Patent Specification for the UK Patent No. 971,700 covering the therapeutic compositions of phenylalkanoic acid derivatives, including ibuprofen, for the relief of pain, fever and inflammation that were developed by Dr John Nicholson and Dr Stewart Adams. The filing of the complete specification was on 12 January 1962.

compounds are related to their effects on the production of prostaglandins were important in understanding the actions of these NSAIDs. However, it is important to note that the discovery of ibuprofen and other NSAIDs did not proceed with the advantage of knowing how aspirin-type drugs worked.

Adams and his colleagues had assayed the anti-erythemic activity of a number of salicylates that had been proposed or shown to have anti-inflammatory or pain-relieving effects in rheumatic patients, including the hydroxylated metabolites of salicylate, most of which had proved to have low or nonexistent activity. These results on the development of salicylates and other NSAID derivatives at that time have been discussed in an extensive review by Adams and Cobb (1967) and also by Rainsford (1984). The stage was therefore set for developing a 'super' aspirin. The UV erythema assay had been validated and, in general, a number of salicylates/benzoates tested most of which had been found to also have comparable (in)activity in patients (Adams and Cobb, 1967).

1.4   COMPOUNDS IN DEVELOPMENT

The case for chemical support set out in the report (No. 848) by Dr Adams was successful and the late Dr John Nicholson, an organic chemist (see later) joined Adams and a testing programme was commenced using the guinea-pig UV erythema.

It was clear from report No. 848 that the first compounds to be made would be salicylates and phthalates. There was great optimism, since such compounds had never been investigated before, that agents more potent than aspirin would emerge. This proved to be so, but sadly they were always more toxic than aspirin. This line of attack was therefore abandoned, but the studies proved invaluable since they indicated the importance of the carboxylic group of aspirin for anti-inflammatory activity. It was therefore decided to examine a range of simple compounds with carboxylic acid moieties. Among these a number of phenoxyalkanoics were found to be more active than aspirin in inhibiting the UV erythema. This group of compounds were originally made by Boots as herbicides and were available in the files at that company (Nicholson, 1982).

It is fascinating to note that two plant growth regulators — an indolylacetic acid and a phenoxyalkanoic acid — were the lead compounds at both Merck and Boots. These eventually led to the development of indomethacin and ibuprofen respectively (Shen, 1971; Nicholson, 1982).

John Nicholson was the chemist who led the team involved in the synthesis of the phenoxy compounds and the other progenitors of ibuprofen. After the screening of over 600 phenoxyalkanoic acids made by Nicholson and his colleagues, two compounds emerged in 1958 with potential anti-inflammatory activity: BTS 7268 with twice the anti-inflammatory activity of aspirin, and BTS 8402 which was 6–10 times more potent (Table 1.1). The ethyl ester of BTS 8402 was prepared on the basis that this might have less gastric intolerance than aspirin but was found inactive in the treatment of rheumatoid

TABLE 1.1

Pharmacological activities of some substituted phenoxypropionic, phenylacetic and propionic acids developed by Boots.
Activities of the compounds are compared with aspirin rated = 1

B.T.S. no.	Structure	Activity (aspirin = 1)		
		Anti-inflammatory	Analgesic	Antipyretic
7268	C_2H_5—C$_6$H$_4$—O–CH(CH$_3$)COOH	2		
8402	biphenyl—O–CH(CH$_3$)COOH	6–10	1–2	0.4
10335	$(CH_3)_3C$—C$_6$H$_4$—CH$_2$COOH	4	4	2–4
10499	cyclohexyl—C$_6$H$_4$—CH$_2$COOH	4	10	4
Ibufenac	$(CH_3)_2CHCH_2$—C$_6$H$_4$—CH$_2$COOH	2–4	2–4	4
Ibuprofen	$(CH_3)_2CHCH_2$—C$_6$H$_4$—CH(CH$_3$)COOH	16–32	30	20

From Adams (1987a); reproduced with permission of the Editor of *Chemistry in Britain*.

arthritis at 1.8 g daily (Nicholson, 1982). As Adams (1987a) queried: 'Did this mean that after seven years our entire programme had been based on a false hypothesis — and if so, what should we do next?'

The turning point came with Adams adopting a newly published American technique for analgesic activity, the Randall–Selitto assay based on the relief of pain from pressure applied to the inflamed paws of rats. Up to this time there was no method of showing an analgesic action of aspirin in animals at reasonable oral doses. Using this technique and an anti-pyretic assay it was discovered that the analgesic activity of BTS 8402 was only comparable with that of aspirin and that its antipyretic activity even lower (Table 1.1). Adams then postulated that to have anti-rheumatic activity these compounds should have the triad of analgesic, antipyretic as well as anti-inflammatory activities; properties that were found in the closely related phenylalkanoic acids (Nicholson, 1982).

Even before the demise of the phenoxyalkanoic acids in the 1960s, Nicholson had moved on to develop phenylalkanoic acids, of which the 4-biphenylalkanoic acids had been found to be very potent (Nicholson, 1982) but also very ulcerogenic in the gastrointestinal tract of dogs. A very interesting decision was made at this point to first develop the some-what less potent phenylacetic acids rather than the propionic acids because it seemed, in view of toxicological data then available, that a safer candidate product could be selected from this less potent group (Nicholson, 1982). In retrospect this approach, prompted by a concern for safety and the belief that the propionics were more toxic than they eventually proved to be, was a wrong decision that cost several years work.

From the phenylacetic acids that were synthesized by Nicholson, three compounds emerged (Table 1.1) that had the triad of therapeutic activity sought by Adams. The first of these, BTS 10335, proved active in rheumatoid arthritis but was abandoned in the first trial because it produced rashes in 5 out of 12 patients (Adams, 1987a). Unfortunately, the development of skin rashes was not a condition that could have been predicted from animal studies then (though today it might be possible to postulate the occurrence of this based on knowledge of drug metabolism and comparative irritancy studies *in vitro* and *in vivo*).

To be sure that the occurrence of the rashes was not due to manufacturing impurities, three members of the Research Department took highly purified BTS 10335 for one week at twice the dose taken by patients. One of the three subjects developed a severe rash. This clearly established that the effect was inherent in the compound.

1.5 IBUFENAC — ALMOST THERE, BUT FOR LIVER TOXICITY

The next candidate selected for clinical trial was ibufenac, BTS 11654, a 4-isobutylacetic acid, which proved effective in clinical trials in rheumatoid arthritis and did not pro-duce rashes. Unfortunately, after prolonged use it produced marked liver toxicity in some patients in the United Kingdom (Adams, 1987a). There had been no evidence of liver toxicity in any of the animal studies performed by Dr Barrie Lessel. Curiously, this side-effect did not occur in Japanese people, for reasons that are still not apparent. Indeed, ibufenac continued to be used successfully in Japan for several years after it was withdrawn in the United Kingdom (Adams, 1987a) whereupon it was superseded by ibuprofen in that country.

1.6 MORE SETBACKS

In the meantime another acetic acid, BTS 10499, with a cyclohexyl moiety in the 4-position, was found effective in rheumatoid arthritis patients but, again, this compound produced rashes and was therefore discarded (Adams, 1987a).

1.7 MORE LEARNING

A key finding emerged from studies carried out by Dr Eric Cliffe on the biodisposition of radiolabelled 4-substituted phenylacetic acids compared with that of the 4-phenylpropionic acids (Adams, 1987a). It emerged that the former were distributed more extensively in the body and accumulated in a number of organs to nothing like the same extent as the 4-phenylpropionic acids (Adams, 1987a). Moreover, some early fears about the gastric ulcerogenicity of the propionics in dogs were allayed when further studies showed that some of these compounds had very long plasma half-lives in dogs. Since it had already been shown by Lessel and Adams that the main ulcerogenic action of these compounds was systemic rather than local (a completely unexpected novel finding), it was possible to predict that the clinical potential of the more potent propionics was better than originally thought.

It was these and later findings of the high toxicity of long half-life phenylpropionics in rats that convinced Adams of the importance of plasma half-life in the safety of NSAIDs, and that one of the major factors relating to the safety of ibuprofen was its short half-life of about 2 h. Many years later, based on these earlier experiences, he published data to show that there is a relationship, clinically, between adverse reactions of NSAIDs and their half-lives (Adams, 1987b, 1988).

1.8 IBUPROFEN

It is ironic that eventually there was a surfeit of active phenylalkanoic acid compounds: activity occurred over a wide chemical range. It was necessary, therefore, to perform extensive biochemical and toxicological studies among a number of preferred compounds before ibuprofen, not the most potent, was chosen as being potentially the safest. This decision was based on a whole range of biological data — pharmacological, biochemical and toxicological — that had by then been collected on the phenylalkanoics, and the decision to choose safety rather than potency has proved to be the correct one.

1.8.1   First clinical trials

The first clinical trials with ibuprofen (RD 13621, *syn.* BTS 13621) were performed by Dr Tom Chalmers of the Rheumatic Diseases Unit at the Northern General Hospital, Edinburgh in six patients with rheumatoid arthritis. His report of 8 February 1966 describes a randomized trial in which ibuprofen was given at two dosage levels of 300 mg or 600 mg daily for one week at a time and the results compared with that from one week's treatment with aspirin 3.6 g/day. The allocation to individual drug treatment was random, but there was no washout period in between. Laboratory investigations were performed at the beginning and end of each week of the trial and included hemoglobin, erythrocyte sedimentation rate, total leukocyte and platelet counts, liver transaminases, prothrombin activity, serum urate, urine analysis and tests for occult blood. The patients were assessed for grip strength, joint tenderness and joint size each day.

The results obtained are shown in Figure 1.9, from which it can be seen that ibuprofen at both 300 mg and 600 mg daily produced improvement in grip strength and that there was a trend towards improvement in pressure tolerance (a measure of joint tenderness) with less marked improvement in joint size. One patient on aspirin 3.6 g daily showed faecal occult blood while all the others showed a weak or negative reaction. There were no differences in laboratory parameters observed with any of the treatments. Dr Chalmers noted in his report: 'The pattern of daily measurements [however] shows that throughout the three weeks of trial there was a trend to slight improvement unrelated to the sequence of treatments. This in turn suggests that RD 13621 was adequate substitution for aspirin in the dosages compared and that there was little difference between the two dosages of RD 13621.'

The side-effects were minor and included one patient having reported flatulent dyspepsia on 300 mg ibuprofen and another on 3.6 g aspirin; significantly, no skin rashes were reported.

In retrospect it is surprising in view of later recognition of the daily dosage of 1200–2400 mg being the most effective range that Chalmers found that 300 and 600 mg/day ibuprofen was as active as 3.6 g/day aspirin. However, these results obtained by Chalmers were a great impetus to the programme.

In fact ibuprofen has never been as potent in humans as the animal data (Table 1.1) suggested (16–32 times that of aspirin), for clinical potency is more in the region of three times that of aspirin (see Chapter 6).

Ibuprofen was originally launched in the United Kingdom in 1969 for the treatment of rheumatoid arthritis at a daily dosage of 600–800 mg, but the results were disappointing. Some clinicians, on the basis of their own experience of good safety, increased this dosage to 1200 mg/day. Later, following extensive clinical trials, this was raised to 1200 mg/day and later to what is now the approved prescription dose in the United Kingdom of 1200–2400 mg/day. In 1974, ibuprofen was launched by Upjohn in the United States as Motrin™ at a daily dose of 1200 mg/day with eventually a top level of 3200 mg/day.

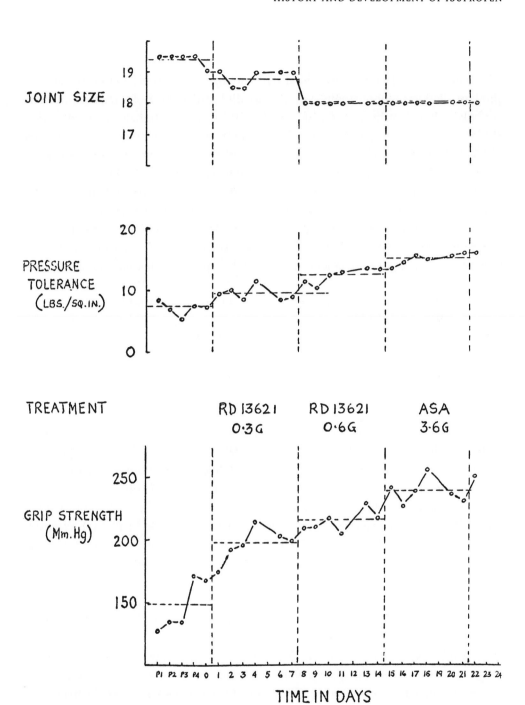

Figure 1.9: Original graphs from the report of Dr Tom Chalmers of the Rheumatic Diseases Unit, Northern General Hospital at Edinburgh, of the responses of a patient to effects of ibuprofen (RD 13621) compared with aspirin.

However, there were still disappointments from some of the earlier clinical investigation at the low dosages of 600–900 mg/day of ibuprofen. Thus, Boardman, Nuki and Dudley Hart (1967) reported that daily dosage with 900 mg ibuprofen failed to produce significant improvement in 20 patients with rheumatoid arthritis, or in 19 patients with osteoarthritis given 600 mg ibuprofen daily. Additionally, in a more extensive series of rheumatic patients, including 5 who were in a single-blind pilot study, 43 in a double-blind trial and 51 with rheumatoid arthritis in an open-label investigation, Thompson, Fox and Newell (1968) found that (a) 600 mg ibuprofen daily was effective in relieving pain and morning stiffness; (b) in a controlled clinical trial 600 mg ibuprofen daily was superior to 3 g daily paracetamol; and (c) ibuprofen given to 55 patients for up to a mean of 38 weeks even up to dosages of 1000 mg daily was effective and without any significant side-effects. This trial was important since it was the first to indicate that ibuprofen could be given to patients unable to take aspirin or other preparations because of dyspepsia.

While there were later reports of variable effects of 300 and 600 mg ibuprofen (Symposium, 1970) it was clear that the drug was safe in these low dosages. In later trials it emerged that higher doses were more effective as well as being relatively safe, especially in the gastrointestinal tract (see review in Chapter 6).

1.8.2   Gastrointestinal safety

Gastrointestinal safety was always a concern in both the pharmacological and clinical studies. In the early clinical trials of ibuprofen 600–900 mg/day only a few subjects had evidence of faecal occult blood and this was much lower than observed in patients who received anti-inflammatory doses of aspirin (Wallden and Gyllenberg, 1970). Cardoe (1970) had noted that 42 arthritic patients who had a history of peptic ulcer disease tolerated ibuprofen when given for 1–24 months, averaging 11 months in all. In this study 34 patients showed 'excellent tolerance' with no indigestion, 3 others had good response, while 5 others had exacerbation of ulcer symptoms. In 45 patients with a history of gastric intolerance, Cardoe (1970) found that there was excellent tolerance in 34, in 5 it was good (only requiring antacids or "alkalis") while in 6 it was poor in those patients who received the drug for 3–24 months. These results are impressive in highlighting the gastrointestinal safety of ibuprofen in patients with susceptibility to ulcer disease even though the doses employed were relatively low by present-day standards. The gastrointestinal blood loss from ibuprofen 800–1800 mg/day was also found by Thompson and Anderson (1970) to be no different from that with paracetamol or placebo, whereas that from calcium aspirin was appreciable. These studies must have given considerable encouragement to those at Boots that at last they had found a replacement for aspirin in rheumatic therapy with much improved gastrointestinal tolerance.

1.9   ACHIEVEMENTS AND REWARDS AT LAST

Throughout this programme of drug discovery involving the examination of over 1500 compounds made specifically for the project, the failure of four clinical candidates, and 15 years' hard work on animal model development and drug synthesis, it was sheer perseverence that lead to the development of ibuprofen. Much of the credit for this success must go to Stewart Adams, the Project Leader, and his small team. His original report in 1956 outlining his hypothesis and proposals for a chemical programme was the foundation on which the whole of the future project was built. The progress with this research and discovery was dotted with successes and many failures. At times the likelihood of the programme proceeding must have been threatened. These days many programmes of this kind might be closed down or lost in the numerous company amalgamations that proceed. However, it is to the credit of the senior management of the Research Department of Boots Pure Drug Company that this research progressed without interference despite what appeared to be frequent failures.

To the people involved, therefore, go our congratulations and admiration. First, to Stewart Adams who studied pharmacy at the University of Nottingham (BPharm, 1945) and later gained a PhD degree in pharmacology at the University of Leeds. He was made a Special Professor at the University of Nottingham in 1977 and awarded the Order of the British Empire in 1987 in recognition of his research culminating in the discovery of ibuprofen.

The late John Nicholson was another key figure who worked closely with Adams for 20 years. He was a quiet, thoughtful and experienced organic chemist. A graduate and postgraduate of Oxford University, he was a precise and talented chemist with a prolific output. It was Nicholson who made the critical decision to move from the phenoxy to phenyl acids and with his colleagues in the Chemistry Division eventually synthesized specifically for the project over 1500 compounds, of which approximately 450 were alkyl-substituted phenylalkanoics. It is a pity that through premature and untimely death he was denied any recognition for his considerable insight and talents in his synthetic efforts and the development of ibuprofen.

On a personal note, Dr Adams has expressed his particular indebtedness to two people. First to Colin Burrows — just the two of them began these studies. He supervised the work in Adams' laboratory with great skill and worked closely with him over the next two decades. Secondly, to Ray Cobb of the Medical Department with whom, particularly in the critical early days when struggling to find a way forward, Adams had many invaluable discussions that continued for many years afterwards.

The Head of the Medical Department, Dr Eric V B Morton, gave much valued enthusiastic support and motivation in the early years of the project and made introductions to a number of leading UK rheumatologists. The key element of personal contact emerges in the philosophical basis and development of ibuprofen. Dr Morton had known Professor

CHAPTER 1

J J R Duthie, who was the Director of the Rheumatic Diseases Unit at the Northern General Hospital in Edinburgh where the first clinical trial of ibuprofen was performed by Dr Chalmers. As can be gleaned from the report by Stewart Adams in 1956, Professor Duthie, then a leading authority on the rheumatic diseases, had given much good advice. His support for the idea of a 'super' aspirin and that aspirin had something 'special', strongly backed by Dr Morton, meant that the plea for chemical support in report No. 848 was accepted and shortly afterwards John Nicholson joined Adams. These personal aspects were obviously of great significance as well as serving to create the basis for the expansion of the project. The enthusiastic participation of physicians, coordinated by Dr J Warwick Buckler, in the early clinical trials in the United Kingdom should also be noted, among them Drs John Golding (Harrogate), Malcolm Thompson (Newcastle), Neil Cardoe (Norwich), Frank Dudley Hart (Westminster) and Watson Buchanan (Glasgow), to name a few. At a very early stage in the life of ibuprofen, Dr Thompson suggested its potential as an OTC alternative to aspirin.

1.10   ULTIMATE RECOGNITION OF SAFETY — OTC STATUS

The recent history of ibuprofen has now progressed to this drug having been approved for non-prescription or over-the-counter (OTC) use in many countries throughout the world, for over a decade and a half in many. This has been a major landmark for the drug in that granting of OTC status has been recognition of its well-established safety record (Paulus, 1990; Rainsford, Roberts and Brown, 1996; Rainsford and Powanda, 1997).

The Boots Company initially applied to the UK Department of Health and Social Security (DHSS), in August 1978 to have ibuprofen, on the basis of its safety record, allowed for non-prescription sale for the treatment of muscular and rheumatic pain, fever and backache with a unit dose of 200 mg and a maximum daily dose in adults of 1200 mg (Adams and Marchant, 1984). However, the Committee on the Safety of Medicines (CSM) of the DHSS provisionally concluded in May 1979 that on the grounds of safety it was unable to recommend to the Ministry to grant a product licence.

A small group under Dr Colin Lewis then proceeded to collect all the data on the safety of ibuprofen and initiated further studies on this aspect. The data thus obtained from 19 000 patients in clinical trials conducted/sponsored by Boots, retrospective analysis of 1957 patients in the United States and adverse drug reaction reports was incorporated in a revised application submitted to the DHSS in April 1982. The CSM decided in December 1982 to consult with interested bodies regarding the possibility of changing the status of ibuprofen from prescription-only to pharmacy sale. Those organizations that were consulted included the Pharmaceutical Society of Great Britain, The Proprietary Association of Great Britain, the medical profession and The Consumers Association. From these consultations, discussions were undertaken in January 1983 between the DHSS and Boots concerning the conditions of licensing the drug for non-prescription use.

TABLE 1.2

Summary of history and developments of the anti-inflammatory project at Boots

1953	Initial thoughts and discussions on a search for aspirin-type drug.
1955	UV erythema in guinea-pig; began preliminary investigations.
1956 (Mar.)	Report No. 848 on UV erythema technique, with recommendations for a chemical programme of work.
1958 (Aug.)	First inhibitors discovered of UV erythema: phenoxy acids.
1958 (Nov.)	RD 8402 (a phenoxy acid) made.
1960	RD 8402 in clinical trial.
1960	RD 10335, RD 10499 and ibufenac made.
1961 (Jun.)	RD 10335 active clinically, but rash in 50% of patients.
1961 (Dec.)	Ibuprofen made.
1962 (May)	Ibufenac active clinically, no rash.
1963 (Mar.)	Clinicians' meeting on ibufenac.
1964	RD 10499 in clinical trial. Active, but rash in 20% of patients.
1964 (Apr.)	Ibuprofen made product candidate.
1964 (Aug.)	Ibufenac started in clinical trials in Japan.
1966 (Feb.)	Ibuprofen shown to be active in clinical trial.
1966 (Apr.)	Ibufenac on UK market.
1967 (Nov.)	Clinicians' meeting on ibuprofen.
1968 (Jan.)	Ibufenac withdrawn UK market because of liver toxicity.
1968 (Mar.)	Ibufenac marketed by Kakenyaku Kako Co. Ltd (Kyoto and Tokyo) in Japan; superseded later by ibuprofen.
1969 (Feb.)	Brufen™ (ibuprofen) launched.
1970	First Symposium on Ibuprofen at the Royal College of Physicians, London.
1983	Approval for ibuprofen OTC in UK ((Nurofen™ launched 8 August 1983).
1984	Approval for ibuprofen OTC in USA.

CHAPTER 1

These discussions included (a) the indications for use of ibuprofen OTC should not exceed those for aspirin, (b) there should be a warning that the drug should not be taken by patients with stomach ulcers, (c) all advertising material should be submitted to the DHSS for approval, and (d) pharmacists should be advised about the product prior to advertising. Adams and Marchant (1984) noted in regard to the warning for gastric ulcer patients that this was not then required for aspirin! The licence was enabled by the amendment to the prescription-only medicine (POM) order on 31 July 1983 (Adams and Marchant, 1984).

Initially the indications for use of the drug in treating dental pain, migraine, period pain and other painful states were approved in the 1970s for prescription use. Later, as safety and efficacy were proved, these indications were extended to OTC use.

Nurofen™, the trade mark brand of ibuprofen, was launched by the Boots subsidiary, Crookes Products Ltd, on 8 August 1983. A year later ibuprofen was given approval by the US Food and Drug Administration for OTC sale on the grounds of proven safety, efficacy being accepted (Paulus, 1990). A submission to the FDA was made by Whitehall Laboratories Division of American Home Products (New York, NY, USA) in association with Boots, and Whitehall Laboratories later marketed ibuprofen as Advil™ under arrangements with Boots.

From the UK and US government viewpoints the granting of OTC status for ibuprofen was a landmark decision. The major issue for the drug regulatory authorities of both governments was the safety of the drug. As one of the earliest prescription drugs to move ('switch') to OTC status, its success and good safety record as an OTC product must have had a significant influence on the decision of health authorities to deregulate many other NSAIDs and other prescription medications.

1.11 WORLDWIDE DEVELOPMENTS

Boots had a long-standing research agreement with The Upjohn Company (Kalamazoo, MI, USA), who in 1967 took up their option and accepted ibuprofen as a product candidate for clinical trial. They proceeded to carry out the necessary additional laboratory and clinical studies for eventual FDA approval in the United States and this was granted in 1974. Thereafter they marketed ibuprofen under the trade mark Motrin™. Upjohn made a valuable contribution to the success of ibuprofen, not to its discovery or development, but on the clinical side where, with their large clinical resources, they were able to explore new indications and higher dosage to an extent that Boots' own limited clinical resources could not have done.

In the 1970s and 1980s both Brufen™ and Motrin™ rapidly found wide acceptance by the rheumatological and other specialists and family/general practitioners as what has probably been regarded as a 'first-line' treatment of pain and inflammation in a wide variety of muscular-skeletal and other conditions.

Numerous other companies now market ibuprofen for OTC and prescription use. Appendix A shows a list of the immense range of ibuprofen products and brand names for the drug that are now available worldwide (the list is by no means complete but does illustrate this point). The extensive commercial development and applications of ibuprofen are a tribute to the pioneers who struggled to develop the fundamental pharmacology and medicinal chemistry leading to ibuprofen; The Boots Company who persevered with research and development; and the medical and scientific community who studied the efficacy, safety and actions of the drug.

Much of this chapter has dealt with those involved in the early years of the development of ibuprofen, but it must be remembered that as a drug candidate progresses towards being a product many others become involved. There were increasing demands on those involved in toxicological, metabolic, pharmaceutical and clinical studies (and in the case of ibuprofen for 20 years after its launch), as well as in the development of new synthetic processes for large-scale production (now thousands of tons). Indeed a completely new factory using latest technology was designed and built at Boots for what was a fairly complicated eight-stage manufacturing process.

Among the tributes to the scientific and technical originality and clinical success of Brufen™ and the Research Department of the Boots Company was the highly prestigious Queen's Award for Technological Achievement, which was given to the company in 1985. By this time over 100 million people had received treatment with ibuprofen in 120 countries throughout the world. With over 7000 publications in which research and clinical studies have been reported using this drug, notably also as a standard of comparison, it can truly be considered to be a well-established standard representative of the class of NSAIDs.

ACKNOWLEDGEMENTS

I should like to specially thank Dr Stewart Adams for his generosity and invaluable help in compiling this chapter, for Figures 1.1 to 1.9, and for extracts from laboratory notes and reports that were used to compile the history of the development of ibuprofen.

REFERENCES

ADAMS, S.S. (1956) The testing of non-hormonal anti-rheumatic compounds. *Research Department Report. No. 848, 5 March 1956*, Boots Pure Drug Co. Ltd.

ADAMS, S.S. (1987a) The discovery of Brufen. *Chemistry in Britain* (Dec.), 1193–1195.

ADAMS, S.S. (1987b) Non-steroidal anti-inflammatory drugs, plasma half-lives, and adverse reactions. *Lancet* 2, 1204–1205.

ADAMS, S.S. (1988) NSAIDs, plasma half-lives, and adverse reactions. *Lancet* 1, 653–654.

ADAMS, S.S. and COBB, R. (1958) A possible basis for the anti-inflammatory activity of salicylates and other non-hormonal anti-rheumatic drugs. *Nature* 181, 733.

ADAMS, S.S. and COBB, R. (1963) The effect of salicylates and related compounds on erythema in the guinea-pig and man. In: DIXON, A. ST J., MARTIN, B.K., SMITH, M.J.H. and WOOD, P.H.N. (eds), *Salicylates. An International Symposium*. London, Churchill, 127–134.

ADAMS, S.S. and COBB, R. (1967) Non-steroidal antiinflammatory drugs. In: ELLIS, G.P. and WEST, G.B. (eds), *Progress in Medicinal Chemistry*, 5, London, Butterworth, 59–133.

ADAMS, S.S. and MARCHANT, B. (1984) . . . and the ibuprofen story. *Pharmaceutical Journal* (24 Nov.), 646.

BOARDMAN, P.L., NUKI, G. and DUDLEY HART, F. (1967) Ibuprofen in the treatment of rheumatoid arthritis and osteo-arthritis. *Annals of the Rheumatic Diseases* 26, 560–561.

■ CHAPTER 1 ■

CARDOE, N. (1970) A review of long-term experience with ibuprofen, with special reference to gastric tolerance. *Rheumatology and Physical Medicine* **11**(Suppl.), 28–31.

COLLIER, H.O.J. (1963) Antagonism by aspirin and like-acting drugs of kinins and SRS-A in guinea-pig lung. In: DIXON, A. ST J., MARTIN, B.K., SMITH, M.J.H. and WOOD, P.H.N. (eds), *Salicylates. An International Symposium*. London, Churchill, 120–126.

NICHOLSON, J.S. (1982) Ibuprofen. In: BINDRA, J.S. and LEDNICER, D. (eds) *Chronicles of Drug Discovery*, vol. 1. New York, Wiley, Chap. 7, 149–171.

PAULUS, H.E. (1990) FDA arthritis advisory committee meeting: guidelines for approving nonsteroidal antiinflammatory drugs for over-the-counter use. *Arthritis and Rheumatism* **33**, 1056–1058.

RAINSFORD, K.D. (1984) *Aspirin and the Salicylates*. London, Butterworth.

RAINSFORD, K.D. and POWANDA, M.C. (eds) (1998) *Safety and Efficacy of Non-Prescription (OTC) Analgesics and NSAIDs*. Dordrecht, Kluwer Academic Publishers.

RAINSFORD, K.D., ROBERTS, S.C. and BROWN, S. (1997) Ibuprofen and paracetamol: relative safety in non-prescription dosages. *Journal of Pharmacy and Pharmacology* **49**, 345–376.

Symposium on Ibuprofen at the Royal College of Physicians, London, 1970. *Rheumatology and Physical Medicine* **11**(Suppl.), 1–105.

THOMPSON, M. and ANDERSON, M. (1970) Studies of gastrointestinal blood loss during ibuprofen therapy. *Rheumatology and Physical Medicine* **11**(Suppl.), 104–108.

THOMPSON, M., FOX, H. and NEWELL, D.H. (1968) Ibuprofen in the treatment of arthritis. *Medical Proceedings — Mediense Bydraes, South Africa* **14**, 579–582.

VANE, J.R. (1971) Inhibition of prostaglandin synthesis as a mechanism of action for aspirin-like drugs. *Nature* **231**, 232–235.

WALLDEN, B. and GYLLENBERG, B. (1970) A comparative study of ibuprofen and calcium-acetylsalicylic acid in rheumatoid arthritis with particular reference to biochemical parameters and side-effects. *Rheumatology and Physical Medicine* **11**(Suppl.), 83–87.

WILHELMI, G. (1949) Ueber die pharmakologischen Eigenschaften von Irgapyrin, einem neuen Präparat aus der Pyrazolreihe. *Schweizer Medizinische Wochenschrift* **79**, 577.

The Medicinal Chemistry of Ibuprofen

KENNETH J NICHOL

Formerly Head of Medicinal Chemistry, Research Department,
Boots Pharmaceuticals, Nottingham, UK

Contents

2.1   INTRODUCTION

Ibuprofen is an original pharmaceutical compound that was invented in the Research Laboratories of the (then) Boots Pure Drug Company Ltd in Nottingham, UK. It is now one of the major pharmaceuticals in the world as well as a source of scientific and academic interest in the noncommercial sphere. Previous reviews of aspects of the discovery, chemistry, pharmacology and clinical use of ibuprofen include those by Adams (1992), Adams and Cobb (1967), Buckler and Adams (1968), Juby (1974), Nicholson (1980) and Shen (1972).

2.2   THE DISCOVERY OF IBUPROFEN

In 1952 the research programme of Boots Pure Drug Co. (later Boots Pharmaceuticals) underwent a radical realignment under the new Research Director Dr (later Sir) Gordon Hobday when attention was concentrated on 'diseases of civilisation', in which was included rheumatic conditions. Pharmacologist Stewart Adams was charged with leading the programme to find medicines effective in these diseases. At that time the drug treatment was either aspirin or the corticosteroids, which had been introduced in the early 1950s. The latter, though clinically effective, often gave rise to severe side-effects, particularly in long-term dosage. Aspirin also had its share of side-effects, notably a marked tendency to cause gastric irritation, in severe cases leading to serious ulceration, but in spite of this was known to be effective in rheumatic patients. Stewart Adams decided that aspirin should be the starting point for the project and set about assessing the vast literature on the compound (the review by Adams and Cobb (1967) includes a survey of salicylates and related compounds). A paper in an obscure journal (Harris and Fosdick, 1952) provided the first faint clue; the authors suggested, on not the most convincing experimental evidence, that the alleviation of pain in inflamed tissue by aspirin was due not only to its well recognized antipyretic effect but also to a parallel oedema-reducing effect. It was also the belief of many rheumatologists that aspirin indeed had some specific effect in the rheumatic condition. Unfortunately, there were no laboratory tests that would demonstrate either this property or the analgesic effect of aspirin; the first task of the project group was the development of a reliable test system. The method described by Wilhemi (1949) was used as the basis and after several years of development became the standard method for screening compounds for anti-inflammatory activity, being capable of demonstrating the activity of aspirin at nontoxic doses (Adams and Cobb, 1958). The method (Adams, 1960) involved exposing the shaved skin of albino guinea-pigs to UV light 30 minutes after dosing with aspirin (which was the positive control) or the experimental compound, and assessing the degree of erythema, on a scale of 1 to 4 (aspirin = 1) after 2 hours.

Once a reliable screening method, now referred to as the UVE screen, had been established (and continued to be developed and improved over the next decade) the way was clear for meaningful testing of compounds. Not surprisingly, the first substances examined were derivatives of aspirin, some of which were commercially available. For other analogues Stewart Adams teamed up with Dr John Nicholson, an experienced and able chemist, who was destined to be the other major player in the discovery story. From April 1957 to September 1958 numerous derivatives and analogues of aspirin were synthesized and tested. Although most were inactive, and a few were little better than aspirin, the main structure–activity conclusion was that a carboxylic acid group, an aromatic ring and possibly an oxygen substituent were desirable for aspirin-like activity. Not an earth-shattering conclusion, it was recognized, but QSAR, computer graphics and receptor theory were far in the future. The standard practice in drug research was to test analogues of wider structural diversity, and here help came from an unrelated area. The Agricultural Research group at Boots had been investigating a range of phenoxyalkanoic acids as potential herbicides and samples of many of the compounds were available. The UVE test had by now been improved to cater for rapid screening of compounds and over the following year 300 analogues were examined. Almost immediately the team was rewarded with success, compound (1) having activity twice that of aspirin.

(1)

More than 600 2-phenoxypropionic acids were tested, many of which were specifically synthesized for the project, the most potent in the UVE screen being 2-(4-biphenylyl)propionic acid, 6–10 times the potency of aspirin (Table 2.1), no other analogue having more than twice that of aspirin. The structure–activity relationships that arose from these results played an important role in the future progression of the project. Table 2.1 lists the compounds more active than aspirin.

4-Substitution, particularly by alkyl or phenyl groups, in the aromatic ring was favoured, 3- and 2-monosubstituted analogues being inactive. With the exception of the 3-methyl-4-isobutyl compound, further substitution in the ring reduced or abolished activity; halogen, alkoxy, alkylthio, alkylsulphonyl, nitro, cyano, amino and substituted amino substituted analogues were poorly active or inactive.

The 4-biphenylyl compound (Table 2.1, compound 4) was selected for a clinical trial in 1960; mindful of the adverse gastric effects of aspirin, believed to be due to the carboxylic acid group, the team elected to use the ethyl ester instead of the acid. To their surprise and dismay, the compound was totally inactive when given to rheumatoid patients at 1.8 g/day. This setback represented the first major crisis point in the project as it cast doubts on the relevance of the UVE test to the human disease condition. The question whether 8402 was similar in properties to aspirin after all brought the realization that the UVE test only measured the anti-inflammatory activity of compounds, whereas aspirin also

TABLE 2.1

Pharmacological potencies of substituted 2-phenoxypropionic acids

$$R \quad \underset{}{\overset{CH_3}{\overline{}}} \quad O \cdot CH \cdot CO_2H$$

Compound	R	UVE[a]
1	4-s-Butyl	2
2	4-Isopropyl	2
3	4-Ethyl	2
4	4-Phenyl	6–10
5	3-Methyl-4-isobutyl	2
6	4-t-Butyl	2
7	4-Isobutyl	2

[a] Guinea pig UV erythema: aspirin = 1.

possessed analgesic and antipyretic properties. A test for the former had recently been published by Randall and Sellitoe (1957); when this was introduced into the testing programme, it was shown that 8402 had comparatively lower analgesic effect (Table 2.2).

A third test to measure antipyretic activity was added and again 8402 had low potency. The decision was thereupon taken that anti-inflammatory activity in the UVE screen was only the first indication of potential and that all three activities should be represented in compounds to be taken forward for trial.

With its most potent member now discarded, the phenoxypropionic acid series was of no further interest. Even before this juncture, John Nicholson had been looking for wider variants of the chemical type to synthesize. Merely replacing the ether oxygen by other linking groups held no promise — phenylthiopropionic acids were inactive and anilino analogues were more toxic. Replacement by a bond was a better option, as a publication by Cavallini (Cavallini *et al.*, 1957) suggested (but without biological evidence) that biphenyl-substituted alkanoic acids had potential as antirheumatic drugs. A programme of synthesis of phenylacetic and phenylpropionic acids was started, initially aimed at analogues of the most active phenoxypropionics, and almost immediately active compounds emerged (Nicholson, 1980). Work quickly concentrated on the phenylacetics because the phenyl-propionics were significantly ulcerogenic in the dog, routes of synthesis were at this time more straightforward for the acetic acids, and the 4-methyl and 4-t-butyl analogues in the propionic acid series were no more potent than the corresponding acetic acid analogues. Pharmacological results were very encouraging: the phenylacetics were generally more potent than the phenoxy analogues, they were active in all three screens and activity was found in many more compounds. By 1961 it was possible to select three compounds — 10335, 10449 and 11654 — from this group for clinical trials (Table 2.2).

TABLE 2.2
Pharmacological properties of research compounds taken to clinical testing

Compound	Structure	UVE[a]	RFA[b]	AP[c]	Clinic	Side-effects
8402	biphenyl–O·CH(CH$_3$)·CO$_2$H	6–10	1–2	< 1	Inactive	
10335	Me$_3$C–C$_6$H$_4$–CH$_2$·CO$_2$H	4	4	2–4	Active	Skin rash
10449	cyclohexyl–C$_6$H$_4$–CH$_2$CO$_2$H	4	10	4	Active	Skin rash
11654 (Ibufenac)	Me$_2$CH·CH$_2$–C$_6$H$_4$–CH$_2$CO$_2$H	2–4	2–4	4	Active	Hepatotoxicity[d]
13621 (Ibuprofen)	Me$_2$CH·CH$_2$–C$_6$H$_4$–CH(CH$_3$)·CO$_2$H	16–32	30	20	Active	(Negligible)

[a] UV erythema. [b] Rat foot analgesia. [c] Rat Antipyrexia. [d] Not evident in clinical trials.
All numerical values relative to aspirin = 1.

All three were effective as antirheumatics in patients, but 10335 and 10449 gave rise to skin rashes and were abandoned. 11654, however, was well tolerated and effective even in patients with a history of gastric intolerance to other drugs. At this point the goal of clinical efficacy and freedom from gastric side-effects seemed to have been attained. Further trials confirmed the promise of the compound, which, with the nonproprietary name of ibufenac, was marketed as Dytransin in 1964. Unfortunately, the product was withdrawn following a low incidence of hepatotoxicity (which had not been evident in laboratory tests or clinical trials) in patients on long-term use. (Dytransin continued to be used in Japan for several years without significant problems, giving rise to a notable example of ethnic difference in side-effects profile.)

The abandonment of ibufenac was the second major crisis point in the project: phenylacetic acids had been eliminated by reason of side-effects in three clinically effective compounds not detected in laboratory testing. Although a further series of active compounds, the phenylpropionic acids, was available for evaluation it was now critical that some assurance could be provided that these compound types possessed a more acceptable side-effects profile.

The original reason for not chosing the phenylpropionics was because they appeared to be more ulcerogenic in the dog. Laboratory examination now revealed that subcutaneous administration of these compounds in dogs produced gastric ulcers, leading to the totally unexpected and novel conclusion that the ulcerogenic activity was systemic rather than local. Furthermore, it transpired that the plasma half-lives of the compounds in dogs were much longer than in other species (Mills *et al.*, 1973). These facts in conjunction indicated that the dog was anomalous in this respect and that there was more likelihood of the phenylpropionics being considered as potential products.

Studies with radiolabelled compounds showed that in both rat and dog the concentration of the propionic acids in plasma and tissues was very much less than for the acetic acids, significantly so in the two areas, skin and liver, where clinical problems had been manifest (Table 2.3).

The way was now clear for clinical testing of the propionic acids. The only problem was an embarrassment of riches, there being a considerable number of compounds with an acceptable level and profile of activity (Table 2.4).

Most of the active compounds were subjected to extended laboratory and preclinical testing. The process was lengthy and cautious, taking almost 3 years, but eventually 13621 was chosen as having the best overall spread of properties (Adams *et al.*, 1969a). (Interestingly, this compound was actually the third example of a phenylpropionic acid synthesized in the project, in which approximately 150 analogues were made.) Clinical trials commenced in 1966. The compound was effective at doses of 600 mg/day without the side-effects seen with ibufenac and was introduced to the UK market in 1969 under the trade name Brufen (nonproprietary name ibuprofen). Here the story of the discovery ends. Ibuprofen is now a major pharmaceutical product, marketed in most countries and

CHAPTER 2

TABLE 2.3

Concentration (μg/g) of ^{14}C compound in rat and dog tissues (17 h post dose)

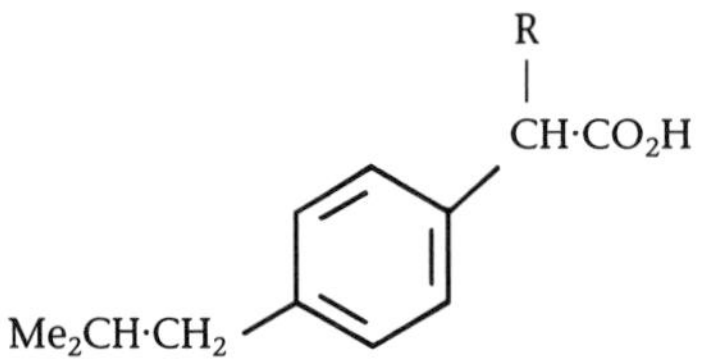

R
|
CH·CO₂H

(structure)

Me₂CH·CH₂

	Rat[a]		Dog[b]	
	R = H	R = Me	R = H	R = Me
Plasma	28	1	16	9
Liver	28	2	35	8
Skin	430	15	NR[c]	NR[c]

[a] 20 mg/kg p.o. twice daily, 4 weeks.   [b] 8 mg/kg p.o. twice daily, 2 weeks.   [c] NR not recorded.

TABLE 2.4

Pharmacological potencies of 2-(4-substituted-phenyl)propionic acids

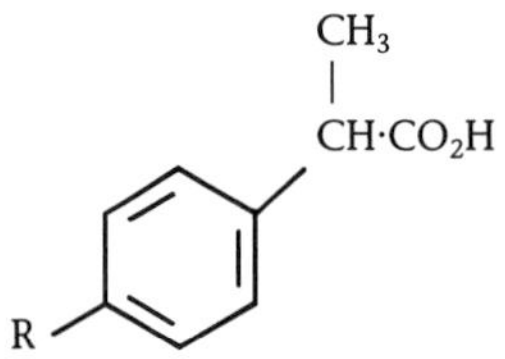

CH₃
|
CH·CO₂H

(structure)

R

Substituent	UVE[a]	RFA[b]	AP[c]
Me₃C—	4	2–4	2
Me₂CH·CH₂—	16–32	8–16	20
Cyclohexyl	32–64	32–64	20
MeEtCH—	8	4–8	
Butyl	4–8	8–16	
Me₂CH—	4	2	
Et₂MeC—	4–8	4	
Propyl	8–16	4	
Me₂CH·CH₂·CH₂—	8		
Cyclopentyl	8		
Cycloheptyl	8		
PhO—	32	16	
Me₂CH·O—	8	4	
PhS—	8–16	8	
CH₂=CH·CH₂O—	8–16	16	
PrO—	4–8		
Me·CH=CH·CH₂O—	2–4		
PrS—	4–8		

[a,b,c] Abbreviations as in Table 2.2.
Potencies relevant to aspirin = 1.

with an annual production of the drug substance approaching 10 000 tonnes per annum. For a succinct summary of post-launch events the reader is recommended Stewart Adams' account (1992).

2.3 SYNTHETIC ROUTES TO IBUPROFEN

As the programme for the synthesis of phenylpropionic acids followed immediately (in reality the two programmes slightly overlapped) that concerned with phenylacetic acids, for which reliable methods of synthesis had been worked out, it is not surprising that Boots project chemists investigated first the simple methylation of the acid side-chain (reaction 1).

Reagents: (i) NaNH$_2$/MeI

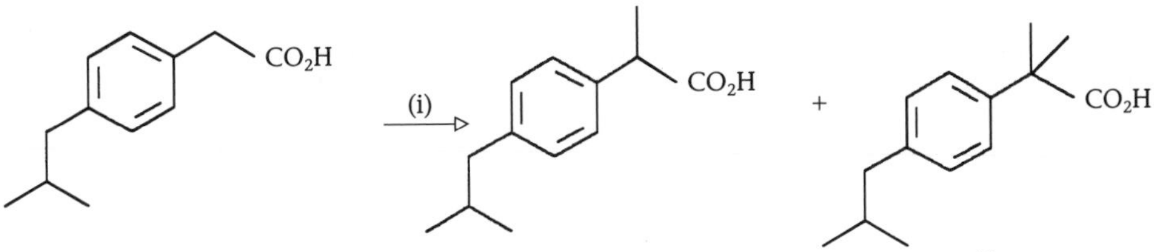

Although providing material for initial screening, the product required rigorous purification to remove unmethylated (2) or dimethylated (4), or frequently both. Compound (4) was readily obtained in a pure form by exhaustive methylation and was found to be inactive in the UVE screen. A more satisfactory route (reaction 2) involved the conversion of the ethyl ester of (2) to the phenylmalonic ester followed by methylation and hydrolysis (Nicholson and Adams, 1964, 1965) although unless the methylation step proceeded 100% the product was contaminated with the acetic acid (2).

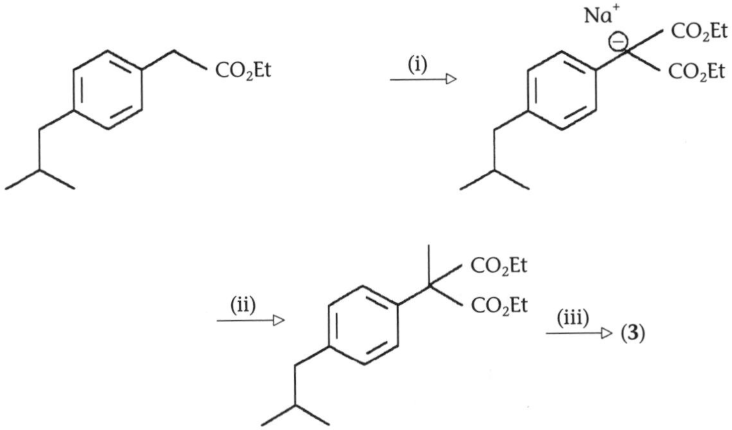

Reagents: (1) Et$_2$CO$_3$/NaOEt; (ii) MeI; (iii) HCl aq

■ CHAPTER 2 ■

■ 33

Although the methylation procedure rapidly lost favour as more reliable routes were found, it has featured in some novel applications. An interesting use of solid support techniques (Backes and Ellman, 1994) involves the coupling (reaction 3) of a phenylacetic acid (via its pentafluorophenyl ester) to the sulfonamide-containing resin (5) and treating the resulting acylsulfonamide with lithium dimethylamide to give the tri-anion (6). Methylation occurs at the enolic α-carbon and hydrolysis yields the phenylpropionic acid.

(R) represents the resin backbone

Reagents: (i) Pentafluorophenyl arylacetate; (ii) lithium dimethylamide; (iii) MeI; (iv) CH_2N_2; (v) NaOH aq

Attention in Boots Chemistry Research turned to one of the intermediates in the synthesis of ibufenac, 4-isobutylacetophenone (7), as a possible intermediate in the synthesis of propionic acids. Reaction with hydrogen cyanide (or an equivalent reagent) yielded a cyanhydrin ((8), R = H, or an acyl equivalent) that could be transformed into ibuprofen by hydrolysis followed or preceded by hydrogenolysis (reaction 4).

Over the years many varieties of this sequence have been evolved, many appearing in the patent literature as ibuprofen gained in importance and competitors sought an exploitable preparative route. The reaction between (7) and HCN was rarely efficient (50%) and subsequent routes, using more complex reagents, aimed at improving this yield. Formation

(4)

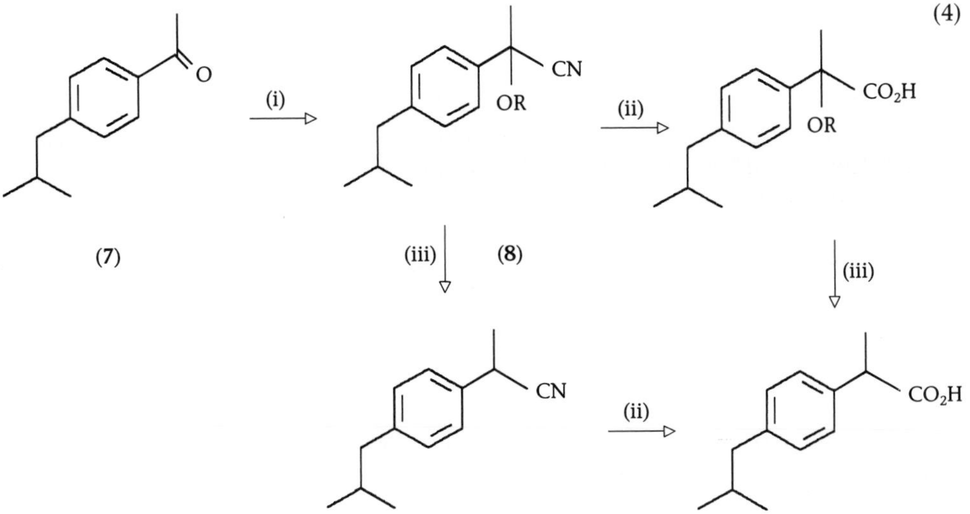

(7)   (8)   (3)

Reagents: (i) HCN or equivalent; (ii) hydrolysis; (iii) hydrogenation

of (8) has been accomplished in good yields using $Me_3SiCN/ZnCl_2/Ac_2O/FeCl_3$ (R = Ac), and $LiCN/(EtO)_3POCl$ (R = $PO(OEt)_3$).

Reagents effecting the hydrogenolysis step were typically $SnCl_2$, red phosphorus/I_2 and Pd-C/H_2 (see e.g. Hiyama, 1986; Harasawa *et al.*, 1984).

A more efficient and reliable method employed 4-isobutylacetophenone in the Darzens glycidic ester synthesis where reaction with ethyl chloroacetate and sodium alkoxide gave (9) in good yield. Hydrolysis followed by oxidation of the resultant aldehyde (the Boots process used silver oxide) provided ibuprofen in excellent yield (reaction 5) (Dytham, 1969). This route was used by Boots for many years in the commercial production of ibuprofen, consistently giving good yields of high purity product.

(5)

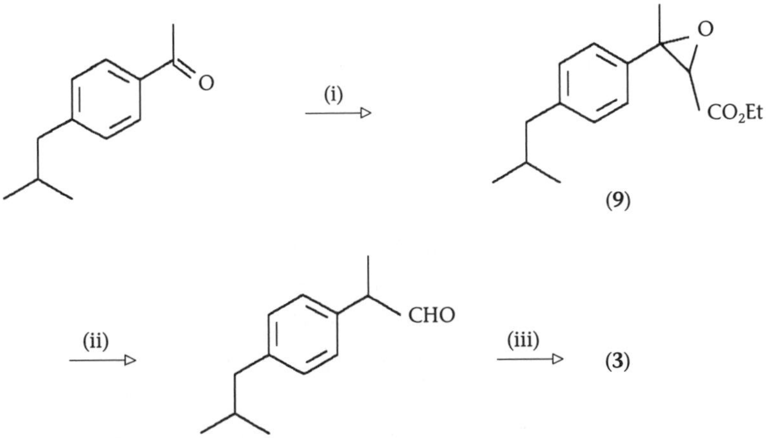

(9)

(3)

Reagents: (i) $ClCH_2 \cdot CO_2Et/NaOEt$; (ii) NaOH aq. /HCl/heat; (iii) AgO

Large-scale manufacture of ibuprofen now tends towards processes akin to heavy chemicals or the petrochemical industry, using reactions such as the catalyzed carboxylation of olefins (Wu, 1994) (reaction 6).

(6)

Reagents: (i) CO (500 psig), MeOH, PPh$_3$, PdCl$_2$, CuCl$_2$

These and many other synthetic pathways have been used to prepare ibuprofen since its market introduction. A comprehensive review (Rieu *et al.*, 1986) categorizes routes to arylpropionic acids generally, many of which are directly aimed at ibuprofen and most others potentially so. Although ibuprofen is by medicines standards a small and relatively simple molecule, it is remarkable that so many variants of synthetic access have been devised. Much of this is undoubtedly due to its importance in medicine, attracting the attentions of competitive producers, but also may be due to its being the archetypical 'profen', the origin of a class of pharmaceuticals.

Possessing one functional group and an inert hydrocarbon moiety, ibuprofen presents a very simple target for synthetic strategies. The real challenge, however, particularly from the commercial viewpoint, has been to manufacture ibuprofen free from significant impurities and by a route that is economic in cost and materials. The elimination of the acetic acid compound (ibufenac), positional isomers such as 21 (R = isobutyl) and structural isomers of the isobutyl chain were significant pieces of work. (At one point Boots chemists devised a production process for isobutylbenzene by the reaction of benzyl-sodium with 2-chloropropane, as commercial material contained significant amounts of *n*-butylbenzene.)

Interesting among the wealth of synthetic routes are those that could be termed academic, devised more to demonstrate a methodology rather than any hope of a commercial process. Two such pieces of work illustrate the point. An elegant use of organoboranes, for example (reaction 7), allows sequentially the isobutyl and the propionic acid moieties to be attached to a benzene ring (Riviera *et al.*, 1992).

Reacting 4-bromophenyl with *t*-butyl-9-BBN gave 4-isobutylphenol which, as the triflate ester, coupled with isopropenyl-9-BBN furnishing 1-methyl-4-isobutylstyrene (**10**). Hydroboration and oxidation with molecular oxygen gave the phenylpropan-1-ol (**11**), readily oxidized by platinum and molecular oxygen to ibuprofen in overall yield of 39%.

(7)

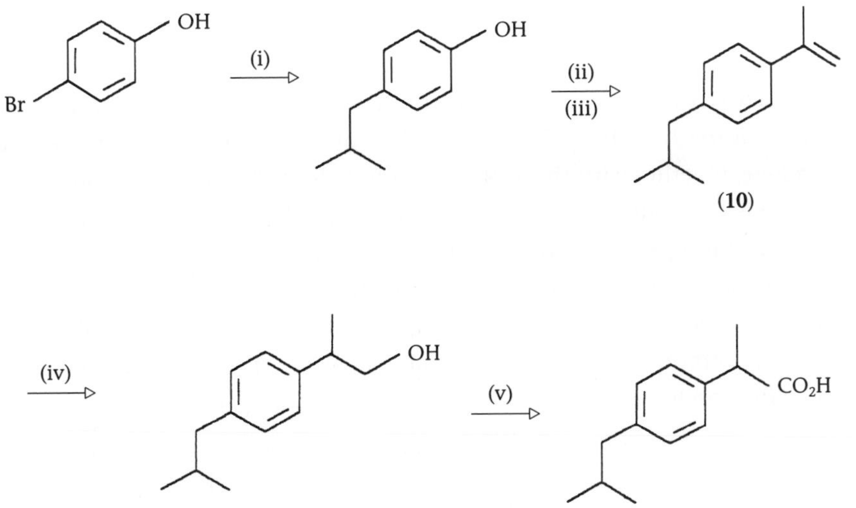

(10)

(11)   (3)

Reagents: (i) But-9-BBN/Pd(PPh$_3$)$_4$; (ii) (CF$_3$SO$_2$)$_2$O; (iii) 2-propenyl-9-BBN/Pd(PPh$_3$)$_4$;
(iv) (MeS)$_2$B/O$_2$; (v) Pd(OH)$_2$/O$_2$
[9-BBN = 9-borobicylo[3.3.1]nonane]

An intriguing application of a 'super base', a mixture of n-butyllithium and potassium
t-butoxide, demonstrates a one-pot synthesis of ibuprofen from p-xylene (Faig and
Schlosser, 1991) involving three consecutive metallations at benzylic carbons and three
subsequent electrophilic reactions (reaction 8). The overall 'one-pot' yield is 52%, which
rises to 69% if each intermediate is isolated and purified. The difference in yield is surprisingly small considering the potential for competing side-reactions. A detailed impurity
analysis of the sequence might provide interesting information on the site-specificity of
the individual steps.

(8)

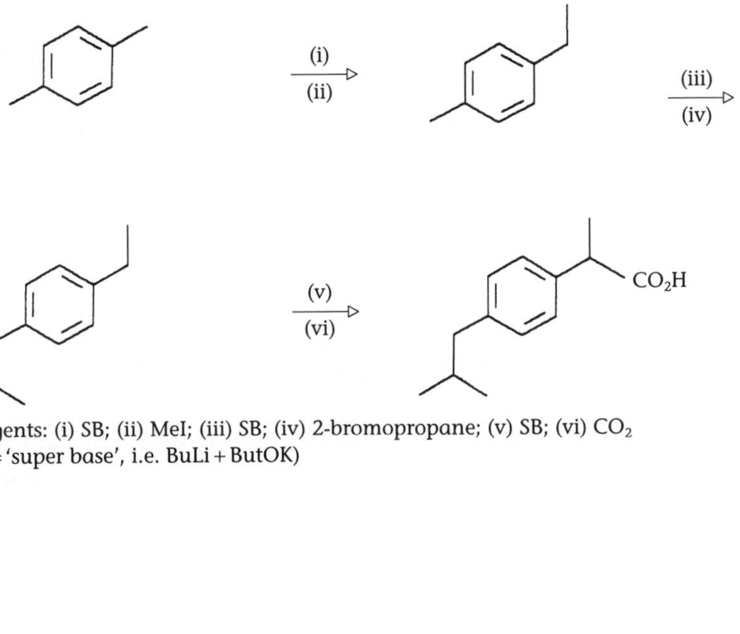

Reagents: (i) SB; (ii) MeI; (iii) SB; (iv) 2-bromopropane; (v) SB; (vi) CO$_2$
(SB = 'super base', i.e. BuLi + ButOK)

2.4   BIOLOGICAL ACTIVITIES OF IBUPROFEN ANALOGUES

The structure–activity comparisons of many of the compounds prepared and tested in the Boots laboratories have been discussed by Nicholson (1980). Some of these results are repeated here, together with those of other compounds that have been produced in other locations. For the purposes of this section the term 'ibuprofen analogues' is largely restricted to phenylpropionic acids, omitting fused-ring compounds such as naproxen and the biphenylpropionic acids such as flurbiprofen.

The carboxylic acid group appears to be essential for good activity, particularly when separated by one carbon atom from the aromatic nucleus, although some activity has been reported for 3-arylpropionic and 4-arylbutyric acids (see e.g. Juby, 1974).

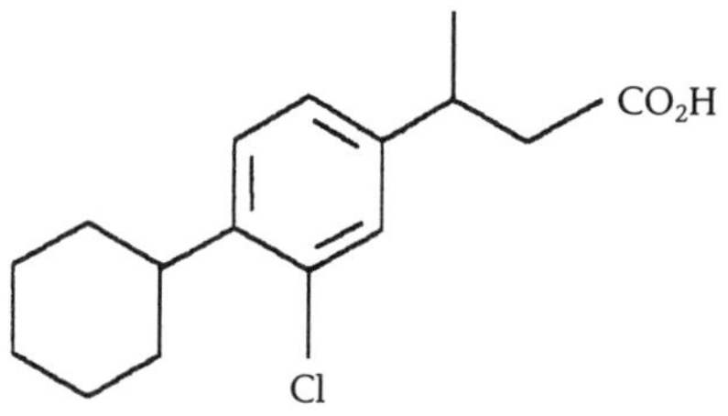

(12) 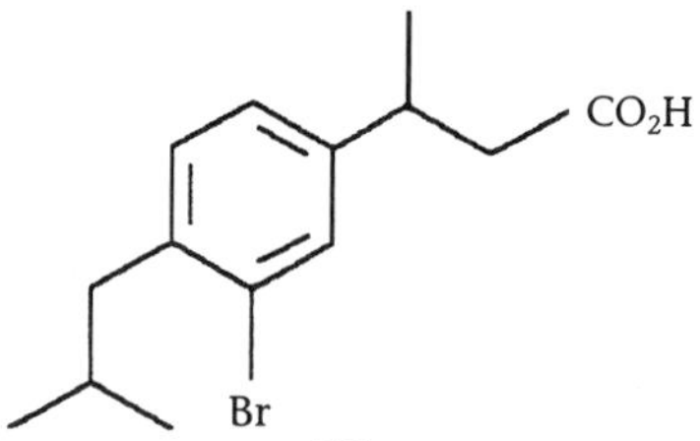   (13)

Homologues such as (12) (Redel *et al.*, 1970) are weakly active (and toxic) in the rat paw oedema test while (13) (Kuchar *et al.*, 1978) was less active than ibuprofen in inhibiting kaolin-induced oedema.

Primary alcohols (14) have potency similar to the corresponding acids, to which they are probably oxidized *in vivo*.

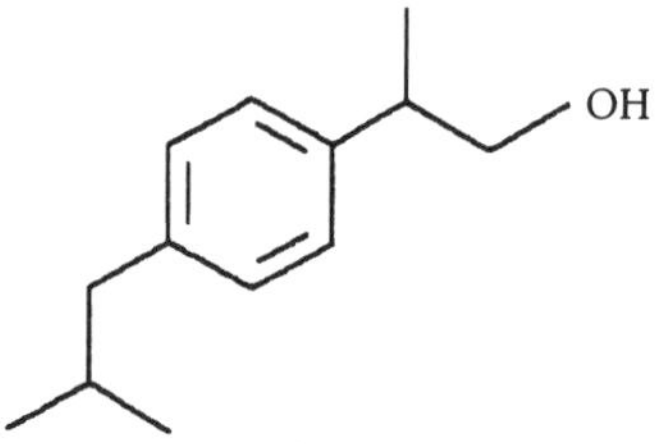

(14) 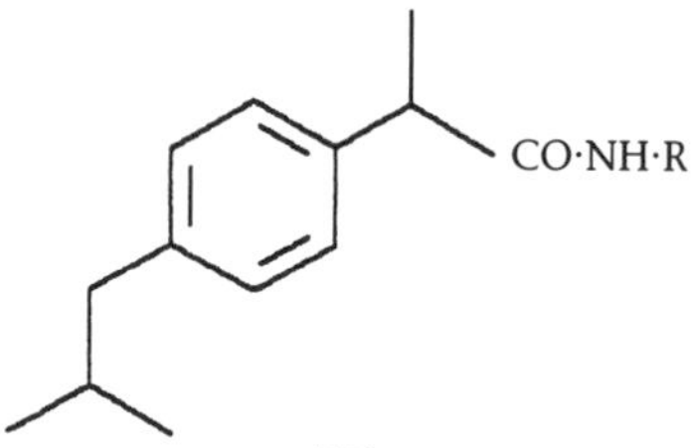   (15)

Amides (15) (R = H or alkyl) are less active; the hydroxamic acid ibuproxam ((15), R = OH) is reported to be better tolerated than ibuprofen and may be, by hydrolysis, acting partly as a slow-release form. Esters of ibuprofen are hydrolyzed to the acids *in vivo*.

Compounds (16) and (17) bearing groups thought of as carboxylic acid isosteres were inactive in the UVE test; (17) is reported (Valenti *et al.*, 1983) to have peripheral analgesic properties similar to those of ibuprofen.

(16)   (17)

The optimum α-substituent in the acid side-chain is usually methyl (18), although a few α-ethyl analogues, e.g. butibufen (19) (Carretero *et al.*, 1978) have been claimed to have good activity.

(18)   (19)

In general, compounds (18) where R = Me were several times more potent in the UVE test than those where R = H (Nicholson, 1980). It is likely that the introduction of a methyl group, in creating two enantiomers, provides a chiral binding group of the correct size to fit the putative prostaglandin synthetase receptor site.

Variation of substitution in the phenyl ring provides a wide range of active compounds. Boots chemists initially concentrated upon alkyl and cycloalkyl substituents, primarily in the 4-position as these were the groups conferring best activity in the related phenylacetic and phenoxypropionic acid series (Table 2.4). This decision was quickly justified when the third and fourth compounds synthesized (4-isobutyl and 4-cyclohexyl) became leading contenders for product status. Little activity was found in the 2- and 3- substituted analogues at that time.

The 4-cyclohexyl compound (20) (R = H) was 4–8 times more potent than the corresponding cyclopentyl or cycloheptyl analogues but was eventually discarded as a potential product on consideration of its possible ulcerogenic potential. Interestingly, the S-(+) enantioner of a chloro analogue (20) (R = Cl) was also reported to have very high potency (Shen, 1972) but was eventually abandoned owing to gastric intolerance and renal papillary necrosis (Sarett, 1971).

(20)   (21)

CHAPTER 2

3-Substitution in the benzene ring has been successful in some cases. The 4-phenoxy and 4-benzoyl compounds did not achieve product candidate status, but the 3-phenoxy ((21), R = O·Ph) fenoprofen (Lilly) and 3-benzoyl ((21), R = CO·Ph) ketoprofen (Rhone-Poulenc-Rorer) are marketed products.

The 4-(2-thenoyl) compound (22) (suprofen) was sufficiently active to be marketed but the oral dosage form was withdrawn because of adverse side-effects.

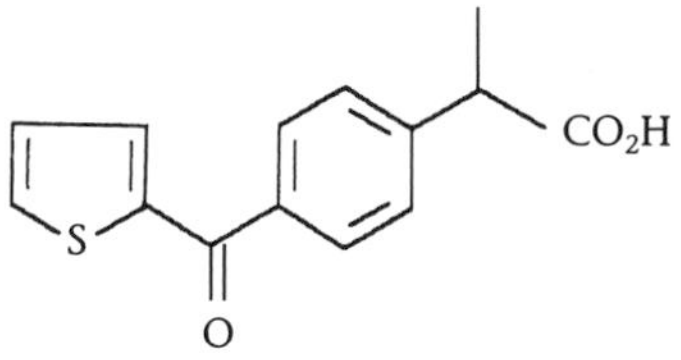

(22)

A range of 4-(substituted)amino compounds (23) proved to possess good anti-inflammatory activity (Dumaitre *et al.*, 1979); the most active compound ((23), R = methallyl) compared well with ibuprofen and is marketed as alminoprofen (Bouchera).

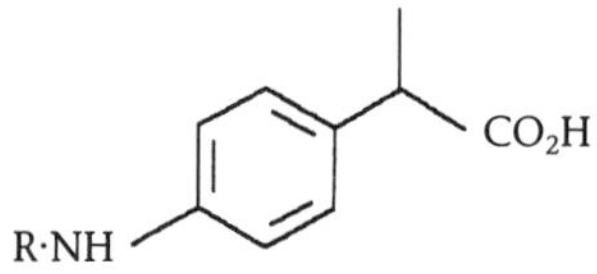

(23) 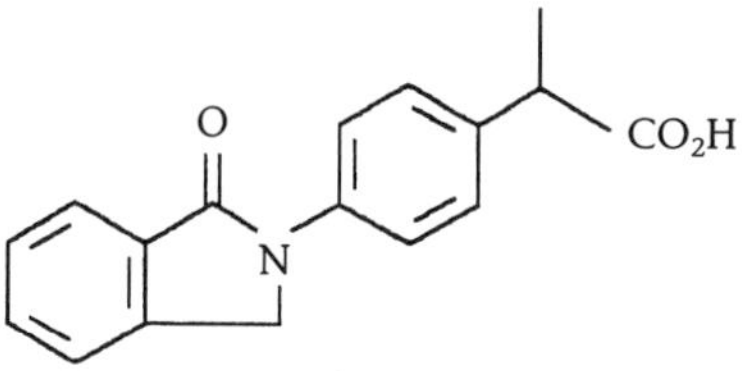 (24)

Two compounds with N-linked heterocycles in the 4-position, indoprofen (24) and pirprofen (25) have exhibited good antirheumatic activity in clinical use but both have been withdrawn by reason of side-effects.

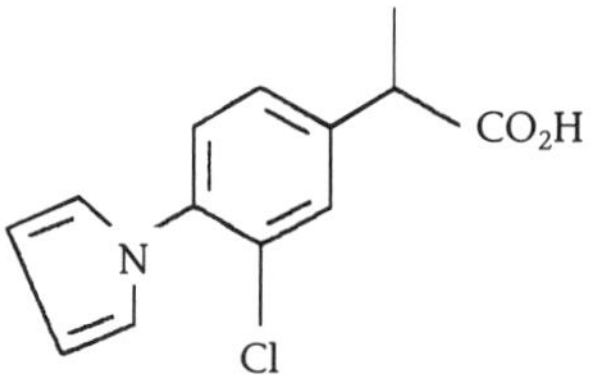

(25) 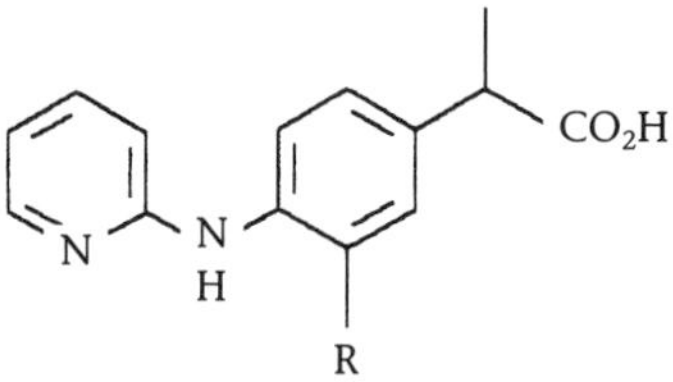 (26)

4-(2-Pyridylamino) compounds (26) (R = H or Cl) are reported (Hino *et al.*, 1983) to be superior to ibuprofen. Other nitrogen-substituted analogues include the azo compound (27) (Crossley, 1988) and the cinnamamide (28) (Nakagawa *et al.*, 1986), both claimed to have anti-inflammatory properties.

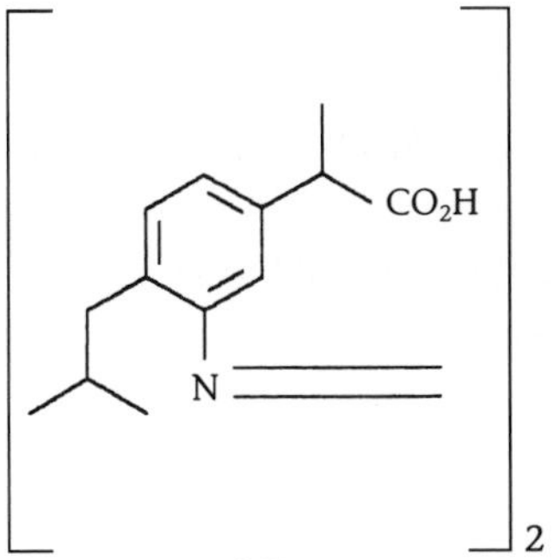

(27)

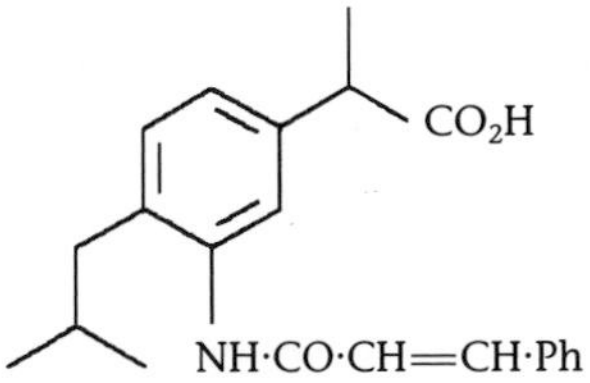

(28)

Few monocyclic ring variants are of note. The cyclohex-1-ene compound (a tetrahydro ibuprofen) (29) was devoid of anti-inflammatory activity but possessed fibrinolytic properties (Vincent *et al.*, 1973) while (29) (R = cyclohexyl) was a potent adjuvant arthritis inhibitor in the rat (Vincent *et al.*, 1972).

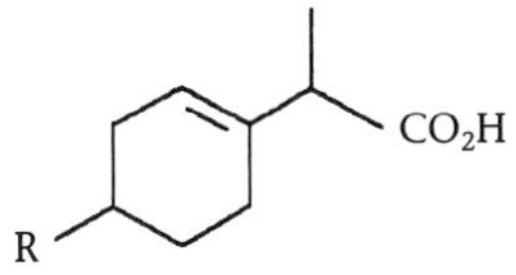

(29)

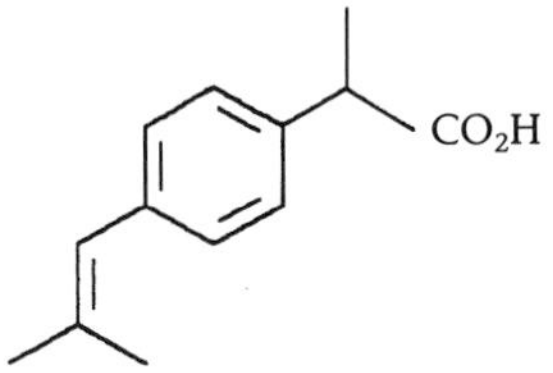

(30)

Functionalization of the 4-isobutyl group of ibuprofen has received little attention. Metabolites A, B, C and D (see Section 2.5) are inactive. The 4-(2,2-dimethylvinyl) analogue (30) is reported to have activity similar to that of ibuprofen (Amano *et al.*, 1986).

2.5 METABOLITES OF IBUPROFEN

2.5.1 Metabolites and enantiomer inversion

Ibuprofen possesses a relatively simple molecular structure, with no group such as ester or amide that is readily hydrolyzed. First pass metabolism would therefore be most likely to lead to oxygenated products while retaining the initial carbon skeleton.

Early investigations into the metabolism of ibuprofen (Adams *et al.*, 1967) revealed that there were two principal metabolites, designated A and B, in the urine of normal human subjects. They were readily isolated, having retained the acidic group of the dosed compound, and were shown by elemental analysis and spectroscopy to possess the structures (31) and (32).

CHAPTER 2

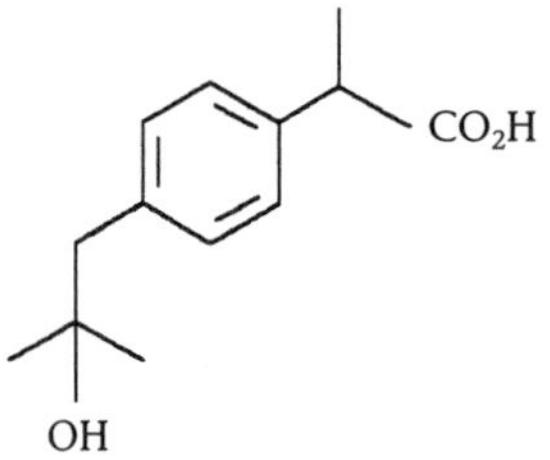

(31) 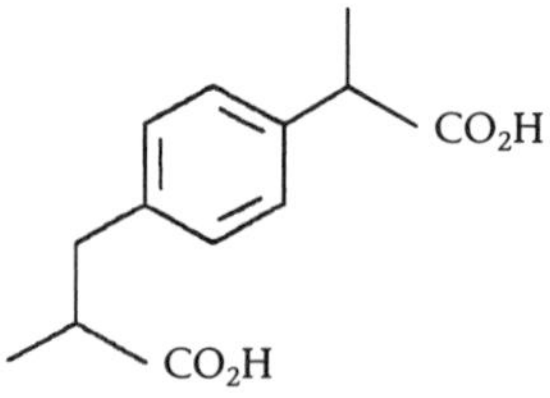   (32)

Although the racemate had been dosed, both metabolites were found to have (+) rotation. This was not considered too unusual for (32) as a second chiral centre had been created, but this was not the case for (31), which might have been expected to retain its racemic nature. It was suspected that this effect may have been due to a difference in the metabolism of the two enantiomers of ibuprofen, but the reality was more fundamental. When ibuprofen enantiomers were dosed to man, both (+) and (−) isomers yielded (+) metabolites (Mills *et al.*, 1973). The inescapable conclusion was that the poorly active (−) enantiomer was at least partially converted to the active (+) isomer in man. An extensive study by Wechter and Kaiser (Wechter *et al.*, 1974) conclusively demonstrated the point. When the (+) isomer, now believed to have the *S* configuration, was dosed, metabolite A was almost entirely *S*, and B was essentially 50/50 *S/S* and *S/R*, there being no specificity in configuration in the formation of the new chiral centre. When the *R* enantiomer was dosed, however, the metabolite A fraction contained similar proportions of *S* and *R* while the metabolite B fraction consisted of all four possible diastereoisomers *SR*, *SS*, *RS* and *RS*. Furthermore, unaltered ibuprofen excreted was largely of the *S* configuration.

Although the (+) and (−) isomers of ibuprofen had similar potency in the guinea-pig UVE test, the (+) form was considerably more potent in the *in vitro* inhibition of prostaglandin synthetase (Adams *et al.*, 1976).

The metabolites A and B originally found in urine of man (Adams *et al.*, 1967) were later (Mills *et al.*, 1973) found in the urine of rat, baboon and dog, although in widely varying amounts. Metabolites A and B were shown to be inactive in the UVE test (Adams *et al.*, 1969a). By 1969, two further metabolites had been detected (Adams *et al.*, 1969b). Their structures (33), (34) were assigned by Brooks and Gilbert (1974) in a GC-MS study involving the amides of metabolites with (*R*)-(+)-1-phenylethylamine.

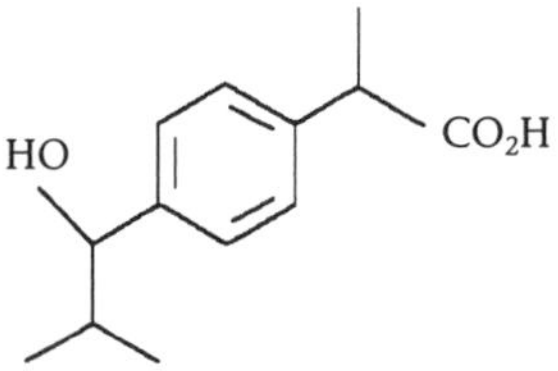

(33) 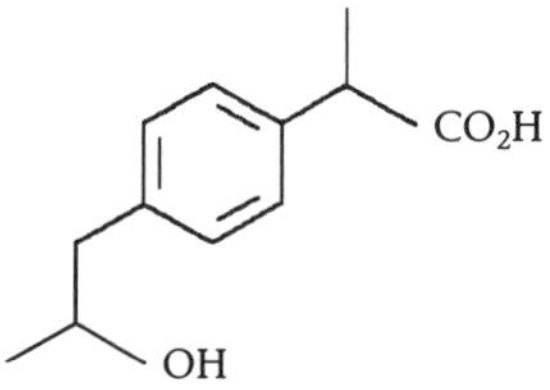   (34)

Thus ibuprofen has been proved to be metabolized at each of the carbon atoms of the isobutyl group. The 4'-carboxylic acid (35) is the principal metabolite in anephric subjects, and has been found in trace amounts in normal volunteers. (The rapid clearance of metabolites A, B, C and D presumably prevents its accumulation.) (Pettersen, 1978) To date no hydroxylation of the phenyl ring or of the propionic acid group has been detected. The ketone (36) is similarly not found.

2.5.2   Synthesis of metabolites

Once the structure of the metabolites of ibuprofen had been determined, it was advantageous to devise synthetic routes since obtaining them by extraction from urine was not a preferred source of supply. Metabolite A may be prepared (Kurz and Houser, 1981) by a novel 1,6-eliminative cleavage of an epoxide (37) derived from ibuprofen by bromination, dehydrobromination and oxidation. Treatment of (37) with potassium t-butoxide yielded the acrylic acid (38) which, on hydrogenation, provided the racemic metabolite A (reaction 9). The synthesis of metabolites C and E has been reported (Teien et al., 1981).

Reagents: (i) ButOK; (ii) H_2/Pd-C

Metabolite C was readily obtained by reduction of the ketone (36), which was formed in low yield by oxidation of ibuprofen (reaction 10).

(10)

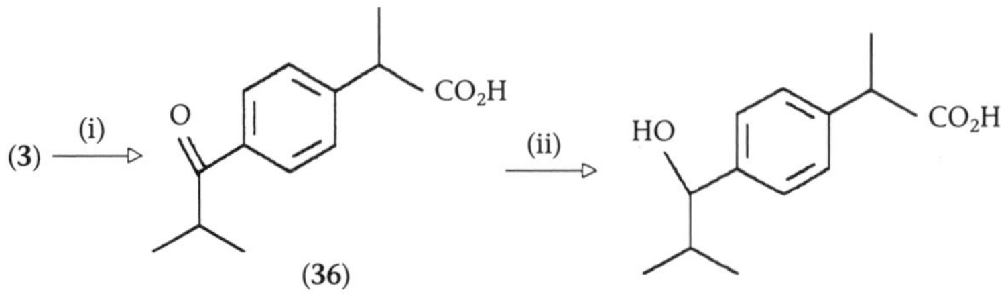

(3) →(i) → (36) →(ii) →

Reagents: (i) KMnO₄; (ii) NaBH₄

The dimethyl ester of (35) was obtained as in reaction (11). The low yield following chromatographic purification suggests that dimethylated products were also formed.

(11)

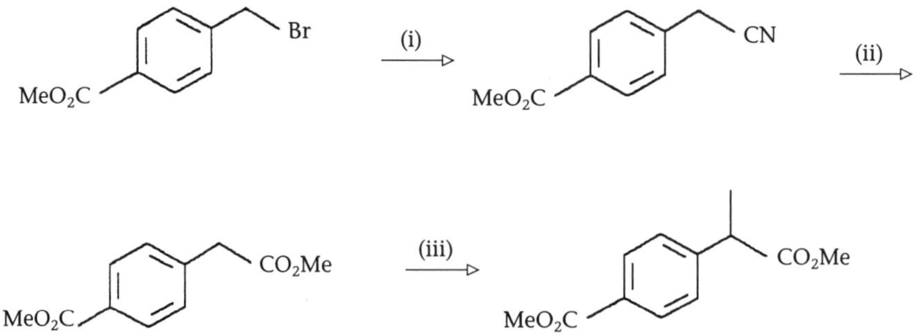

Reagents: (i) KCN/18-**crown**-6; (ii) HBr/MeOH, H₂O; (iii) LiN(CMe)₂/MeI

2.6 IBUPROFEN ENANTIOMERS

The ibuprofen molecule possesses a chiral centre in the propionic acid group and therefore can exist two isomeric forms or optical isomers, whose chemical properties are identical but which have equal optical rotations of opposite sign. The (+) form (originally described as *d*- or *dextro*-) has been shown (Ghislandi *et al.*, 1982) to have the *S*-configuration and is now always referred to as (*S*)-(+)-ibuprofen. Analogously the (–) (*l*- or *laevo*-) form is the (*R*)-(–) enantiomer.

Ibuprofen has been marketed since 1969 as the racemic substance. In the last decade there has been considerable debate whether only single enantiomers of chiral pharmaceuticals should be permitted. It is rightly pointed out that in many pharmacologically active chiral compounds the two optical isomers have widely different biological effects, see e.g. Jamali *et al.* (1989). In the case of ibuprofen, there seems not to be a compelling case for restricting to the active (*S*)-(+) as the racemate has been in use for two decades without serious problems, and no adverse effects have been convincingly attributed to the (*R*)-(–) isomer. Nevertheless, the matter has generated high interest in the (*S*)-(+) form and numerous patents have been issued claiming its use in medicine while synthetic routes to the isomers have proliferated. These latter have been collated in a comprehensive review (Sonawane, 1992). It is worth noting that few if any of the methods are truly selective for either isomer, at best yielding a product enriched in the target enantiomer.

Essentially there are two broad types of approach, the first separating the racemate into its component enantiomers and the second synthesizing either enantiomer using stereoselective synthetic procedures. The classical method of resolution of a racemic acid involves fractional crystallization of a salt of the racemate with a single, pure enantiomer of an organic amine. Natural alkaloids have been traditional, although synthetic amines are now more favoured because of cost, availability, reliability and variety. Ibuprofen may be resolved using (R)- or (S)-2-phenylethylamine (Hardy et al., 1994).

Esters of racemic ibuprofen may be selectively hydrolyzed using enzymes (Ahmar et al., 1989), to provide one enantiomer as the acid and the other as unchanged ester, separated by standard procedures (reaction 12). This method be of use on a laboratory scale, but the high dilution and long reaction times may restrict use in commercial production. Progress may depend upon developments in immobilized enzyme technology.

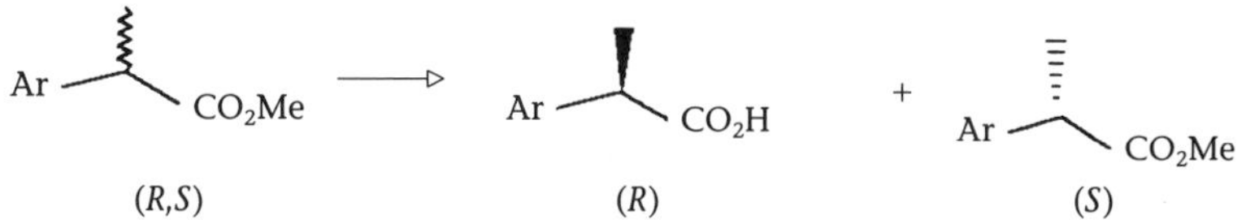

(12)

$$Ar \overset{\xi}{\underset{}{\diagup}} CO_2Me \longrightarrow Ar \overset{}{\underset{}{\diagup}} CO_2H + Ar \overset{}{\underset{}{\diagup}} CO_2Me$$

(R,S)   (R)   (S)

To date there is no laboratory method which mimics the *in vivo* inversion of (R)-ibuprofen to the S isomer.

Stereochemical synthetic procedures for constructing the ibuprofen molecule are frequently variants of methods used to prepare the racemic molecule and fall into three broad categories. The first involves use of a chiral catalyst to create a chiral centre in a reaction between nonchiral reactants. A simple example is the hydrogenation of the acrylic acid (**39**) in the presence of a chiral catalyst (Grosselin, 1991) (reaction 13).

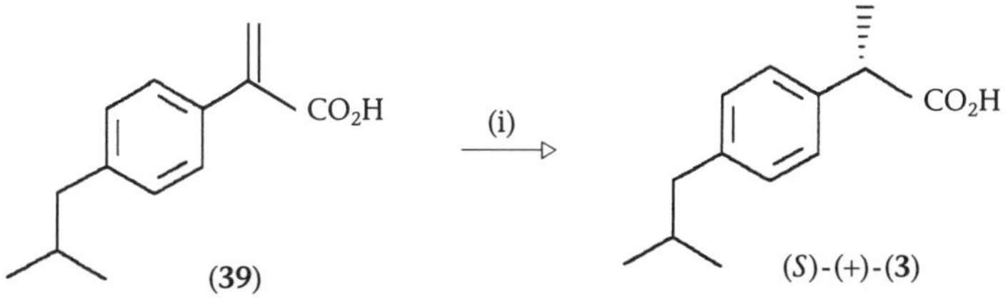

(13)

(39)   (S)-(+)-(3)

Reagents: (i) Rh catalyst/H_2

The second category includes construction of ibuprofen from a chiral synthon as in the alkylation-type reaction of a lactic acid enantiomer (**40**) with isobutylbenzene (reaction 14).

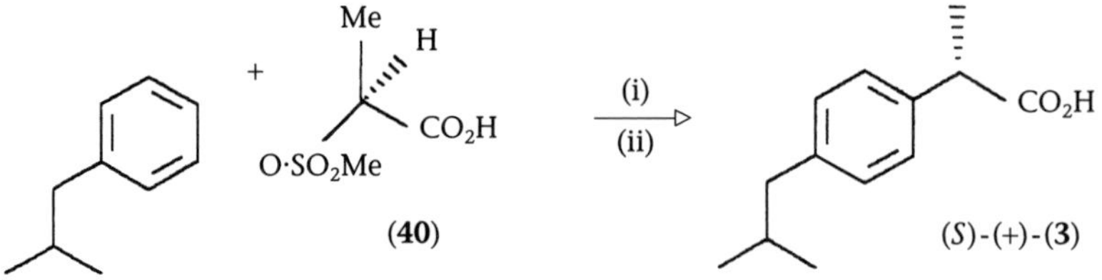

(14)

(40)   (S)-(+)-**(3)**

Reagents: (i) AlCl$_3$; (ii) NaOH aq

Third is induction of chirality using a sacrificial chiral reactant (i.e. one which covalently bonds to other reactants but is wholly or partly removed at a later stage). Typical is the reaction of the keten (**41**) with a cyclic chiral alcohol and subsequent hydrolysis (reaction 15).

(15)

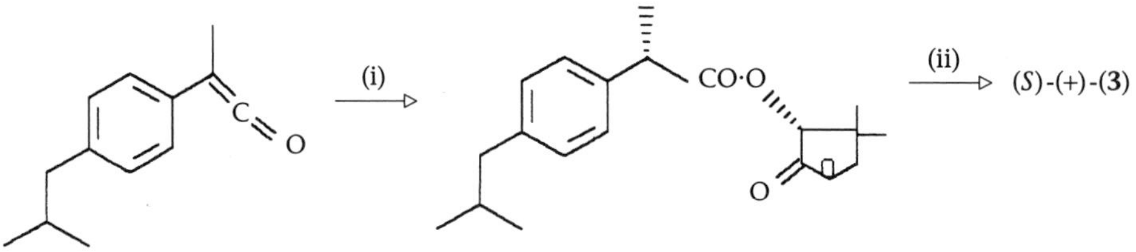

(41)

Reagents: (i) (S)-pantolactone; (ii) LiOH/heptane/MeCN/H$_2$O

Liquid chromatography over chiral adsorbents provides a useful method for obtaining small quantities of very pure material (Booth and Wainer, 1996).

2.7   PHYSICOCHEMICAL ASPECTS

The chromatographic assay of ibuprofen and its metabolites and their stereoisomers is usually preceded by derivatization to amides, typically using one of the enantiomers of 1-phenylethylamine (Vangiessen and Kaiser, 1975). A range of amides was studied (Wainer and Doyle, 1983; Nicoll-Griffith, 1987) for use in HPLC assays on Pirkle-type chiral columns. The glucuronide ester metabolites of ibuprofen were investigated using HPLC in conjunction with high-field ^{1}H NMR (Spraul *et al.*, 1993).

Conformational analysis (Smeyers *et al.*, 1985) and quantum mechanical studies (Smeyers *et al.*, 1989) have been performed on ibuprofen and analogues. Octanol/water partition data and chromatographic data (La Rotonda *et al.*, 1983) and pH solubility and partition coefficients (Chiarni and Tartarini, 1984) have been reported.

ACKNOWLEDGEMENTS

Thanks are particularly due to Dr Ian Hunneyball, Director of Research, Knoll Pharmaceuticals, Nottingham for allowing use of library facilities and access to original data from Boots Pharmaceuticals concerning the research programme that led to the discovery of ibuprofen.

REFERENCES

ADAMS, S.S. (1960) Analgesic-antipyretics. *Journal of Pharmacy and Pharmacology* **12**, 251.

ADAMS, S.S. (1992) The propionic acids: a personal perspective. *Journal of Clinical Pharmacology* **32**, 317.

ADAMS, S.S. and COBB, R. (1958) A possible basis for the anti-inflammatory activity of salicylates and other nonhormonal antirheumatic drugs. *Nature* **181**, 773–774.

ADAMS, S.S. and COBB, R. (1967) Nonsteroidal anti-inflammatory drugs. In: ELLIS, G.P. and WEST, B.B. (eds), *Progress in Medicinal Chemistry* 5. Amsterdam, Elsevier, 59–138.

ADAMS, S.S., CLIFFE, E.E., LESSEL, B. and NICHOLSON, J.S. (1967) Some biological properties of 2-(4-isobutylphenyl)propionic acid. *Journal of Pharmaceutical Science* **56**, 1686.

ADAMS, S.S., McCULLOUGH, K.F. and NICHOLSON, J.S. (1969a) The pharmacological properties of ibuprofen, an anti-inflammatory analgesic and antipyretic agent. *Archives Internationales de Pharmacodynamie et de Therapie* **173**, 115.

ADAMS, S.S., BOUGH, R.G., CLIFFE, E.E., LESSEL, B. and MILLS, R.F.N. (1969b) Absorption, distribution and toxicity of ibuprofen. *Toxicology and Applied Pharmacology* **15**, 310.

ADAMS, S.S., BOUGH, R.G., CLIFFE, E.E., DICKINSON, W., LESSEL, B., McCULLOUGH, K.F., MILLS, R.F.N., NICHOLSON, J.S. and WILLIAMS, G.A.H. (1970) Some aspects of the pharmacology, metabolism, and toxicology of ibuprofen. *Rheumatology and Physical Medicine, Supplement, Symposium on Ibuprofen*, 9–26.

ADAMS, S.S., BRESLOFF, P. and MASON, C.G. (1976) Pharmacological differences between the optical isomers of ibuprofen: evidence for metabolic inversion of the (−)-isomer. *Journal of Pharmacy and Pharmacology* **28**, 256.

AHMAR, A., GIRARD, C. and BLOCH, R. (1989) Enzymatic resolution of methyl 2-alkyl-2-arylacetates. *Tetrahedron Letters* **30**, 7053.

AMANO, T., KOSHIWAKA, K., OGAWA, T., SANO, T., OHUCHI, Y., TAMAMI, T., HATAYAMA, K., HIGUCHI, S., AMANUMA, F. and SOTA, K. (1986) Synthesis and anti-inflammatory activity of alkylphenylpropionic acids. *Chemical and Pharmaceutical Bulletin* **34**, 4653–4662.

BACKES, B.J. and ELLMAN, J.A. (1994) Carbon–carbon bond-forming methods on solid support. Utilization of Kenner's 'safety-catch' linker. *Journal of the American Chemical Society* 11171.

BOOTH, T.D. and WAINER, I.W. (1996) Investigation of the enantioselective separations of α-alkylarylcarboxylic acids on an amylose tris(3,5-dimethylphenylcarbamate) chiral stationary phase using quantitative structure–enantioselective retention relationships. Identification of a conformationally driven chiral recognition mechanism. *Journal of Chromatography A* **737**, 157.

■ CHAPTER 2 ■

BROOKS, C.J.W. and GILBERT, M.T. (1974) Studies of urinary metabolites of 2-(4-isobutylphenyl)propionic acid by gas–liquid chromatography–mass spectrometry. *Journal of Chromatography* 99, 541–551.

BUCKLER, J.W. and ADAMS, S.S. (1968) The phenylalkanoic acids. Laboratory and clinical studies. *Medical Proceedings* 574.

CARRETERO, J.M., MARTIN, J.L. and RON, A. (1978) Butibrufen, a novel nonsteroidal anti-inflammatory compound. *European Journal of Medicinal Chemistry* 13, 77–80.

CAVALLINI, G., MASSANINI, E., NARDI, D. and D'AMBROSIO, R. (1957) Further research on biphenyl, stilbene and diphenylethane derivatives — potential anticholesterinemic, antirheumatic drugs. VII. *Journal of the American Chemical Society* 79, 3514.

CHIARINI, A. and TARTARINI, A. (1984) pH-Solubility relationship and partition coefficients for some anti-inflammatory arylaliphatic acids. *Archiv der Pharmazie* 317, 268.

CROSSLEY, R. (1988) Preparation of azobis(benzeneacetic acids) as inflammation inhibitors. *GB Patent* 2203434 (John Wyeth and Brother Ltd).

DUMAITRE, B., FOUQUET, A., PERRIN, C., CORNU, P.J., BOUCHERLE, A., PLOTKA, P., DOMAGE, G. and STREICHENBERGER, G. (1979) Synthèse de quelques dérivés des acides amino-4-phénylacétique et (amino-4-phényl)-2-propionique possédant des activités anal-gésiques et anti-inflammatoires. *European Journal of Medicinal Chemistry* 14, 207.

DYTHAM, R.A. (1969) Improvements in the preparation of phenylalkanoic acids. *GB Patent* 1160725 (Boots Pure Drug Co. Ltd).

FAIGL, F. and SCHLOSSER, M. (1991) A one-pot synthesis of ibuprofen involving three con-secutive steps of superbase metalation. *Tetrahedron Letters* 32, 3369–3370.

GHISLANDI, V., LA MANNA, A., AZZOLINO, O., GAZZANIGA, A. and VERCESI, D. (1981) Con-figurational relationships in antiphlogistic hydratropic acids. *Il Farmaco (Edizion Scientifico)* 37, 81.

GROSSELIN, J.-M. (1991) Preparation of optically active 2-aryl propionic acids — especially ketoprofen — by hydrogenation of 2-aryl-acrylic acids in 2-phase solvent in presence of chiral rhodium complex with water-soluble ligand. *French Patent* 2651494 (Rhone-Poulenc Sante).

HARDY, R., COE, P.F., HIRST, A. and O'DONNELL, H.O. (1994) Preparation of substantially pure enantiomers of phenylpropionics acids. *WO Patent* 94 12460 (Boots Co. plc).

HARRIS, S.C. and FOSDICK, L.S. (1952) Theoretical considerations of the mechanism of antipyretic analgesia. *Northwestern University Bulletin* 53, 6.

HARASUWA, S., NAKAMURA, S., YAGI, S., KURIHARA, T., HAMADA, Y. and SHIOIRI, T. (1984) A new synthesis of some non-steroidal anti-inflammatory agents via cyanophosphates. *Synthetic Communications* 14, 1365.

HINO, K., NAKAMURA, H., NAGAI, Y., UNO, H. and NISHIMURA, H. (1983) Nonsteroidal anti-inflammatory agents. 2. [(Heteroarylamino)phenyl]alkanoic acids. *Journal of Medical Chemistry* **26**, 222.

HIYAMA, T., INOUE, M. and SAITO, K. (1986) A facile route to [±]-2-arylpropionic acids. *Synthesis* 645.

JAMALI, F., MEHVAR, R. and PASUTTO, F.M. (1989) Enantioselective aspects of drug action and disposition: therapeutic pitfalls. *Journal of Pharmaceutical Sciences* **78**, 695.

JUBY, P.F. (1974) Aryl- and heteroalkanoic acids and related compounds. In: SCHERRER, R.A. and WHITEHOUSE, M.W. (eds), *Antiinflammatory Agents*, vol. 1. London, Academic Press, 91–127.

KAISER, D.G., VANGIESSEN, G.J., REISCHER, R.J. and WECHTER (1976) Isomeric inversion of ibuprofen (*R*)-enantiomer in humans. *Journal of Pharmaceutical Sciences* **65**, 269.

KUCHAR, M., BRUNOVA, B., REJHOLEC, V. and GRIMOVA, J. (1978) Quantitative relationships between the structure and the anti-inflammatory activity of aryl-*n*-butyric acids. *European Journal of Medicinal Chemistry* **13**, 363.

LA ROTONDA, M.I., AMATO, G., BARBATO, F., SILIPO, C. and VITTORIA, A. (1983) Relationships between octanol-water partition data, chromatographic indices and their dependance on pH in a set of nonsteroidal anti-inflammatory drugs. *Quantitative Structure-Activity Relationships* **2**, 163.

KURZ, R.R. and HOUSER, D.J. (1981) A 1,6-eliminative epoxide cleavage in the sythesis of an ibuprofen metabolite. *Journal of Organic Chemistry* **46**, 202.

MILLS, R.F.N., ADAMS, S.S., CLIFFE, E.E., DICKINSON, W. and NICHOLSON, J.S. (1973) The metabolism of ibuprofen. *Xenobiotica* **3**, 589.

NAKAGAWA, A., TSUJI, M. and MIZOTA, T. (1986) Preparation of phenylalkanoic acid derivatives as antiinflammatory agents. *Japanese Patent* 61271262 (Hisamitsu Pharmaceutical Co.).

NICHOLSON, J.S. (1980) In: BINDRA, J.S. and LEDNICER, D. (eds) *Chronicles of Drug Discovery*, vol. 1. Chichester, Wiley, 148–171.

NICHOLSON, J.S. and ADAMS, S.S. (1964) Anti-inflammatory agents. *GB Patent* 971700 (Boots Pure Drug Co. Ltd).

NICHOLSON, J.S. and ADAMS, S.S. (1965) Anti-inflammatory agents. *GB Patent* 1012480 (Boots Pure Drug Co. Ltd).

NICHOLL-GRIFFITH, D.A. (1987) Stereoelectronic model to explain the resolution of enantiomeric ibuprofen amides on the Pikle chiral stationary phase. *Journal of Chromatography* **402**, 179–187.

PETTERSON, J.E., ULSAKER, G.A. and JELLUM, E. (1978) Studies on the metabolism of 2,4'-isobutylphenylpropionic acid (ibuprofen) by gas chromatography and mass spectrometry. Dialysis fluid, a convenient medium for studies on drug metabolism. *Journal of Chromatography* **145**, 413.

■ CHAPTER 2 ■

RANDALL, L.O. and SELITTO, J.J. (1957) A method for measurement of analgesic activity on inflamed tissue. *Archives Internationales de Pharmacodynamie et de Therapie* **111**, 409.

REDEL, J., BROUILHET, H., BAZELY, N., JOUANNEAU, M. and DELBARRE, F. (1970) Préparation et activité anti-inflammatoire des acides *p*-cyclohexylphénylpropioniques. *Comptes Rendus de l'Academie de Sciences Paris (D)* **270**, 224.

RIEU, J.-P., BOUCHERLE, A., COUSSE, H. and MOUZIN, G. (1986) Methods for the synthesis of anti-inflammatory 2-aryl propionic acids. *Tetrahedron* **42**, 4095–4131.

RIVERA, I., COLBERG, J.C. and SODERQUIST, J.A. (1992) Ibuprofen and naproxen via organoboranes. *Tetrahedron Letters* **33**, 6919–6922.

SARETT, L.H. (1971) Introduction: International Symposium on Inflammation and Therapy — Experiences with Indomethacin. *Arzneimittel-Forschung* **21**, 1759–1761.

SHEN, T.Y. (1972) Perspectives in nonsteroidal anti-inflammatory agents. *Angewandte Chemie, International Edition* **11**, 460–472.

SMEYERS, Y.G., CUELLAR-RODRIGUEZ, S., GALVES-RUANO, E. and ARIAS-PEREZ, M.S. (1985) Conformational analysis of some α-phenylpropionic acids with anti-inflammatory activity. *Journal of Pharmaceutical Sciences* **74**, 47.

SMEYERS, Y.G., HERNANDEZ-LAGUNA, A., MUNOZ-CARO, C., AGUILERA, J., GALVES-RUANO, E. and ARIAZ-PEREZ, M.S. (1989) Quantum mechanical study and nuclear magnetic resonance measurements of some α-arylcarboxyalkyl acids as anti-inflammatory agents. *Journal of Pharmaceutical Sciences* **78**, 764.

SONANWANE, H.R., BELLUR, N.S., AHUJA, J.R. and KULKARNI, D.G. (1992) Recent developments in the synthesis of optically active α-arylpropanoic acids: an important class of non-steroidal antiinflammatory agents. *Tetrahedron* A **3**, 163–192.

SPRAUL, M., HOFMANN, M., DVORTSAK, P., NICHOLSON, J.K. and WILSON, I.A. (1993) High-performance liquid chromatography coupled to high-field proton nuclear magnetic resonance spectroscopy: application to the urinary metabolites of ibuprofen. *Analytical Chemistry* **65**, 327–330.

TEIEN, G., ULSAKER, G.A. and PETTERSEN, J.E. (1981) Synthesis of metabolites of 2-(4-isobutylphenyl) propionic acid — ibuprofen. *Acta Pharmaceutica Suecica* **18**, 233–238.

VALENTI, P., RAMPA, A., FABBRI, G., GIUTSI, P. and CIMA, L. (1983) *Tetrahedron* Tetrazole analogues of ibuprofen and flurbiprofen. *Archiv der Pharmazie* **316**, 752–755.

VANGIESSEN, G.J. and KAISER, D.G. (1975) GLC (Gas–liquid chromatographic) determination of ibuprofen [*dl*-2-(*p*-isobutylphenyl)propionic acid] enantiomers in biological specimens. *Journal of Pharmaceutical Sciences* **64**, 798–801.

VINCENT, M., REMOND, G. and POIGNANT, J.P. (1972) *dl*-α-[4-Cycloalkyl(hexen-1-yl)] alkanoic acids and derivatives as anti-inflammatory and antiarthritic compounds. *Journal of Medicinal Chemistry* **15**, 75.

VINCENT, M., REMOND, G., DESNOYERS, P. and LABAUME, J. (1973) *dl*-α-[4-Cycloalkyl(hexen-1-yl)] alkanoic acids and derivatives as fibrinolytic and thrombolytic compounds. *Journal of Medicinal Chemistry* **16**, 710.

WAINER, I.W. and DOYLE, T.D. (1983) Application of high-performance liquid chromatographic chiral stationary phases to pharmaceutical analysis: structural and conformational effects in the direct enantiomeric resolution of α-methylarylacetic acid anti-inflammatory agents. *Journal of Chromatography* **284**, 117–124.

WECHTER, W.J., LOGHLAND, D.G., REISCHLER, R.J., VANGIESSEN, G.J. and KAISER, D.G. (1974) Nature and mechanism of the inversion of *R*(–) *p*-iso-butyl hydratropic acid. *Biochemical and Biophysical Research Communications* **61**, 833.

WILHELMI, G. (1949) Ueber die Pharmakologischen Eigenschaften von Irgaprin, einen neuen Preparat aus der Pyrazolreihe. *Schhweizerische Medizinische Wochenschrift* **79**, 577.

WU, T.C. (1994) Olefinic process for preparing aryl-substituted aliphatic carboxylic esters [e.g., ibuprofen methyl ester]. *US Patent* 5315028 (Ethyl Corp.).

CHAPTER 2

3

The Pharmaceutics of Ibuprofen

F HIGTON

Boots Healthcare International, Nottingham, UK

Contents

Ibuprofen (2-(4-isobutylphenyl)propionic acid) was the first of the propionic acid NSAIDs to be marketed successfully. Owing to the presence of a single asymmetric carbon atom, the molecule exists as the (S)-(+) (dextro) or (R)-(−) (laevo) isomer. Conventional ibuprofen occurs as a racemic mixture of the two isomers, but almost all the prostaglandin synthetase inhibition activity resides with the (S)-(+) isomer.

This chapter will focus exclusively on the properties and formulations relating to racemic ibuprofen and its derivatives. Since much of the most up-to-date information on new dosage formats and formulations is to be found in the patent literature, that source has been used extensively. It should be noted, however, that the references are to patent applications and this does not necessarily mean that the patent has been subsequently granted, nor that it is still in force.

3.1 PHYSICAL AND CHEMICAL CHARACTERISTICS OF IBUPROFEN

Ibuprofen is a white crystalline, slightly waxy solid with a slight odour and a strong and characteristic taste. The drug also produces a burning sensation or 'kick' in the back of the throat when swallowed, adding to the difficulty of producing formulations with acceptable taste characteristics. The chemical formula is shown in Figure 3.1. The raw material is available from a number of commercial sources, the major suppliers being Knoll Pharmaceuticals and the Albemarle Corporation. Supplies are also available, at the time of writing, from Francis and from Indian sources. Since the various suppliers use differing routes of synthesis, the impurity profiles vary. The Knoll material is currently produced at two sites, Nottingham, UK and Bishop, Texas, USA. The Albemarle material is produced at a single site, Orangeburg, South Carolina. The major impurities arising from the synthesis are shown in Table 3.1. Romero (1991) studied ibuprofen from a number of sources — Boots (now Knoll), Ethyl (now Albemarle) Francis and Cheminor — and concluded that even though the material from different sources did not show major differences in physicochemical properties and that different polymorphs were not present, the materials behaved differently during processing, especially with respect to the quantity of granulation solution required to achieve a suitable end point, and that tablets with differing compact strengths and friabilities were produced. While this work does not indicate that any source of material is necessarily superior, it does indicate that great care must be exercised in changing from one source to another and emphasizes the importance of careful preformulation studies.

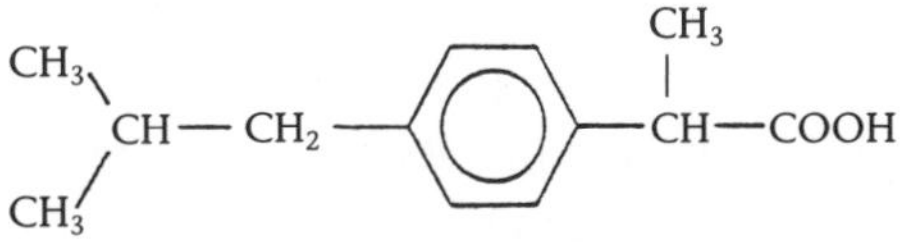

Figure 3.1: The chemical structure of ibuprofen.

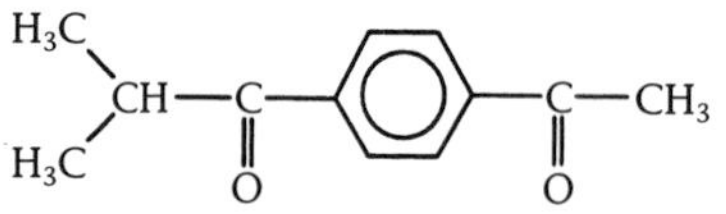

Figure 3.2: The chemical structure of 4-isobutyrylacetophenone (ibap).

TABLE 3.1

Major impurities found in ibuprofen, and their typical values

Compound	Typical value (µg/g)
Knoll (Nottingham source)	
2-(4-Methylphenyl)propionic acid	up to 100
2-(4-Isobutylphenyl)propionamide	1000
2-(4-*n*-Propylphenyl)propionic acid	up to 500
2-(3-Isobutylphenyl)propionic acid	500
2-(4-*n*-Butylphenyl)propionic acid	up to 500
Albemarle	
2-Hydroxy-2-(4-isobutylphenyl)propionic acid	less than 500
2-(3-Isobutylphenyl)propionic acid	~600
2-(4-*n*-Butylphenyl)propionic acid	3000
Di-isobutylisatropic acid	less than 500
1,3-Di-(isobutylphenyl)butane	less than 200
1,3-Di-(isobutylphenyl)-1-butanone	less than 200

TABLE 3.2

The particle size-related physical characteristics of commonly available grades of ibuprofen (Knoll)

	Available grades		
	Ibuprofen 25	Ibuprofen 38	Ibuprofen 50
Particle size (µm)[a]	20–33	33–45	45–60
Bulk density (g/cm³)	0.2–0.4	0.25–0.5	0.4–0.6
Tap density (g/cm³)	0.4–0.6	0.5–0.7	0.6–0.8

[a] By Malvern Laser Particle Size Analyser.

Under adverse storage conditions, ibuprofen-containing dose forms can produce a number of breakdown products, of which the major degradation product is 4-isobutyrylacetophenone (ibap). The structure of ibap is shown in Figure 3.2 and this compound is a useful marker for chemical deterioration of a product. The major impurities arising from synthesis of ibuprofen and the major breakdown product are resolvable by high-performance liquid chromatography. The particle size-related physical characteristics of ibuprofen are shown in Table 3.2 for the Knoll material and in Table 3.3 for material sourced from Albermarle. The chemical specifications as defined in the EP and the USP are given in Tables 3.4 and 3.5 respectively.

TABLE 3.3

The particle size-related physical characteristics of commonly available grades of ibuprofen (Albemarle)

	Available grades		
	Ibuprofen 20	Ibuprofen 40	Ibuprofen 70
Particle size (µm)[a]	17–27	30–50	55–85
Bulk density (g/cm³)	0.25	0.36	0.44
Tap density (g/cm³)	0.47	0.58	0.64

[a] First figure, 15% centile; second figure, 85% centile.

TABLE 3.4

Ibuprofen chemical specifications: European Pharmacopoeia, 3rd edition (1997)

Test	Specification
Characters	Complies
Identification tests	
Test A: Melting point	Complies with A and C or A, B and D
Test B: UV spectra	
Test C: IR spectra	
Test D: Thin-layer chromatography	
Appearance of solution	Clear and colourless
Optical rotation	−0.05 to +0.05°
Related substances (by liquid chromatography)	Complies
Heavy metals	Limit 10 µg/g
Loss on drying	not more than 5000 µg/g
Sulfated ash	not more than 1000 µg/g
Assay	98.5–101%

TABLE 3.5

Ibuprofen chemical specifications: US Pharmacopeia, 23rd edition, Suppl. 5 (1996)

Test	Specification
Identifcation tests	
Infrared absorption	Complies
UV absorption	Complies
HPLC	Corresponds to standard preparation
Chromatographic purity (HPLC)	Complies
Heavy metals	Limit 20 µg/g
Residue on ignition	Not more than 5000 µg/g
Water	Not more than 1%
Organic volatile impurities	Complies
Assay	97–103%
Limit of 4-isobutylacetophenone (ibap)	Limit 1000 µg/g

CHAPTER 3

TABLE 3.6

Solubilities of ibuprofen in organic solvents

Solvent	Approximate solubility[a]
Acetone	> 10
Ethanol	> 10
Octanol	33.0
Hexane	3.3
Distilled water	< 0.1

Source: Knoll Pharmaceuticals.
[a] Approximate solubility of ibuprofen at ambient temperature (% wt/vol).

Ibuprofen is sparingly soluble in hexane and freely soluble in ethanol, octanol, dimethyl sulfoxide and chloroform. Solubilities in various organic solvents are given in Table 3.6. The relationship of solubility and pH is shown in Figure 3.3. The pH profile of solubility indicates that the solubility of ibuprofen increases sharply with pH, the drug being largely insoluble at low pH values but readily soluble at alkaline pH. This has a significant bearing on aspects of formulation and also on the pH conditions that are selected for the dissolution testing of ibuprofen-containing solid dosage forms.

Potentiometric determination of the dissociation constant of ibuprofen gives a pK_a value of 4.54. Extensive experimentation has demonstrated the absence of polymorphism in ibuprofen and storage at relative humidities of 0, 31%, 58%, 86%, 94% and 100% for 3 months showed no weight change, indicating that ibuprofen is essentially nonhygroscopic.

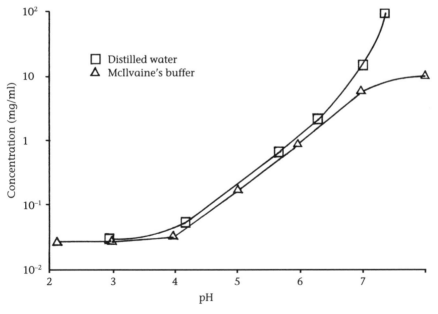

Figure 3.3: Ibuprofen solubility versus pH.

As shown elsewhere in this volume, the absorption and elimination of ibuprofen in humans are rapid, with peak serum levels being achieved in 1 to 2 hours in fasted subjects, and the drug exhibits a half-life of approximately 2 hours. These parameters can, however, be substantially modified by means of formulation. The presence of food reduces both the T_{max} and the C_{max} but total absorption is essentially unaffected.

Thus, when considering the pharmaceutics of ibuprofen, a number of properties of the drug have to be considered, namely, its unpleasant taste and the associated burning or 'kick' in the throat when swallowed, the lack of solubility at low pH and the relatively short half-life. As will be demonstrated later, the material possesses only moderate compaction properties, a significant fact since tablets are still the predominant dose form for ibuprofen.

3.2 PRODUCTS AVAILABLE WORLDWIDE

Since the market for ibuprofen is well developed, especially in the prescription field, a number of improvements and alternative dosage forms have been developed over the years.

Table 3.7 shows the distribution of dosage forms in some of the major western European markets and the United States. Some care needs to be exercised when interpreting the data. Sales cover both prescription and nonprescription business. The data for the United Kingdom and the United States cover pharmacy and grocery outlets and sources of the Netherlands data include pharmacy, grocery and foodstore outlets. The German data are derived from studies in Germany prior to reunification and arise from East and West German pharmacies and West German drugstores and unlicensed outlets.

Despite the relative sophistication of the ibuprofen market, examination of the availability of dosage forms shows that tablets still predominate. Most of the tablets are either sugar or film coated. A number of capsules, oral syrups or suspensions and topical preparations are also available. Oral drops, which enable the dose to be finely controlled, are specific to the Italian market.

TABLE 3.7
Availability of dosage forms in major European territories and the United States
(% of total sales by dosage format)

Dosage form	UK	France	Germany	Italy	Netherlands	Belgium	Spain	USA
Tablets	82	95	76	88	98	89	89	97
Effervescent[a]	0.3	–	0.3	–	–	0.6	–	–
Capsules	–	4	1	–	–	0.6	6.5	1
Controlled release[b]	0.5	–	–	2.5	–	–	–	–
Oral liquids	2	–	–	–	1.3	–	–	2.1
Oral drops	–	–	–	4	–	–	–	–
Topicals	16	–	21	1.5	0.4	10	–	–

[a] Tablets or granules.   [b] All formats.

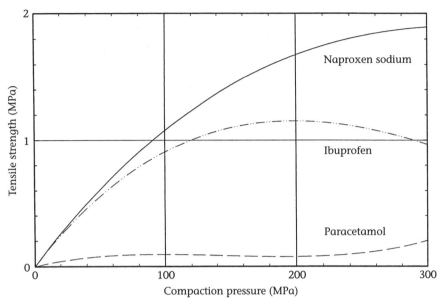

Figure 3.4: Compaction properties of ibuprofen.

3.3 SOLID DOSE PRESENTATIONS

As previously discussed, analysis of the market data shows that tablets are the predominant dosage form. Ibuprofen shows moderate compaction characteristics, as indicated in Figure 3.4.

The data show the properties of ibuprofen compared to paracetamol (which is normally regarded as having poor compaction properties) and sodium naproxen, which possesses good compressibility. Tensile strength of the tablet is derived from the equation

$$TS = \frac{2\,CS}{\pi\,dt}$$

where CS is crushing strength in newtons (measured by diametral crushing at a strain rate of 1 mm/min), d is the compact diameter in mm and t is the compact thickness in mm. The data were generated on a compaction simulator using settings pertinent to a conventional rotary tablet press. Compaction problems are compounded by the relatively high dose of the drug (200 or 400 mg) and a typical compressed core may comprise 90% drug. Notwithstanding this, it is well known in the industry that it is possible to prepare such tablets on a commercial basis using conventional wet granulation techniques.

A survey of the patent literature shows that several attempts have been made to improve upon the basic granulation process. Franz (1986) produced a wet granulation process for the preparation of a tablet containing about 90% of ibuprofen together with croscarmellose sodium and small quantities of other tableting aids. The patent claims that the resulting tablets are stable and show good bioavailability and processing characteristics; also, owing to their high bulk density they can accommodate a high level of ibuprofen for a given tablet size.

Haldar (1988) and co-workers used a fluid-bed granulation technique to prepare ibuprofen tablets and investigated the effect of process variables and excipient levels on tablet characteristics and showed that both the type and level of binder and the processing variables require careful optimization in order to achieve the desired product characteristics. Denton claims two fluid-bed granulated formulations for ibuprofen, thereby offering a simpler (and less expensive) method of production. The first (Denton, 1989) utilizes a combination of ibuprofen and any internally cross-linked alkali metal carboxymethylcellulose, and the latter (Denton and Salpekar, 1992) uses poly(vinyl pyrrolidone) (PVP) (applied partially in a dry mix prior to spraying and partially in the spray-granulation solution). The PVP formulation also yields a tablet with a relatively high drug content of around 90%.

Ho and Blank (1989a) spray dried a dispersion of ibuprofen, pre-gelled starch and a wetting agent to produce a granule showing good flow characteristics and compression properties that in turn produced a stable tablet with superior dissolution and bioavailability. Some workers have also made use of the relatively low melting point of ibuprofen (75°C) to produce solid dose formulations. Deboeck and co-workers (1990) melted a mixture of the drug with fatty acid glycerides or polyglycides and glycerides to produce a eutectic. This was then filled into hard gelatine capsules. Danz used the process of direct melt extrusion to produce a material which could be directly tableted (Danz *et al.*, 1995), and Rittner melted pure ibuprofen and in the presence of seed materials cooled the mass on to a roller or belt cooler resulting in particles that could be directly compressed (Rittner *et al.*, 1990).

Attempts have also been made to improve the various tableting parameters of ibuprofen by modifying the crystal form of the drug. Gordon and Amin (1984) claimed that ibuprofen with what the authors describe as an essentially equant or hexagonal habit exhibits superior flow and improved compaction properties and that the resulting tablets show significantly reduced dissolution time, whilst Goddard and Knesel (1992) patented a process for producing elongated crystals that are also claimed to give superior flow characteristics. Two groups of workers at the Boots Company plc used crystallization techniques to produce, in one case, agglomerates comprising ibuprofen and starch that possessed good tableting properties (Atkin *et al.*, 1993), and in the second, aggregates of crystals showing improved flow and yielding tablets with good dissolution characteristics (Allan *et al.*, 1987).

Lohner and Posselt (1986) patented a liquid-fill soft gelatin capsule where the ibuprofen was dissolved in a poly(oxyethylene)–poly(oxypropylene) polymer. The inventors claim that the speed of absorption is increased since the drug is in solution. Despite the fact that one would expect the ibuprofen to precipitate in the acid medium of the stomach, available data suggest that adding the drug essentially in solution decreases the T_{max}.

CHAPTER 3

Fritsch and Growinghol (1990) claim an effervescent granule comprising a soluble salt of ibuprofen and a combination of bicarbonate and an organic acid, and Carcano (1995) developed a fluidized-bed process involving aqueous granulation followed by rapid drying to also produce an effervescent product that is claimed to show good physical stability.

It can therefore be seen that there is considerable recent activity based around the development of more efficient and more cost-effective conventional solid dose formats.

3.3.1 Sustained release preparations

The pharmacological properties of ibuprofen make it an ideal model drug for the application of various sustained release technologies. The T_{max} is of the order of 1.5 h and the half-life of the drug in the body of the order of 2 h.

A number of techniques are reported in both the literature and patent filings to extend the duration of action by delaying the release of the drug. These usually involve the coating of the drug directly, the coating of granules, pellets or the final solid dose unit, or the incorporation of the drug in a matrix which, *in vivo*, slowly releases the drug through the processes of erosion and/or diffusion. The different modes of action of the various types of sustained release dosage forms are illustrated in Figure 3.5.

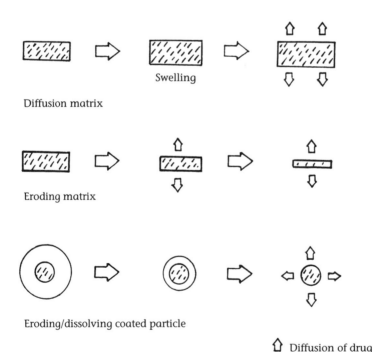

Figure 3.5: Mechanisms of release of drug from sustained release formats.

Much interest has been expressed, usually through the patent literature, in cellulose and its derivatives as a medium for achieving controlled or sustained release. Shaikh and co-workers (1987) investigated granules and compressed tablets utilizing various grades and quantities of ethylcellulose and ibuprofen and indomethacin as model drugs. The drugs were added as a solid dispersion. *In vitro* dissolution testing indicated that the granules released their drug according to zero-order kinetics, whereas the tablets appeared to be diffusion controlled. Perhaps not surprisingly, the greater the content of ethylcellulose the more retarded was the drug release, but the viscosity grade of the polymer also exerted a significant, though lesser effect. Ojantakanen *et al.* (1992) prepared hard gelatin capsules of ibuprofen using hydroxypropylmethylcelluloses (HPMC) and anionic sodium carboxymethylcelluloses (NaCMC) as excipients. Both materials produced retarded release, that of the former greater than the latter. The viscosity grade of the NaCMC had no significant effect. Various workers have, however, claimed specific grades and levels of cellulose derivatives as release-controlling agents, e.g. Mohar *et al.* (1988) (hydroxypropylmethylcellulose with a specific methoxyl and hydroxypropoxyl content); Chen and Defesche (1989) (ethylcellulose, dimethylaminoethyl methacrylate and methacrylic acid ester copolymer or high-viscosity hydroxypropylmethylcellulose co-precipitated with the drug); Gaylord and Nigalaye (1989) (a combination of cellulose ethers and an alkali metal carboxylate); and Kokubo and Maruyaman (1994) (hydroxypropylmethylcellulose of tightly specified methoxyl and hydroxypropyl contents, particle size and viscosity grade.)

The use of xanthan (or other similar gums) is claimed by Pankhania *et al.* (1987). Blagbrough *et al.* (1989) showed in volunteers suffering from osteoarthritis and rheumatoid arthritis that acceptable blood levels were achieved with a single 1.6 g dose, and Wilson *et al.* (1989) used a gamma scintographic technique to explain the dual plasma level peak that is associated with this formulation (Figure 3.6). Scintography revealed that the tablet remained intact (releasing the drug by a combination of diffusion and erosion) until it reached the ascending and transverse colon where it broke up and started to disintegrate.

Variants of xanthan gum formulations have been claimed by Bongiovann *et al.* (1992) using xanthan gum and cellulose derivatives and by Balchwal (1993), who claim to be able to tailor the release of drugs with a combination of xanthan and locus bean gums.

Other sustained-release bases include gel-forming dietary fibre (Kuhrts, 1992), sugar esters of 10–15-carbon fatty acids (Jansen and Hendrickx, 1987), polyanhydrides (Domb and Maniar, 1991) and a mixture of water-soluble and water-insoluble casein salts that the patentees (Nuernberg *et al.*, 1994) also claim gives a two-stage delayed release pattern.

An alternative approach that has been adopted by a number of workers is to mix the drug with various excipients and present it in the form of a beadlet, which is then coated with polymers that dissolve in the intestine so delaying the release. The mechanism for dissolving the coating is usually (but not exclusively) pH related. Coating materials quoted in the patent literature include cellulose butyrate phthalate or cellulose hydrogenphthalate

CHAPTER 3

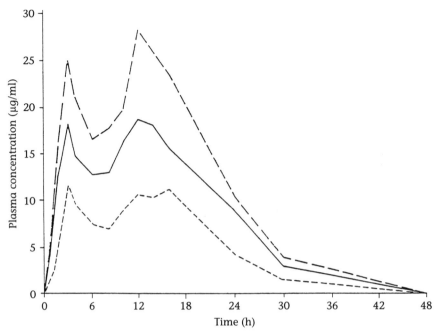

Figure 3.6: Mean plasma concentration profiles of ibuprofen in volunteers following administration of different single doses of a sustained release formulation: — —, 2400 mg; —, 1600 mg; – – –, 800 mg.

(Heinicke and Morella, 1994), neutral acrylic resin (Barry *et al.*, 1988), high-viscosity PVP (Giudice and Ravelli, 1982) and ethylcellulose or shellac in combination with starch or talc (Taisho, 1990). Complex physical presentations are also quoted. European patent EP-212747 (Kelm *et al.*, 1987) describes a propionic acid derivative-containing core granule with a first coating of acrylic polymer enteric material, a second coat of methacrylic acid polymer and finally a top coat containing additional NSAID and hydrophilic excipients. The effect of this is to give immediate release of part of the drug, thereby overcoming a disadvantage that can be encountered with ibuprofen sustained release formulations. Slowing the release of the drug to extend the period of activity delays the onset of action and an unacceptable time may elapse before the patient obtains effective pain relief.

This difficulty has also been addressed by producing a tablet (possibly in the form of a bilayer tablet) containing an immediate release and a sustained release moiety (Radebaugh *et al.*, 1988; Schneider *et al.*, 1990; Conte *et al.*, 1995).

3.4   LIQUIDS AND SEMI-SOLIDS

Liquid presentations of ibuprofen offer advantages to certain patients and consumers over conventional solid dose forms. It has been estimated that 8% of the adult population experience difficulty in swallowing tablets or capsules and it is usually easier to dose a small child with a syrup or suspension rather than with a tablet. Paediatric products have been available since the late 1970s and have been available in the United Kingdom with OTC (P) status since 1994. The suitability and safety of ibuprofen for paediatric use has been discussed in the literature (Reekie, 1990; Anon, 1991). Preparation of a liquid presentation of ibuprofen is, however, not without its pharmaceutical difficulties. The most challenging is that of taste. It has already been indicated that ibuprofen has an unpleasant flavour and produces a burning sensation or 'kick' in the throat when swallowed. Because of this it is better to produce a liquid presentation of ibuprofen in the form of a suspension. In such a presentation, the ibuprofen is essentially kept out of solution and the flavour impact is reduced. Other methods of addressing the taste-masking of ibuprofen will be considered later.

Having identified that the suspension is the preferred dose form, the major problem is then to find a suspension system that will produce a physically stable product. Hashem *et al.* (1987) investigated a number of suspending agents using mefenamic acid, flufenamic acid, glafenine azapropazone and ibuprofen as model compounds and showed that a combination of 1% each of veegum, sorbitol and algin gave a stable suspension as indicated by a relatively high suspension volume on storage. The resulting suspension was also easily remixed on inversion and gave good *in vitro* release.

Kimura *et al.* (1992) compared the bioavailability of a suspension using 2% hydroxypropylmethylcellulose as the suspending agent, a 'dry syrup' in the form of a sucrose-based powder taken with water and a conventional tablet and showed both the suspension and the dry syrup to show a superior rate of dissolution. This was also reflected in speed of absorption *in vivo* in dogs. Haas (1989) patented an ibuprofen syrup formulation containing a relatively low level of stabilizer that is, it is claimed, adapted to form a molecular film around the ibuprofen particle, and Khan and Lampard (1987) have developed a formulation in which a suspension is formed *in situ* when a powder mix is added to water.

3.5   TASTE-MASKING OF IBUPROFEN

While it is not solely in the liquid dosage formulations that the taste of ibuprofen is a disadvantage, it is for these dose forms that the problem is heightened. A tablet or capsule can be swallowed without the patient detecting the flavour and this can be aided by coating the dose form to offer additional taste-masking.

Figure 3.7 shows the time intensity curve for the two major taste components of ibuprofen (bitterness and the burning sensation). The results are derived from work using a small number of laboratory workers (K A Khan, 1997, personal communication). From these data it is clearly seen that part of the problem of poor taste of ibuprofen is caused by the persistent nature of the bitterness and part by the delayed onset of the burning sensation. For reference, the taste profile of a typical, conventional flavouring agent has been

CHAPTER 3

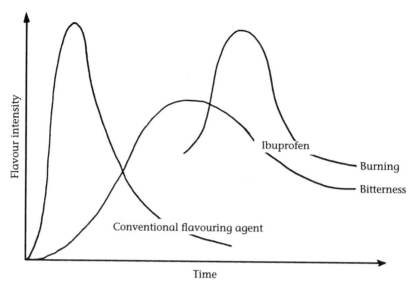

Figure 3.7: The taste intensity versus time curve for ibuprofen (K A Khan, personal communication, 1997).

superimposed on the graph, indicating the shorter period over which the conventional flavour is effective. For this reason the usual taste-masking techniques using flavouring agents are only partially effective for ibuprofen. With the exception of Geyer and Tuliani (1995), most workers have addressed the problem of taste-masking of ibuprofen by coating the drug or granule, embedding the drug in a base that partially prevents contact between the drug and the organs of taste, using a dose form that allows the ibuprofen to be diluted, or maintaining the drug in a form that avoids the ibuprofen entering the solution phase. Geyer and Tuliani, however, claim a novel form of ibuprofen itself, which they describe as neomorphic and which contains a high level of amorphic ibuprofen. This is claimed to have a markedly less unpleasant taste compared with conventional crystalline ibuprofen.

The patent literature relating to the coating of drug particles with materials that offer taste protection is extensive. Mapelli claims a core drug coated with a polymeric membrane soluble at a pH $\geq$ 5 and an acidic component that helps to prevent the membrane dissolving in the oral cavity (Mapelli *et al.*, 1991). Taisho (1996) claims a drug core coated initially with a gastric-soluble coat, then with a coat of water-soluble macromolecules. Workers at American Home Products have used a spray drying technique combining the ibuprofen with plasticized ethylcellulose (Ho and Blank, 1989b), ethylcellulose (or related cellulose derivatives) and colloidal silica (Reuter and Harrison, 1989a) or cellulose acetate phthalate (CAP) and colloidal silica (Reuter and Harrison, 1989b). The modified use of CAP is also claimed by other workers (Powell and Calanchi, 1991; Ghanta and Guisinger, 1995). Other coating materials claimed include hydroxypropylmethylcellulose phthalate

(Patell, 1990), dimethylaminoethyl methacrylate and neutral methacrylic acid in combination with cellulose acetate (Hoy and Roche, 1996) or with a cellulose ester (Hoy and Roche, 1993) and the combination of a pseudocolloid and fumaric acid (Gergely *et al.*, 1986). The use of inert clays as immediate coating agents is also claimed (Hsiao, 1989). Two workers (Shen, 1991; Mehta, 1992) claim polymer coatings that are resistant to chewing, enabling the coated material to be incorporated into chewable tablets, and Lukas and Morella (1992) coated micocapsules to produce very small particles with a smooth continuous coating, which can also be embedded into a chewable matrix. Fauvelle *et al.* (1989) report a dosage form comprising small spheroids (300–500 μm) that are coated to efficiently mask the taste. The resulting product is intended to be spread on food. The taste-masking of the product (promoted as Sparklets) is excellent, but the mouth feel is gritty and although the product is fully bioavailable the time to maximum concentration is delayed compared to that with conventional tablets.

This is a problem common to many of the taste-masking solutions that use coating techniques, and this is not surprising since many of the materials used are those that are also used for producing sustained release formulations.

Other attempts at taste-masking involve the formation of various β-cyclodextrin complexes (Hunter and Yau, 1989; Coutel *et al.*, 1990; Grattan, 1993) or hydroxypropyl-β-cyclodextrin complexes (Motola *et al.*, 1991) using ibuprofen or its salts or compounds. Further approaches involve the imbedding of ibuprofen, usually in the form of coated particles in various substrates. These include a freeze-dried matrix (Gole *et al.*, 1995), a chewable tablet (Denick *et al.*, 1994), a tri-layer tablet (Taisho, 1988) and a chewing gum (Reiner and Seneci, 1996).

Pankhania and Lewis (1988) showed that combination of ibuprofen with aluminium hydroxide produced significant taste-masking. Taste-masking by dilution was achieved in both effervescent (Carcano and Costa, 1990; Ehrenhoefer, 1995) and noneffervescent presentations (Haas, 1989; Gregory *et al.*, 1991). But the most commonly used approach for a liquid presentation is to produce a suspension of the drug. By keeping the drug out of solution, the adverse taste effects are avoided. This has been achieved by the use of the insoluble aluminium salt of ibuprofen (Upjohn, 1979) or by adjusting the pH of the product to between 3.5 and 5.0 so that the drug is essentially insoluble (Mody and Mogavero, 1988; Motola *et al.*, 1990; Gowan, 1991; Paris and Sinturel, 1995).

Using one or more of these techniques it is possible to produce a palatable presentation of ibuprofen, thereby improving patient compliance and reducing the need to consider alternative active ingredients.

3.6 SUPPOSITORIES

Examination of Table 3.7 indicates that suppositories do not represent a significant dose form for ibuprofen, although products are available in some territories. The two major problems to be overcome when formulating suppositories are to ensure that the drug is released from the suppository matrix and secondly to ensure that local irritation is not produced. Work in healthy volunteers using ibuprofen solutions and suspensions showed that the rectal route was a viable route of administration (Eller *et al.*, 1989). Ibuprofen was dosed as the sodium salt (in solution) and as the aluminium salt (in suspension). The suspension showed a slower T_{max} than the solution and perhaps surprisingly the rectal route was slower than the oral route. Notwithstanding these results, the study showed that the rectal route is viable and may be useful for conditions where the patient is unable to take medication by mouth.

3.7   TOPICAL PRESENTATIONS

The concept of treating certain conditions (notably strains, sprains, rheumatic and muscular pain) by applying a topical preparation to, or close to, the affected area is attractive. It offers the patient a less invasive approach, hopefully with fewer side-effects. However, the major problem in formulating such a presentation is that of penetrating the skin, one of the main functions of the skin being to exclude foreign substances from the body. All the NSAID topical products currently available claim to work locally rather than systemically and where trials have been conducted involving the measurement of plasma levels of NSAID, these levels are significantly lower than would be expected if a systemic presentation had been used. It should also be noted that not all regulatory authorities are convinced that such products are efficacious, and at the time of writing the FDA have not licensed any topical NSAIDs.

Several workers have used *in vitro* methods to compare the skin-penetrating ability of different products, or to examine the effects exerted by different excipients. Shaikh *et al.* (1984) deposited different doses of ibuprofen onto full-thickness cadaver skin and, using a diffusion cell, measured the penetration of ibuprofen over 11, 24 and 49 h periods. In this model the external skin surface was exposed to environmental conditions, thus more closely mimicking the situation *in vivo* compared to conventional diffusion cells. This work showed that the higher the dose the greater the penetration. However, penetration was not directly-dose dependent (that is, a 50-fold increase in drug applied produced less than a 50-fold increase in penetration). When the deposited drug film (in this case the model drug was flurbiprofen) was replaced by a 10% solution of the drug, after an initial lag period, the penetration rate increased 4-fold. These workers also demonstrated that occlusion does not enhance absorption from the skin surface but does increase the penetration of drug already present in the stratum corneum, and that the addition of *N*-methyl-2-pyrrolidone acts as a penetration enhancer, increasing the penetration of ibuprofen 3-fold.

Valenti *et al.* (1990) examined the release of ibuprofen from three carriers *in vitro* and concluded that, of the three formulations tested, the aqueous gel gave the best results.

Comparison of a commercially available oil-in-water cream and a modified cellulose gel produced a similar conclusion (Treffel 1993a). When two different cream products were compared with two commercially available gels (Treffel and Gabard, 1993b), it was concluded that the gels released significantly more ibuprofen into the epidermis, and furthermore that the 10% gel released a greater amount than a 5% gel of broadly similar formulation.

All the trials so far considered illustrate the differing abilities of the various formulations to release ibuprofen from the carrier into the epidermis. This, however, does not necessarily mean that the drug will subsequently reach the target area.

Muktadir *et al.* (1986) investigated eight different bases and studied their abilities to release ibuprofen into an aqueous medium. The two formulations with the best release rate — a water-washable formulation base comprising white petroleum, stearyl alcohol, lanolin, isopropyl esters of lanolin fatty acids, GMS-SE, poly(oxyethylene monostearate), glycerin and sodium bicarbonate and a hydrophilic formulation comprising essentially white petroleum, stearyl alcohol, propylene glycol, sodium lauryl sulfate and water — were applied to the shaved backs of rabbits and the blood plasma levels were measured. The absorption rate constant for the hydrophilic formulation (which showed the lower release rate *in vitro* of the two formulations) was higher than that for the water-washable formulation. The elimination constants for the two formulations were similar. Addition of 10% dimethyl sulfoxide (a well-recognized absorption enhancer) to the formulations increased the serum levels and absoption from the hydrophilic base, whereas it slightly reduced the availability from the water-washable base. These results indicate that absorption enhancers need to be tailored to specific formulations if their benefits are to be maximized.

Guinea-pig studies (Berner and Wagener, 1987; Giese 1990) were used to investigate the distribution of ibuprofen resulting from the application of a commercially available cream. These showed that within 20 min significant ibuprofen levels were found in the subcutaneous tissues and in the muscles. The plasma concentrations were about one-tenth those of the tissues. Two hours after application the tissue levels had increased by a further 50%, but greater percentage increases were seen in the plasma, and trials in the same species using radioactively labelled ibuprofen showed that the drug appeared in the plasma 90 min after application and that ibuprofen could be detected throughout the skin and muscle.

Studies have been conducted in healthy volunteers (Kleinbloesem *et al.*, 1994) comparing plasma levels of ibuprofen arising from the application of a hydrogel formulation (quantity of ibuprofen applied 500 mg) and ingestion of a standard tablet (400 mg). The latter gave a 5-fold C_{max}, and a 4-fold area under the curve compared to the former. It also showed a slightly lower elimination half-life. A similar technique was also used to compare three highly differentiated formulations (Seth, 1993) viz. a hydro-alcoholic gel, a hydrophilic ointment and an oil-in-water emulsion (cream). The gel was superior in all

CHAPTER 3

parameters studied (C_{max}, T_{max} and area under the curve). Detailed information regarding distribution has also been obtained by tissue biopsy from patients undergoing knee surgery (Eve *et al.*, 1992). Ibuderm was applied to 12 patients and the levels of ibuprofen in skin, subcutaneous adipose tissue, muscle, deep fascia and synovium were determined. Ibuprofen was present in all tissues studied at a broadly similar level with the exception of the skin, where levels were 50-fold higher. Following application of Trauma-Dolgit Gel (Berner *et al.*, 1989), ibuprofen levels were measured in the subcutis, tendons, muscle and within the joint capsule. The data show that there is considerable penetration into the muscles and the joint capsule, and it is claimed that this increases the efficacy of the cream compared with a standard product of the same drug content. The plasma level is very low compared to that which would result from oral administration.

However, when interpreting such data consideration should also be given to the binding affinities of the different tissues. Menzel and Kolarz (1992) have studied these and have demonstrated that muscle has the highest binding affinity for ibuprofen and tendon the lowest.

Patent activity has been extensive in this area, indicating that there is still a need to produce an effective product that performs well in use. Standard topical applications include a combination of ibuprofen, medium chain-length triglycerides and poly(oxyethylene) fatty acid esters which it is claimed is effective at a lower drug level than in a standard cream (Gruber *et al.*, 1983); ibuprofen in an oil-in-water suspension with a preferred pH of 5–5.8 for which superior skin penetration is claimed (Agisim *et al.*, 1992), an emulsion cream containing a high concentration of the drug in the hydrophilic phase which aids release from the carrier (Campbell and Seth, 1992); and a combination incorporating menthol and benzyl alcohol and a glycol which again is claimed to improve skin penetration (Smith *et al.*, 1991).

Various adhesive patch formulations, in which the drug is either admixed with the adhesive or contained in a separate layer, are also the subject of patent applications (Lohmann and Co., 1987; Hisamitsu, 1992, 1993; Kyukyu Yakuhin Kogyo, 1993; Rolf and Sjoblom, 1995; Math and Sawaya, 1995; Hirano and Tsuruta, 1996). Patches aid dose control, provide a format that is more convenient for the consumer to use, and allow easy removal should the patient wish to discontinue treatment.

In summary, for topical therapy it is possible by careful formulation to produce a composition that will penetrate the skin and establish reasonable levels in the affected tissues. Gel formulations appear to be more effective at achieving skin penetration than conventional creams and it is possible to add penetration enhancers, but these need to be carefully tailored to the specific formulation. Data to prove conclusively that topical products give clinical benefit are difficult to generate and at least one major regulatory authority does not yet accept that topical NSAID formulations are efficacious. The most commonly available topical presentation is the gel format, although there is extensive patent activity involving the development of patches.

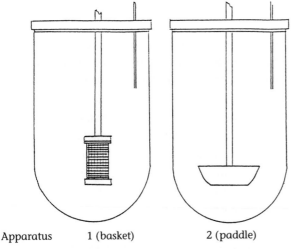

Apparatus   1 (basket)   2 (paddle)

Figure 3.8: Dissolution apparatus (basket and paddle types).

3.8 *IN VITRO/IN VIVO* TESTING

For many years the pharmaceutical industry has endeavoured to produce an inexpensive, accurate, repeatable and relevant test for drug dosage forms, especially solid dose formats, to ensure that commercially available products release the drug *in vivo* in a consistent and effective manner. The technique that most closely mimics normal use is to administer the drug to healthy volunteers and measure drug plasma levels. Such techniques are widely used for basic research into the pharmacokinetics of drugs but are obviously unsuitable for routine analysis, being expensive, time-consuming and ethically unacceptable where suitable *in vitro* methods exist. Even *in vivo* tests are problematic in that patient-to-patient variation within a test group can be marked, extrapolation of results from one set of volunteers or patients to another is unsafe and the plasma level of drug does not necessarily correlate with the pharmacological effect. Notwithstanding these various difficulties, bioavailability testing using volunteers forms the standard against which *in vitro* methods are judged.

It is generally accepted that dissolution testing, involving the dissolving of the product in a suitable buffered medium, with controlled mixing, under sink conditions, currently offers the most acceptable means of determining drug release on a routine basis. When determining test methods for ibuprofen-containing products, the solubility of the drug has to be considered if sink conditions are to be achieved. Since ibuprofen is essentially insoluble at low pH, neutral or slightly alkaline media are normally employed. The European Pharmacopoeia describes two types of apparatus for dissolution testing but does not define specific conditions for individual monographs (Figure 3.8). The United States

Pharmacopeia in the monographs for individual products defines apparatus type, method of stirring, speed of stirring and dissolution medium.

Extrapolation of results from test to test where different dissolution apparatus or conditions are used is unsound; therefore a clear understanding of the specific test conditions used is essential when reviewing published data. Early studies using three strengths of commercially available ibuprofen tablets, from two sources, compared *in vivo* results from healthy volunteers with dissolution data obtained using two different dissolution methods (Stead *et al.*, 1983). Both dissolution methods used the USPXX rotating basket method. The first utilized a speed of rotation of 100 rpm and 900 ml of phosphate buffer pH 6.9, and the second a speed of 200 rpm and a dissolution medium of 500 ml of 0.1 mol/l HCl topped with 400 ml of *n*-hexane to provide sink conditions. In the latter case the basket was immersed in the aqueous medium and the interface between the aqueous and organic layer was stirred.

The *in vivo* data showed that one source of tablets available in strengths of 200 mg and 400 mg (source B) showed clear dose proportionality as indicated by the area under the curve, that is the 400 mg tablet produced an area approximately twice that of the 200 mg tablet. However, the other source (source A) available as 100 mg, 200 mg and 300 mg tablets gave broadly similar areas under the curve, irrespective of strength, indicating decreasing availability at higher strengths.

When the percentage of drug dissolved was plotted against time for the tablets from source A, using data obtained from the dissolution study conducted at pH 6.9, there appeared to be some correlation with the *in vivo* data since the 200 mg tablet released the drug faster than the 300 mg, which was again faster than the 400 mg. However the test also appeared to discriminate against the two strengths of tablet from source B where no *in vivo* differences were seen.

The study at acidic pH, using the mixed organic and inorganic medium, proved problematic in that some of the higher-strength tablets failed to disintegrate properly in the acidic medium and the transfer of drug into the organic layer was low. The authors concluded that suitable predictive bioavailability tests were unlikely to become available in the foreseeable future. This paper is important since it emphasizes two key points relating to the dissolution and bioavailability of ibuprofen. First, at the time of publication (1982) commercially available products existed that showed poor availability *in vivo* and, secondly, while it was possible to devise an *in vitro* dissolution method that would differentiate between nonequivalent formulations it was also possible to produce a method that would identify *in vitro* differences that simply do not exist *in vivo*.

It is, however, quite clear that the formulation of an ibuprofen-containing solid dose form can significantly effect the absorption of the drug in man, and this has been confirmed by *in vivo* studies performed by a number of groups of workers (Gillespie *et al.*, 1982; Kallstrom *et al.*, 1988; Palva *et al.*, 1985; Karttunen *et al.*, 1990).

TABLE 3.8

Comparison of the USP dissolution methods for ibuprofen tablets

	Pre-November 1996[a]	Post-November 1996[b]
Apparatus	1 (basket)	2 (paddle)
Speed	150 rpm	50 rpm
Buffer	Phosphate pH 7.2	Phosphate pH 7.2
Volume	900 ml	900 ml
Time	30 min	60 min
Q value	70%	80%

[a] USP 23rd edn (1995).   [b] USP 2rd edn, Suppl. 5 (1996).

Vidgren *et al.* (1991) used the USP dissolution method that was in effect prior to November 1996 (USP rotating basket, 150 rpm and phosphate buffer pH 7.2) to compare two commercially available film-coated tablets and an effervescent formulation and compared the results with the outcome of a bioavailability study in healthy volunteers. Differences in the rate of drug release were detected *in vitro*, with the effervescent tablet showing the faster rate of release. However, *in vivo* results showed the preparations to be broadly similar, although one of the film-coated tablets gave a higher peak plasma concentration and a faster T_{max} than the other two formulations. This is perhaps surprising since the dissolved effervescent tablet is effectively in solution and it is generally thought that solutions give faster *in vivo* absorption.

The authors speculate that the effervescent product did not give faster absortion owing to the recrystallization of the ibuprofen in the acidic medium of the stomach. This then produced a poorly absorbed suspension rather than a true solution.

As has already been indicated, the USP dissolution method for ibuprofen was changed with effect from November 1996. Conditions for the two methods are shown in Table 3.8. Dash *et al.* (1988) compared the results obtained from the two methods applied to two batches of commercially available ibuprofen tablets. The two batches (A and B) met all the requirements of the USP, including the dissolution method incorporated in the monograph prior to November 1996 (method 1), but behaved differently when subjected to testing using the USP method post November 1996 (method 2). Batch B showed an acceptable profile using both methods, whereas batch A gave poor dissolution, with marked tablet-to-tablet variation, when tested using method 2. When the two batches were subjected to *in vivo* testing in volunteers, both showed acceptable and similar profiles. It would therefore appear from this work that the USP, in modifying the monograph for the dissolution testing of ibuprofen, has produced a procedure that is more discriminating, but that the differences detected are not meaningful in the *in vivo* situation. This would argue for the retention of the pre-November 1996 method (method 1) as the preferred method for release of the tablets commercially.

CHAPTER 3

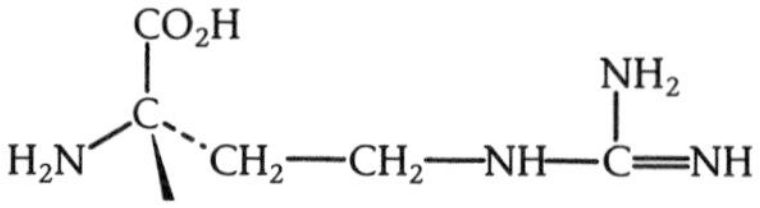

Figure 3.9: The chemical structure of L-arginine (L-2-amino-5-guanidinovaleric acid).

3.9 IBUPROFEN SALTS AND DERIVATIVES

The absorption profile of ibuprofen having been established *in vivo*, several attempts have been made to modify the way in which the drug behaves. We have already considered work to extend the time over which the drug exerts its pharmacological action in the section on sustained release preparations, but efforts have also been made to speed the onset of action and develop products that give faster pain relief.

One way to achieve this has been the development of salts and derivatives of ibuprofen. Such materials include alkali metal salts, ibuprofen lysinate and a mixture of ibuprofen and arginine. It can be argued that such combinations will, by virtue of their increased solubility, show superior onset of activity.

Fini and co-workers studied five NSAIDs and four derivatives, the four derivatives being the sodium salt (Na) the *N*-(2-hydroxyethyl)piperazinium derivative (PE), the *N*-methylglucosammonium derivative (MGA), and the arginate (Arg) and they compared the solubilities at different pHs with those of the free acid (Fini *et al.*, 1985). For ibuprofen at all pH values the sodium salt showed superior solubility and at all the pH values studied all the derivatives were superior to the free acid in terms of solubility.

The use of the combination of arginine (Figure 3.9) and ibuprofen, in a molar ratio between 1.1 and 1.5, is claimed in the patent literature (Bonadeo *et al.*, 1995) and the patentees indicate that the resulting combination shows remarkable chemical and physical stability. Furthermore, when sodium bicarbonate is added, the resulting product, it is claimed, achieves a T_{max} of around 15 min as opposed to 1.5 h obtained with conventional tablets containing the free acid (Gazzaniga *et al.*, 1988). Ibuprofen/arginine combinations are marketed in Switzerland under the trade name of Spedifen and marketing authorizations also exist in a number of other European territories.

Clinical work demonstrating the efficacy of the combination against other NSAIDs and against placebo was presented to the XVII National Congress on Pain, in June 1994 at Perugia, Italy, and the pharmacokinetic data in healthy volunteers of two strengths of tablet (equivalent to 200 mg and 400 mg of free acid) has been published (Ceppi Monti *et al.*, 1992) supporting claims for the speed of absorption.

The other derivative of ibuprofen that is commercially available as a licensed product is ibuprofen lysinate, whose structure is shown in Figure 3.10. The product is available as Saren (Bracco, Italy), Dolormin (J and J, Germany) and Imbrun (Merckle GmbH Blaubeuren, Germany). The lysinate is a white crystalline powder, soluble in water 1 in 5.

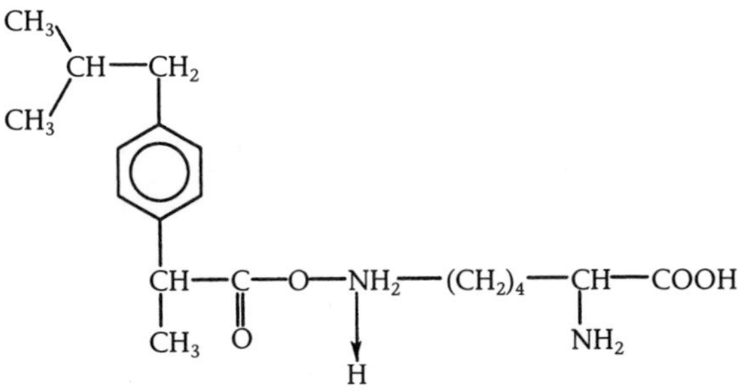

Figure 3.10: The chemical structure of ibuprofen lysinate.

When a single tablet of 500 mg of ibuprofen lysinate (equivalent to 290 mg of free acid) (Saren) was administered to healthy volunteers, the T_{max} occurred between 30 and 60 min after dosing and at 30 min the plasma ibuprofen level was twice that obtained with a conventional 300 mg ibuprofen tablet (Anon, 1978).

Geisslinger et al. (1989) generated in vitro and in vivo data for the film-coated lysinate tablets Imbrun, and compared their performance with that of a conventional sugar-coated tablet containing the free acid (Dolgit). Dissolution studies were conducted using the USPXXI apparatus (rotating basket) at 150 rpm with 900 ml of artificial juice at pH values of 1.2, 2.5, 4.0 and 7.2. Both products showed excellent dissolution at pH 7.2 (greater than 90% dissolved in 15 min) and both also showed poor dissolution at pH 1.2 and pH 2.5 (less than 30% in 30 min), but the difference was seen at pH 4.0 where the free acid gave poor dissolution and the lysinate gave excellent dissolution. When the absoption of the two formulations was compared in fasting volunteers, both formulations were equally bioavailable, although the lysinate showed an appreciably faster T_{max} (lysinate 0.55 h and free acid 0.89 h). It is likely that the major part of this effect arises from the difference between the lysinate and the free acid rather than the difference between sugar-coated and film-coated tablets.

Martin et al. (1990) also studied Imbun tablets and compared their performance against that of intravenous injections of ibuprofen free acid. This work showed that the ibuprofen from the lysinate is totally bioavailable and that the Imbun tablets produced peak plasma concentration approximately 0.75 h after dosing, somewhat slower than the findings of Geisslinger. It would therefore appear that, compared to conventional formulations containing the free acid, the rate of absorption of ibuprofen can be significantly improved by presenting the drug as the lysinate.

However, there remain a number of problems associated with the use of derivatives of ibuprofen. Since tablets are still the most popular dose form for ibuprofen-containing products, the compaction characteristics of the drug and its derivatives are important commercially. Figure 3.11 shows the relationship between tensile strength of compacts and applied compaction pressure, determined using a compaction simulator. It will be seen from these data that sodium ibuprofen possesses poor compaction characteristics.

CHAPTER 3

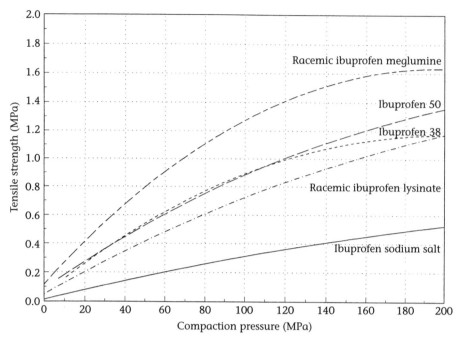

Figure 3.11: Compaction properties of ibuprofen salts, derivatives and mixtures.

Those of the lysinate are broadly similar to those of ibuprofen free acid. A further problem associated with derivatives is that of equivalent weights. Table 3.9 shows the weight of the derivative or combination that is equivalent to 200 mg of free acid. Some of these significantly increase the weight of 'drug' that has to be incorporated into the dose form. This can increase the bulk of the product significantly and produce a final dosage form that is difficult to swallow, especially at the higher doses.

In the case of the lysinate the problem can be obviated by the pretreatment of the drug. Both major suppliers are able to offer ibuprofen lysinate that is roller compacted, aiding the flow of the material and allowing direct compression and thus the ability to produce a smaller tablet.

TABLE 3.9

Approximate weights of ibuprofen derivatives/salts equivalent to 200 mg of ibuprofen free acid

Derivative	Equivalent weight
Ibuprofen free acid	200 mg
Sodium ibuprofen dihydrate	256 mg
Ibuprofen plus arginine	453 mg
Ibuprofen lysinate	340 mg

Lastly, in all cases, the cost of derivatives is more expensive than that of the free acid on a dose-for-dose basis. Partly this arises because of the relatively small quantities that are produced commercially but also, in the case of the amino acid derivatives, from the relatively high cost of the feedstocks.

Notwithstanding these problems, such derivatives and combinations do allow the speed of absorption of ibuprofen to be increased and potentially offer the ability to produce faster relief of pain.

3.10   SUMMARY

Ibuprofen is a proprionic acid NSAID with anti-inflammatory, analgesic and antipyretic properties and such is its safety profile that it is widely available over the counter for the treatment of self-limiting conditions. Its physical characteristics allow it to be successfully formulated into a number of dose forms, but account has to be taken of its poor solubility at low pH and its adverse taste characteristics.

In a conventional tablet format, when studied in fasting volunteers, the drug will typically exhibit a half-life of 2 h and a T_{max} of approximately 1.5 h, but by careful modification of the formulation it is possible to extend the duration of action of the drug and by the use of mixtures, salts or derivatives, the rate of absorption can be significantly increased. *In vivo* performance can be predicted from *in vitro* dissolution testing, but it is important that the test method selected is such that it does not falsely discriminate between formulations that show similar pharmacokinetic properties *in vivo*.

It is likely that, despite the appearance of other NSAIDS on the scene, ibuprofen will continue to be a well-accepted analgesic and will be the subject of significant future work to further improve its acceptability and usefulness.

REFERENCES

AGISIM, G.R., BLANK, R.G., CHEN, G.Y. and MODY, D.S. (1992) Novel topical analgesic prepn. contg. Ibuprofen — in solid form has increased transdermal penetration. Patent, EP-499399.

AKHTER, S.A. and BARRY, B.W. (1985) Absorption through human skin of ibuprofen and flurbiprofen; effect of dose variation, deposited drug films, occlusion and the penetration enhancer N-methyl-2-pyrrolidone. *Journal of Pharmacy and Pharmacology* **37**, 27–37.

ALLAN, K., BOGAN, D.W., CHEN, J.R. and SLATER, R.M. (1987) Aggregation of Ibuprofen crystals to form granules — having improved flow properties, for formulations having good dissolution properties. Patent, EP-241126.

ANON (1978) Solufen. *Drugs of Today* **14**(3), 96.

ANON (1991) Junifen suspension — ibuprofen for febrile children. *Drug and Therapeutics Bulletin* **29**(3), 11–12.

ATKIN, G.J., DREW, P. and TURNER, J.L. (1993) Pharmaceutical compsns. prodn. in the form of homogeneous agglomerates — by mixing specified amts. of 2-(4-isobutylphenyl) propionic acid and starch. Patent, WO9304676.

BALCHWAL, A.R. (1993) Locust bean gum as granulating and binding agent for tablets. Patent, EP-360562.

BARRY, B.W., YORK, P. and MULLEY, B.A. (1988) Sustained release Ibuprofen formulation — comprises granules contg. drug and microcrystalline cellulose core with coating of water-swellable acrylic polymer, etc. Patent, EP-255404.

BERNER, V.G. and WAGENER, H.H. (1987) Zur perkutanen Kinetik von Ibuprofen aus einer Cremezubereitung. *Arzneimittel-Forschung/Drug Research* **37**(11), 808.

BERNER, G., ENGELS, B. and VOGTLE-JUNKERT, U. (1989) Perkutane Ibuprofen-Therapie mit Trauma-Dolgit Gel. *Medwelt* **40**, 1024–1027.

BLAGBOROUGH, I.S., DAYKIN, M.M., DOHERTY, M., PATRICK, M. and SHAW, N.P. (1989) Synovial fluid and plasma levels of extended release ibuprofen in osteo and rheumatoid arthritis. *Journal of Pharmacy and Pharmacology* **41**(suppl.), 144.

BONADEO, D., GAZZANIGA, A., STROPPOLO, F. and VIGANO, L. (1995) New liq. compsn. for oral use contg. arginine and Ibuprofen — useful as analgesic, anti-pyretic and anti-inflammatory. Patent, WO9500134.

BONGIOVANN, G., CALANCHI, M.M. and MARCONI, M.G.R. (1992) Pharmaceutical dosage form — comprising hard gelatin capsule contg. mini-tablets formed from active ingredient and xanthan gum matrix. Patent, WO9204013.

CAMPBELL, L.A. and SETH, P.L. (1992) High concn. Ibuprofen forming soln. in hydrophilic solvents and adding to oil/water emulsion. Patent, US5104656.

CARCANO, M. (1995) Prepn. of effervescent and soluble granules contg. active principle — by feeding controlled moisture content air flow through mixt. of acid and basic cpds. onto which water spray is directed. Patent, EP-673644.

CARCANO, M. and COSTA, M. (1990) Effervescent Ibuprofen compsns. — contg. Ibuprofen and its sodium salt, sodium bicarbonate and citric acid. Patent, EP-351353.

CEPPI MONTI, N., GAZZANIGA, A., GIANESELLO, V., STROPPOLO, F. and LODOLA, E. (1992) *Arzneimittel-Forschung/Drug Research* **42**, 556–559.

CHEN, J.R. and DEFESCHE, C. (1989) Sustained release ibuprofen granules — comprise homogeneous mixt. with polymer providing slow release at gastric and intestinal pH. Patent, EP-297866.

CONTE, U., GIUNCHEDI, P. and MAGGI, L. (1995) Multilayered controlled release oral solid pharmaceutical comprises first layer contg. active material, excipients and additives, and second layer contg. same or different active material. Patent, WO9501781.

COUTEL, A., COURTEILLE, F., VANHOEVE, M. and COUTEL-EGROS, A. (1990) Compsns. contg. inclusion cpd. of cyclodextrin — that breaks down easily in water or saliva having no unpleasant taste. Patent, WO9014089.

DANZ, P., FRANK, G., HUERNER, I., MAASZ, J. and WALTER, R. (1995) Directly tabletable drug granulate prodn. — by melt extruding mixt. of low melting drug and auxiliaries then comminuting, esp. for aryl:propionic acid derivs. Patent, DE4418837.

DASH, B.H., BLANK, R.G., SCHACHTEL, B.P. and SMITH, A.J. (1988) Ibuprofen tablets dissolution versus bioavailability. *Drug. Dev. and Ind. Pharm.* **14**(11), 1584.

DEBOECK, A.M., MAES, P. and BAUDIER, P. (1990) Eutectic mixtures for oral administration — contg. non-steroid anti-inflammatory agent and fatty acid glyceride(s). Patent, EP-349509.

DENICK, J., LECH, S. and SCHOBEL, A.M. (1994) Palatable, chewable compsn. for treatment of cold and sinus symptoms — contain high proportion of silicon dioxide to overcome the unpleasant taste of the active ingredients. Patent, WO9428870.

DENTON, L.E. (1989) Ibuprofen granules for tableting — contg. alkali metal carboxymethyl cellulose, lubricant, cellulose and starch. Patent, WO8902266.

DENTON, L.E. and SALPEKAR, A.M. (1992) Granulation compsn. prepn. contg. ibuprofen — with short disintegration and dissolution. Patent, US5104648.

DOMB, A.J. and MANIAR, M. (1991) Branched polyanhydride polymers for controlled delivery of substances — is prepd. by polymerisation of dicarboxylic acid and specified branching agent. Patent, WO9118940.

EHRENHOEFER, F. (1995) Effervescent compsns. — comprising ibuprofen salt, separate from effervescent granules contg. citric acid, dissolves rapidly to produce a clear soln. with a neutral taste. Patent, CH-684929.

ELLER, M.G., WRIGHT, C. and DELLA-COLETTA, A.A. (1989) Absorption kinetics of rectally and orally administered ibuprofen. *Biopharmaceutics and Drug Disposition* **10**, 269–278.

EVE, M.D., DANDY, D.J., CRAWFORD, F.E. and GUY, G.W. (1992) Tissue and plasma levels of ibuprofen following application of a topical application (Ibuderm) in twelve patients undergoing major knee surgery. Presentation at the *Vth World Conference on Clinical Pharmacology and Therapeutics, Yokohama Japan.*

FAUVELLE, F., NICOLAS, P., BOYER, J.F., TOD, M., PERRET, G. and PETITJEAN, O. (1989) Pharmacokinetic advantages of an original oral medicament form: Sparklets, *Fundamental and Clinical Pharmacology* **3**(2), 181.

FINI, A., ZECCHR, V. and TARTARINI, A. (1985) Dissolution profiles of NSAID carboxylic acids and their salts with different counter ions. *Pharmaceutica Acta. Helvetiae* **60**, 4.

FRANZ, R.M. (1986) Dry granulate compsn. contg. ibuprofen and croscamellose sodium — useful for formulating compressed tablets and filled capsules contg. high level of ibuprofen. Patent, EP-172014.

CHAPTER 3

FRITSCH, C. and GROWINGHOL, W. (1990) Effervescent ibuprofen compsns. — comprising acid and granules contg. ibuprofen salt and carbonate. Patent, EP-369228.

GAYLORD, N.G. and NIGALAYE, A. (1989) Sustained release solid drug dosage unit form — contains drug nonionic cellulose ether and alkali metal carboxylate. Patent, EP-322222.

GAZZANIGA, A., GIANESELLO, W., STROPPOLO, F. and VIGANO, L. (1988) Water soluble analgesic Ibuprofen formulation — contains L-arginine and sodium bicarbonate to reduce gastric irritation. Patent, GB2193093.

GEISSLINGER, G., DIETZEL, K., BEZLER, H., NUERNBERG, B. and BRUNE, K. (1989) Therapeutically relevant differences in the pharmacokinetical and pharmaceutical behaviour of Ibuprofen lysinate as compared to Ibuprofen acid. *International Journal of Clinical Pharmacology, Therapeutics and Toxicology* **27**(7), 324–328.

GERGELY, G., GERGELY, I. and GERGELY, T. (1986) Pharmaceutical compsns. contg. irritant substance — coated with pseudo-colloid and fumaric acid. Patent, WO8602834.

GEYER, R.P. and TULIANI, W. (1995) Analgesic, antipyretic or anti-inflammatory compsn. — contg. Ibuprofen in neomorphic, mainly amorphous, form, having improved taste and causing less gastric irritation. Patent, WO9501321.

GHANTA, S.R. and GUISINGER, R.E. (1995) Taste-masked microcapsules — with a high payload of NSAID drug, e.g. Ibuprofen. Patent, WO9505166.

GIESE, U. (1990) Absorption and distribution of ibuprofen from a cream formulation after dermal administration to guinea-pigs. *Arzneimittel-Forschung/Drug Research* **40**(1), 76.

GILLESPIE, W.R., DISANTO, A.R., MONOVICH, R.E. and ALBERT, K.S. (1982) Relative bioavailability of commercially available Ibuprofen oral dosage forms in humans. *Journal of Pharmaceutical Sciences* **71**, 1034–1038.

GIUDICE, V. and RAVELLLI, V. (1982) Sustained release Ibuprofen composn. — comprises spheroids of inert core, active ingredient layer and sustained release outer coating. Patent, EP-61217.

GODDARD, L.E. and KNESEL, G.A. (1992) Prepn. of crystalline ibuprofen — having larger average particle length and improved flow properties. Patent, WO9208686.

GOLE, D.J., REO, J., ROCHE, E.J. and WILKINSON, P.K. (1995) Freeze-dried pharmaceutical dosage forms for oral use — consists of taste-masked porous matrix of water-soluble or water-dispersible carrier material. Patent, EP-636365.

GORDON, R.E. and AMIN, S. (1984) Ibuprofen with crystal habit equant or hexagonal in shape with advantageous properties for economic tablet prepn. Patent, EP-120587.

GOWAN, W.G. (1991) Aq. pharmaceutical suspension for taste masking compsn. — comprises pharmaceutical active, xanthan gum, pregelatinised starch and polyoxyethylene sorbitan mono-oleate. Patent, EP-405930.

GRATTAN, J. (1993) Use of ibuprofen-beta-cyclodextrin complex for hot water admin. — obtd. by crystallisation from aq. soln. Patent, WO9320850.

GREGORY, S.P., JOZSA, A.J. and KALDAWI, R.E. (1991) Masking unpleasant taste of water-soluble Ibuprofen salts by incorporation of alkali metal bicarbonate, alkali metal monohydrogen phosphate or alkali metal tribasic citrate. Patent, EP-418043.

GRUBER, K., LOHNER, M., POSSELT, K. and WAGENER. H. (1983) Anti-inflammatory and analgesic medicaments for external application — contg. Ibuprofen dissolved in triglyceride(s), glyceryl monostearate, polyoxyethylene stearate and polyoxyethylene fatty acid ester. Patent, EP-87062.

HAAS, R.T. (1989) Liq. Ibuprofen compsns. for treating pain, etc. — comprising Ibuprofen compsn. dissolved in aq. medium contg. bicarbonate compsn. for a clear, stable prod. Patent, WO8903210.

HAAS, R.T. (1987) Stable liq. Ibuprofen syrup compsn. — for treating pain and inflammation. Patent, US4684666.

HALDAR, R., GANGADHARAN, B., MARTIN, D. and MEHTA, A. (1988) Fluidized bed granulation of ibuprofen. *Pharmaceutical Research* 5(10), 8255.

HASHEM, F., RAMADAN, E. and EL-SAID, Y. (1987) Effect of suspending agents on the characteristics of some anti-inflammatory suspensions. *Pharmazie* 2, 727.

HEINICKE, G.W. and MORELLA, A.M. (1994) Pelletised, sustained release compsm., partic. for anti-inflammatory drugs comprises core element contg. low aq. solubility form active ingredient, binder and core seed and core coating contg. enteric polymer, etc. Patent, WO9403160.

HIRANO, M. and TSURUTA, K. (1996) Patch contg. anti-inflammatory with carboxy gp. — and menthol, with fatty acid salt to prevent esterification and increase penetration. Patent, WO9608245.

HISAMITSU PHARM CO. LTD (1992) Anti-inflammatory plaster for high bioavailability — contains styrene-isoprene-styrene block copolymer crotamiton and anti-inflammatory. pref. 4-biphenylacetic acid, etc. Patent, JP04321624.

HISAMITSU PHARM CO. LTD (1993) Percutaneous plaster having good percutaneous absorption — contains styrene-isoprene-styrene block copolymer cross-linked by irradiation. Patent, JP05139962.

HO, Y.T.R. and BLANK, R.G. (1989a) Directly compressible ibuprofen compsn. — comprises spray-dried aq. dispersion of ibuprofen, pre-gelatinised starch, disintegrant and wetting agent. Patent, EP-298666.

HO, V.T.R. and BLANK, R.G. (1989b) Therapeutic taste-neutral powder form of Ibuprofen — obtd. by spraying-drying dispersion of Ibuprofen and ethyl cellulose in water contg. dissolved or suspended. Patent, EP-322137.

HOY, M.R. and ROCHE, E.J. (1993) Taste masking coating for chewable medicament tablets comprises a blend of methylaminoethyl methacrylate-methacrylic acid ester and a cellulose ester. Patent, EP-523847.

HOY, M.R. and ROCHE, E.J. (1996) Chewable medicament tablet — has taste-masking polymer blend coating. Patent, US5489436.

HSIAO, C. (1989) Taste concealing pharmaceutical dosage unit — comprises sub-dosage units having inner core pellet coated with active agent and 1st layer of clay and 2nd layer of resin. Patent, US4874613.

HUNTER, C. and YAU, D. (1989) New complexes of beta-cyclodextrin with ibuprofen salts — contg. more ibuprofen than cyclo dextrin, of improved organoleptic profile and bio-availability. Patent, EP-346006.

JANSEN, F.H. and HENDRICKX, J. (1987) Sustained release pharmaceutical tablets esp. contg. ibuprofen — have sugar ester of higher fatty acid and other ingredients present. Patent, EP-230332.

KALLSTROM, E., HEIKINHEIMO, M. and QUIDING, H. (1988) Bioavailability of three commercial preparations of Ibuprofen. *Journal of International Medical Research* 16, 44–49.

KARTTUNEN, P., SAANO, V., PARONEN, P., PEURA, P. and VIDGOREN, M. (1990) Pharmacokinetics of Ibuprofen in man: a single dose comparison of two over-the-counter, 200 mg preparations. *International Journal of Clinical Pharmacology, Therapeutics and Toxicology* 28, 251–255.

KELM, G.R., WHALEN, S.D. and KEETER, W.E. (1987) Analgesic propionic acid cpd. particles with multilayer coating — giving immediate release then sustained release. Patent, EP-212747.

KHAN, K.A. (1997) Personal communication.

KHAN, K.A. and LAMPARD, J.F. (1987) Powder or tablet compsn. contg. Ibuprofen — and a water-insoluble hydrophilic polymer to give an improved suspension of Ibuprofen in water. Patent, EP-228164.

KIMURA, S., IMAI, T., UENO, M. and OTAGIRI, M. (1992) Phamaceutical evaluation of ibuprofen fast-absorbed syrup containing low-molecular-weight gelatin. *Journal of Pharmaceutical Sciences* 81(2), 141–144.

KLEINBLOESEM, C., AL-HAMDAN, Y., FORGO, I. *et al.* (1994) Pharmacokinetics of Ibuprofen after administration of a topical hydrogel formulation. *British Journal of Clinical Pharmacology* 37(5), 520.

KOKUBO, H. and MARUYAMA, N. (1994) Sustained release tablets for regulating speed of medicinal substance comprise hydroxypropyl-methyl cellulose particles. Patent, JP06305982.

KUHRTS, E.H. (1992) Prolonged release drug tablet formulation using gel-forming fibre — uses gas generating couple to disintegrate fibre and allow leaching of drug for e.g. analgesic, vitamin(s), minerals etc. Patent, US5096714.

KYUKYU YAKUHIN KOGYO KK (1993) Nonsteroidal transdermal patch for therapeutic system — comprises drug, mixt. of triethylene glycol and terpene(s), and water-absorptive, pressure-sensitive adhesive base. Patent, JP05155762.

LOHMANN and CO. (1987) Planar device for trans-dermal, controlled drug delivery — with regions of adhesive and material reservoir at the same level. Patent, WO8706144.

LOHNER, M. and POSSELT, K. (1986) Soft gelatin capsules which contain ibuprofen — contain soln. of ibuprofen in polyoxyethylene-polyoxypropylene polymer or in mixt. of polyalkylene glycol and surfactant. Patent, EP-178436.

LUKAS, S. and MORELLA, A.M. (1992) Pharmaceutical free-flowing powder for analgesics etc. — comprises microcapsules composed of drug-contg. core with coating contg. water-insol. polymer. Patent, CA2068366.

MAPELLI, L.G., MARCONI, M.G. and ZEMA, M. (1991) Polymer coated pharmaceutical formulations — for masking taste of oral drugs, comprise acidic component for reducing dissolution in oral activity. Patent, WO9116043.

MARTIN, W., KOSELOWSKE, G., TOBERICH, H., KERKMANN, T.H., MANGOLD, B. and AUGUSTIN, J. (1990) Pharmacokinetics and absolute bioavailability of ibuprofen after oral administration of ibuprofen lysine in man. *Biopharmaceutics and Drug Disposition* 11, 265–278.

MATH, M. and SAWAYA, A. (1995) Ibuprofen transdermal patches — contg. adhesive and cationic acrylate copolymers and diethyl phthalate. Patent, WO9531193.

MEHTA, A.M. (1992) Chewable taste-masked pharmaceutical compsns. — of active agent core and high and low temp. film forming polymers mixt. Patent, US5084278.

MENZEL, J. and KOLARZ, G. (1992) Bindungsvermogen von Ibuprofen an humanes Gewebe. *Arzneimittel-Forschung/Drug Research* 42(1), 318.

MODY, D.S. and MOGAVERO, A. (1988) Taste masked paediatric Ibuprofen compsn. — contg. suspension stabilisers, taste masking agent and citric acid. Patent, US4788220.

MOHAR, M., KREMZAR, L., JERALASTRU, Z. *et al.* (1988) Sustained release tablets with hydroxypropyl-methylcellulose carrier — also contg. microcrystalline cellulose, and opt. glycerol ditripalmito-stearate lubricant. Patent, EP-284849.

MOTOLA, S., MOGAVERO, A., AGISIM, G.R. and PANOPOULOS, P.N. (1990) Buffered, low pH formulations of Ibuprofen — avoid bitter after taste and throat bite. Patent, EP-390369.

MOTOLA, S., AGISIM, G.R. and MOGAVERO, A. (1991) Palatable ibuprofen aq. soln. contains hydroxypropyl-beta-cyclodextrin — to form inclusion complex to mask ibuprofen taste, and sweetener to mask acid taste. Patent, US5024997.

CHAPTER 3

MUKTADIR, A., BABAR, A., CUTIE, A.J. and PLAKOGIANNIS, F.M. (1986) Medicament release from ointment bases: III. Ibuprofen: *In vitro* release and *In vivo* absorption in rabbits. *Drug Dev. and Ind. Pharm.* **12**(14), 2521–2540.

NUERNBERG, E., RITSERT, S. and SEILLER, E. (1994) Prodn. of retard pharmaceutical formulations, esp. for memantine comprises using casein salts as matrix for controlled two-stage release. Patent, EP-582186.

OJANTAAKANEN, S., HANNULA, A.-M., MARVOLA, M. and KLINGE, E. (1992) Sustained release ibuprofen capsules containing hydrophilic polymers as diluents. *Pharmaceutisch Weekblad Scientific Edition*, **14**(5), 35.

PALVA, E.S., KONNO, K. and VENHO, V.M.K. (1985) Bioavailability of ibuprofen from three preparations marketed in Finland. *Acta Pharmaceutica Fennica*, **94**, 31–35.

PANKHANIA, M.G. and LEWIS, C.J. (1988) Pharmaceutical ibuprofen compsn. — contains aluminium hydroxide to mask the ibuprofen taste. Patent, EP-264187.

PANKHANIA, M.G., MELIA, C.D. and LAMPARD, J.F. (1987) Solid sustained release pharmaceutical compsn. — contg. a pharmacologically active ingredient and xanthan gum as sustained release carrier. Patent, EP-234670.

PARIS, L. and SINTUREL, C. (1995) New compsn. comprising an aq. Ibuprofen dispersion — uses a gel and avoids the bitter taste; it has analgesic and anti-inflammatory use. Patent, WO9517177.

PATELL, M.K. (1990) Masking unpleasant taste of pharmaceuticals, esp. Ibuprofen by wet granulating blend with hydroxypropyl-methyl-cellulose phthalate aq. soln. Patent, EP-366101.

POWELL, T.C. and CALANCHI, M.M. (1991) Taste-masked microencapsulated nonsteroidal anti-inflammatory drugs — encapsulated with cellulose acetate phthalate and with high drug pay-load. Patent, EP-413533.

RADEBAUGH, G.W., JULIAN, T.N. and GLINECKE, R. (1988) Shaped and compressed sustained pharmaceutical compsn. — contains ethylcellulose and povidone as excipients, pharmaceutically active cpd. and granulating agent. Patent, WO8808299.

REEKIE, R.M. (1980) Paediatric ibuprofen — an overview. *British Journal of Clinical Practice* **4**(8 Suppl.), 70–72.

REINER, A. and SENECI, A. (1996) Tablet with chewing gum base and contg particles of active ingredient — opt microencapsulated or coated with protective laquer of cellulose deriv or polyethylene glycol. Patent, WO9603111.

REUTER, G.L. and HARRISON, M.M. (1989a) Therapeutic taste-neutral powder form of Ibuprofen — obtd. by spray-drying suspension of colloidal silica in lower alkanol soln. of Ibuprofen and cellulose material. Patent, US4835187.

REUTER, G.L. and HARRISON, M.M. (1989b) Therapeutic taste-neutral powder form of Ibuprofen — obtd. by spray-drying suspension of colloidal silica in lower alkanol soln. of Ibuprofen and cellulose acetate phthalate. Patent, US4835186.

RITTNER, S., STUVEN, U., STEIDL, D. *et al.* (1990) Ibuprofen particles for direct tableting prepn. — by solidifying melt then comminution to free flowing particles. Patent, EP-362728.

ROLF, D. and SJOBLOM, U.E.K. (1995) Non-occlusive, medication-contg. adhesive patch — comprising a porous backing layer and a pressure-sensitive hydrocolloid gel reservoir contg. medication. Patent, EP-674913.

ROMERO, A.J., LUKAS, G. and RHODES, C.T. (1991) Influence of different sources on the processing and biopharmaceutical properties of high-dose ibuprofen formulations. *Pharmaceutica Acta Helvetiae* **66**, 34–43.

SCHNEIDER, G., STANISLAUS, F., HOFER, J.M., HEESE, G.U. and HUBER, H.J. (1990) Controlled release medicaments — contg. drug in both retard and enteric form, used for oral admin. of anti-inflammatory analgesic and antipyretic agents. Patent, EP-348808.

SETH, P.L. (1993) Percutaneous absorption of ibuprofen from different formulations. *Arzneimittel-Forschung/Drug Research* **43**(11), 898.

SHAIKH, N.A., ABIDI, S.E. and BLOCK, L.H. (1987) Evaluation of ethylcellulose as a matrix for prolonged release formulations. II. Sparingly water-soluble drugs: Ibuprofen and indomethacin. *Drug Dev. and Ind. Pharm.* **13**(14), 2495–2518.

SHEN, R. (1991) Ibuprofen as chewable taste masked tablet — has controlled release using methacrylic acid copolymer elastic coating in microcapsules. Patent, WO9115194.

SMITH, J.F., VAUGHAN, D.P. and HENDERSON, K.M. (1991) Ibuprofen menthol compsn. for topical application — opt. contg. benzyl alcohol and/or glycol for rheumatic pain and inflammation. Patent, WO9104733.

STEAD, J.A., FREEMAN, M., JOHN, E.G., WARD, G.T. and WHITING, B. (1983) Ibuprofen tablets: dissolution and bioavailability studies. *International Journal of Pharmaceutics* **14**, 59–72.

TAISHO PHARM CO. LTD (1996) Stable masked granules used for drugs — contain core substances with bitter taste, coating layer of gastric soluble macromolecule and coating layer of water soluble macromolecule. Patent, JP08040881.

TAISHO PHARMACEUT KK (1988) Triple-layer ibuprofen-contg. tablet — has layer contg. ibuprofen between 2 layers of excipient to mask unpleasant taste. Patent, J63301817.

TAISHO PHARMACEUT KK (1990) Release-controlled compsns. comprises core of Ibuprofen and layer contg. water insol polymer and powder. Patent, J02003608.

TREFFEL, P. and GABARD, B. (1993a) Feasibility of measuring the bioavailability of topical ibuprofen in commercial formulations using drug content in epidermis and a methyl nicotinate skin inflammation assay. *Skin Pharmacology* **6**, 268–275.

TREFFEL, P. and GABARD, B. (1993b) Ibuprofen epidermal levels after topical application *in vitro* effect of formulation, application time, dose variation and occlusion, *British Journal of Dermatology* **129**, 286–291.

UPJOHN (1979) Stable suspension of aluminium salts of Ibuprofen without the bitter taste of the acid and other salts. Patent, US4145440.

VALENTI, M., BANDI, G.L., PASSAROTTI, C. and FOSSATI, A. (1990) Utilizzazione del simulatore di assorbimento cutaneo 'Sartorius' per la messa a punto di forme farmaceutiche trans-dermiche contenenti FANS. *Bolletino Chimico Farmaceutico — Anno* **129**, 247.

VIDGREN, M., SAANO, V., PARONEN, P., PEURA, P., ROMPPANEN, T. and KEINANEN, T. (1991) *In vitro* dissolution and pharmacokinetic evaluation of two film-coated and an effervescent tablet of ibuprofen. *Acta Pharmaceutica Fennica* **100**, 275–280.

WILSON, C.G., WASHINGTON, N., GREAVES, J.L. *et al.* (1989) Biomodal release of ibuprofen in a sustained release formulation: a scintigraphic and pharmacokinetic open study in healthy volunteers under different condition of food intake. *International Journal of Pharmaceutics* **50**, 155–161.

The Pharmacokinetics of Ibuprofen in Humans and Animals

DION R BROCKS[1] AND FAKHREDDIN JAMALI[2]*

[1]College of Pharmacy, Western University of Health Sciences, Pomona, CA, USA;
[2]Faculty of Pharmacy and Pharmaceutical Sciences, University of Alberta, Edmonton, AB, Canada T6G 2N8

Contents

The pharmacokinetic properties of ibuprofen have been studied intensely. It was the first 2-arylpropionic acid (2-APA) nonstereoidal anti-inflammatory drug (NSAID) developed and marketed for treatment of arthritic disorders, and in many countries it has been granted non-prescription status for treatment of pain and fever. Consequently, it enjoys widespread use on a worldwide basis.

Ibuprofen is chiral (Figure 4.1) and is administered clinically as the racemate. Similar to all other available 2-APA derivatives (Jamali, 1988), the S enantiomer possesses the majority of the pharmacological activity, as measured by inhibition of prostaglandin synthesis (Adams *et al.*, 1976). A great deal of interest has recently been directed towards ibuprofen and some other 2-APAs owing to a unique metabolic process that they undergo, called chiral inversion. In this process, which was first reported for (R)-ibuprofen in the early to mid-1970s (Mills *et al.*, 1973; Wechter *et al.*, 1974; Kaiser *et al.*, 1976; Adams *et al.*, 1976), the largely inactive R enantiomer is enzymatically converted to the active S enantiomer in a unidirectional manner. Chiral inversion is both a species- and drug-specific, biochemically mediated pathway of metabolism, and has been much studied since the early 1980s (Hutt and Caldwell, 1983; Jamali, 1988). This metabolic route raises some interesting considerations regarding not only the analysis and interpretation of pharmacokinetic data, but also the relationship between plasma concentrations and pharmacological activity or side-effects. Much effort and debate have been expended in an attempt to make sense of the biochemical basis of chiral inversion, and the anatomical site(s) where the process occurs.

4.1 ANALYTICAL METHODS

Because the enantiomers of ibuprofen differ greatly in their pharmacological and pharmacokinetic properties, it is important to adopt stereospecific assay methodology. This should not create difficulties for investigators, as over the past 20 years there have been several stereospecific GC and HPLC analytical methods published for the quantitation of ibuprofen enantiomers in biological fluids (Table 4.1). The first method was published by Vangiessen and Kaiser (1975), in which the authors derivatized the ibuprofen enantiomers at the site of the carboxylic acid moiety with *l*-α-methylbenzylamine, to form amide diastereomers. These enantiomeric diastereomers were then resolved using

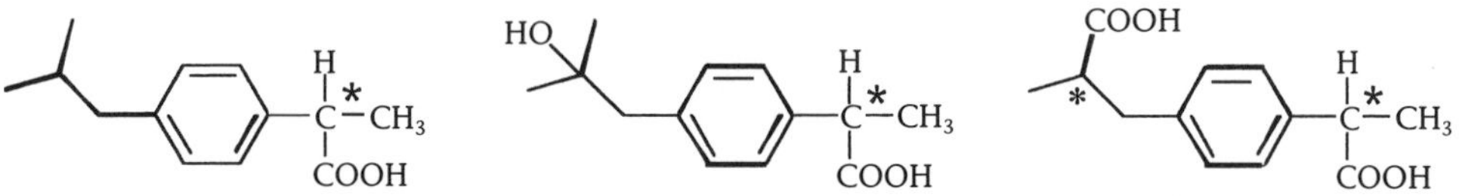

| Ibuprofen | Hydroxyibuprofen | Carboxyibuprofen |

Figure 4.1: Structure of ibuprofen and its major metabolites. Chiral centre denoted by asterisk.

TABLE 4.1

Stereospecific assays available for the quantification of ibuprofen enantiomers in human specimens

Method	Specimen	Chromatographic method used for chiral resolution[a]	Sample volume (ml)	Stated lower limit of quantitation (mg/l)	Reference
GC-MS	Plasma/synovial fluid	PD	0.2	0.003	Jack et al. (1992)
HPLC-FL	Plasma	PD	0.5	0.1	Lemko et al. (1993)
HPLC-UV	Plasma	PD	0.5	0.1	Mehvar et al. (1988)
HPLC-UV	Plasma/urine	PD	0.5	0.25	Wright et al. (1992)
GC-FID	Plasma/urine	PD	1.0	1.0	Vangiessen and Kaiser (1975)
HPLC-UV	Plasma	CSP	0.5	1.0	Naidong and Lee (1994)
HPLC-UV	Plasma/urine/bile	PD and CSP	Plasma 0.5 Urine/bile 1.0	0.1	Geissinger et al. (1989a)
HPLC-UV	Urine	PD	0.5–1.0	6.0	Rudy et al. (1990)
GC-NPD	Plasma/urine	PD	1.0	0.075	Singh et al. (1986)
GC-MS	Plasma	PD	0.1–0.2	0.1	Zhao et al. (1994)
HPLC-UV	Plasma	CSP	0.5	1.0	Naidong and Lee (1994)
HPLC-UV	Urine	CSP	1.0	6.25	Nicoll Griffith et al. (1988)
HPLC-UV	Plasma	PD	1.0	0.5	Lee et al. (1984)
HPLC-UV	Plasma	PD	0.5	1.0	Avgerinos and Hutt (1987)
HPLC-UV	Plasma	CSP	0.5	0.1	Menzel-Soglowek et al. (1990)

[a] PD, precolumn derivatization; CSP, chiral stationary phase.

conventional gas chromatography. Similarly to the first method of Vangiessen and Kaiser (1975), most of the available methods utilize precolumn derivatization with a homochiral reagent to form diastereomers of the ibuprofen enantiomers, which are then resolved on a conventional HPLC or GC column. Chiral HPLC stationary phases have also been used for resolving ibuprofen enantiomers, without the need for derivatization (Table 4.1).

Some investigators have attempted to justify why stereospecific analysis of ibuprofen may not be necessary. For example, Brown *et al.* (1992) conducted a pharmacokinetic study of ibuprofen in febrile children, using nonstereospecific methodology. They gave five reasons why the use of a nonstereospecific assay may not be necessary for the study of a pharmacokinetic–pharmacodynamic relationship between ibuprofen and antipyretic response. None of the reasons given is compelling. For example, the authors suggested that a nonstereospecific assay is not required since the relative antipyretic potency of the enantiomers is not known. It is certain, however, that one will not gain insight into the relative potencies of the enantiomers if a nonstereospecific assay is used. Any justification for the validity of pharmacokinetic results can be easily avoided by using a stereospecific analytical method, of which there are currently an ample number from which to use.

4.2 ABSORPTION OF IBUPROFEN

Ibuprofen is usually given as its acid form, although salt and ester formulations are available in some countries (Reynolds, 1993). For routine clinical use, the oral route is mostly used for administration of ibuprofen. Usual oral doses of 1.2–1.8 g daily are administered in divided doses to adult patients, typically in the form of tablets. In some patients doses reaching up to 2.4–3.2 g/day may be employed. In children, usual doses of 20–40 mg/kg may be given as divided oral doses. There are some 5% cream or gel formulations available also (Reynolds, 1993).

Most oral formulations of ibuprofen display almost complete systemic bioavailability, regardless of their rate of absorption. Hall *et al.* (1993) administered matching oral and intravenous doses of ibuprofen to healthy volunteers, and based on mean AUC the absolute bioavailability was over 92% for each enantiomer (Table 4.2). Cheng *et al.* (1994) also administered matching i.v. and oral doses of ibuprofen, and reported the absolute bioavailabilities of the *R* and *S* enantiomers to be 83.6% and 92.0%, respectively. In general, different formulations may exhibit differences in the rate of absorption, and accordingly the values of t_{max} and C_{max} are formulation dependent (Table 4.2).

In general, when the *R* enantiomer is administered alone, the t_{max} value of the formed (*S*)-ibuprofen lags behind that of its antipode, probably owing to the time required for the formation of the *S* enantiomer due to chiral inversion (Table 4.2). In general, this observation also appears to be valid for the comparison of the t_{max} of the *S* and *R* enantiomers after administration of the racemate (Table 4.2). In one study it was noted that when the

CHAPTER 4

TABLE 4.2

Summary of pharmacokinetics of ibuprofen enantiomers in clinical studies

Study participants	No.	Age (years)	Dose (mg)	C_{max} (mg/l) S	R	t_{max} (h) S	R	AUC_{0-t} (mg/l)·h S	R	$t_{1/2}$ (h) S	R	CL/F (l/h)[a] S	R	V_d/F (l)[a] S	R	Reference
Healthy	8	28	800 rac	–	–	–	–	–	–	3.0	4.2	5.04	6.42	12.6	41.0	Rudy et al. (1995)
			800 rac q 8h	–	–	–	–	–	–	3.7	6.4	5.04	8.70	11.5	70.0	
Elderly	14	73	800 rac	–	–	–	–	–	–	2.8	4.2	5.64	7.02	15.7	42.0	Rudy et al. (1995)
			800 rac q 8h	–	–	–	–	–	–	3.9	8.4	5.28	7.56	14.3	94.0	
Elderly renal insufficiency	13	75	800 rac	–	–	–	–	–	–	3.3	3.5	4.98	6.24	15.9	28.0	Rudy et al. (1995)
			800 rac q 8h	–	–	–	–	–	–	4.3	5.5	5.28	7.68	17.4	56.0	
Healthy	8	(19–37)	600 rac	30	27.5	1.44	–	107	74.2	2.6	2.7	–	4.04	–	15.7	Jamali et al. (1988b)
			600 rac	31.5	23.5	2.75	–	122	73.9	2.6	2.8	–	4.06	–	16.6	
			600 rac	23.9	20.3	1.42	–	90.8	56.9	2.4	2.0	–	5.27	–	15.4	
			600 rac	26.7	17.3	2.83	–	100	51.5	2.2	2.2	–	5.83	–	18.8	
Healthy (oriental)	10	60	800 rac	–	–	–	–	287	240	3.3	3.1	–	1.67	–	7.5	Chen and Chen (1995)
Nerve root compression patients	46	51	800 rac	26.1	20.7	1.5	1.5	85.5(t=8)	65.5(t=8)	2.5	1.7	–	–	–	–	Bannwarth et al. (1995)
Healthy	10	19–30	400 rac i.v.	–	–	–	–	71.7	67.7	2.8	3.3	–	3.19	–	15.2	Hall et al. (1993)
			400 rac oral	–	–	–	–	70.3	62.8	2.3	2.8	4.59	3.55	15.0	14.4	
Healthy	11	(0.5–1.0)	7.6 rac mg/kg sol	9.7	11.8	2.9	2.9	31.5	36.6	1.6	1.5	–	1.14	–	2.85	Rey et al. (1994)
Arthritis	24	–	400 S	21.8	–	2.3	–	77.3	–	1.9	–	5.42	–	14.9	–	Geisslinger et al. (1993)
			600 rac	20.3	17.7	2.4	2.3	86.2	67.6	2.1	2.0	–	5.06	–	14.6	

Healthy	11	–	600 rac	38	25	1.3	1.2	127	74.0	2.1	1.7	–	4.05	–	9.64	Levine et al. (1992)
			600 rac with food	29	19	1.6	1.5	116	59.0	2.1	1.7	–	5.08	–	12.7	
Healthy	12	(18–34)	400 rac	8.7	7.7	6	4.4	58(t=12)	42.0	2.8	2.2	–	4.76	–	15.1	Cox et al. (1988)
Healthy			400 rac	17	18	1.3	1.2	58(t=12)	50.0	2.2	1.4	–	4.00	–	8.1	
Healthy	6	33	50 rac sol	–	–	–	–	7.5	6.4	2.8	2.2	–	3.92	–	12.5	Jamali et al. (1992)
			100 rac sol	–	–	–	–	13.3	11.5	2.9	2.2	–	4.35	–	13.8	
			200 rac sol	–	–	–	–	23.5	20.9	2.1	1.7	–	4.78	–	11.7	
			400 rac sol	–	–	–	–	42.6	36.6	2.1	1.9	–	5.46	–	15.0	
			600 rac sol	–	–	–	–	70.6	61.1	2.2	2.6	–	4.91	–	18.4	
			600 rac tab	–	–	2.17	–	70.8	52.7	2.0	2.1	–	5.69	–	17.3	
			1200 rac sol	–	–	–	–	126	106	2.2	2.5	–	5.66	–	20.4	
Healthy	12	(20–29)	300 R sol	7.63	34.9	1.375	0.4	48.7	97.5	2.8	1.8	–	3.08	–	8.0	Smith et al. (1994)
			300 S sol	29.7	–	0.4583	–	69.2	–	1.7	–	4.33	–	–	–	
			600 rac sol	29.0	29.6	0.6333	0.6	98.6	78.8	2.4	1.7	–	3.81	–	9.3	
			300 R + 600 S sol	49.8	30	0.525	0.5	149	75.3	2.2	1.7	–	–	–	–	
Healthy	8	29	600 S	–	–	–	–			–	–	–	–	4.93	–	Rudy et al. (1991)
			600 R	–	–	–	–			–	–	–	7.80	–	–	
			800 rac	–	–	–	–			–	–	5.24	6.78	–	–	
Healthy	12	24	600 rac	16.2	14	2.1	1.7	78.9	50.5	3.1	3.2	–	6.80	–	33.0	Oliary et al. (1992)
Healthy	5	25	400 rac q 8h	14.3	10.6	2.3	1.6	48.0	31.1	2.5	2.2	–	7.34	–	24.5	Walker et al. (1993)
			1200 rac	35.4	25.4	1.8	1.8	186	106	3.2	3.2	–	3.77	–	17.4	
Healthy	8	52	600 rac	23.3	23.4	1.8	1.8	94.5	73.5	1.8	1.7	–	4.08	–	10.0	Li et al. (1993)
Healthy	8	52	400 S	26.8	–	1.8	–	101	–	1.6	–	3.96	–	9.14	–	
Cirrhosis	8	56	600 rac	14.2	19.5	1.1	1.2	81.6	87.1	3.4	3.1	–	3.44	–	15.4	
	8	52	400 S	24.9	–	2.1	–	144	–	2.6	–	2.78	–	10.4	–	

TABLE 4.2 (*continued*)

Study participants	No.	Age (years)	Dose (mg)	C_{max} (mg/l) S	R	t_{max} (h) S	R	AUC_{0-t} (mg/l)·h S	R	$t_{1/2}$ (h) S	R	CL/F (l/h)[a] S	R	V_d/F (l)[a] S	R	Reference
Osteoarthritis	45	58	300 rac	11.1	10.5	2.0	1.9	42.9	27.7	2.0	1.7	6.93	5.94	20.0	14.6	Rudy et al. (1992)
			300 q.i.d × 3 days	12.7	12.0	2.1	2.3	54.4	35.9	3.1	2.8	5.27	4.96	23.6	20.0	
			600 rac	13.8	16.4	1.9	2.3	74.3	56.6	3.5	2.3	7.46	5.79	37.7	19.2	
			600 rac q.i.d. × 3 days	18.2	18.7	2.0	1.6	81.4	55.5	3.0	2.9	7.24	6.50	31.3	27.2	
Arthritis	8	50	800 rac mg q 8h	26	24	1.3	1.1	93	67	1.98	1.78	–	5.97	–	15.3	Cox et al. (1991)
Healthy	12	(19–40)	200 S	–	–	–	–	–	–	1.77	–	3.91	–	8.8	–	Cheng et al. (1994)
			200 R	–	–	–	–	–	–	–	1.82	–	3.00	–	7.4	
			400 rac	–	–	–	–	–	–	–	1.74	–	3.52	–	7.8	
Arthritis	21	57	300 rac q.i.d.	–	–	–	–	67.2	–	–	–	–	–	–	–	Bradley et al. (1992)
	24	58	600 rac q.i.d.	–	–	–	–	98.7	–	–	–	–	–	–	–	
Healthy female	8	24	6 mg/kg R	–	36.9	–	0.7	55.4	97.3	–	1.7	–	3.83	–	10.2	Knights et al. (1995)
Healthy male	8	21	6 mg/kg R	–	33.8	–	0.5	67.9	97.4	–	1.7	–	4.42	–	12.2	
Healthy male	6	–	400 mg	19.0	17.8	1.64	1.59	75.0	52.2	2.18	1.33	–	4.00	–	7.46	Suri et al. (1997)
Febrile children	17	(1–11.3)	6 mg/kg liquid	13.9	13.4	1.11	0.7			2.3	1.5	–	1.24 ml/min/kg	–	0.158 l/kg		Kelley et al. (1992)

Subject	n	Age	Dose													Reference
Healthy	4	(31–45)	400 S	–	–	–	–	93.1	–	1.7	–	4.46	–	10.5	–	Lee et al. (1985)
			400 R	–	–	–	–	59.3	101	–	2.0	–	4.06	–	9.9	
			800 rac	–	–	–	–	128	82.3	2.5	1.7	–	5.26	–	11.5	
Arthritic	8	58	400–800 rac b.i.d.–t.i.d.	–	–	–	–	–	–	2.3	1.6	–	5.94	–	0.16 l/kg	Day et al. (1988)
Healthy	11	(25–47)	300 S	19.1	–	1.44	–	65.7	–	2.1	–	4.87	–	14.7	–	Geisslinger et al. (1990)
			300 R	6.51	21.6	2.1	1.1	34.4	55.7	2.2	2.1	–	5.96	–	18.1	
			600 rac	16.4	14.3	1.8	1.5	91.7	54.3	2.3	2.3	–	5.66	–	18.7	
Healthy	4	(25–47)	150 S	9.14	–	1.35	–	39.2	–	1.9	–	4.12	–	11.0	–	Geisslinger et al. (1990)
			500 S	27.3	–	1.97	–	117	–	2.2	–	4.59	–	14.8	–	
Healthy	6	(21–42)	800 rac	28.5	27.1	1.625	1.4	108	75.2	2.3	1.6	–	5.32	–	12.5	Evans et al. (1990)
Healthy	4	(23–28)	200 rac	11.3	10	1.13	1.1	43.7	23.9	1.9	1.9	–	4.19	–	11.2	
			400 rac	16.9	14.1	1.87	1.4	75.4	41.8	3.4	3.2	–	4.78	–	22.3	
			800 rac	31.6	24.4	1.89	1.6	141	73.6	2.0	2.1	–	5.44	–	16.7	
			1200 rac	47.7	29.5	2.19	1.8	216	86.1	2.0	4.2	–	6.97	–	42.6	
Healthy	8	(25–47)	300 S	18.7	–	1.4	–	67.2	–	2.2	–	5.03	–	16.0	–	Geisslinger et al. (1989b)
			300 R	6.4	19.8	2.1	1.0	32.4	57.2	2.2	1.8	–	5.55	–	14.4	
			600 rac	16.8	14.8	1.9	1.7	89.8	57.0	2.4	2.3	–	5.37	–	17.8	

a If not presented in paper, mean parameters for R enantiomer calculated by us using the relationships $\overline{CL/F} = \dfrac{Dose_R}{AUC_R}$ and $\overline{V_d/F} = \dfrac{\overline{t_{1/2,R}} \cdot \overline{CL_R}}{0.693}$.

b rac = racemate; sol = solution; tab = tablet; liq = liquid.

S enantiomer is given alone, the peak concentrations are higher and attained more rapidly than when the S enantiomer is given in the form of the racemate (Geisslinger *et al.*, 1990). The importance of the observation was outlined by pointing out that for analgesia a rapid onset of action is desired. As a possible explanation for the difference in t_{max}, the authors suggested formulation differences caused by the introduction of the R enantiomer, as it is known that a racemate is not simply a mixture of two enantiomers, but rather a compound possessing different physicochemical properties from pure enantiomer (Dwivedi *et al.*, 1992). Stereochemically pure enantiomers of ibuprofen exhibit approximately 2-fold greater solubility and faster dissolution than the racemate (Dwivedi *et al.*, 1992). An explanation not offered by the Geisslinger *et al.* (1990) was that the delay in C_{max} after racemate was due to the time required for generation of the S enantiomer by chiral inversion of R enantiomer.

As elaborated later in this chapter, in the presence of a presystemic inversion process, it would be anticipated that the percentage of the dose systemically available as the therapeutically active S enantiomer would be higher than that after an immediate release dosage form containing the same amount of racemic compound (Jamali *et al.*, 1988; Mehvar and Jamali, 1988b).

The effect of food on the absorption of ibuprofen enantiomers has been assessed in healthy male volunteers given 600 mg of ibuprofen with or without a standard high fat-content meal (Levine *et al.*, 1992). Compared to fasted conditions, there was no discernible effect of the meal on the rate or extent of ibuprofen absorption. This information is of particular usefulness as it has been recommended that ibuprofen be taken with food to reduce the frequency or intensity of upper gastrointestinal side-effects.

Alternate routes of nonparenteral administration of ibuprofen have been explored. For example, in one study, eight healthy volunteers were given a solution and a suspension formulation of ibuprofen rectally in a randomized fashion (Eller *et al.*, 1989). Compared to oral administration, rectal solution resulted in a similar extent of bioavailability. In contrast, the rectal suspension yielded an extent of absorption only approximately 60% that of the same formulation when given orally. Rectal administration of both formulations yielded lower (62–67%) C_{max} values. The t_{max} was longer for suspension than solution for both routes of administration. It was concluded that rectal administration of ibuprofen offers a viable alternative to the oral route, and may be of special benefit in patients with adult respiratory distress syndrome.

4.3 DISTRIBUTION

4.3.1 Protein binding

Similarly to other NSAIDs, ibuprofen displays extensive (99%) binding to plasma proteins (Lin *et al.*, 1987). Consequently, most studies have reported a relatively low volume of distribution of the drug (Table 4.2) of approximately 10–20 l in adult patients and volunteers.

Nonlinear pharmacokinetics have been reported for ibuprofen, and have been attributed to saturation of plasma protein binding. In one study, the pharmacokinetics of (R+S)-ibuprofen were studied in 15 healthy caucasian males (mean age 25 years) after administration of single doses of 400, 800 or 1200 mg of racemate (Lockwood *et al.*, 1983). A deviation from linearity in the dose vs total bound + unbound ibuprofen AUC relationship was noted over this range of doses, although the relationship between dose and AUC of unbound drug was linear. Since there was no change in the percentage of the dose recovered in urine, which ranged from 77% to 85% between the three dose levels, a decrease in bioavailability was not suggested. Rather, the plateau was attributed to saturation of plasma protein binding at the higher dose levels, with a compensatory increase in CL of total drug.

In a stereospecific assessment, Evans *et al.* (1989b) administered a single 800 mg oral tablet of ibuprofen to six healthy volunteers, and serial blood samples were obtained for 10 h. Using equilibrium dialysis and radioactively labelled ibuprofen, the plasma protein binding of ibuprofen enantiomers was studied. The unbound fraction of the *R* enantiomer (0.45%) was significantly less than that of the *S* enantiomer (0.77%) in the patient samples. Based on the individual data presented, the mean unbound *S*:*R* AUC ratio was significantly greater (2.2) than that of mean total (bound + unbound) drug (1.4). The unbound concentration of each enantiomer was influenced by the presence of its antipode, suggesting the possibility of a pharmacokinetic interaction between the enantiomers. These results were corroborated by Paliwal *et al.* (1993), who found that in subjects given 300 mg of *R* enantiomer, 600 mg racemate, or 300 mg *R*+600 mg *S*, plasma (R+S)-ibuprofen concentration greater than 30 mg/l resulted in a parallel progressive rise in the unbound fraction of both enantiomers (Figure 4.2). Interestingly, in the absence of administered antipode, the unbound concentrations of both enantiomers appeared to increase in an approximately linear manner with increasing concentration. There also appeared to be an interaction between the enantiomers at the level of protein binding (Figure 4.2).

The acyl glucuronides of several NSAIDs have been shown to exhibit irreversible binding to albumin, which is the major plasma binding protein for NSAIDs (Zia-Amirhosseini *et al.*, 1995). Ibuprofen glucuronide may also cause the formation of irreversibly bound drug–protein adducts *in vitro* (Castillo *et al.*, 1995). The reaction required the presence of ibuprofen glucuronide; parent drug added alone did not generate adduct formation. Over a 24 h incubation period, 1.5% to 1.7% of the available ibuprofen was covalently bound to plasma proteins. Enantiomer binding was not studied in this experiment. The potential toxicological significance of this binding has yet to be specifically addressed, although it has been postulated that such covalent binding might precipitate immunologically mediated toxicity. Compared to some other NSAIDs, most notably of the aryl-alkyl acid class, the degree of covalent binding of ibuprofen to protein is low.

CHAPTER 4

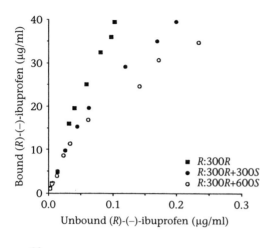

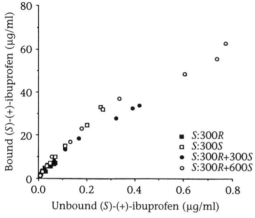

Figure 4.2: Bound–unbound relationship between ibuprofen enantiomers in a representative healthy subject after administration of different doses of ibuprofen. (From Paliwal *et al.* (1993), with permission.)

4.3.2 Tissue distribution

Synovial fluid

The synovial membrane has been postulated to be the site of action of NSAIDs (Wallis and Simkin, 1983), and several studies have in turn examined synovial fluid concentrations of ibuprofen and its enantiomers. Day *et al.* (1988) and Cox *et al.* (1988) studied the kinetics of ibuprofen enantiomers in synovial fluid of arthritic patients requiring aspiration of synovial effusions of the knee. Day *et al.* (1988) reported in their patients that the CL of (*R*)-ibuprofen ranged from 61 to 109 ml/min, whereas that of the *S* enantiomer, assuming 60% inversion, ranged from 66 to 185 ml/min. The t_{max} in synovial fluid was longer than in plasma for both enantiomers, and concentrations in synovial fluid were generally lower

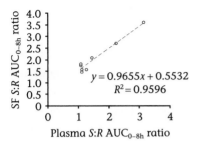

Figure 4.3: Relationship between S:R AUC$_{0-8h}$ ratios in synovial fluid (SF) and plasma of 8 arthritic patients. (Plotted from data of Cox *et al.* (1991).)

than in corresponding plasma samples. Trough plasma concentrations (i.e. 8–12 h post dose) were generally much higher in synovial fluid than in plasma. Delayed and extended uptake of ibuprofen into the synovial cavity was offered to explain the therapeutic efficacy of ibuprofen when given every 12 h, even though plasma concentrations decline rapidly with a $t_{1/2}$ of often less than 2 h.

The findings of Cox *et al.* (1988) paralleled those of Day *et al.* (1988). The t_{max} in synovial fluid of both enantiomers lagged approximately 2 h behind that in serum. The mean S:R ratio of AUC in synovial fluid was 2.1 compared to 1.6 in plasma; a linear relationship was present between this ratio in the two fluids (Figure 4.3). Maximum synovial fluid concentrations lagged behind those in plasma or serum. Hence, the authors suggested the use of trough serum or plasma ibuprofen concentrations in concentration vs effect studies, to ensure attainment of post-distributive ibuprofen levels at the site of action (Cox *et al.*, 1988).

Elmquist *et al.*, 1994 described two methods of calculating the synovial exit rate constants, and used ibuprofen as an example for use of these methods. Using nonstereospecific literature data, they calculated transfer rate constants from synovial fluid to plasma ranging from 0.29 h^{-1} to 0.45 h^{-1}, and mean transit times in synovium of 2.22 to 3.44 h.

The protein binding of ibuprofen is greater in plasma than in synovial fluid (Wanwimolruk *et al.*, 1983), which is to be expected on the basis of the lower concentrations of albumin in synovial fluid.

Blister fluid

Owing to clinical and practical considerations, limitations are involved in the collection of serial synovial fluid samples from arthritic patients for pharmacokinetic assessments of NSAIDs at their site of action (Walker *et al.*, 1993; Seideman *et al.*, 1994). Blister fluid, which shares similarities to synovial fluid particularly from the perspective of albumin concentrations, has been proposed as a suitable surrogate site to mimic the time course and amount of drug present in the synovium. In one study involving arthritic patients with knee effusions and induced suction blisters, serial plasma, synovial and blister fluid

CHAPTER 4

samples were collected and assayed for ibuprofen enantiomer content after single 1200 mg doses of racemate (Seideman *et al.*, 1994). The mean AUC values of the enantiomers were of similar magnitude in synovial and blister fluids. The rate constants for entry of the two enantiomers into the synovial cavity were very similar (~0.35 h^{-1}). There were significant differences between the two enantiomers in their entry into the extracellular compartments and exit from the blister compartment. The t_{max} values of ibuprofen enantiomers in synovial and blister fluids were closely related, but between patients there was a poor relationship between magnitude of the ibuprofen concentrations in the two fluids. Specifically, in some patients blister fluid concentrations were much higher than in synovial fluid, whereas in other patients synovial fluid concentrations were higher. Although blister fluid might be useful for relating the time course of pharmacological effect of ibuprofen in an individual patient, it might not be as useful a tool for quantifying the magnitude of the effect owing to the lack of correlation between concentrations in the two fluids.

Cerebrospinal fluid

Because of the involvement of the CNS in the antipyretic and analgesic properties of NSAIDs, the CNS uptake of ibuprofen enantiomers has been studied (Bannwarth *et al.*, 1995). The authors studied 46 patients (30 M, 16 F; mean age 51 years) with normal plasma protein levels who were admitted to hospital for treatment of nerve-root compression. The subjects were given 800 mg of ibuprofen followed by simultaneous collection of plasma and cerebrospinal fluid samples for determination of ibuprofen enantiomer concentration. The AUC_{0-8h} of the R and S enantiomers in CSF were 0.9% and 1.5% of those in plasma, respectively. This was in line with the higher unbound fraction of the S enantiomer in plasma (Paliwal *et al.*, 1993). Peak ibuprofen enantiomer concentrations occurred in CSF later than in plasma, and the delay was attributed to passive transport of drug into the CSF. More drug was present in the CSF than could be accounted for on the basis of the unbound concentration in plasma, leading the authors to speculate on the presence of protein binding in the CSF. Interestingly, the mean $S{:}R$ AUC ratio of ibuprofen enantiomers in CSF (2.1) was similar to that of unbound drug in plasma (2.3), but higher than that of total drug in plasma (1.3). Similar trends were present for C_{max}. This finding in CSF is in line with the higher plasma unbound concentration of the S enantiomer as compared with the antipode (Paliwal *et al.*, 1993).

Breast milk and saliva

Excretion of ibuprofen into breast milk is negligible; approximately 1 mg of a racemic dose of 400 mg is excreted per day into the breast milk (Albert *et al.*, 1984). This is expected on the basis of the high degree of acidic nature and plasma protein binding of ibuprofen.

Secretion into saliva is also reported to be negligible (Albert *et al.*, 1984).

Binding to other tissues

Because NSAIDs are indicated for connective-tissue disease, it is relevant to understand the ability of these drugs to bind to those tissues. For practical reasons, however, human tissue disposition studies are difficult to perform *in vivo*. Nevertheless, some information regarding the distribution of ibuprofen to human tissue is available from *in vitro* and *post mortem* studies. *In vitro* experiments with human connective tissue have shown that radioactively labelled ibuprofen can bind to skin, muscle, subcutaneous, tendon and joint capsule tissues (Menzel and Kolarz, 1992). Of these tissues, binding was highest in muscle and lowest in tendon tissue. Actin was found to be the primary component through which ibuprofen bound itself to muscle tissues. Tissue concentrations of ibuprofen have been determined in a 26-year-old man who died from overdose with the drug (Kunsman and Rohrig, 1993). Using an HPLC assay, it was determined that high concentrations of the drug were present in the liver and blood. Brain concentrations were approximately 20% of those in the liver.

The process responsible for chiral inversion of ibuprofen, namely the formation of an ibuprofen-acyl CoA thioester, is related to fatty acid metabolism. As part of this process, at least in the rat, Williams *et al.* (1986) have shown that (*R*)-ibuprofen can replace endogenous fatty acids in triacylglycerols, and thus be incorporated into adipose tissue. (*S*)-Ibuprofen, however, could not form these entities (Carbaza *et al.*, 1996). It has been suggested that these hybrid triglycerides could have possible toxicological sequelae (Williams *et al.*, 1986), although definitive proof supporting this hypothesis has yet to be brought forth.

4.4 CLEARANCE

Both enantiomers of ibuprofen possess a relatively short terminal elimination $t_{1/2}$ of approximately 2 h (Table 4.2). With increasing dose a plateau is evident in the AUC vs dose relationship (Figure 4.4) and, as discussed above, this has been attributed to a saturation of plasma protein binding at higher dose levels. Based on the linear relationship between dose and unbound plasma AUC (Lockwood *et al.*, 1983; Evans *et al.*, 1990), it would appear that the intrinsic metabolic rate of unbound ibuprofen remains constant over a wide range of doses.

Two studies have assessed the relationship between single doses of ibuprofen and AUC of the enantiomers (Figure 4.4). Evans *et al.* (1990) studied the relationship between dose and AUC of ibuprofen in four healthy volunteers given a tablet formulation. The AUC vs dose relationship of the *S* enantiomer was approximately linear after administration of the racemate. Nonlinearity, however, was visible in the AUC vs dose relationship of the *R* enantiomer. In contrast, the AUC vs dose relationship of unbound drug was linear for both enantiomers. These findings are in line with the competitive protein binding displacement results of Paliwal *et al.* (1993). Jamali *et al.* (1992) found, after administration

CHAPTER 4

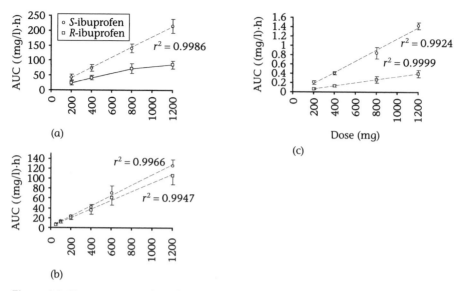

Figure 4.4: Dose proportionality of ibuprofen enantiomers. Figures were drawn from the mean data presented in each paper. (a) AUC of total (bound + unbound) enantiomer in plasma vs administered dose (Evans *et al.*, 1990); (b) AUC of total (bound + unbound) enantiomer in plasma vs administered dose (Jamali *et al.*, 1992); (c) AUC of unbound enantiomer in plasma vs administered dose (Evans *et al.*, 1990).

of racemate, that mean S to mean R AUC ratios from the dose range of 50 mg to 1200 mg of solution formulation were relatively constant (Table 4.2; Figure 4.4), ranging from 1.12 to 1.19. Although the overall mean AUC vs dose relationship appeared to be linear for both enantiomers (Figure 4.4), there was some suggestion towards a change of CL with increasing dose in some of the subjects.

Smith *et al.* (1994) assessed the influence of competitive and nonlinear binding enantiomers on stereoselective disposition of ibuprofen by random administration of four treatments of ibuprofen to 12 healthy subjects. The CL of total R enantiomer in plasma was enhanced in the presence of the S enantiomer, although the CL of unbound R enantiomer in plasma remained unaffected by the presence of its antipode. This observation was in accordance with the findings of displacement of R enantiomer by (*S*)-ibuprofen from plasma proteins (Paliwal *et al.*, 1993), and by the dose ranging study by Evans *et al.* (1990). After repeated doses, the nonlinearity in AUC of (*S*)-ibuprofen may be more readily apparent. Bradley *et al.* (1992) have reported nonlinearity in the AUC of (*S*)-ibuprofen after repeated doses of 300 mg q.i.d. and 600 mg q.i.d. in arthritic patients. In an earlier study of another NSAID, flurbiprofen, an interaction between the enantiomers was reported in both rats (Jamali *et al.*, 1988) and humans (Berry *et al.*, 1989). The clearance of (*R*)-flurbiprofen was doubled when it was administered as the racemate as compared with the optically pure enantiomer.

4.4.1 Metabolism of ibuprofen

Metabolic fate of ibuprofen

Ibuprofen is extensively metabolized in humans to pharmacologically inactive metabolites (Figure 4.1). After administration of radiolabelled compound as part of a 200 mg q 6h dosage regimen, to humans, less than 1% of the total dose has been reported as being excreted into the urine as unchanged or acyl glucuronidated ibuprofen (Mills *et al.*, 1973). Other investigators have found a greater recovery of drug in urine as acyl glucuronidated ibuprofen. For example, Lee *et al.* (1985) determined that 1.5% and 12.5% of the administered dose of (R)- and (S)-ibuprofen, respectively, was excreted in the urine as acylglucuronide after administration of 400 mg of each enantiomer. Rudy *et al.* (1991) also found a higher percentage of acyl glucuronide in urine than Mills *et al.*, with 8.9% of the racemic dose recovered in urine over 24 h. Hence, it would appear that the report of Mills *et al.* (1973) underestimated the extent of glucuronidation of ibuprofen. Compared to the NSAIDs pirprofen and flurbiprofen, *in vitro* hepatic glucuronidation of ibuprofen occurs at a slower rate across a number of animal species, including Gunn rat, dog, monkey, rabbit, mouse and human. The only species in which the rate of microsomal glucuronidation exceeded that of pirprofen and flurbiprofen was in cat (Magdalou *et al.*, 1990).

In plasma, the majority of the circulating ibuprofen-related material is present in the form of parent compound. Oxidative metabolism appears to be the major fate of ibuprofen, followed by acyl-glucuronidation of the oxidized metabolites. The major reported metabolites of ibuprofen are 2-[4-(2-carboxypropyl)phenyl]propionic acid and 2-[4-(2-hydroxy-2-methylpropyl)phenyl]propionic acid (Figure 4.1), each of which are products of structural modification of the isobutyl portion of the parent compound (Mills *et al.*, 1973). These two metabolites account for 35% and 26%, respectively, of the total urinary metabolite recovery over 24 h (Mills *et al.*, 1973). Other less prevalent hydroxylated metabolites of ibuprofen have also been characterized in human urine (Brooks and Gilbert, 1974). One unique metabolic product of (S)-ibuprofen is in fact the S enantiomer, as described below.

Hall *et al.* (1993) reported that the formation CL of the major metabolites of ibuprofen were larger for the S enantiomer than the R enantiomer, after both intravenous and oral dosing. For all metabolites, the mean formation CL values were slightly higher after oral as compared to intravenous dosing.

Conjugation of xenobiotic carboxylic acids with amino acids is a common biotransformation reaction. This reaction is known to be facilitated by the formation of CoA thioesters, which are also implicated in the chiral inversion process. Shirley *et al.* (1994) found that this route comprised a minor route in the biotransformation of ibuprofen; following a single 400 mg dose of ibuprofen to four healthy subjects, less than 2% of the 24 h urinary recovery consisted of taurine conjugate, and no glycine conjugate was detectable. The majority of this material possesses the S configuration. Studies involving rat

CHAPTER 4

liver mitochondria showed that this formation of the conjugate occurred primarily in the mitochondria, and required the preliminary formation of the CoA thioester.

Sanins *et al.* (1990) have shown that the relative proportions of the hydroxy- and carboxyibuprofen metabolites formed by isolated rat hepatocytes are in line with the respective urinary recoveries in studies *in vivo*. Glucuronidation was a minor pathway of metabolism by rat hepatocytes.

Chiral inversion

Chiral inversion is a unique metabolic pathway which influences the disposition of ibuprofen and some other 2-arylpropionic acid NSAIDs, including fenoprofen and ketoprofen. This pathway is of particular interest because in most species it involves a unidirectional conversion of a fraction of the dose of largely inactive (*R*)-ibuprofen to active (*S*)-ibuprofen. Because the extent of inversion can have a direct impact on the therapeutic and toxicological profile of ibuprofen enantiomers, a consideration of factors that may modify the extent of inversion is important. Inversion also imparts an influence on the interpretation of CL of the *S* enantiomer, and on the meaning of CL of (*R+S*)-ibuprofen when nonstereospecific assay methodology is used. It is important to note that many chiral NSAIDs are not subject to chiral inversion, and when it does occur its extent may vary between different species.

Mills *et al.* (1973) provided the first data suggesting chiral inversion of ibuprofen in humans. In healthy volunteers it was noted that the specific rotation of recovered urinary metabolites was more positive than expected after administration of purified *R*-(−)-ibuprofen. After administration of individual enantiomers to humans, it was noted that after *R*, but not *S* enantiomer, considerable amounts of antipode were detectable in plasma (Lee *et al.*, 1985; Figure 4.5). This provided evidence for unidirectional nature of the inversion process of ibuprofen in humans.

The fraction of the dose of (*R*)-ibuprofen subject to inversion has been estimated to range between 35% and 70% in humans (Lee *et al.*, 1985; Geisslinger *et al.*, 1989 and 1990; Hall *et al.*, 1993; Rudy *et al.*, 1991; Cheng *et al.*, 1994). It has been reported by both Smith *et al.* (1994) and Hall *et al.* (1993) that for the partial clearances of non-inversion processes, the *S* enantiomer is cleared more rapidly from plasma than the *R* enantiomer.

In earlier studies, the fraction of *R* enantiomer inverted to (*S*)-ibuprofen, and CL of the *S* enantiomer, were determined by administration of optically pure enantiomer (Lee *et al.*, 1985; Figure 4.5). A drawback to this approach is that the enantiomers are known to inter-act with one another at the level of plasma protein binding (Paliwal *et al.*, 1993). Hence, administration of a single enantiomer might not truly reflect the clinical situation in which both enantiomers are initially present. Rudy *et al.* (1991) described two unique methods to determine the CL and V_d of (*S*)-ibuprofen, by co-administration of a small amount of deuterated (*S*)-ibuprofen with a dose of the *R* enantiomer or racemate, and by determination of the stereoisomeric composition of the major urinary metabolites

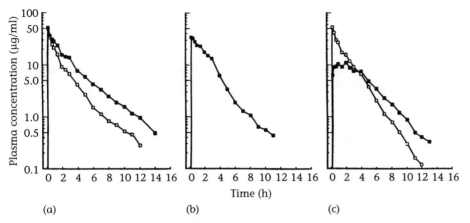

Figure 4.5: Plasma concentrations of (*R*)- (open symbols) and (*S*)-ibuprofen (filled symbols) after administration of (a) 800 mg racemate, (b) 400 mg (*S*)-ibuprofen and (c) 400 mg (*R*)-ibuprofen. (From Lee *et al.* (1985), with permission.)

of ibuprofen after administration of racemate. Young subjects were administered single oral doses of (*R*)-(600 mg) or racemic (800 mg) ibuprofen, co-administered with a 10 mg dose of deuterium-labelled (*S*)-ibuprofen. The deuterated material was differentiated from the nondeuterated material using GC-MS analysis, and its time course in plasma was assumed to represent the time course of (*S*)-ibuprofen which was not formed by inversion of the *R* enantiomer. The three different methods used, namely administration of pure (*S*)-ibuprofen, co-administration of deuterated (*S*)-ibuprofen with racemate and *R* enantiomer, and determination of urinary metabolites, were compared. The range of calculated mean fractional inverted values using the different methods were similar, ranging from 0.48 to 0.66. The urinary metabolite method yielded values for fraction inverted that were significantly higher than those derived from the deuterated (*S*)-ibuprofen method. Incomplete urine collection of metabolite and possible inversion of *R* metabolites were given as possible causes for the difference. Although the authors thoroughly described the possible difficulties with the (*S*)-ibuprofen-only approach, they did not mention possible liabilities of the deuterated (*S*)-ibuprofen approach, which include the assumption that the plasma protein binding and metabolic CL are unaffected by the presence of the deuterium label (i.e., no isotope effect).

In general, in humans and most other species, but not all (Jamali *et al.*, 1997, Chen *et al.*, 1991), the chiral inversion of NSAIDs is unidirectional from *R* to *S*. Sanins *et al.* (1990) studied the metabolism of ibuprofen by isolated rat hepatocytes after incubation with (*R*)- or (*S*)-ibuprofen, hydroxyibuprofen and carboxyibuprofen stereoisomers. When *S* enantiomer was added to the media, there was no measurable rise in the concentrations of (*R*)-ibuprofen; this was in line with the unidirectional nature of inversion from *R* to *S* enantiomer in humans.

CHAPTER 4

4.4.2 Consequences of chiral inversion on ibuprofen clearance calculations using nonstereospecific calculations

Using nonstereospecific analysis, the following relationship has been proposed to describe the total body clearance of $(R+S)$-ibuprofen after administration of the racemate:

$$CL_{R+S} = \frac{\text{Dose}_{R+S} \cdot F}{\text{AUC}_{R+S}} \tag{4.1}$$

Since most estimates have placed the bioavailability of racemic ibuprofen near 1, both enantiomers would appear to be completely absorbed with a minimum of hepatic first pass effect. Hence, for ibuprofen the term for F may be dropped from equation (4.1). It has been recognized that the calculation of CL of (S)-ibuprofen is not straightforward when R enantiomer is administered owing to the formation of the S enantiomer from the R enantiomer. As such, using the administered dose of S enantiomer in the calculation of CL will cause an underestimation of true CL of (S)-ibuprofen after racemate. It may also be shown that the CL_{R+S} as calculated above is subject to error, as follows.

Assuming presystemic inversion processes (Jamali *et al.*, 1988b), and equal absorption characteristics for each enantiomer, one may calculate the CL of ibuprofen enantiomers after administration of racemate as follows:

$$CL_R = \frac{\left(\frac{1}{2}\text{Dose}_{R+S}\right) \cdot \left(1 - f_{\text{inv}}^{\text{pre}}\right)}{\text{AUC}_R} \tag{4.2}$$

and

$$CL_S = \frac{\left(\frac{1}{2}\text{Dose}_{R+S}\right) \cdot \left(1 + f_{\text{inv}}^{\text{pre}}\right)}{\text{AUC}_S} \tag{4.3}$$

where $f_{\text{inv}}^{\text{pre}}$ indicates the fraction of the administered dose of R enantiomer inverted to S enantiomer via the presystemic inversion process. Therefore, the CL of racemate is as follows:

$$CL_{R+S} = \frac{\left(\frac{1}{2}\text{Dose}_{R+S}\right) \cdot \left[\left(1 - f_{\text{inv}}^{\text{pre}}\right) + \left(1 + f_{\text{inv}}^{\text{pre}}\right)\right]}{\text{AUC}_{R+S}} = \frac{\text{Dose}_{R+S}}{\text{AUC}_{R+S}} \tag{4.4}$$

Therefore, the conventional calculation of CL_{R+S} is appropriate when only presystemic inversion is a factor. There is much evidence, however, to support the involvement of a systemic inversion process (Hall *et al.*, 1993). Assuming that both processes are involved, the following relationships represent the CL of the individual enantiomers after administration of racemate:

$$CL_R = \frac{\left(\frac{1}{2}\text{Dose}_{R+S}\right) \cdot \left(1 - f_{\text{inv}}^{\text{pre}}\right)}{\text{AUC}_R} \tag{4.6}$$

$$CL_S = \frac{\left(\frac{1}{2}\text{Dose}_{R+S}\right) \cdot \left(1 + f_{\text{inv}}^{\text{pre}} + f_{\text{inv}}^{\text{sys}}\right)}{AUC_S} \tag{4.7}$$

$$CL_{R+S} = \frac{\left(\frac{1}{2}\text{Dose}_{R+S}\right) \cdot \left[\left(1 - f_{\text{inv}}^{\text{pre}}\right) + \left(1 + f_{\text{inv}}^{\text{pre}} + f_{\text{inv}}^{\text{sys}}\right)\right]}{AUC_{R+S}} = \frac{\left(\frac{1}{2}\text{Dose}_{R+S}\right) \cdot \left(2 + f_{\text{inv}}^{\text{sys}}\right)}{AUC_{R+S}} \tag{4.8}$$

where $f_{\text{inv}}^{\text{sys}}$ indicates the fraction of the administered dose of R enantiomer inverted to S enantiomer via systemic processes. Thus, it is apparent that CL_{R+S} should include the portion of the dose attributed by the systemic inversion process, irrespective of the presence of presystemic inversion. In the presence of a systemic inversion process, the S enantiomer derived from chiral inversion is actually a product of systemic CL of the R enantiomer, a situation that is analogous to the case of enterohepatic recirculation. As such, an underestimation of the true CL_{R+S} occurs if the fraction of the dose of R enantiomer inverted by systemic clearance to S enantiomer is not taken into account. This is the case when the conventional calculation of CL_{R+S} (equation 4.1) is used in conjunction with non-stereospecific data.

Mechanism of chiral inversion

The mechanism behind the chiral inversion of ibuprofen has been studied intensely. Wechter *et al.* (1974) proposed that the inversion process was linked to enzymes involved in lipid metabolism, and required the substrates CoA and ATP for initiation. Since then, the biochemical requirements for enzymatic chiral inversion of ibuprofen have received considerable attention. In rat liver homogenates, the chiral inversion process requires the presence of ATP and CoA (Knihinicki *et al.*, 1989). Menzel *et al.* (1994) later showed that rat liver mitochondria require, as the first step of chiral inversion, the formation of an ibuprofenyl–adenylate complex. The formation of this intermediate was stereospecific for the R enantiomer; incubations with (*S*)-ibuprofen failed to show complex formation in the presence of cofactors. The authors concluded that CoA thioester formation was dependent on the prior formation of the adenylate intermediate, and that this reaction was specific for the R enantiomer (Figure 4.7).

Using deuterated (*R*)-ibuprofen, Chen *et al.* (1990) found that in male Wistar rats the inversion process was associated with loss of a deuterium atom in the α-methine position, but not in the trideuterated α-methyl positions. Sanins *et al.* (1991) also studied the pharmacokinetics of (*R*)-ibuprofen as unlabelled and labelled drug. Using GC-MS, the authors determined that as part of the inversion process, the α-methine (C-2) hydrogen atom of ibuprofen is lost, the phenyl hydrogen atoms are retained, and the presence of (*S*)- and (*R*)-ibuprofen proved that epimerization could be bidirectional. However, the absence of R enantiomer after administration of (*S*)-ibuprofen *in vivo* indicated the presence of a highly stereospecific step for the formation of ibuprofenyl-CoA.

CHAPTER 4

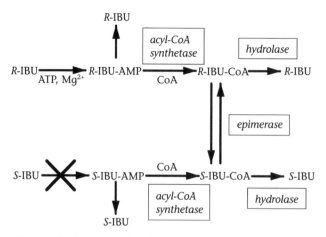

Figure 4.6: Biochemical mechanism of inversion process as proposed by Menzel *et al.* (1994).

Tracy and Hall (1991) have shown that ibuprofenyl-CoA is rapidly epimerized in the presence of homogenized rat liver. After only a 3-second incubation of thioester with liver homogentate, epimerization was apparent. It was also demonstrated that the use of indirect HPLC assays, in which alkali is used to hydrolyze the ibuprofenyl-CoA thioesters, caused inadvertent epimerization of ibuprofen (17%). The same group (Tracy and Hall, 1992; Tracy *et al.*, 1993) later created (*R*)- and (*S*)-ibuprofenyl-CoA thioesters and measured hydrolysis and epimerization rates. Whole liver was collected from rats and humans, and prepared whole liver homogenated, and separated microsomal, mitochondrial, and cytosolic fractions. Since epimerization of the ibuprofen-CoA thioesters was equal in both directions, and since *in vivo* the inversion process is unidirectional, these results indicated that formation of the thioester intermediate is the basis for stereoselectivity of ibuprofen.

When (*S*)-ibuprofen was incubated with rat liver homogenates, Tracy *et al.* (1993) found an absence of (*S*)-ibuprofenyl-CoA. This indicated stereoselectivity in synthetase activity. In the presence of the *S* enantiomer, (*R*)-ibuprofenyl-CoA formation was inhibited, but only at supraphysiological concentrations of *S* enantiomer. Medium and long-chain acyl-CoA synthetases were implicated in the CoA thioester formation process.

Knights and Jones (1992) found that both (*S*)- and (*R*)-ibuprofen could inhibit the formation of palmitoyl-CoA formation by rat liver microsomal long-chain fatty acid CoA ligase. The inhibition kinetics by (*R*)-ibuprofen were competitive in nature, with a k_i of 36 μmol/l. The k_i of inhibition by *S* enantiomer was 52 μmol/l, and the inhibition kinetics were of a mixed nature. Brugger *et al.* (1996) also examined the contribution of rat liver microsomal long-chain acyl-CoA synthetases to the formation of ibuprofenoyl-CoA synthetase. Both palmitic acid and (*S*)-ibuprofen were observed to have a profound effect on the formation of ibuprofenoyl-CoA formation. The k_m (inhibitory constant) for palmitic acid was much lower (13.5 μmol/l) than that of (S)-ibuprofen (405 μmol/l). Both inhibitions were competitive in nature. Using SDS gel electrophoresis, it was apparent that the enzyme responsible for the formation of both palmitic acid-CoA and (R)-ibuprofen-CoA thioesters had the identical molecular mass of 72 kDa. The results strongly suggested that the same enzyme was responsible for the formation of both products.

The effects of ibuprofen enantiomers on rat hepatocellular acyl-CoA levels and respiration and metabolism were studied by Knights and Drew (1992). After incubation of hepatocytes with (S)-ibuprofen, there were no changes observed in the hepatocellular concentrations of acyl-CoA. In contrast, (R)-ibuprofen caused a dose-dependent significant decrease in the concentrations of hepatocyte CoA levels. Both enantiomers caused increases in the hepatocyte lactate:pyruvate concentration ratio, and in the β-hydroxybutyrate:acetoacetate ratio. The increase in lactate:pyruvate concentrations was somewhat greater in the presence of (R)-ibuprofen. Changes were also observed in mitochondrial respiration and uncoupling of oxidative phosphorylation in the presence of either enantiomer, although the changes appeared more marked in the presence of the R enantiomer.

The ability of hepatoma cells from human and rat has been assessed (Menzel-Soglowek et al., 1992). Both cell types were found to cause chiral inversion of (R)-ibuprofen. Species specificity was noted, as the fraction of (R)-ibuprofen inverted was higher in the incubations involving rat hepatoma cells than human HEP G2 hepatoma cells. It was stated that the use of these hepatoma cells may provide a useful alternative to isolated rat liver perfusions and isolated hepatocytes owing to their simplicity of use.

Although much of this work has implied the unidirectional nature of chiral inversion, the observation of chiral inversion of (S)-ibuprofen to antipode in some species underscores the species-dependent nature or kinetics of this metabolic pathway (Chen et al., 1991).

Anatomical site of chiral inversion

The anatomic location of the enzymes responsible for the unidirectional chiral inversion of the R to the S enantiomer has been the focal point of debate among some pharmaceutical scientists. This is an important issue because it has implications from the perspective of both therapeutic and pharmacokinetic bioequivalence of oral formulations. This possibility was first raised by Jamali et al. (1988b) after studying the relative bioavailability of ibuprofen enantiomers from two 600 mg formulations. The mean t_{max} of total (R+S)-ibuprofen was significantly different between the two products, suggesting a difference in rate of absorption. Following administration of the product with the higher t_{max}, the S:R ratio of AUC was significantly greater than the corresponding less rapidly absorbed product. A plateau in the S:R ratio of ibuprofen enantiomers was observed 6–8 h after administration of the doses. The authors suggested the involvement of a presystemic inversion process, likely of

CHAPTER 4

gastrointestinal origin. Therefore, the ibuprofen content in less rapidly absorbed formulation would be exposed to the inverting enzymes for a longer period of time, which could, in turn, explain the higher AUC of (S)-ibuprofen after its administration.

By use of simulations, Mehvar and Jamali (1988) later hypothesized that a systemic inversion process should cause a continuous progression of the $S:R$ ratio with the passing of time. A plateau in the relationship, as seen in the study of Jamali *et al.* (1988b), would therefore suggest the presence of a single presystemic, extrahepatic inversion process. It was also predicted that there should be a difference in the half-lives of the enantiomers if systemic processes were responsible for the inversion, and in the paper by Jamali *et al.* (1988b) there were no significant differences noted between the enantiomers in $t_{1/2}$, further supporting the possible involvement of a presystemic process for the inversion of ibuprofen. In fact, many of the available pharmacokinetic studies have indicated a similarity in the elimination rate contants between the enantiomers of ibuprofen. Half-life, however, is not only a function of inversion processes, and is influenced by both distribution and clearance via other metabolic processes, which could account for this observation.

Hall *et al.* (1993) published a study, the results of which were claimed to exclude the possibility of presystemic gastrointestinal inversion. Ten healthy subjects were administered intravenous or oral doses of 400 mg racemic ibuprofen. The authors infused ibuprofen intravenously over a period of 1 h. They also attempted to determine the fractional CL of the R enantiomer attributable to inversion by two methods. These included the co-administration and calculation of CL of deuterated (S)-ibuprofen enantiomer from serum, in addition to stereospecific measurement of urinary recovery of intact drug and metabolite. The assumptions influencing these calculations were that the metabolites themselves did not undergo inversion, and the absence of an isotope effect on the pharmacokinetics of labelled (S)-ibuprofen. The authors found no significant differences between the AUC of (S)- or (R)-ibuprofen between the intravenous and oral routes of administration (Table 4.2; Figure 4.7), and their two independent calculations of CL of (R)-ibuprofen by inversion were nearly identical. The absolute bioavailabilities of (R)- and total (R+S)-ibuprofen were nearly complete after oral administration. The authors presented values indicating that over 50% of the CL of the R enantiomer was attributable to the inversion process. Although it did not reach statistical significance, the mean S to mean R ratio of AUC was higher after oral (1.12) than that following i.v. (1.06) administration. The presence of inversion after intravenous administration proved the involvement of a systemic process in chiral inversion of ibuprofen.

A prerequisite for significant chiral inversion in the gastrointestinal tract would be sufficiently long gastrointestinal residence time for the process to occur (i.e. a long t_{max}). Rate of absorption is a critical consideration in a study intended to establish the presence or absence of a presystemic chiral inversion process (Mehvar and Jamali, 1988). In fact, Hall *et al.* (1993) utilized a relatively rapidly absorbed formulation (mean $t_{max} = 1.5$ h),

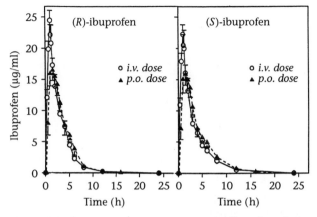

Figure 4.7: Plasma concentration vs time profiles after administration of oral and intravenous doses of 400 mg racemate. (From Hall *et al.* (1993), with permission.)

with a correspondingly short gastrointestinal residence time. This would consequently minimize the contribution of presystemic inversion in the gastrointestinal tract. Based on the results of the intravenous dose utilized in this study, there is no doubt that a systemic process is involved in the inversion process of (*R*)- to (*S*)-ibuprofen. However, based on the study design used, the possibility of presystemic inversion by the intestinal tract cannot be ruled out.

Other studies have also attempted to study presystemic inversion of ibuprofen. For example, Smith *et al.* (1994) mentioned that as the percentage of (*R*)-ibuprofen in the dosage form increased, the $t_{1/2}$ of the *S* enantiomer similarly increased, thus ruling out the possibility of presystemic inversion. The authors, however, utilized a solution dosage form in this study, with a short t_{max} and correspondingly low gastrointestinal residence time. Other authors have also concluded the lack of a presystemic inversion process for ibuprofen (Cheng *et al.*, 1994), at the same time utilizing a rapidly absorbed formulation in the study design.

Jamali *et al.* (1992) published an additional study that sought to examine the influence of absorption rate on the amount of ibuprofen inverted. The authors also performed an *in vitro* experiment to establish the presence of inversion activity in human intestinal tissue. Using a randomized crossover design, the authors administered matching 600 mg doses of racemate as tablet and solution formulation to six healthy volunteers. As expected, absorption after administration of the solution doses was rapid, t_{max} being attained in less than 15 min. In contrast, for the 600 mg tablet formulation, the mean t_{max} was 2.2 h. The *S:R* ratio of AUC was significantly higher after tablet (1.35) than after 600 mg as solution (1.16). This observation was in line with the previous study of Jamali *et al.* (1988b), and with the concept of presystemic inversion by the gastrointestinal tract. An additional experiment was conducted, in which segments of ileal and colonic tissues

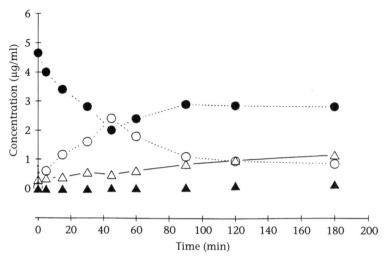

Figure 4.8: *In vitro* inversion of (*R*)-ibuprofen after incubation with human colon tissue. Key: triangles, (*S*)-ibuprofen; circles, (*R*)-ibuprofen; open symbols, unchanged enantiomer; filled symbols, conjugated enantiomer. (From Jamali *et al.*, 1992, with permission.)

resected from cancer patients were exposed to (*R*)-ibuprofen *in vitro*. Within 3 h between 20% and 33% of the *R* enantiomer was found to invert to (*S*)-ibuprofen; in the absence of gut tissue, no such inversion was observed (Figure 4.8). This provided definitive proof of the ability of the gastrointestinal tract to facilitate chiral inversion. From this study it was concluded that inversion of ibuprofen occurred both systemically, presumably by the liver, and presystemically by intestinal tissue. Sattari and Jamali (1994) and Berry and Jamali (1991) obtained similar results using rat intestine for (*R*)-ibuprofen and (*R*)-fenoprofen, respectively.

Jeffrey *et al.* (1991) used perfused tissue preparations to examine the extent of inversion of (*R*)-ibuprofen by rat liver and intestinal tissues. The dose was administered either via vascular perfusate into gut (duodenum/jejunum, jejunum, or ileum) and liver tissue, or via the gut lumen. There was no evidence of inversion by the rat intestinal preparations when (*R*)-ibuprofen was administered via the gut lumen. In this study a rapidly absorbed solution was placed into the gut lumen, with t_{max} being achieved by 10–20 min in duodenal and jejunal tissues, and 20–30 min in ileal tissue. As stated above, this would considerably minimize the contribution of the process of presystemic intestinal inversion.

One study has been published in which two tablet formulations with markedly different absorption rates have been studied. Using a crossover design, Cox *et al.* (1998) determined the pharmacokinetics and relative bioequivalence of ibuprofen enantiomers in 11 subjects after administration of a single dose of two formulations (generic, Apotex, Canada and Motrin, Upjohn, Canada) containing 400 mg of ibuprofen. The formulations possessed noticeable differences in their plasma profiles, with both ibuprofen enantiomers from

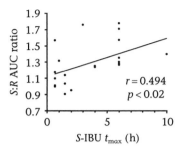

Figure 4.9: Relationship between $S{:}R$ AUC ratio and t_{max}. (Plotted from data of Cox *et al.* (1988).)

the Motrin tablet being absorbed more rapidly than from the generic form. There were no significant differences in the extent of absorption of the S enantiomer from the dosage forms, although the systemic availability of the R enantiomer was significantly less from the less rapidly absorbed generic formulation.

Although the primary objective of this study (Cox *et al.*, 1988) was to compare the bioavailability of the two administered formulations using a stereospecific assay, we have retrospectively noted additional observations from the raw data. A weak but statistically significant linear relationship was present between the $S{:}R$ AUC ratio and t_{max} of the S enantiomer (Figure 4.9). Although the $S{:}R$ ratios of AUC were not significantly different between the formulations using Student's t-test for paired samples, in 8 of the 11 subjects the $S{:}R$ ratio was higher for the more slowly absorbed formulation. For the more slowly absorbed formulation it was also of note that the t_{max} of the S enantiomer was longer than that of the R enantiomer in 7 of the 11 subjects, and in no subject was the S enantiomer t_{max} shorter than that of the R enantiomer. The difference in t_{max} between enantiomers in that formulation was statistically significant ($p < 0.05$). In contrast, for the rapidly absorbed formulation, the t_{max} of the S enantiomer was longer than that of the R enantiomer in only two of the subjects, and the difference did not attain statistical significance. The $S{:}R$ ratios of t_{max} were 1.09 and 1.38, and of C_{max} were 0.96 and 1.21 for the rapidly and slowly released formulations of ibuprofen, respectively. These differences can be explained by a presystemic gastrointestinal inversion process. The ratios may be nearer unity for the rapidly absorbed formulation because insufficient time may have been permitted for the presystemic process to occur. Hepatic first pass effect would not be expected to be a relevant factor in this observation, because ibuprofen is a slowly cleared drug (plasma CL < 5% of hepatic blood flow).

Using simulations (Figure 4.10) with SAAMII (SAAM Institute, Redmond, WA, USA) we have examined the influence of rate of absorption on the relative t_{max} of ibuprofen enantiomers in the presence and absence of presystemic inversion, using rate constants generated by Hall *et al.* (1993) for inversion and noninversion processes (Figure 4.10). A range of k_a values was used for the purposes of the simulations. For each simulation using a different k_a value, the value of k_a was kept the same for each enantiomer. If only systemic

CHAPTER 4

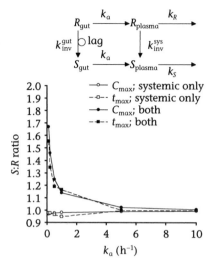

Figure 4.10: Simulation to illustrate the influence of k_a on the $S:R$ ratios of C_{max} and t_{max}. The absorption rate constant was varied, and the values of k_R and k_S were set to 0.08 and 0.354 h^{-1}, respectively as reported by Hall et al. (1992). The k_{inv}^{sys} (systemic inversion rate constant) and k_{inv}^{gut} (presystemic inversion) were set to 0.13 h^{-1}; in the case of systemic inversion only, k_{inv}^{gut} was set to a value of zero.

inversion occurs, the t_{max} would be virtually the same for each enantiomer irrespective of the k_a value. In contrast, in the presence of presystemic inversion, as the absorption rate (k_a) declines, considerable differences begin to appear between the enantiomers in C_{max} and t_{max}. This is in agreement with the data of Cox *et al.*, in which the absorption rate of the slowly released product was less than in any other published stereoselective pharmacokinetic study of ibuprofen enantiomers.

Chen *et al.* (1991) studied epimerization of (R)- and (S)-ibuprofenyl-CoA in various rat tissue homogenates. Both enantiomer-CoA thioesters were observed to undergo epimerization in a variety of subcellular tissue preparations, although the rate of inversion was greatest in rat liver and kidney homogenates. Epimerization activity was also observed in intestine, muscle, lung, and heart tissues, although at a much lower rate of catalysis.

Using three different formulations of ibuprofen with a range of absorption rates, Sattari and Jamali (1994) studied the chiral inversion of ibuprofen in the Sprague–Dawley rat. The $S:R$ ratio of AUC was significantly increased with the more slowly released formulation ($S:R = 7.3$) compared to the rapidly released formulations ($S:R \cong 3.5$). The t_{max} of the slowly absorbed formulation was 2.3 h compared to < 1 h for the rapidly absorbed formulations. Using everted rat gut preparations, inversion of ibuprofen was observed to occur in intestinal tissue. The inversion was greatest in ileal and jejunal tissues.

Reichel *et al.* (1995) developed antibodies to rat liver (R)-ibuprofenyl-CoA epimerase in rabbits, which in turn were used to obtain purified epimerase enzyme. Using these techniques, a protein of molecular mass 42 kDa was identified as being the epimerase enzyme. Using Western blotting techniques the tissue localization of (R)-ibuprofenyl-CoA epimerase was determined. Concentrations of the enzyme were highest in rat liver, kidney, heart, lung and ileal tissue. Using incubation experiments of (R)-ibuprofen in homogenized rat tissues, preformed (R)-ibuprofenyl-CoA thioesters were significantly inverted to (S)-ibuprofen in liver, kidney, ileum, and heart tissues. (R)-Ibuprofen was only significantly inverted to S enantiomer in the presence of liver tissue, however. In guinea-pigs the data were similar to those in the rat, with the exception that both homogenized liver and kidney tissues were capable of significantly inverting (R)-ibuprofen to antipode.

Hall *et al.* (1992) studied the chiral inversion of ibuprofen in isolated perfused rabbit lung preparations in the presence and absence of bovine serum albumin. It was found that, in the absence of protein binding, lung tissue can facilitate the chiral inversion of ibuprofen and fenoprofen. When bovine serum albumin was added to the perfusate, there was no detectable inversion of R to S enantiomer for either ibuprofen or fenoprofen. Hence, although inversion by lung tissue was possible, *in vivo* the contribution of the pulmonary route to the overall inversion process would be minimal. The authors commented on the possible corollary between these results and those involving intestinal gut preparations (e.g. Berry and Jamali, 1991; Jamali *et al.*, 1992; Sattari and Jamali, 1994) in which inversion was observed in those tissues. The implication would be that, since plasma proteins were not added to the intestinal preparations, the results may be valid from the standpoint of physiological relevance. However, these were not perfusion studies, so the need for plasma proteins in intestinal incubation medium would be questionable. Furthermore, in a study of fenoprofen inversion by everted gut preparations, inversion was much greater on the mucosal side of the membrane (Berry and Jamali, 1991). This suggests that the bulk of presystemic inversion of NSAID by intestinal tissue occurs prior to drug transfer into the splanchnic blood flow. Consequently, plasma protein binding may not be a critical factor in determining the extent of presystemic intestinal inversion.

We believe that the available evidence is in support of a presystemic process as a component of chiral inversion of ibuprofen. This has more recently been reconfirmed in both rats (Adeyeye and Chen, 1997) and humans (Aiba *et al.*, 1997). The relative importance of the presystemic inversion to the overall chiral inversion of ibuprofen and other NSAIDs has not been quantified in a systematic manner. However, it would be anticipated that the longer the t_{max} of the administered formulation, the greater would be the contribution of presystemic inversion to the total amount of inversion. Study designs that utilize rapidly absorbed dosage forms do little towards clarifying the issue. From the perspective of clinical usage of ibuprofen, most preparations exhibit rapid absorption under fasting conditions, and consequently presystemic inversion by the intestine should not significantly impact on the overall amount of inversion in the majority of patients. This is borne out

CHAPTER 4

by the lack of evidence of significant presystemic intestinal inversion in numerous studies in which rapidly absorbed formulations were studied. There may be certain clinical conditions, however, associated with reduced rates of intestinal motility and transit, in which presystemic intestinal inversion could conceivably become significant. These include pregnancy, co-administration of drugs such as anticholinergics or narcotic analgesics, and pathophysiological states, each associated with reduced gastrointestinal motility.

Hepatocellular site of inversion

Knihinicki *et al.* (1991) synthesized both *S*- and *R*-CoA thioesters, then incubated them in the presence of whole rat liver homogenate, or with rat liver fractions containing either mitochondria or microsomal proteins. In each of the homogenates and fractions studied, there was evidence of bidirectional epimerization of the preformed ibuprofen-CoA thioesters. Differences were observed in the localization of racemase and hydrolases in the subcellular fractions studied. The degree of racemization and hydrolysis of the (*S*)- and (*R*)-ibuprofen-CoA thioesters seemed to be equal in the mitochondrial and microsomal fractions. In the microsomal fraction, however, racemization appeared to be less than that in the mitochondrial fraction. In comparison, the rate of hydrolysis of the *S*-CoA thioester appeared to be less than that of its antipode in the microsomal fraction.

Tracy and Hall (1992) have demonstrated that inversion of (*R*)-ibuprofen was fastest in mitochondria, followed by microsomal and then cytosolic fractions. In the cytosolic fraction, inversion activity exceeded that of hydrolytic activity.

4.5 INTERSPECIES DIFFERENCES IN PHARMACOKINETICS OF (*R*)- AND (*S*)-IBUPROFEN

As is the case for most drugs, interspecies differences in ibuprofen pharmacokinetics and metabolism have been reported. In most species the metabolites of ibuprofen formed are similar, and include hydroxyibuprofen and carboxyibuprofen. Chiral inversion of ibuprofen occurs in many species, and with the exception of one study (Chen *et al.*, 1991), the inversion process has mostly been observed to occur in a unidirectional manner from the *R* to the *S* enantiomer.

Interspecies differences are present in the plasma protein binding of ibuprofen. At clinically relevant plasma concentrations, the bound fraction of (*R+S*)-ibuprofen *in vitro* is 95% in baboon, 96% in Sprague–Dawley rat, and over 99% in human and dog plasma (Mills *et al.*, 1973). In male Wistar rats the V_{dss} values of the *R* and *S* enantiomers are 0.57 and 0.96 l/kg, respectively (Knihinicki *et al.*, 1990), and are higher than those reported in humans (Table 4.2). In dogs the V_{dss} is approximately 0.14 and 0.18 l/kg, respectively, for the *R* and *S* enantiomers (Beck *et al.*, 1991), and is similar to human values. These V_{dss}

findings in rat and dog are in line with the plasma protein binding results of Mills *et al.* (1973).

Tracy *et al.* (1993) performed incubations with ibuprofen and whole liver homogenates, and showed that the formation of ibuprofenyl-CoA thioesters was 4-fold more efficient in the rat than human. However, overall the extent of inversion appears to be similar between the two species. The amount of inversion in the rat may be compensated by a faster rate of non-inversion metabolic processes (e.g. oxidation and glucuroconjugation). Rat microsomal protein had double the V_{max}/k_m of mitochondrial protein, which was in accordance with the known hepatocellular distribution of the synthetase enzyme. No synthetase activity was present in cytosolic fractions of rat.

In rabbits (Williams *et al.*, 1991), it was found that as the ibuprofen dose was increased, the arterial CL of both enantiomers declined significantly (24% for (*S*)-ibuprofen, and 28% for (*R*)-ibuprofen). This was similar to other findings in rats, in which saturation of metabolism to hydroxy- and carboxymetabolites of ibuprofen was reported (Shah and Jung, 1987). This was unlike the situation in humans, in which saturable plasma protein binding leads to a dose-related increase in plasma CL of total bound + unbound drug. In rabbits the fraction of the dose of (*R*)-ibuprofen inverted to *S* enantiomer was 0.30–0.33, which is less than that observed in humans.

Chen *et al.* (1991) studied inversion of ibuprofen in Wistar rats, Hartley guinea-pigs, Dutch male rabbits and healthy human volunteers. Single blood samples were obtained from each animal, and the stereochemical composition of ibuprofen and hydroxylated metabolite in the samples was determined. Differences were noted between species in the *R:S* ratios, although the times used for sampling differed between animals. It was of note that after administration of *S* enantiomer, there were significant levels of *R* enantiomer detected in the plasma of guinea-pigs. In rats and rabbits, there were also noticeable, although lesser, amounts of *R* enantiomer in plasma. These findings suggest that the inversion process may be bidirectional in some species or strains of rats, rabbits and guinea-pigs, but not in others.

Ahn *et al.* (1991a) reported that the pharmacokinetics of ibuprofen were stereoselective in beagle dogs. The fractional chiral inversion of (*R*)-ibuprofen was 0.73, a value similar to that reported for humans. Significant inversion was likewise observed in bile duct-cannulated dogs after administration of i.v. or intraduodenal dosing of (*R*)- and (*S*)-ibuprofen (Beck *et al.*, 1991). No evidence of chiral inversion by the gastrointestinal tract was present in this study; the fraction of drug inverted was 72% and 70% for the i.v. and i.d. routes, respectively, which is in accordance with human values. A solution dosage form with rapid absorption was utilized, and this was recognized by the authors as perhaps having minimized the degree of presystemic intestinal inversion. In the dog, almost all of the urinary and biliary recovery of enantiomer was as the *S*-configuration (Beck *et al.*, 1991).

CHAPTER 4

Unlike another 2-APA NSAID, flurbiprofen (Berry and Jamali, 1989), there is no pharmacokinetic interaction at the level of plasma protein binding between ibuprofen enantiomers when given together to male Wistar rats (Knihinicki *et al.*, 1990). The fraction of (*R*)-ibuprofen inverted in the Wistar rat was estimated to be between 0.5 and 0.7, similar to human values.

Hutt *et al.* (1993) have provided evidence suggesting stereoselective metabolism of racemic ibuprofen to hydroxyibuprofen by the microbial species *Verticillium lecanii*. It could not be determined from the study whether chiral inversion of ibuprofen had occurred, as pure *R* enantiomer was not used in the experiments.

4.6   EXCRETION OF IBUPROFEN

The urinary excretion of unchanged ibuprofen is negligible; the primary route of elimination of ibuprofen is mediated via oxidative drug metabolism (Mills *et al.*, 1973). In most studies, urinary recovery of ibuprofen-related material is over 80% (Evans *et al.*, 1990; Hall *et al.*, 1993). Acyl-glucuronidated ibuprofen accounts for approximately 10–13% of the urinary excretion of ibuprofen metabolite. Hydroxyibuprofen and carboxyibuprofen account for approximately 25% and 45% of the total urinary excretion of ibuprofen-related material, respectively (Lee *et al.*, 1985; Evans *et al.*, 1990).

The biliary elimination of ibuprofen after administration of a single 600 mg dose has been studied in three patients (2F; 1M) with cholangiodrainage from the common bile duct (Schneider *et al.*, 1990). Bile constituted a minor pathway of elimination of ibuprofen and its major metabolites. Less than 2% of the dose was recovered in the bile as the sum of parent drug, glucuronide and phase I metabolite species. In contrast, an average of 50% of the total administered dose was recovered in urine from the same patients over the same time period.

To gain insight regarding the renal excretion of ibuprofen enantiomers, Ahn *et al.* (1991b) studied the excretion of ibuprofen enantiomers in the isolated perfused rat kidney. After surgical implantation of catheters in the ureter and the artery of the right kidney, the organ was excised and placed in a recirculating perfusion apparatus. Bolus doses of individual ibuprofen enantiomer were introduced into the recirculating perfusate to permit initial concentrations of 10 µg/ml or 100 µg/ml (*n* = 4 per dose). An increase was found in the perfusate flow after ibuprofen at both dose levels. Although the plasma unbound fraction of (*S*)-ibuprofen was 10–17% greater than that of the *R* enantiomer, the renal clearance of conjugated *R* enantiomer was over 2-fold greater than that of the *S* enantiomer. When corrected for unbound fraction and glomerular filtration rate, the extraction ratio of (*R*)-ibuprofen was 3.9-fold higher than that of the *S* enantiomer. This indicated that the kidneys possessed glucuroconjugative activity. There was no evidence for chiral inversion by the isolated perfused rat kidneys.

4.7 RELATIONSHIP BETWEEN EFFECT AND PLASMA CONCENTRATIONS

4.7.1 Therapeutic effects

Owing to the nature of rheumatoid arthritis, it is difficult to obtain a precise relationship between plasma concentrations and efficacy because of the somewhat subjective nature of the major symptoms of the disease. There are, however, scoring methods available to rate symptoms such as pain, stiffness and general sense of well-being, which are of use in establishing a relationship between pharmacokinetics and pharmacodynamics. In one placebo-controlled trial (Grennan *et al.*, 1983), the effects of increasing doses of ibuprofen (placebo, 200 mg, 400 mg, or 600 mg q.i.d) were studied in 21 patients with established rheumatoid arthritis (age 20–65 years). The authors recorded assessments of articular index, pain index, pain score, and thermographic index. For pharmacokinetic analysis, nonstereospecific methods were used. Evidence was present for a saturation of plasma protein binding, on the basis of increased unbound fraction with increasing dose, and a plateau in the AUC vs dose relationship. A plateau also appeared to be present in the pharmacodynamic measurements, as there were no significant improvements in articular index, pain index, or pain score between the doses of 1600 mg to 2400 mg. Saturation of tissue receptors at doses greater than 1600 mg was suggested. Although the possible confounding influence of chiral inversion was not discernible owing to the assay method used, it was suggested that pharmacodynamic variability exceeds the variability in the pharmacokinetics of (R+S)-ibuprofen, and that doses of greater than 1600 mg might not be of much clinical utility in most patients.

In a double-blinded study, Bradley *et al.* (1992) examined the relationship between serum concentrations of (S)-ibuprofen and clinical response after repeated administration of 300 or 600 mg of the racemate q.i.d. There was no relationship apparent between the trough serum concentrations and pain score in the study patients. Relationships were, however, present between S enantiomer serum trough concentrations and AUC, and efficacy as measured by disability health assessment questionnaire and physician global assessment. A placebo control group was not included in the study. The authors suggested that trough serum concentrations of the (bound + unbound) S enantiomer provides a suitable endpoint for measurement of an ibuprofen concentration vs effect relationship.

Surgery to remove the third molar tooth has been accepted as a standard test for assessing analgesia. Using this model, there appears to be a positive relationship between plasma concentration and analgesic activity of ibuprofen (Laska *et al.*, 1986). Attainment of an ibuprofen (S+R) concentration range of 11–30 μg/ml 1 h post-dose was needed for complete pain relief in 50% of patients. In a recent study, Suri *et al.* (1997) administered ibuprofen and flurbiprofen to healthy volunteers. Dental pain was invoked by applying electric current to a healthy front tooth of each subject. Pain measurement was ranked using two methods, either by each subject's classification using a subjective measurement scale, or by tooth pulp evoked potentials. The pain measurement data was then linked to the plasma S enantiomer concentration data by use of a one-compartment model with an effect compartment incorporated into the equation. The estimated concentrations in the effect compartment were then used in the E_{max} model to determine EC_{50} and k_{e0} values. For both drugs, the time of maximal pain relief lagged behind that of plasma t_{max} values. The EC_{50} and k_{e0} for ibuprofen differed noticeably between the two methods used for pain assessment. Using the evoked potential method, the EC_{50} was almost 3-fold lower (8.7 mg/l) than that of the pain rating method (24.4 mg/l). A similar magnitude of difference was observed for k_{e0}. The use of the effect compartment in the model seemed to diminish the hysteresis present in the concentration vs effect relationship, compared to the use of plasma concentration data.

4.7.2 Toxic effects

In an attempt to determine the influence of predisintegration of ibuprofen tablets on gastrointestinal (GI) side-effects, 30 healthy volunteers were given, in a parallel design, 800 mg ibuprofen t.i.d ($n = 10$/group) as intact tablet, predisintegrated tablet in water, or as predisintegrated tablet in orange juice (Friedman et al., 1990). There were no significant differences in indices of absorption (t_{max} and C_{max}) between the three groups, although the extent of absorption measured by AUC was significantly lower for the ibuprofen in orange juice group. From the vantage point of side-effects and endoscopic findings, predisintegration caused more adverse GI effects than whole tablet. It was suggested that there may be an inverse relationship between absorption rate and mucosal damage, and that the damage elicited from the predisintegrated formulations was of local origin, rather than the systemic prostaglandin synthesis inhibition widely believed to be the most important causative factor in the generation of mucosal damage.

The relationship between the plasma concentrations of (S)-ibuprofen and its antiplatelet response was studied in four healthy subjects after single doses of 200, 400, 800 and 1200 mg of ibuprofen (Evans et al., 1991). The inhibition of thromboxane B_2 (TxB_2) production by ibuprofen concentration data were fitted to the sigmoid E_{max} model, and unbound plasma concentrations of (S)-ibuprofen were used to assess the relationship (Figure 4.11). By exposing whole blood to the enantiomers of ibuprofen and racemate, it was established that the R enantiomer was devoid of TxB_2 inhibitory activity over the concentration range 0.5–10 mg/l. Serum TxB_2 concentrations fell in a manner inversely related to the rise in plasma ibuprofen concentrations. The inhibitory effect became more pronounced with an increase in dose. The unbound plasma concentration data fit well to the TxB_2 inhibitory data using the sigmoid E_{max} model. Increasing the dose of ibuprofen resulted in more prolonged inhibition of TxB_2 production.

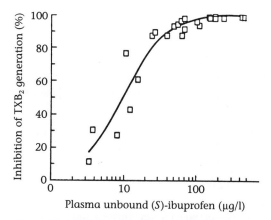

Figure 4.11: Relationship between thromboxane B_2 generation and unbound (S)-ibuprofen plasma concentrations. Solid line represents predicted relationship based on sigmoidal E_{max} model. (From Evans *et al.* (1991), with permission.)

4.8   PHARMACOKINETICS IN SPECIAL POPULATIONS

Febrile children and infants

Ibuprofen is available in liquid dosage formulations for administration to paediatric patients requiring analgesia and antipyresis. Several studies have thus examined the pharmacokinetics of ibuprofen in paediatric patients. In one study, the pharmacokinetics of racemic ibuprofen were studied in 17 febrile children aged 3.1 to 9.6 years (Nahata *et al.*, 1991). Doses of 5 or 10 mg/kg of liquid formulation were administered, and a nonstereospecific assay method was used to measure serum drug concentrations. Between the two doses, the C_{max} was approximately dose proportional (28.4 vs 43.6 mg/l at 5 or 10 mg/kg, respectively), and there were no significant differences in t_{max}, CL or $t_{1/2}$. The t_{max} was attained in 1.2 h, oral CL was ~1.3 ml/min/kg, and $t_{1/2}$ was 1.6 h. Brown *et al.* (1992) also studied two strengths of ibuprofen in febrile children, and the AUC of (R+S)-ibuprofen was similarly approximately dose proportional between 5 and 10 mg/kg. The CL/F and V_d/f of (R+S)-ibuprofen were higher in children < 2.5 years of age than in those > 2.5 years.

The pharmacokinetics of ibuprofen enantiomers were studied in 18 febrile children (Kelley *et al.*, 1992). In these patients, mean CL/F and V_d/F were 1.24 ml/min/kg and 0.16 l/kg, respectively, for (R)-ibuprofen. Although CL/F and V_d/F values of 1.24 ml/min/kg and 0.248 l/kg, respectively, were given for the S enantiomer, their derivation was based on fraction inverted data derived from adult volunteers (0.6), which may or may not be valid. The authors calculated a larger value of V_d for the S enantiomer, which may indicate that, as in adults, the unbound fraction of (S)-ibuprofen in plasma is greater than its antipode. The authors noted counterclockwise hysteresis curves when the mean temperature

CHAPTER 4

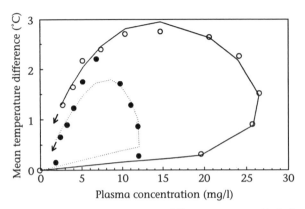

Figure 4.12: Mean temperature difference vs mean (*S+R*)-ibuprofen (open symbols) and acetaminophen plasma concentrations. (From Kelley *et al.* (1992), with permission.)

difference before and after the ibuprofen dose was plotted vs the plasma concentration of both enantiomers and total ibuprofen (Figure 4.12). It is known that a lag-time is present for the attainment of maximal CSF levels and perhaps in the brain (Bannwarth *et al.*, 1995), which could be responsible for the hysteresis observed here.

The single dose pharmacokinetics of ibuprofen (8 mg/kg) were studied in 38 febrile children ranging in age from 0.25 to 10.4 years (Kauffman and Nelson, 1992). The results from pharmacokinetic analysis were used to examine the pharmacokinetic-antipyretic relationship. The authors observed a 1–3 h lag time between peak plasma concentrations of ibuprofen and maximal temperature decrease. There were no discernible relationship between the age of the patients and the pharmacokinetics of ibuprofen. Older children (≥ 6 years) had a significantly lower response and onset of response than infants (≤ 1 year). There was no mention of the children aged 1 to 6 years of age. The authors suggested, as a possible cause of the greater efficacy of ibuprofen in infants, the greater surface area:body weight ratio in infants relative to older children, which in turn might improve heat dissipation and antipyretic response to ibuprofen. Another possible cause mentioned was a greater *R* to *S* inversion of ibuprofen in infants relative to older children. Other possibilities not mentioned were a reduced CL of the *S* enantiomer by non-inversion processes in infants relative to older children, and perhaps greater penetration or binding of ibuprofen in the CNS, where the hypothalamic thermoregulatory system is located, in infants. Given the findings of Chen and Chen (1995) in Taiwanese patients, it is of note that in this study most (89.8%) of the children enrolled were black.

Postoperative paediatric patients

The pharmacokinetics of ibuprofen were studied in 11 infants (6–18 months of age; 7 M and 4 F) given ibuprofen for postoperative analgesia (Rey *et al.*, 1994). The patients were given a mean dose of 7.6 mg/kg as syrup. The CL/F and V_d/F of $(R+S)$-ibuprofen were reported to be 0.11 l/h/kg and 0.2 l/kg, respectively, and were similar to those values reported in adults (Table 4.2). Interestingly, the plasma concentrations of the R enantiomer exceeded those of the S enantiomer in these infants. Possible reasons included a higher $S:R$ CL ratio in these patients as compared to adults, or diminished R to S enantiomer inversion. The authors suggested the possible need for a higher dosage in this population owing to the relatively low plasma concentrations of the active S enantiomer relative to the R enantiomer.

Juvenile arthritis

Makela *et al.* (1981) have studied the nonstereoselective pharmacokinetics of ibuprofen in 33 patients (mean age 11 years; 18 girls, 15 boys) with juvenile rheumatoid arthritis. The patients received a mean dose of 12.4 mg/kg t.i.d. The formulation administered was not specified. Analysis of post dose, serial serum samples indicated that t_{max} occurred between 1 and 2 h post dose. Mean C_{max} was 31 mg/l, and in 12 subjects mean $t_{1/2}$ was 2.3 h. In synovial fluid samples obtained from the same patients, t_{max} was reached in 5–6 h, and peak concentrations were 13 mg/l. The synovial fluid concentrations 12 h after dosing were higher than those in corresponding serum samples. It was concluded that a dose of approximately 40 mg/l provides sufficiently high levels of ibuprofen in the synovial fluid of patients with juvenile rheumatoid arthritis for therapeutic effect to occur.

Children with cystic fibrosis

Ibuprofen has been evaluated for its anti-inflammatory properties in order to reduce the inflammatory response associated with *Pseudomonas* pulmonary infections in children with cystic fibrosis. In a pharmacokinetic study (Konstan *et al.*, 1991), 19 patients with CF and 4 healthy subjects were enrolled who ranged in age from 6 to 12 years. When daily doses of 300, 400, or 600 mg were administered for 1 month to four children with CF in a randomized crossover sequence, the AUC appeared to rise in accordance with the increase in dose. The $t_{1/2}$ was approximately 90 min at each dose level, and $V_d$area of $(R+S)$-ibuprofen was approximately 0.2–0.3 l/kg. Compared to 4 healthy children, the patients with CF appeared to attain much lower plasma concentrations of ibuprofen, as assessed using C_{max} (27.3% less) and AUC (46.0% less). The mean t_{max} was approximately the same for both patients with CF and healthy subjects. The calculated $V_d$area$/F$ was ~50% higher in patients with CF than healthy children. Possible causes of the altered pharmacokinetics of ibuprofen in the presence of CF include an increase in unbound fraction in plasma, a decrease in bioavailability, or an increase in intrinsic metabolic CL.

■ CHAPTER 4 ■

Elderly adults

In a dose-proportionality assessment involving 17 healthy elderly subjects (mean age 70 years), over the dose range of single doses of 400 mg to 1200 mg ibuprofen, there was an increase in $(R+S)$-ibuprofen CL/F of approximately 50% (Albert *et al.*, 1984). There was also an increase in CL/F of unbound drug, although it was much less marked than for total unbound + bound drug (16.9%). The V_d/F also increased for total but not for unbound drug with an increase in dose, suggesting a saturation of plasma protein binding with increasing dose, and a subsequent increase in CL and V_d of total drug. The results were similar to those observed in young healthy volunteers.

Kendall *et al.* (1990) studied 58 patients with arthritis entered in a study to determine the pharmacokinetics of a $(R+S)$-ibuprofen after administration of a sustained release dosage form. There were two groups of subjects, an elderly group (mean 71 years) and a young group (mean 49 years). Patients were given two 800 mg sustained release tablets. There was no difference between the two age groups in extent of absorption. Indices of rate of absorption were not summarized or reported. However, at steady-state, plasma concentration vs time profiles were similar, and there appeared to be somewhat higher mean C_{max} in the elderly patients. Mean t_{max} appeared to occur at 6 h post dose in both age groups.

In general, it would appear that ageing by itself does not cause significant changes in the pharmacokinetics of ibuprofen and its enantiomers.

Rheumatic disease

In general, arthritis per se does not appear to influence the pharmacokinetics of ibuprofen (Table 4.2). Geisslinger *et al.* (1993) undertook a study to compare variability in the disposition of (S)-ibuprofen following administration as the individual S-enantiomer (400 mg) and as the racemate (600 mg $R+S$) to patients with rheumatoid arthritis. There were no significant differences between the S enantiomer (400 mg) when given alone as compared to racemate (300 mg). AUC was higher for S than R when given as racemate, although there were no significant differences between the enantiomers in their $t_{1/2}$. The authors suggested, since variability in the pharmacokinetics of the S enantiomer were not different in the two treatment groups, that chiral inversion did not impart much additional variability in the kinetics of the S enantiomer. They suggested that the range in their CL/F data for the R enantiomer was higher than that of the S enantiomer. The authors concluded by stating that there was substantial interindividual variability in the kinetics of ibuprofen enantiomers in arthritic subjects, and that the degree of variability was similar between arthritic patients and healthy subjects. They also suggested, based on the similarities in variability of (S)-ibuprofen between the two groups, that administration of the pure S enantiomer was not likely to confer any therapeutic advantage over racemate. The study results are not definitive since a crossover design was not used, although the authors did attempt to match subjects for age, body weight and creatinine clearance.

Rudy *et al.* (1992) studied the pharmacokinetics of ibuprofen in 45 patients with osteoarthritis after single and repeated administration of 300 or 600 mg of the racemate. The CL did not appear to be dependent on the dose administered. The patients displayed greater variability in CL of (*R*)-ibuprofen, and in $t_{1/2}$ of both enantiomers, than reported previously in healthy subjects. In these patients, over 70% of the total dose was recovered in urine as unchanged drug plus metabolites, which was consistent with that observed in healthy volunteers. Using the metabolite data, the authors calculated the fraction of the dose of *R* enantiomer inverted to range from 35% to 85% with a mean overall value of 65%. This was also consistent with previous reports involving healthy volunteers.

Bradley *et al.* (1992) found that body weight and creatinine clearance were inversely related to the variability observed in serum ibuprofen concentrations in their study involving patients with osteoarthritis.

Renal insufficiency

In order to examine the effect of a number of disease states known to have effects on renal hemodynamics on the stereoselective pharmacokinetics of ibuprofen, 32 patients and 10 age-matched control subjects were recruited (Chen and Chen, 1995). The pharmacokinetics of ibuprofen enantiomers were studied after the ingestion of 800 mg of the racemate. Compared to the control group, the plasma concentrations of the *S* enantiomer were significantly higher in most of the groups of patients. Significant increases were observed in (*S*)-ibuprofen concentrations in the patients with diabetes, hypertension, hyperlipidemia, coronary artery disease, congestive heart failure and chronic renal failure. No such increases were discernible in those patients with hyperuricemia or cerebral vascular disease. In contrast, in most patients there was no associated increase in the plasma concentrations of the *R* enantiomer. It was not possible to clearly differentiate the effects of one specific disease on the pharmacokinetics of the drug, however, as patients mostly were afflicted with more than one of these disease states. Using multiple regression analysis, the authors identified age and advanced hypertension as independent factors that could cause an increase in AUC of the *S* enantiomer. Indices of absorption (C_{max}, t_{max}) were not described, probably owing to the relatively sparse sample collection schedule used over the first 4 h.

Seven anephric patients undergoing hemodialysis treatment were given 800 mg of ibuprofen t.i.d for 2 weeks (Antal *et al.*, 1986). After the last dose was administered, dialysis was initiated and venous and arterial blood samples were obtained and the plasma was assayed for drug. There was little difference noted in the plasma concentrations between the arterial and venous sides of the dialyzer, and little change in the calculated *k* values. There were significant accumulations noted for two inactive metabolites, however. The authors confirmed, as might be expected for a highly metabolized drug with extensive plasma protein binding, that hemodialysis does not influence the pharmacokinetics of ibuprofen.

CHAPTER 4

Rudy *et al.* (1995) studied the pharmacokinetics of ibuprofen enantiomers in 31 elderly patients with varying degrees of renal function after single and repeated doses of 800 mg ibuprofen given every 8 h. A single 10 mg dose of deuterated (*S*)-ibuprofen was co-administered with the dose of ibuprofen before each pharmacokinetic determination. A control group of 8 young healthy volunteers was also included in the study for comparative purposes (age 24–34 years).

There was no difference between the three groups in the fraction of *R* enantiomer inverted to (*S*)-ibuprofen. Significant increases were noted in the unbound serum concentrations of *S* but not of *R* enantiomer. A diminished unbound CL of (*S*)-ibuprofen was also noted in the renally impaired patients compared to the healthy volunteers, resulting in 45% greater steady-state serum concentrations. No effect was noticed in total body CL, owing to the combination of decreased unbound CL and increased unbound fraction. Although Chen and Chen (1995) found that renal impairment caused increases in plasma concentrations compared to healthy control subjects, Rudy *et al.* (1995) noted that the patients used in the two studies may have differed in clinical status and in their racial make-up.

Rudy *et al.* (1995) reported relatively large values of V_d for the *R* enantiomer, mean values of which were approximately 1 l/kg and > 1 l/kg at steady-state in the elderly patients and young volunteers, respectively. After a single dose, the calculations of V_d of the *R* enantiomer were also higher (0.62 l/kg) than other studies that reported the V_d of both ibuprofen enantiomers to be ~0.2 l/kg. These large values are not in line with the protein binding results of this and other studies, as it is the *R* enantiomer that is more avidly bound than the *S* enantiomer. As such, the *S* enantiomer might be expected to have a somewhat larger V_d than the *R* enantiomer. These anomalous values were not discussed by the authors.

Hepatic disease

The influence of liver disease on the pharmacokinetics of ibuprofen enantiomers was studied in 8 male patients with moderate cirrhosis (Li *et al.*, 1993). A group of healthy age-matched control volunteers (6M, 2F) was also studied for comparative purposes. Each subject was given a single 400 mg dose of ibuprofen. The authors found a number of statistically significant differences between the patients and healthy volunteers. Both C_{max} and t_{max} of the *R* enantiomer were significantly reduced in the patient group, although there was no difference between the two groups in the extent of absorption. The $t_{1/2}$ was significantly longer in the patients for both enantiomers. For both enantiomers there were significant reductions in the amount of parent and acyl-glucuronidated species in the urine.

After administration of the individual *S* enantiomer, the patients and control groups differed significantly in the $t_{1/2}$ and extent of absorption. Cirrhotic patients had a longer $t_{1/2}$ and an increased AUC of (*S*)-ibuprofen compared to healthy subjects.

The $R{:}S$ concentration ratios were consistently higher in the cirrhotic patients than in the control subjects. On this basis, and because of the lower (S)-ibuprofen concentrations attained after racemate, the authors suggested the possibility of reduced presystemic inversion in cirrhotic patients. The possible influence of altered protein binding was also mentioned, which is a critical consideration for ibuprofen owing to its extensive binding by albumin, the concentrations of which may be decreased in chronic liver diseases. The longer $t_{1/2}$ of both enantiomers, coupled with lower urinary recovery of drug and acyl glucuronide from 0 to 12 h post dose suggests a reduced metabolic CL in cirrhotic patients.

Cox *et al.* (1985) studied the inversion of ibuprofen in normal and fatty isolated perfused rat livers. The percentage CL of the R enantiomer attributed to chiral inversion was the same in normal and fatty livers (58–59%).

Burn patients

Serious burn injury is associated with a number of pathophysiological alterations in circulatory status, fluid balance, renal and hepatic function, and plasma protein binding, all of which may influence drug disposition. In a study involving 10 burn patients given 10 mg/kg of ibuprofen as oral suspension, a relatively wide range in $t_{1/2}$ was reported. A wide range in C_{max} was reported, although the timing of drug administration in relation to meals was not standardized. There was no apparent relationship between size of burn and plasma concentrations. The authors suggested that higher doses might be necessary in some patients with burns, since total plasma concentrations of ibuprofen were somewhat lower than expected for maximum effectiveness (10–20 mg/l). Unbound drug concentrations were not measured, however, which might indicate a different conclusion regarding the dose requirement in this patient population, considering that for some other drugs, such as phenytoin, plasma protein binding may be decreased in burn patients owing to decreased albumin concentrations (Bowdle *et al.*, 1980).

Effect of gender and race

Many of the available clinical studies have involved both male and female subjects, and upon examination of the data there does not appear to be an influence of gender on the pharmacokinetics of ibuprofen. Knights *et al.* (1995) detected no significant difference in any pharmacokinetic parameter between males and females given 6 mg/kg of (R)-ibuprofen. There has, however, been the suggestion of an effect of race on ibuprofen kinetics. Compared to other studies, very high values of AUC of both enantiomers were reported in all of the patient groups studied by Chen and Chen (1995). Racial differences might distinguish this study from others, as it involved oriental subjects. In contrast, most of the available North American, European and Australian studies have utilized caucasian patients and volunteers. Small and Wood (1989) have reported a difference between black and white subjects in the pharmacokinetics of ibuprofen after administration of H_2 antagonists (see below). Further study is warranted to examine possible differences between races in the pharmacokinetics of ibuprofen enantiomers.

Experimental induced diabetes mellitus caused a significant reduction in the elimination of ibuprofen in hepatocyte preparations (Xiaotao and Hall, 1995). Differences were present in the elimination of (S)- and (R)-ibuprofen in control rat liver hepatocytes against those from streptozotocin-treated rats and Zucker diabetic fatty rats. The fractional inversion of (R)-ibuprofen was significantly higher in streptozotocin-treated rats and Zucker diabetic fatty rats than in control rats. There was, however, no increase in ibuprofenyl-CoA synthetase activity in liver homogenates between the control and diabetic rats, indicating that the enhanced inversion in diabetes was attributable to increased hepatocellular CoA levels.

4.9 DRUG INTERACTIONS

4.9.1 Anti-ulcer medications

Owing to the gastrointestinal side-effects of NSAIDs, anti-ulcer medications such as histamine H_2-receptor antagonists are occasionally coadministered with ibuprofen. Hence, the potential exists for drug interactions with ibuprofen. Cimetidine, a known inhibitor of some cytochrome P450 isoenzymes, was administered in doses of 200 mg q.i.d to 6 healthy male volunteers for 25 h before ibuprofen 800 mg (Evans *et al.*, 1989a). Cimetidine was continued for 36 h after the dose of ibuprofen. Cimetidine co-administration had no detectable effect on the pharmacokinetics of ibuprofen enantiomers or on the unbound fraction of ibuprofen enantiomers in plasma. The lack of an effect of cimetidine and nizatidine on ibuprofen pharmacokinetics has also been reported by Forsyth *et al.* (1988).

Stephenson *et al.* (1988) studied the effects of two H_2 antagonists, cimetidine and ranitidine, on the pharmacokinetics of ibuprofen 600 mg in 12 healthy young subjects (mean age 25 years). There was no stereospecific analysis. Similarly to other studies (Evans *et al.*, 1989a; Forsyth *et al.*, 1988), there were no significant differences in the pharmacokinetics of ibuprofen when it was administered alone compared to co-administration of cimetidine or ranitidine. These study results were reanalyzed later to look for possible racial differences, and the results were reported (Small and Wood, 1989). No differences were observed between 6 black (3M, 3F) and white (3M, 3F) subjects in AUC, $t_{1/2}$, or CL/F. There were, however, significant differences in the effect of cimetidine and ranitidine on the indices of absorption, namely C_{max} and t_{max}. Compared to that in white patients, the C_{max} was significantly higher in black patients after co-administration of both H_2 antagonists. The increase in mean C_{max} in black subjects was on the order of 23–42%. There was also the suggestion of a shorter t_{max} in the black patients after co-administration of H_2 antagonists. The clinical relevance of this observation is not known.

Gontarz *et al.* (1987) studied the pharmacokinetics of 400 mg ibuprofen in 8 healthy volunteers with and without co-administration of antacid. The antacid was a combination of aluminium and magnesium hydroxides. The authors reported a lack of effect of this antacid on ibuprofen pharmacokinetics. Neuvonen *et al.* (1991) also studied the effect of co-administration of magnesium hydroxide alone on racemic ibuprofen pharmaco-kinetics in 6 healthy women volunteers (Neuvonen *et al.*, 1991). Each subject was given single doses of 400 mg ibuprofen tablets with or without 850 mg of magnesium hydroxide in a randomized crossover fashion. Magnesium hydroxide resulted in a decreased mean t_{max} and significantly increased C_{max} of ibuprofen (~31% higher), with no significant change in overall extent of absorption as assessed using $AUC_{0-24 h}$. This finding was specific for ibuprofen; ketoprofen and diclofenac, which were also assessed, were not affected by co-administration of magnesium hydroxide. The differences in findings from those of Gontarz *et al.* (1987) were attributed to the opposing effects of aluminium and magnesium hydroxides on gastric emptying rate. The authors suggested that magnesium hydroxide be co-administered when ibuprofen is being used for the alleviation of pain.

Berardi *et al.* (1988) have shown that altering gastric pH by administration of raniti-dine does not influence the release characteristics of a sustained release formulation of ibuprofen, or the pharmacokinetics of ibuprofen after immediate release tablets.

Small *et al.* (1991) recruited 12 healthy subjects aged 23 years to assess the possible effects of misoprostol and ranitidine on the pharmacokinetics of racemic ibuprofen. In random fashion each subject received 600 mg of ibuprofen alone, with 200 µg of misoprostol, or with 150 mg of ranitidine. Neither anti-ulcer drug impacted on the C_{max}, t_{max}, AUC or $t_{1/2}$ of (*R+S*)-ibuprofen.

Sucralfate is another anti-ulcer drug sometimes co-administered with ibuprofen. On three occasions, 11 healthy male subjects were administered single 600 mg doses in a random fashion (Levine *et al.*, 1992). Ibuprofen was given alone, or with the last dose of a 2-day course of 1 g sucralfate q.i.d. Sucralfate did not affect the extent of ibuprofen absorption. With respect to the speed of absorption, co-administration of sucralfate caused a significant reduction in the C_{max} of both enantiomers compared to the fasted state. This was attributed to a delay in absorption rather than a reduced rate of absorption, however, because there was no difference in the rate of absorption as assessed by non-linear least-squares best fit estimates.

Zidovudine

Ibuprofen may be of use as an analgesic and anti-inflammatory agent in hemophiliac HIV(+) patients with chronic painful arthropathy (Ragni *et al.*, 1992). There have been reports of increased frequency of hemathroses and hematomas in patients receiving con-current treatment with zidovudine and ibuprofen. As part of a study designed to study this potential interaction more thoroughly, a repeated-dose pharmacokinetic assessment of ibuprofen was conducted in 10 hemophiliac HIV(+) male patients in the presence and absence of zidovudine (Ragni *et al.*, 1992). There was no discernible effect of zidovudine

CHAPTER 4

treatment on the steady-state pharmacokinetics of $(R+S)$-ibuprofen. There did seem to be an enhanced effect of ibuprofen on prolongation of bleeding time, and decreased platelet adhesiveness and platelet aggregation. A pharmacokinetic explanation for the findings cannot be ruled out on the basis of these results, however, as unbound drug concentration was not measured, nor was stereospecific analysis used to quantify enantiomer concentrations; (S)-ibuprofen possesses essentially all of the platelet function modifying activity.

Codeine

In combination, codeine did not appear to influence the pharmacokinetics of single dose, orally administered ibuprofen in young healthy volunteers (Kaltenbach et al., 1994). There were no changes in rate or extent of absorption of ibuprofen.

Antihyperlipidemic drugs

Bile acid sequestering resins, which are used in the treatment of type II hyperlipoproteinemia, may decrease the gastrointestinal absorption and increase the CL of some acidic drugs. To test for the presence of a drug interaction between bile salt sequestering agents and ibuprofen, 6 healthy male volunteers were given 400 mg ibuprofen with and without single doses of either 10 g colestipol or 8 g cholestyramine in a randomized three-way crossover study (Al-Meshal et al., 1994). Compared to the control group, colestipol had no effect on ibuprofen pharmacokinetics as assessed using nonstereospecific methodology. In contrast, co-administration of cholestyramine caused a significant delay in the attainment of t_{max} from 1.25 h under control conditions to 2.25 h. The C_{max} and AUC of ibuprofen were also significantly reduced after the co-administration of cholestyramine, although $t_{1/2}$ was unaffected. The authors concluded that cholestyramine, perhaps owing to the presence of quaternary amine groups in its resin structure, causes reductions in both the extent and the rate of ibuprofen absorption. Caution has been advised in the co-administration of ibuprofen with methotrexate owing to the possibility of reduced tubular secretrion, glomerular filtration, protein binding displacement, and decreased hepatic metabolism of methotrexate (Brouwers and de Smet, 1994; Krough, 1995).

Owing to its high degree of binding to plasma proteins, ibuprofen has the potential to competitively interfere with the binding of other drugs. For example, ASA appears to cause a displacement of ibuprofen and other NSAIDs from plasma proteins (Albert and Gernaat, 1984). However, pharmacodynamic consequences are not expected for this sort of interaction owing to the compensatory effect of CL on the displaced unbound drug, resulting in unchanged plasma unbound drug.

Because clofibric acid can enhance the activities of CoA, it was possible that it could influence the chiral inversion of ibuprofen. Using rat liver homogenates, Knights et al. (1991) demonstrated that long-chain CoA ligase activities were increased by 50–100% after 5 days of dosing rats with clofibric acid. The mean chiral inversion of (R)-ibuprofen was increased 68% after pretreatment of rats with clofibric acid.

Roy-De Vos *et al.* (1996) also studied the effects of clofibrate on the chiral inversion of ibuprofen in the rat. Inversion of (*R*)-ibuprofen was studied in isolated perfused rat livers and hepatocytes both with and without pretreatment with clofibric acid (280 mg/kg/day). Control liver preparations and livers exposed acutely to clofibrate during liver perfusion were also studied. In the perfusion experiments involving individual *R* enantiomer, clofibrate caused a substantial increase in the amount of (*S*)-ibuprofen formed via chiral inversion. This was the case for both acute administration and 3 days pretreatment with clofibrate, although the amount of *S* formed was greater in the pretreated livers. There was no antipode formed when *S* enantiomer alone was infused into rat liver. In hepatocytes incubated with (*R*)-ibuprofen, inversion increased with the amount of clofibric acid placed in the incubation medium. Interestingly, as the hepatocyte incubations progressed, there was a decrease in the CoA concentrations measured in those preparations containing (*R*)-ibuprofen only, an increase in those containing clofibric acid, and no change when both (*R*)-ibuprofen and clofibric acid were present together.

Oral contraceptive steroids

Hormonal factors may influence certain biotransformation reactions in the body. Knights *et al.* have reported the lack of effect of oral contraceptives on the pharmacokinetics of (*R*)-ibuprofen in female subjects given 6 mg/kg of (*R*)-ibuprofen. The AUC of the formed (*S*)-ibuprofen was similarly not affected by co-administration of oral contraceptives. Because much of the dose of *R* enantiomer is inverted to (*S*)-ibuprofen, the authors suggested that it was likely that the pharmacokinetics of the *S* enantiomer would not be affected by oral contraceptives.

Other drugs

The fractional chiral inversion and mean residence time of ibuprofen enantiomers in isolated rat hepatocytes was found to be influenced by the presence of other agents, including the antiepileptic agent valproic acid (Xiaotao and Hall, 1993). Valproic acid caused increases in the MRT of both ibuprofen enantiomers. At the same time, there was a decrease observed in the AUC of ibuprofenyl-CoA. Barbiturates are known to induce the metabolism of ibuprofen in several species, including the rat (Mills *et al.*, 1973), dog, and monkey (Magdalou *et al.*, 1990).

Effect of ibuprofen on the pharmacokinetics of other drugs

Ibuprofen has been reported to cause increases (up to 66%) in the serum concentrations of lithium when ingested concurrently (Ragheb, 1990). The increase appears to be more consistent and of greater magnitude in elderly patients. Erythrocyte concentrations of lithium are also increased in the presence of ibuprofen (Kristoff *et al.*, 1986). The increase in concentrations appears to occur in the presence of normal renal function, and has been hypothesized to be secondary to a tubular prostaglandin-dependent mechanism. Another case report has linked an ibuprofen-induced reduction in renal function to baclofen toxicity in a 64-year-old man with spinal injury (Dahlin and George, 1984). For the same reason, caution has been advised in the co-administration with cyclosporin (Brouwers and de Smet, 1994).

4.10 CONCLUSIONS

Ibuprofen is the prototypical 2-APA NSAID, and continues to enjoy use throughout the world for its antiarthritic, analgesic and antipyretic properties. Similarly to other NSAIDs, ibuprofen shares the properties of high extent of metabolism, low CL, extensive binding to plasma proteins, and low volume of distribution. Except for the upper end of the therapeutic range of concentrations, the drug exhibits linear pharmacokinetics. It would be a challenge indeed to name a currently available chiral drug that has had as much attention directed towards its stereospecific pharmacokinetics as has ibuprofen. In general the plasma concentrations of (S)-ibuprofen are predominant except in adults with liver cirrhosis and infants recovering from minor genitourinary surgery. Although unidirectional chiral inversion processes influence the kinetics of ibuprofen and some other 2-APA derivatives (fenoprofen, ketoprofen), it is important to recognize that the process varies in importance between different NSAIDs, does not seem to occur at all for some 2-APA NSAIDs (e.g. flurbiprofen), and is also species specific. There is no doubt of the contribution of a systemic process to the inversion of ibuprofen, and the liver has been implicated as an important site for this process. There is also evidence for a presystemic inversion process in the intestinal tract. Although the findings have been disputed by some scientists, possible deficiencies in those studies, most notably the use of rapidly absorbed dosage forms, may have masked the presence of a presystemic process. Pathophysiological changes seem to have little or moderate influence on the pharmacokinetics of ibuprofen. Although there is some evidence for a dose–response relationship for ibuprofen in patients with rheumatoid arthritis, a definitive therapeutic range of concentrations has not been established. A greater understanding of the relationship between toxic effects with serum enantiomer concentrations may be helpful in the clinical use of the drug.

REFERENCES

ADAMS, S.S., BRESLOFF, P. and MASON, C.G. (1976) Pharmacological differences between the optical isomers of ibuprofen: Evidence for metabolic inversion of the (–) isomer. *Journal of Pharmacy and Pharmacology* 28, 256–257.

ADEYEYE, C.M and CHEN, F.F. (1997) Stereoselective disposition of suspensions of conventional wax–matrix sustained release ibuprofen microspheres in rats. *Pharmaceutical Research* 14, 1811–1816.

AHN, H.Y., AMIDON, G.L. and SMITH, D.E. (1991a) Stereoselective systemic disposition of ibuprofen enantiomers in the dog. *Pharmaceutical Research* 8, 1186–1190.

AHN, H.Y., JAMALI, F., COX, S.R., KITTAYANOND, D. and SMITH, D.E. (1991b) Stereoselective disposition of ibuprofen enantiomers in the isolated perfused rat kidney. *Pharmaceutical Research* **8**, 1520–1524.

AIBA, T., TSE, M.M., BENET, L.Z. and LIN, E.T. (1997) Effect of dosage formulation on stereoisomeric inversion of ibuprofen in human volunteers. *Pharmaceutical Research* **14**, S608.

ALBERT, K.S. and GERNAAT, C.M. (1984) Pharmacokinetics of ibuprofen. *American Journal of Medicine* **77**, 40–46.

ALBERT, K.S., GILLESPIE, W.R., WAGNER, J.G., PAU, A. and LOCKWOOD, G.F. (1984) Effect of age on the clinical pharmacokinetics of ibuprofen. *American Journal of Medicine* **77**, 47–50.

AL-MESHAL, M.A., EL-SAYED, Y.M., AL-BALLA, S.R. and GOUDA, M.W. (1994) The effect of colestipol and cholestyramine on ibuprofen bioavailability in man. *Biopharmaceutics and Drug Disposition* **15**, 463–471.

ANTAL, E.J., WRIGHT, C.E., BROWN, B.L., ALBERT, K.S., AMAN, L.C. and LEVIN, N.W. (1986) The influence of hemodialysis on the pharmacokinetics of ibuprofen and its major metabolites. *Journal of Clinical Pharmacology* **26**, 184–190.

AVGERINOS, A. and HUTT, A.J. (1987) Determination of the enantiomeric composition of ibuprofen in human plasma by high-performance liquid chromatography. *Journal of Chromatography* **415**, 75–83.

BANNWARTH, B., LAPICQUE, F., PEHOURCQ, F. *et al.* (1995) Stereoselective disposition of ibuprofen enantiomers in human cerebrospinal fluid. *British Journal of Clinical Pharmacology* **40**, 266–269.

BECK, W.S., GEISSLINGER, G., ENGLER, H. and BRUNE, K. (1991) Pharmacokinetics of ibuprofen enantiomers in dogs. *Chirality* **3**, 165–169.

BERARDI, R.R., DRESSMAN, J.B., ELTA, G.H. and SZPUNAR, G.J. (1988) Elevation of gastric pH with ranitidine does not affect the release characteristics of sustained release ibuprofen tablets. *Biopharmaceutics and Drug Disposition* **9**, 337–347.

BERRY, B.W. and JAMALI, F. (1989) Enantiomeric interaction of flurbiprofen in the rat. *Journal of Pharmaceutical Sciences* **78**, 632–634.

BERRY, B.W. and JAMALI, F. (1991) Presystemic and systemic chiral inversion of (R)-(−)-fenoprofen in the rat. *Journal of Pharmacology and Experimental Therapeutics* **258**, 695–701.

BOWDLE, T.A., NEAL, G.D., LEVY, R.H. and HEIMBACH, D.M. (1980) Phenytoin pharmacokinetics in burned rats and plasma binding of phenytoin in burned patients. *Journal of Pharmacology and Experimental Therapeutics* **213**, 97–99.

BRADLEY, J.D., RUDY, A.C. and KATZ, B.P. *et al.* (1992) Correlation of serum concentrations of ibuprofen stereoisomers with clinical response in the treatment of hip and knee osteoarthritis. *Journal of Rheumatology* **19**, 130–134.

CHAPTER 4

BROOKS, C.J.W. and GILBERT, M.T. (1974) Studies of urinary metabolites of 2-(4-isobutylphenyl)propionic acid by gas–liquid chromatography–mass spectrometry. *Journal of Chromatography* 99, 541–551.

BROUWERS, J.R.B.J. and DE SMET, P.A.G.M. (1994) Pharmacokinetic–pharmacodynamic drug interactions with nonsteroidal anti-inflammatory drugs. *Clinical Pharmacokinetics* 27, 462–485.

BROWN, R.D., WILSON, J.T., KEARNS, G.L., EICHLER, V.F., JOHNSON, V.A. and BERTRAND, K.M. (1992) Single dose pharmacokinetics of ibuprofen and acetaminophen in febrile children. *Journal of Clinical Pharmacology* 32, 231–241.

BRUGGER, R., ALIA, B.G., REICHEL, C. *et al.* (1996) Isolation and characterization of rat liver microsomal (R)-ibuprofenoyl-CoA synthetase. *Biochemical Pharmacology* 52, 1007–1013.

CARBAZA, A., SUESA, N., TOST, D. *et al.* (1996) Stereoselective metabolic pathways of ketoprofen in the rat: incorporation into triacylglycerols and enantiomeric inversion. *Chirality* 8, 163–172.

CASTILLO, M., LAM, Y.W.F., DOOLEY, M.A., STAHL, E. and SMITH, P.C. (1995) Disposition and covalent binding of ibuprofen and its acyl glucuronide in the elderly. *Clinical Pharmacology and Therapeutics* 57, 636–644.

CHEN, C.S., CHEN, T. and SHIEH, W.R. (1990) Metabolic stereoisomeric inversion of 2-arylpropionic acids. On the mechanism of ibuprofen epimerization in rats. *Biochimica et Biophysica Acta* 1033, 1–6.

CHEN, C.S., SHIEH, W.R., LU, P.H., HARRIMAN, S. and CHEN, C.Y. (1991) Metabolic stereo-isomeric inversion of ibuprofen in mammals. *Biochimica et Biophysica Acta* 1078, 411–417.

CHEN, C.Y. and CHEN, C.S. (1995) Stereoselective disposition of ibuprofen in patients with compromised renal hemodynamics. *British Journal of Clinical Pharmacology* 40, 67–72.

CHENG, H., ROGERS, J.D., DEMETRIADES, J.L., HOLLAND, S.D., SEIBOLD, J.R. and DEPUY, E. (1994) Pharmacokinetics and bioinversion of ibuprofen enantiomers in humans. *Pharmaceutical Research* 11, 824–830.

CONE, J.B., WALLACE, B.H., OLSEN, K.M., CALDWELL, F.T. JR., GURLEY, B.J. and BOND, P.J. (1993) The pharmacokinetics of ibuprofen after burn injury. *Journal of Burn Care and Rehabilitation* 14, 666–669.

COX, J.W., COX, S.R., VANGIESSEN, G. and RUWART, M.J. (1985) Ibuprofen stereoisomer hepatic clearance and distribution in normal and fatty in situ perfused liver. *Journal of Pharmacology and Experimental Therapeutics* 232, 636–643.

COX, S.R., BROWN, M.A., SQUIRES, D.J., MURRILL, E.A., LEDNICER, D. and KNUTH, D.W. (1988) Comparative human study of ibuprofen enantiomer plasma concentrations produced by two commercially available ibuprofen tablets. *Biopharmaceutics and Drug Disposition* 9, 539–549.

Cox, S.R., Gall, E.P., Forbes, K.K., Gresman, M. and Goris, G. (1991) Pharmacokinetic of the (R)-(–) and (S)-(+) enantiomers of ibuprofen in the serum and synovial fluid of arthritis patients. *Journal of Clinical Pharmacology* **31**, 88–94.

Dahlin, P.A. and George, J. (1984) Baclofen toxicity associated with declining renal clearance after (R)-ibuprofen. *Drug Intelligence and Clinical Pharmacy* **18**, 805–808.

Day, R.O., Williams, K.M., Graham, G.G., Lee, E.J., Knihinicki, R.R. and Champion, G.D. (1988) Stereoselective disposition of ibuprofen enantiomers in synovial fluid. *Clinical Pharmacology and Therapeutics* **43**, 480–487.

Dwivedi, S.K., Sattari, S., Jamali, F. and Mitchell, A.G. (1992) Ibuprofen racemate and enantiomers: phase diagram, solubility and thermodynamic studies. *International Journal of Pharmaceutics* **87**, 95–104.

Eller, M.G., Wright, C. and Della-Coletta, A.A. (1989) Absorption kinetics of rectally and orally administered ibuprofen. *Biopharmaceutics and Drug Disposition* **10**, 269–278.

Elmquist, W.F., Chan, K.K.H. and Sawchuk, R.J. (1994) Transsynovial drug distribution: synovial mean transit time of diclofenac and other nonsteroidal anti-inflammatory drugs. *Pharmaceutical Research* **11**, 1689–1697.

Evans, A.M., Nation, R.L. and Sansom, L.N. (1989a) Lack of effect of cimetidine on the pharmacokinetics of (R)-(–)- and (S)-(+)-ibuprofen. *British Journal of Clinical Pharmacology* **28**, 143–149.

Evans, A.M., Nation, R.L., Sansom, L.N., Bochner, F. and Somogyi, A.A. (1989b) Stereoselective plasma protein binding of ibuprofen enantiomers. *European Journal of Clinical Pharmacology* **36**, 283–290.

Evans, A.M., Nation, R.L., Sansom, L.N., Bochner, F. and Somogyi, A.A. (1990) The relationship between the pharmacokinetics of ibuprofen enantiomers and the dose of racemic ibuprofen in humans. *Biopharmaceutics and Drug Disposition* **11**, 507–518.

Evans, A.M., Nation, R.L., Sansom, L.N., Bochner, F. and Somogyi, A.A. (1991) Effect of racemic ibuprofen dose on the magnitude and duration of platelet cyclo-oxygenase inhibition: relationship between inhibition on thromboxane production and the plasma unbound concentration of (S)-(+)-ibuprofen. *British Journal of Clinical Pharmacology* **31**, 131–138.

Forsyth, D.R., Jayasinghe, K.S. and Roberts, C.J. (1988) Do nizatidine and cimetidine interact with ibuprofen? *European Journal of Clinical Pharmacology* **35**, 85–88.

Friedman, H., Seckman, C., Lanza, F., Royer, G., Perry, K. and Francom, S. (1990) Clinical pharmacology of predisintegrated ibuprofen 800 mg tablets; an endoscopic and pharmacokinetic study. *Journal of Clinical Pharmacology* **30**, 57–63.

Geisslinger, G., Dietzel, K. and Loew, D. *et al.* (1989a) High-performance liquid chromatographic determination of ibuprofen, its metabolites and enantiomers in biological fluids. *Journal of Chromatography* **491**, 139–149.

CHAPTER 4

GEISSLINGER, G., STOCK, K.P., BACH, G.L., LOEW, D. and BRUNE, K. (1989b) Pharmacological differences between (R)-(–)- and (S)-(+)-ibuprofen. *Agents and Actions* **27**, 455–457.

GEISSLINGER, G., SCHUSTER, O., STOCK, K.P., LOEW, D., BACH, G.L. and BRUNE, K. (1990) Pharmacokinetics of (S)-(+)- and (R)-(–)-ibuprofen in volunteers and first clinical experience of (S)-(+)-ibuprofen in rheumatoid arthritis. *European Journal of Clinical Pharmacology* **38**, 493–497.

GEISSLINGER, G., STOCK, K.P., LOEW, D., BACH, G.L. and BRUNE, K. (1993) Variability in the stereoselective disposition of ibuprofen in patients with rheumatoid arthritis. *British Journal of Clinical Pharmacology* **35**, 603–607.

GONTARZ, N., SMALL, R.E., COMSTOCK, T.J., STALKER, D.J., JOHNSCON, S.M. and WILLIS, H.E. (1987) Effect of antacid suspension on the pharmacokinetics of ibuprofen. *Clinical Pharmacy* **6**, 413–416.

GRENNAN, D.M., AARONS, L., SIDDIQUI, M., RICHARDS, M., THOMPSON, R. and HIGHAM, C. (1983) Dose–response study with ibuprofen in rheumatoid arthritis: clinical and pharmacokinetic findings. *British Journal of Clinical Pharmacology* **15**, 311–316.

HALL, S.D., HASSANZADEH-KHAYYAT, M., KNADLER, M.P. and MAYER, P.R. (1992) Pulmonary inversion of 2-arylpropionic acids: influence of protein binding. *Chirality* **4**, 349–352.

HALL, S.D., RUDY, A.C., KNIGHT, P.M. and BRATER, D.C. (1993) Lack of presystemic inversion of (R)- to (S)-ibuprofen in humans. *Clinical Pharmacology and Therapeutics* **53**, 393–400.

HUTT, A.J. and CALDWELL, J. (1983) The metabolic chiral inversion of 2-arylpropionic acids — a novel route with pharmacological consequences. *Journal of Pharmacy and Pharmacology* **35**, 693–704.

HUTT, A.J., KOOLOOBANDI, A. and HANLON, G.W. (1993) Microbial metabolism of 2-arylpropionic acids: chiral inversion of ibuprofen and 2-phenylpropionic acid. *Chirality* **5**, 596–601.

JACK, D.S., RUMBLE, R.H., DAVIES, N.W. and FRANCIS, H.W. (1992) Enantiospecific gas chromatographic–mass spectrometric procedure for the determination of ketoprofen and ibuprofen in synovial fluid and plasma: application to protein binding studies. *Journal of Chromatography* **584**, 189–197.

JAMALI, F. (1988) Pharmacokinetics of enantiomers of chiral nonsteroidal anti-inflammatory drugs. *European Journal of Drug Metabolism and Pharmacokinetics* **13**, 1–9.

JAMALI, F., BERRY, B.W., TEHRANI, M.R. and RUSSELL, A.S. (1988a) Stereoselective pharmacokinetics of flurbiprofen in humans and rats. *Journal of Pharmaceutical Sciences* **77**: 666–669.

JAMALI, F., SINGH, N.N., PASUTTO, F.M., RUSSELL, A.S. and COUTTS, R.T. (1988b) Pharmacokinetics of ibuprofen enantiomers following oral administration of tablets with different absorption rates. *Pharmaceutical Research* **5**, 40–43.

JAMALI, F., MEHVAR, R., RUSSELL, A.S., SATTARI, S., YAKIMETS, W.W. and KOO, J. (1992) Human pharmacokinetics of ibuprofen enantiomers following different doses and formulations: intestinal chiral inversion. *Journal of Pharmaceutical Sciences* **81**, 221–225.

JAMALI, F., LOVLIN, R. and ABERG, G. (1997) Bi-directional chiral inversion of ketoprofen in CD-1 mice. *Chirality* **9**, 29–31.

JEFFREY, P., TUCKER, G.T., BYE, A., CREWE, H.K. and WRIGHT, P.A. (1991) The site of inversion of (*R*)-(–)-ibuprofen: studies in rat using in-situ isolated perfused intestine/liver preparations. *Journal of Pharmacy and Pharmacology* **43**, 715–720.

KAISER, D.G., VANGIESSEN, G.J., REISCHER, R.J. and WECHTER, W.J. (1976) Isomeric inversion of ibuprofen (*R*)-enantiomer in humans. *Journal of Pharmaceutical Sciences* **65**, 269–273.

KALTENBACH, M.L., MOHAMMED, S.S., MULLERSMAN, G., PERRIN, J.H. and DERENDORF, H. (1994) Pharmacokinetic evaluation of two ibuprofen-codeine combinations. *International Journal of Clinical Pharmacology and Therapeutics* **4**, 210–214.

KAUFFMAN, R.E. and NELSON, M.V. (1992) Effect of age on ibuprofen pharmacokinetics and antipyretic response. *Journal of Pediatrics* **121**, 969–973.

KELLEY, M.T., WALSON, P.D., EDGE, J.H., COX, S. and MORTENSEN, M.E. (1992) Pharmacokinetics and pharmacodynamics of ibuprofen isomers and acetaminophen in febrile children. *Clinical Pharmacology and Therapeutics* **52**, 181–189.

KENDALL, M.J., JUBB, R. and BIRD, H.A. *et al.* (1990) A pharmacokinetic comparison of ibuprofen sustained-release tablets given to young and elderly patients. *Journal of Clinical Pharmacy and Therapeutics* **15**, 35–40.

KNIGHTS, K.M. and DREW, R. (1992) The effects of ibuprofen enantiomers on hepatocyte intermediary metabolism and mitochondrial respiration. *Biochemical Pharmacology* **44**, 1291–1296.

KNIGHTS, K.M. and JONES, M.E. (1992) Inhibition kinetics of hepatic microsomal long chain fatty acid-CoA ligase by 2-arylpropionic acid nonsteroidal anti-inflammatory drugs. *Biochemical Pharmacology* **43**, 1465–1471.

KNIGHTS, K.M., ADDINALL, T.F. and ROBERTS, B.J. (1991) Enhanced chiral inversion of (*R*)-ibuprofen in liver from rats treated with clofibric acid. *Biochemical Pharmacology* **41**, 1775–1777.

KNIGHTS, K.M., MCLEAN, C.F., TONKIN, A.L. and MINERS, J.O. (1995) Lack of effect of gender and oral contraceptive steroids on the pharmacokinetics of (*R*)-ibuprofen in humans. *British Journal of Clinical Pharmacology* **40**, 153–156.

KNIHINICKI, R.D., WILLIAMS, K.M. and DAY, R.O. (1989) Chiral inversion of 2-arylpropionic acid nonsteroidal anti-inflammatory drugs — I: *In vitro* studies of ibuprofen and flurbiprofen. *Biochemical Pharmacology* **24**, 4389–4395.

KNIHINICKI, R.D., DAY, R.O., GRAHAM, G.G. and WILLIAMS, K.M. (1990) Stereoselective disposition of ibuprofen and flurbiprofen in rats. *Chirality* **2**, 134–140.

CHAPTER 4

KNIHINICKI, R.D., DAY, R.O. and WILLIAMS, K.M. (1991) Chiral inversion of 2-arylpropionic acid nonsteroidal anti-inflammatory drugs — II: Racemization and hydrolysis of (R)- and (S)-ibuprofen-CoA thioesters. *Biochemical Pharmacology* **42**, 1905–1911.

KONSTAN, M.W., HOPPEL, C.L., CHAI, B. and DAVIS, P.B. (1991) Ibuprofen in children with cystic fibrosis: pharmacokinetics and adverse effects. *Journal of Pediatrics* **188**, 956–964.

KRISTOFF, C.A., HAYES, P.E., BARR, W.H., SMALL, R.E., TOWNSEND, R.J. and ETTIGI, P.G. (1986) Effect of ibuprofen on lithium plasma and red blood cell concentrations. *Clinical Pharmacy* **5**, 51–55.

KROUGH, C.M.E. (ed.) (1995) *CPS: Compendium of Pharmaceuticals and Specialties*, 30th edn. Ottawa, Canadian Pharmaceutical Association.

KUNSMAN, G.W. and ROHRIG, T.P. (1993) Tissue distribution of ibuprofen in a fatal overdose. *American Journal of Forensic and Medical Pathology* **14**, 48–50.

LASKA, E.M., SUNSHINE, A., MARRERO, I., OLSON, N., SIEGEL, C. and McCORMICK, N. (1986) The correlation between blood levels of ibuprofen and clinical analgesic response. *Clinical Pharmacology and Therapeutics* **40**, 1–7.

LEE, E.J.D., WILLIAMS, K.M., GRAHAM, G.G., DAY, R.O. and CHAMPION, G.D. (1984) Liquid chromatographic determination and plasma concentration profile of optical isomers of ibuprofen in humans. *Journal of Pharmaceutical Sciences* **73**, 1542–1544.

LEE, E.J.D., WILLIAMS, K., DAY, R., GRAHAM, G. and CHAMPION, D. (1985) Stereoselective disposition of ibuprofen enantiomers in man. *British Journal of Clinical Pharmacology* **19**, 669–674.

LEMKO, C.H., CAILLE, G. and FOSTER, R.T. (1993) Stereospecific high-performance liquid chromatographic assay of ibuprofen; improved sensitivity and sample processing efficiency. *Journal of Chromatography* **619**, 330–335.

LEVINE, M.A.H., WALKER, S.E. and PATON, T.W. (1992) The effect of food or sucralfate on the bioavailability of (S)-(+) and (R)-(–) enantiomers of ibuprofen. *Journal of Clinical Pharmacology* **32**, 1110–1114.

LI, G., TREIBER, G., MAIER, K., WALKER, S. and KLOTZ, U. (1993) Disposition of ibuprofen in patients with liver cirrhosis: stereochemical considerations. *Clinical Pharmacokinetics* **25**, 154–163.

LIN, J.H., COCCHETTO, D.M. and DUGGAN, D.E. (1987) Protein binding as a primary determinant of the clinical pharmacokinetic properties of nonsteroidal anti-inflammatory drugs. *Clinical Pharmacokinetics* **12**, 402–432.

LOCKWOOD, G.F., ALBERT, K.S. and GILLESPIE, W.R. *et al.* (1983) Pharmacokinetics of ibuprofen in man. I. Free and total area/dose relationships. *Clinical Pharmacology and Therapeutics* **34**, 97–103.

MAGDALOU, J., CHAJES, V., LAFAURIE, C. and SIEST, G. (1990) Glucuronidation of 2-arylpropionic acids pirprofen, flurbiprofen, and ibuprofen by liver microsomes. *Drug Metabolism and Disposition* **18**, 692–697.

MAKELA, A.L., LEMPIAINEN, M. and YLIJOKI, T. (1981) Ibuprofen levels in serum and synovial fluid. *Scandinavian Journal of Rheumatology* **39**(Suppl. 6), 15–17.

MEHVAR, R. and JAMALI, F. (1988) Pharmacokinetic analysis of the enantiomeric inversion of chiral nonsteroidal anti-inflammatory drugs. *Pharmaceutical Research* **5**, 76–79.

MEHVAR, R., JAMALI, F. and PASUTTO, F.M. (1988) Liquid-chromatographic assay of ibuprofen enantiomers in plasma. *Clinical Chemistry* **24**, 493–496.

MENZEL, J. and KOLARZ, G. (1992) Binding affinity of ibuprofen in human tissues. *Arzneimittelforschung* **42**, 325–327.

MENZEL, E.J. and KOLARZ, G. (1994) Binding capacity of ibuprofen to muscle proteins. *Arzneimittelforschung* **44**, 341–343.

MENZEL, S., WAIBEL, R., BRUNE, K. and GEISSLINGER, G. (1994) Is the formation of (R)-ibuprofenyl-adenylate the first stereoselective step of chiral inversion? *Biochemical Pharmacology* **48**, 1056–1058.

MENZEL-SOGLOWEK, S., GEISSLINGER, G. and BRUNE, K. (1990) Stereoselective high-performance liquid chromatographic determination of ketoprofen, ibuprofen and fenoprofen in plasma using a chiral alpha 1-acid glycoprotein column. *Journal of Chromatography* **532**, 295–303.

MENZEL-SOGLOWEK, S., GEISSLINGER, G., MOLLENHAUER, J. and BRUNE, K. (1992) Metabolic chiral inversion of 2-arylpropionates in rat H4IIE and human HEP G2 hepatoma cells. *Biochemical Pharmacology* **43**, 1487–1492.

MILLS, R.F.N., ADAMS, S.S., CLIFFE, E.E., DICKINSON, W. and NICHOLSON, J.S. (1973) The metabolism of ibuprofen. *Xenobiotica* **3**, 589–598.

NAHATA, M.C., DURRELL, D.E., POWELL, D.A. and GUPTA, N. (1991) Pharmacokinetics of ibuprofen in febrile children. *European Journal of Clinical Pharmacology* **40**, 427–428.

NAIDONG, W. and LEE, J.W. (1994) Development and validation of a liquid chromatographic method for the quantitation of ibuprofen enantiomers in human plasma. *Journal of Pharmaceutical and Biomedical Analysis* **4**, 551–556.

NEUVONEN, P.J. (1991) The effect of magnesium hydroxide on the oral absorption of ibuprofen, ketoprofen and diclofenac. *British Journal of Clinical Pharmacology* **31**, 263–266.

NICOLL-GRIFFITH, D.A., INABA, T., TANG, B.K. and KALOW, W. (1988) Method to determine the enantiomers of ibuprofen from human urine by high-performance liquid chromatography. *Journal of Chromatography* **428**, 103–112.

CHAPTER 4

OLIARI, J., TOD, M., NICOLAS, P., PETITJEAN, O. and CAILLE, G. (1992) Pharmacokinetics of ibuprofen enantiomers after single and repeated doses in man. *Biopharmaceutics and Drug Disposition* **13**, 337–344.

PALIWAL, J.K., SMITH, D.E., COX, S.R., BERARDI, R.R., DUNN-KUCHARSKI ,V.A. and ELTA, G.H. (1993) Stereoselective, competitive, and nonlinear plasma protein binding of ibuprofen enantiomers as determined in vivo in healthy subjects. *Journal of Pharmacokinetics and Biopharmaceutics* **21**, 145–161.

RAGHEB, M. (1990) The clinical significance of lithium–nonsteroidal anti-inflammatory drug interactions. *Journal of Clinical Psychopharmacology* **10**, 350–354.

RAGNI, M.V., MILLER, B.J., WHALEN, R. and PTACHCINSKI, R. (1992) Bleeding tendency, platelet function, and pharmacokinetics of ibuprofen and zidovudine in HIV(+) hemophilic men. *American Journal of Hematology* **40**, 176–182.

REICHEL, C., BANG, H., BRUNE, K., GEISLLINGER, G. and MENZEL, S. (1995) 2-Arylpropionyl-CoA epimerase: partial peptide sequences and tissue localization. *Biochemical Pharmacology* **50**, 1803–1806.

REY, E., PARIENTE-KHAYAT, A. and GOUYET, L. *et al*. (1994) Stereoselective disposition of ibuprofen enantiomers in infants. *British Journal of Clinical Pharmacology* **38**, 373–375.

REYNOLDS, J.E.F. (ed.) (1993) Ibuprofen. In *Martindale, The Extra Pharmacopeia*, 13th edn. London, Pharmaceutical Press.

ROY-DE VOS, M., MAYER, J.M., ETTER, J.C. and TESTA, B. (1996) Clofibric acid increases the unidirectional chiral inversion of ibuprofen in rat liver preparations. *Xenobiotica* **26**, 571–582.

RUDY, A.C., ANLIKER, K.S. and HALL, S.D. (1990) High-performance liquid chromatographic determination of the stereoisomeric metabolites of ibuprofen. *Journal of Chromatography* **528**, 395–405.

RUDY, A.C., KNIGHT, P.M., BRATER, D.C. and HALL, S.D. (1991) Stereoselective metabolism of ibuprofen in humans: administration of *R*-, *S*- and racemic ibuprofen. *Journal of Pharmacology and Experimental Therapeutics* **259**, 1133–1139.

RUDY, A.C., BRADLEY, J.D., RYAN, S.I., KALASINSKI, L.A., XIAOTAO, Q. and HALL, S.D. (1992) Variability in the disposition of ibuprofen enantiomers in osteoarthritis patients. *Therapeutic Drug Monitoring* **14**, 464–470.

RUDY, A.C., KNIGHT, P.M., BRATER, D.C. and HALL, S.D. (1995) Enantioselective disposition of ibuprofen in elderly patients with and without renal impairment. *Journal of Pharmacology and Experimental Therapeutics* **273**, 88–93.

SANINS, S.M., ADAMS, W.J., KAISER, D.G., HALSTEAD, G.W. and BAILLIE, T.A. (1990) Studies on the metabolism and chiral inversion of ibuprofen in isolated rat hepatocytes. *Drug Metabolism and Disposition* **18**, 527–533.

SANINS, S.M., ADAMS, W.J. and KAISER, D.G. *et al.* (1991) Mechanistic studies on the metabolic chiral inversion of (*R*)-ibuprofen in the rat. *Drug Metabolism and Disposition* 19, 405–410.

SATTARI, S. and JAMALI, F. (1994) Evidence of absorption rate dependency of ibuprofen inversion in the rat. *Chirality* 6, 435–439.

SCHNEIDER, H.T., NUERNBERG, B., DIETZEL, K. and BRUNE, K. (1990) Biliary elimination of non-steroidal anti-inflammatory drugs in patients. *British Journal of Clinical Pharmacology* 29, 127–131.

SEIDEMAN, P., LOHRER, F., GRAHAM, G.G., DUNCAN, M.W., WILLIAMS, K.M. and DAY, R.O. (1994) The stereoselective disposition of the enantiomers of ibuprofen in blood, blister and synovial fluid. *British Journal of Clinical Pharmacology* 38, 221–227.

SHAH, A. and JUNG, D. (1987) Dose-dependent pharmacokinetics of ibuprofen in the rat. *Drug Metabolism and Disposition* 15, 151–154.

SHIRLEY, M.A., GUAN, X.G., KAISER, D.G., HALSTEAD, G.W. and BAILLIE, T.A. (1994) Taurine conjugation of ibuprofen in humans and in rat liver in vitro. Relationship to metabolic chiral inversion. *Journal of Pharmacology and Experimental Therapeutics* 269, 1166–1175.

SINGH, N.N., PASUTTO, F.M., COUTTS, R.T. and JAMALI, F. (1986) Gas chromatographic separation of optically active anti-inflammatory 2-arylpropionic acids using (+)- or (–)-amphetamine as derivatizing reagent. *Journal of Chromatography* 378, 125–135.

SMALL, R.E. and WOOD, J.H. (1989) Influence of racial differences on effects of ranitidine and cimetidine on ibuprofen pharmacokinetics. *Clinical Pharmacy* 8, 471–472.

SMALL, R.E., WILMOT-PATER, M.G., McGEE, B.A. and WILLIS, H.E. (1991) Effects of misoprostol or ranitidine on ibuprofen pharmacokinetics. *Clinical Pharmacy* 10, 870–872.

SMITH, D.E., PALIWAL, J.K., COX, S.R., BERARDI, R.R., DUNN-KUCHARSKI, V.A. and ELTA, G.H. (1994) The effect of competitive and nonlinear plasma protein binding on the stereoselective disposition and metabolic inversion of ibuprofen in healthy subjects. *Biopharmaceutics and Drug Disposition* 15, 545–561.

STEPHENSON, D.W., SMALL, R.E. and WOOD, J.H. *et al.* (1988) Effect of ranitidine and cimetidine on ibuprofen pharmacokinetics. *Clinical Pharmacy* 7, 317–321.

SURI, A., GRUNDY, B.L., DERENDORF, H. (1997) Pharmacokinetics and pharmacodynamics of enantiomers of ibuprofen and flurbiprofen after oral administration. *International Journal of Clinical Pharmacology and Therapeutics* 35, 1–8.

TRACY, T.S. and HALL, S.D. (1991) Determination of the epimeric composition of ibuprofenyl-CoA. *Analytical Biochemistry* 195, 24–29.

TRACY, T.S. and HALL, S.D. (1992) Metabolic inversion of (*R*)-ibuprofen: epimerization and hydrolysis of ibuprofenyl-coenzyme A. *Drug Metabolism and Disposition* 20, 322–328.

TRACY, T.S., WIRTHWEIN, D.P. and HALL, S.D. (1993) Metabolic inversion of (*R*)-ibuprofen: formation of ibuprofenyl-coenzyme A. *Drug Metabolism and Disposition* 21, 114–120.

■ CHAPTER 4 ■

VANGIESSEN, G.J. and KAISER, D.G. (1975) GLC determination of ibuprofen [*dl*-2-(*p*-isobutylphenyl)propionic acid] enantiomers in biological specimens. *Journal of Pharmaceutical Sciences* 5, 798–801.

WALKER, J.S., KHIHNICKI, R.D., SEIDEMAN, P. and DAY, R.O. (1993) Pharmacokinetics of ibuprofen enantiomers in plasma and suction blister fluid in healthy volunteers. *Journal of Pharmaceutical Sciences* 82, 787–790.

WALLIS, W.J. and SIMKIN, P.A. (1983) Antirheumatic drug concentrations in human synovial fluid and synovial tissue: observations on extravascular pharmacokinetics. *Clinical Pharmacokinetics* 8, 496–522.

WANWIMOLRUK, S., BROOKS, P.M. and BIRKETT, D.J. (1983) Protein binding of nonsteroidal anti-inflammatory drugs in plasma and synovial fluid of arthritic patients. *British Journal of Clinical Pharmacology* 15, 91–94.

WECHTER, W.J., LOUGHHEAD, D.G., REISCHER, R.J., VANGIESSEN, G.J. and KAISER, D.G. (1974) Enzymatic inversion at saturated carbon: nature and mechanism of the inversion of (R)-(–) *p*-iso-butyl hydratropic acid. *Biochemical and Biophysical Research Communications* 61, 833–837.

WILLIAMS, K., DAY, R., KNIHINICKI, R. and DUFFIELD, A. (1986) The stereoselective uptake of ibuprofen enantiomers into adipose tissue. *Biochemical Pharmacology* 35, 3403–3405.

WILLIAMS, K.M., KNIHINICKI, R.D. and DAY, R.O. (1991) Pharmacokinetics of the enantiomers of ibuprofen in the rabbit. *Agents and Actions* 34, 381–386.

WRIGHT, M.R., SATARI, S., BROCKS, D.R. and JAMALI, F. (1992) Improved high performance liquid chromatographic assay method for the enantiomers of ibuprofen. *Journal of Chromatography* 583, 259–265.

XIAOTAO, Q. and HALL, S.D. (1993) Modulation of enantioselective metabolism and inversion of ibuprofen by xenobiotics in isolated rat hepatocytes. *Journal of Pharmacology and Experimental Therapeutics* 266, 845–851.

XIAOTAO, Q. and HALL, S.D. (1995) Enantioselective effects of experimental diabetes mellitus on the metabolism of ibuprofen. *Journal of Pharmacology and Experimental Therapeutics* 274, 1192–1198.

ZHAO, M.J., PETER, C., HOLTZ, M.C., HUGENELL, N., KOFFEL, J.C. and JUNG, L. (1994) Gas chromatographic spectrometric determination of ibuprofen enantiomers in human plasma using (R)-(–)-2,2,2-trifluoro-1-(9-anthryl)ethanol as derivatizing reagent. *Journal of Chromatography B, Biomedical Applications* 656, 441–446.

ZIA-AMIRHOSSEINI, P.Z., HARRIS, R.Z., BRODSKY, F.M. and BENET, L.Z. (1995) Hypersensitivity to nonsteroidal anti-inflammatory drugs [letter]. *Nature Medicine* 1, 2–4.

Pharmacology and Toxicology of Ibuprofen

K D RAINSFORD

Division of Biomedical Sciences and Biomedical Research Centre,
Sheffield Hallam University, Pond Street, Sheffield S1 1WB, UK

Contents

Ibuprofen is typical of the class of nonsteroidal anti-inflammatory drugs (NSAIDs) and has anti-inflammatory, analgesic and antipyretic activities (Dollery, 1991). In contrast to aspirin, ibuprofen only has relatively weak antithrombotic activity (Thilo *et al.*, 1974; Thomas *et al.*, 1982; Furst, 1994). This is because not only does it not exhibit anticoagulant effects but also it is a weak inhibitor of platelet aggregation in humans (Royer *et al.*, 1985), whereas the prolonged, irreversible, inhibition of platelet cyclooxygenase I (COX-1) results in sustained inhibition of thromboxane production observed with aspirin (Rainsford, 1984). This difference is important for it probably underlies, in part, the relatively low incidence of gastrointestinal (GI) bleeding and ulceration observed with ibuprofen in comparison with aspirin. Moreover, this low GI ulcerogenicity and renal toxicity of ibuprofen distinguish this drug from all other NSAIDs. The modest reversible inhibitory effects on COX isoenzymes combined with the pharmacokinetics of this drug probably account for the relatively high safety profile of ibuprofen.

A summary of the principal molecular and cellular effects of ibuprofen in relation to its pharmacological actions is shown in Figure 5.1. Here the link between pharmacokinetics of ibuprofen and the effects on prostaglandin production and other cellular effects of this drug is emphasized.

5.1 BASIC PHARMACOLOGY AND TOXICOLOGY

5.1.2 Acute anti-inflammatory activity

UV erythema

As mentioned in Chapter 1, the discovery of ibuprofen was based on the assay of this and other propionates initially in the guinea-pig UV erythema model (Adams *et al.*, 1969). This model has been suggested by some as being a model for the discovery of 'aspirin-like' drugs. It is an acute anti-inflammatory model and involves exposing the depilated skin of guinea-pigs (or rats, see Table 5.1) briefly (80–90 s) to UV-B irradiation (wavelength 280–320 nm), a major cause of sunburn in humans (Winder *et al.*, 1958; Otterness and Bliven, 1985). Adams and co-workers (1969, 1970) considerably modified the procedures employed in this assay as established by Wilhelmi (1949) and this had important consequences for establishment of the utility of the model (see Chapter 1).

In the early stages of the development of the acute inflammation there is increased vascular permeability and mast cell degranulation with accompanying release of histamine and 5-hydroxytryptamine (5-HT, serotonin) within 10–15 min (Otterness and Bliven, 1985). There follows in the period of 2–6 h considerable production of prostaglandins (PGs) in the UV-irradiated skin (Otterness and Bliven, 1985). Thus, it is not surprising that inhibitors of PG production are detected in this model (Otterness and Bliven, 1985). However, as indicated later (see section 5.1.6 'Effects on prostaglandin production related

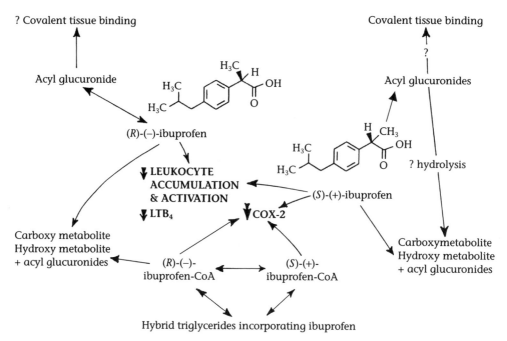

Figure 5.1: Concepts of the principal modes of action in inflammation and related actions of racemic ibuprofen and the relationship to the metabolism of the drug. The major actions of ibuprofen centre on the effects of the (S)-(+) enantiomer in inhibiting cyclooxygenases (COX). In inflammation and in the spinal pathways mediating pain, the effect of the drug is to inhibit the production of prostaglandins by blocking the activity of the inducible COX-2 isoenzyme. Ibuprofen also has actions on leukocyte accumulation and activation; some effects on leukotriene production appear to be ascribed to both (R)-(–) and (S)-(+) isoforms of the drug. These effects on leukocytes may occur at somewhat higher concentrations than the effects on prostaglandin production. Other actions of ibuprofen in regulating the production or activity cytokines may occur in specific conditions; some of these effects may be a consequence of effects on prostaglandin production or on leukocyte functions. The metabolism of the (R)-(–) enantiomer of ibuprofen occurs by the formation of an acyl-coenzyme A (acyl-CoA) intermediate that is derived from fatty acid biosynthesis. The formation of 'hybrid' triglycerides of ibuprofen may occur from this pathway and lead to accumulation of the drug in lipids, including those in membranes. The consequences of this metabolic route of the drug are not known. While acyl glucuronides are among the major end-products of drug metabolism, their reactivity with proteins/peptides and other molecules (as postulated with other NSAIDs that cause liver injury) is probably relatively weak since hepatic injury is rare with this drug.

to pharmacological activities') the irreversible inhibition of COXs seen with aspirin is not a feature of ibuprofen. To some extent it is surprising that ibuprofen proved to be a relatively potent inhibitor of UV erythema in comparison with aspirin (Adams and Cobb, 1963; Adams *et al.*, 1969), especially in the long-term since the prolonged inhibition of skin PGs by aspirin might be expected to lead to more sustained inhibition of UV erythema than with ibuprofen (Table 5.1). However, this explanation does not consider the relative contribution of pharmacokinetics of these drugs to their anti-inflammatory effects. While both drugs will accumulate in the inflamed tissues exposed to UV, it is

TABLE 5.1

Anti-erythema activity of ibuprofen compared with other NSAIDs or analgesics in guinea-pigs or rats

Drug	Guinea-pig					Rat	
	Approx. ED$_{50}$ [a] (mg/kg p.o.) (1)	Relative potency (1)	ED$_{50}$ (mg/kg p.o.) (95% CI) 2 doses (–1 h, 0 h) (2)	Effective dose (mg/kg p.o.) 2 doses (–1 h, 0 h) (3)	ED$_{50}$ (mg/kg p.o.) (4)	Approx. ED$_{50}$ (mg/kg p.o.) (5)	Approx. ED$_{50}$ (mg/kg topical) (5)
Ibuprofen	2.5–5.0	16–32	5.0 (1.7–15.0)		3.0	22.4	0.3
Antipyrine				100			
Aspirin	80	1.0		100–200	115	148	9.2
Diclofenac					9.0		
Flufenamic acid						38.5	10.9
Flurbiprofen					0.2		0.28
Indomethacin			3.0 (1.6–5.6)		6.0	1.3	1.3
Ketoprofen			8.9 (3.0–26.8)		13.0		
Mefenamic acid			35.5 (12.7–99.3)				
Naproxen					3.0		
Paracetamol	[> 240] [b]					> 100	
Phenylbutazone	[10] [b]		20.9 (7.6–57.7)	18.0	8.0	17.2	5.6
Piroxicam					0.25		
Salicylate. Na	[120] [b]			200	9.0		
Sulindac					16.0		
Tolmetin. Na							

[a] Approximate values only since authors point out that dose–response curves are not similar with ibuprofen compared with aspirin.
[b] [ ] denotes effective oral dose.
References: (1) Adams et al. (1969), Adams and Cobb (1963); (2) Tsukada et al. (1978); (3) Winder et al. (1958); (4) Otterness et al. (1979); (5) Law and Lewis (1977).

unlikely that appreciable amounts of aspirin would accumulate there (due to the rapid conversion of aspirin to salicylate); instead salicylate would predominate therein, a weaker reversible inhibitor of PG production. With ibuprofen the plasma clearance of this drug as reflected by the terminal half-time of elimination ($t_{1/2}$) is about 2–3 h in most species (including humans) (Brocks and Jamali, see Chapter 4). In comparison, aspirin has a $t_{1/2}$ of only 10–15 min and the rapid de-esterification to salicylate ($t_{1/2} = 2$–4 h) means that the latter is the predominant component (70–80% total salicylates) in the circulation (Rainsford, 1984).

The bioconversion of racemic or *rac*-ibuprofen leads to production of (*S*)-(+)-ibuprofen from the (*R*)-(–) enantiomer; the former being the more potent PG synthesis inhibitor (Figure 5.1). Hence, metabolism of *rac*-ibuprofen leads to production of the more potent anti-inflammatory component, whereas with aspirin metabolism to salicylate leads to a less active drug being formed. Thus, understanding of the relative *in vivo* potencies of these and other NSAIDs depends on understanding of their pharmacokinetics and especially the amounts of active drug(s) accumulating at sites of action.

Effects of ibuprofen compared with other NSAIDs in UV erythema

Adams and co-workers (1969) observed that ibuprofen was 16–32 times more potent than aspirin in the UV erythema assay. In the UV assay adapted to rats, Law and Lewis (1977) showed that ibuprofen given orally was 7 times more potent than aspirin but was about 1/20 as potent of indomethacin p.o. In the guinea-pig model Tsukada *et al.* (1978) showed that ibuprofen was less potent as an anti-inflammatory agent than was indomethacin. Using the two-dose regime (with the drugs given at –1 and 0 h) Tsukada *et al.* (1978) showed that ibuprofen has a high degree of oral potency, intermediate between those of indomethacin and ketoprofen, although the 95% fiducial limits overlapped (Table 5.1). These results are surprising in relation to their prostaglandin synthesis inhibitory effects since ibuprofen is appreciably less potent than the other two drugs (see Section 5.1.6). Interestingly, Law and Lewis (1977) showed that ibuprofen applied topically in the UV erythema assay in rats was among the most potent of all NSAIDs tested (Table 5.1).

In a variants of the skin inflammation model in which arachidonic acid or PGE_2 are injected subdermally, it has been found that ibuprofen is only slightly less potent than indomethacin (Ohnishi *et al.*, 1982). An ointment of ibuprofen (3%) topically applied proved among the more potent of all NSAIDs in the UV erythema assay in guinea-pigs (Takeuchi *et al.*, 1985). The drug was slightly more potent than topically applied flufenamic acid and appreciably more so than phenylbutazone and hydrocortisone-17-valerate (Takeuchi *et al.*, 1985). Similarly, topically applied ibuprofen was more potent than beta-methasone-17-valearate in the arachidonic acid-induced erythema model in guinea pigs. These results suggest that ibuprofen has high oral and percutaneous anti-inflammatory activity in skin reactions involving PG-related systems.

Carrageenan oedema in rats

This model was originally developed by Winter, Risley and Nuss, in 1962, to assess anti-inflammatory activity of NSAIDs in response to injection of carrageenan into the hind-paws of rats (Winter *et al.*, 1962). It has since been employed extensively in the search for new NSAIDs and in defining their mode of action (Otterness and Bliven, 1985). There has subsequently been development of the carrageenan-induced inflammation in the pleural cavity as a model for quantitation of the fluid exudate, cellular infiltration and inflammatory mediators during the inflammatory response (Vinegar *et al.*, 1976, 1982). The sequence of inflammatory responses differs between these models (Vinegar, 1976, 1982) and this is an important consideration when trying to define the mode of action of NSAIDs.

Essentially, the sequence of inflammatory events in both models begins at about 10–20 min with perivascular accumulation and adhesion of polymorphonuclear leukocytes (PMNs) to capillary walls following the expression of leukocyte and endothelial adhesion molecules. There follows at 1–3 h increased capillary permeability, exudation of plasma components and fluid and the extravasation of blood cells adjacent to the location of the inflammagen (Di Rosa *et al.*, 1971; Bolam *et al.*, 1974; Vinegar *et al.*, 1969, 1976, 1982). The accumulation and activation of PMNs at inflamed sites probably results from the activation of complement production (Vinegar *et al.*, 1982). Also, within the first hour kinins are produced that act on cell receptors and consequently lead to activation of phospholipase A_2 and subsequent release of arachidonate to form prostaglandins (Vinegar *et al.*, 1976, 1982).

Although mast cells accumulate in inflamed sites, it is generally considered that there is little, if any, activation of these cells to release 5-hydroxytryptamine (5-HT; serotonin) and histamine (Van Arman *et al.*, 1965; Bolam *et al.*, 1974; Vinegar *et al.*, 1976, 1982; Horakava *et al.*, 1980). In contrast to the effects of carrageenan, the subplantar or pleural injection of yeast in rats yields appreciable activation of mast cells (Van Arman *et al.*, 1965).

The initial phase of inflammation induced by subplantar injection of carrageenan results only in a small degree of footpad swelling due to accumulation of fluid (oedema). The secondary phase of inflammation following subplantar carrageenan results in much greater footpad swelling than seen in the first phase, peaking at 3–5 h (Vinegar *et al.*, 1976, 1982). In contrast, fluid accumulation following intrapleural injection of this inflammagen is progressive and peaks at about 9 h (Vinegar *et al.*, 1976, 1982). Paw swelling declines progressively over 6–24 h, while pleural effusion extends over a longer period of 24–48 h (Vinegar *et al.*, 1976, 1982). The relative practical advantages of the pleural effusion model are that this allows for sampling of pleural fluid for the determination of cellular accumulation and inflammatory mediators not readily possible with the footpad model, whereas with the latter paw swelling can be readily measured so that it is a faster way to measure anti-inflammatory activity of drugs.

CHAPTER 5

In both, the secondary phase of subplantar and pleural inflammation results in release of lysosomal hydrolases, oxyradicals and prostaglandins (PGs) E_2, $F_{2\alpha}$ and 6-keto-$PGF_{1\alpha}$ (Willis, 1970; Vinegar et al., 1982). Leukocyte COX-2 is induced at 1–3 h in the pleural cavity of rats injected with carrageenan (Harada et al., 1996) and this probably accounts for the amplification of PG production. While the exact period of cytokine production is not well defined, it is likely that interleukins (ILs) 1, 6 and 8 together with tumour necrosis factor-α (TNF-α) are produced during the secondary phase of inflammation (Dunn, 1991). Monocytes also accumulate in this period (Vinegar et al., 1976, 1982) and their activation to macrophages leads to cytokine production.

Prostaglandin production in the region of the cerebral ventricles of the brain has been shown to accompany paw oedema (Bhattacharya and Das, 1984), though this might result from pyrogenic substances present in carrageenan preparations (Vinegar et al., 1976) as well as from the IL-1 released from inflamed sites into the circulation. Recent studies have also shown that carrageenan-induced paw oedema results in increased levels of immunoreactive PGE_2 (reflecting increased COX-2) in the dorsal horn coincident with expression of proteins *jun/fos* from oncogene expression (Malmberg and Yaksh, 1995; Buritova et al., 1996a). The latter gene activation may also reflect production of other inflammatory mediators. Elevated footpad temperature accompanies the oedemogenic response (Vinegar et al., 1969) and this may also result from IL-1 and pyrogenic substances acting on the hypothalamus.

NSAIDs inhibit the second phase of paw swelling with little effect on the first phase (Vinegar et al., 1969). These effects have been ascribed to the drugs' inhibitory actions on prostaglandin production and the accumulation and activation of PMNs (Higgs, 1989). Their relative activities in inhibiting PG production compared with accumulation and activation of leukocytes varies from drug to drug. Where drugs act in the yeast oedema or polymyxin-B models, additional influences on mast cell activation must be invoked (Van Arman et al., 1965; Bertelli and Soldani, 1979). The kaolin oedema model is, in contrast, characterized by profound accumulation of fluid containing prostaglandins and kinins with few leukocytes (Gemmell et al., 1979). These differences in the mediators and cells involved in the expression of the inflammatory responses in these models emphasize the importance of knowing which of these are produced at different phases of the inflammatory process. The drug actions on the various inflammatory mediators will influence the end response of local swelling and pain. Thus, the actions of NSAIDs in these models depends on the type and dose of inflammagen employed and the time course of effects on different phases of inflammation.

Effects of ibuprofen compared with other NSAIDs in carrageenan oedema

The acute anti-inflammatory effects of ibuprofen in the carrageenan paw oedema model show that this drug is appreciably more potent than aspirin and phenylbutazone, but less so than indomethacin (Table 5.2). Under single dose conditions where the drug is given

TABLE 5.2

Anti-oedemic effects of ibuprofen compared with other NSAIDs in paw assays in rats

Drug	Approx. ED$_{50}$ (mg/kg p.o.) (1)	Carrageenan assay					Polymyxin B ED$_{50}$ (mg/kg p.o. at 6 h approx.) (5)
		ED$_{50}$[a] (mg/kg p.o.) (95% CI) (2)	MED (mg/kg) (3)	Relative potency[b] (cf. MED) (3)	Approx.[c] ED$_{35}$ (mg/kg p.o.) (3)	(4)	
Ibuprofen	6	24.3 (10.6–39.2)	0.6	1	9	6–18	150
Aspirin	100–300	69.9 (33.4–146)	39.4	0.02	100	60	300
Fenclofenac		9.1 (4.0–20.7)	23.8	0.03	60		
Flufenamic acid							
Indomethacin	2–6	3.3 (2.1–7.3)	1.0	0.6	3.0	1.3	3–9
Phenylbutazone	17–50	13.8 (6.4–29.7)	7.2	0.08	15	10–30	25

[a] Ibuprofen has a long dose-response curve in this assay.
[b] Potency with respect to ibuprofen = 1.
[c] Drugs given 1 h before subplantar injection of carrageenan.
References: (1) Adams et al. (1969); (2) Shimizu et al. (1975); (3) Atkinson and Leach (1976); (4) Nuss et al. (1976); (5) Bertelli and Soldani (1979).

60 min prior to carrageenan, ibuprofen is about 10 times more potent than aspirin but about one-half to one-third as potent as indomethacin (Table 5.2). Thus, the relative anti-oedemic effects of ibuprofen appear from these data to be comparable with the anti-erythemic activity of the drug.

Otterness, Wiseman and Gans (1979) attempted to determine the relevance of the rat carrageenan paw oedema assay and the guinea-pig UV-erythema assay for predicting clinical dosage in rheumatoid arthritis. They observed that the correlation of the logarithm of the ED_{50} values in these assays for 12 NSAIDs (including ibuprofen) compared with the logarithm of the daily clinical dose of these drugs was better with data from the carrageenan assay than from the UV-erythema test. However, it is of interest that the data for ibuprofen in both these assays appeared well above the regression line, suggesting that this drug may be an outlier.

Using the carrageenan pleural effusion model, Mikami and Miyasaka (1983) showed that ibuprofen 50–100 mg/kg p.o. reduced leukocyte numbers and that 25–100 mg/kg p.o. of the drug reduced exudate volume in rats; this being about the same order of dose for effect as that of phenylbutazone and almost the same as diclofenac. Other NSAIDs exhibited variable responses. Thus, aspirin 50–100 mg/kg p.o. significantly reduced exudate volume but not leukocyte counts. The most potent NSAIDs in this model were indomethacin and ketoprofen, having inhibitory effects on exudate volume and leukocyte accumulation at doses of 1 mg/kg and 2.5–5.0 mg/kg p.o., respectively.

Overall, these results in carrageenan–oedema models show that ibuprofen has acute anti-inflammatory effects that are of intermediate potency and involve reduction of fluid and leukocyte accumulation in the prostaglandin phase of inflammation.

Effects in other oedema models

Gemmell, Cottney and Lewis (1979) compared the effects of 7 NSAIDs and a range of immunoregulatory and other pharmacological agents in four models of paw oedema in rats induced by koalin, zymosan and anti-rat IgG and that from the reversed-passive Arthus reaction (RPA) reaction. All the NSAIDs, except fenclofenac, inhibited the paw oedema reactions in these four models to varying degrees, fenclofenac only inhibiting the RPA (Gemmell et al., 1979). The ED_{50} for ibuprofen in the kaolin oedema model was 163 mg/kg, which was high relative to other NSAIDs (e.g. indomethacin, naproxen and phenylbutazone) but lower than that of aspirin. Ibuprofen was moderately effective in the RPA and zymosan-induced oedema and slightly more potent in the anti-IgG assay. Since these four assays involve complement activation but differ somewhat mechanistically from one another, this is suggestive of a broad spectrum of effects of ibuprofen like that of the NSAIDs (excepting fenclofenac) on this system (Gemmell et al., 1979). Thus, in the zymosan assay there is activation of complement via the alternative pathway (Gemmell et al., 1979). In the kaolin oedema there is participation of prostaglandins, kinins and complement but not amines (Gemmell et al., 1979). The other two assays involve immunological reactions.

In the anti-IgG reactions this antibody would be expected to combine locally in the paw with rat IgG, leading to activation of the complement system by the alternative pathway and resulting in inflammation by anaphylatoxin formation (Gemmell *et al.*, 1979). The RPA also involves complement activation (Gemmell *et al.*, 1979).

In the polymyxin B-induced paw oedema model, where the initial phase is accompanied by release of amines, ibuprofen is about twice as potent as aspirin, slightly less potent than the potent PG synthesis inhibitor ketoprofen, but about 10 times less so than indomethacin (Table 5.2; Bertelli and Soldani, 1979). However, the high doses of ibuprofen and aspirin and shallow slopes of the dose–response curves indicate the drugs are probably not very potent. More pronounced dose–response effects are evident at 6 h during the PG phase of the inflammatory response. Overall, there appear to be relatively weak effects of ibuprofen on the amine phase of inflammation in the polymyxin B model.

5.1.2 Chronic anti-inflammatory activity

Effects in adjuvant arthritis

This animal model is one of a number of *in vivo* systems that resemble rheumatoid and related polyarthritic conditions in humans (Pearson and Wood, 1959; Benslay and Nickander, 1982; Rainsford, 1982a). The joint manifestations of this disease include (a) development of granulation-like tissue and hyperplasia of synovial lining cells to form a pannus-like tissue, (b) mononuclear cell infiltration and activation, and (c) periosteal and, to a lesser extent, other bone and cartilage destruction with accompanying bone nodules (Pearson and Wood, 1959; Rainsford, 1982a). The development of the disease is dependent on (a) the strain of rats employed, (b) the source and preparation of suspending media for the mycobacterial adjuvant, (c) the housing (e.g. under special pathogen free vs open colony conditions) and other environmental conditions, and (d) the timing of administration of the test drugs.

Using the established model of arthritis induced by injection into one of the hind paws of killed *Mycobacterium tuberculosis* in mineral oil in the susceptible Wistar Lewis strain, Atkinson and Leach (1976) showed that when a range of NSAIDs were dosed orally in the period from 21 to 17 days post injection of the adjuvant, ibuprofen was slightly more potent than aspirin but less so than most other NSAIDs in controlling paw and tibiotarsal joint swelling (Table 5.3). These results indicate that ibuprofen is moderately effective as an inhibitor of chronic joint inflammation and bone damage compared with other NSAIDs. Selph *et al.* (1993) found that ibuprofen 50 mg/kg/day given to rats with established adjuvant arthritis consistently lowered fibrinogen levels (a marker of acute-phase reactions) concomitantly with improvement in joint scores. However, joint scores improved with this drug only after day 35, suggesting that it takes a relatively long time for functional improvement to be evident with this disease.

TABLE 5.3

Antiarthritic effects of ibuprofen compared with other NSAIDs in rats in established adjuvant disease

Drug	Approx. ED_{50} (mg/kg) (1)	MED (mg/kg, p.o.) (drug @ days 21–27) (2)	Relative potency[b] (95% CI) (2)	Approx. ED_{50} (mg/kg) (3)
Ibuprofen	45[a]	24.4	1.0 (0.4–2.4)	> 30
Alclofenac			7.3 (3.6–14.2)	
Aspirin		71.7	0.5 (0.3–1.0)	
Benoxaprofen				10
Diclofenac. Na			508 (250–1050)	
Fenclofenac		3.0	8.3 (NS[c])	
Fenoprofen.Ca			7.3 (2.6–20.8)	
Indomethacin	0.3–0.9	0.19	200 (108–367)	1.0
Ketoprofen			317 (142–553)	
Naproxen			36.6 (15–91.7)	30
Phenylbutazone	10–30	2.2	7.1 (3.7–13.3)	30
Piroxicam				0.3–3.0

[a] Doses of 135 mg/kg (Adams et al., 1969) ibuprofen, or 2.7 mg/kg/day indomethacin produced deaths in some rats.
[b] Potency with respect to ibuprofen = 1.
[a] NS = not stated.
References: (1) Adams et al. (1969); (2) Atkinson and Leach (1976); (3) Benslay and Nickander (1982).

Benslay and Nickander (1982) observed that daily oral dosing of 30 mg/kg/day ibuprofen from day 15 post injection (of adjuvant) to day 30 caused statistically significant reduction in hindpaw swelling in both injected and noninjected hindpaws but no significant reduction in radiologically observed bone destruction. Other more potent prostaglandin synthesis inhibitors (e.g. indomethacin, flurbiprofen and piroxicam) produced a dose-related reduction in both swelling and bone destruction, but often this was accompanied by the development of gastrointestinal ulceration or evidence of bleeding (i.e. malaena). Benoxaprofen, an NSAID with relatively weak effects on prostaglandin production but with leukotriene synthesis inhibitory effects, showed dose-related reduction of both soft-tissue paw swelling and bone destruction (Benslay and Nickander, 1982).

In contrast to these results, Maruyama and co-workers (1977) observed that ibuprofen 100 mg/kg/day reduced the joint damage observed radiologically in adjuvant arthritic rats to the extent of appearing almost the same as that in normal (nonarthritic) animals. Similar reduction in joint damage was observed with indomethacin 1 mg/kg/day, phenylbutazone 25 mg/kg/day and aspirin 200 mg/kg/day. The authors also observed a significant reduction in plasma inflammation units and an elevation in the albumin/globulin ratios with 50 mg/kg/day ibuprofen as well as with 1 mg/kg/day indomethacin and 25 mg/kg/day phenylbutazone. The erythrocyte sedimentation rate (ESR) was also slightly reduced with ibuprofen 50 mg/kg/day although this was more pronounced with the other drugs.

Plasma iron concentrations usually decline in adjuvant arthritis as part of the systemic acute-phase response to the disease. Connolly and co-workers (1989) showed that disease-modifying antiarthritic drugs (DMARDs) restore the plasma iron concentrations after 2 weeks treatment in established adjuvant disease. They did not observe a significant improvement with NSAIDs, although there was a clear trend towards a dose-related improvement with ibuprofen 30–100 mg/kg/day that was not seen with the other drugs. This aspect clearly deserves more detailed investigation, especially in view of the importance of iron status in arthritic diseases.

Overall, these results show that while not particularly potent (compared with some other NSAIDs such as indomethacin and phenylbutazone), ibuprofen does effectively control the chronic joint injury and disease manifestations in adjuvant arthritis.

Kaiser and Glenn (1974) observed that ibuprofen and aspirin interacted with one another in the adjuvant arthritis model, the responses of which which depended on whether the drugs were given prophylactically or therapeutically. In the former case the antiarthritic effects were greater with the drug combinations, whereas in the latter the response obtained with the combination was less than that obtained with ibuprofen alone. In attempts to explain these drug interactions the authors determined the plasma levels of the drugs in combination or alone. They observed that aspirin lowered the plasma levels of ibuprofen by 20–65%, whereas ibuprofen had no effects on salicylate levels. Thus it is possible that the effect of aspirin in lowering the plasma ibuprofen levels could explain the diminished response of ibuprofen when in combination with aspirin in the therapeutic but not the prophylactic dosing regime. There is no obvious explanation for the pronounced interaction between aspirin and ibuprofen given in the prophylactic regime.

Other chronic arthritis models

Using an adaptation of the rat adjuvant arthritis model, Sharma and Sharma (1977) studied the effects of anti-inflammatory compounds on the development of adjuvant arthritis in rabbits which enabled the progression of the disease to be examined over a period of 22 weeks, much longer than is generally observed in rats. They observed that ibuprofen 100 mg/kg/day resulted in a significant reduction in joint swelling from week 4 to week 22. A similar reduction was observed with phenylbutazone 100 mg/kg/day. The overall percentage reductions were 60.5% and 57.4%, respectively. The results with the high dose of phenylbutazone are surprising since this drug normally produces gastrointestinal injury in arthritic rats at these doses. The results suggest that phenylbutazone is well tolerated in rabbits. Further investigations of the time course of effects of NSAIDs including ibuprofen are indicated since this model would appear to have particular advantages in view of the prolonged nature of adjuvant disease in rabbits.

CHAPTER 5

TABLE 5.4

Oral analgesic activity of ibuprofen compared with other NSAIDs in rodents

Drug	Mice (PBQ) ED_{50} (mg/kg) (95% CL)[a]				Rat (Randal–Selitto) ED_{50} (mg/kg) (95% CL)			Rat (AA/flex) ED_{50} (mg/kg) (95% CL)	
	(1)	(2)	(3)	(4)	(3)	(2)	(4)	(3)	(4)
Ibuprofen	82.2	14.7	4.9	63 (34–114)	3.2	37	98 (38–250)	11	9 (4–20)
Aspirin	182		120	224 (137–368)	32		276 (127–601)	180	108 (48–243)
Benoxaprofen	25.4								
Diflunisal	55.6		156					6	
Fenclofenac	168								
Fenoprofen.Ca	3.7								
Flurbiprofen									
Indomethacin	19.0	0.6	0.4	3.8 (1.3–11.0)	1.0	9	5.6 (2.6–12)	1.8	0.8 (0.4–1.6)
Ketorolac									
Meclofenamate.Na	9.6								
Mefenamic acid	20.7								
Naproxen	24.1	9.4				14			
Oxaprozin				29 (14–58)			174 (91–330)		89 (35–222)
Phenylbutazone	129		32	244 (176–337)			112 (54–285)	7	12 (5–28)
Piroxicam	0.44		1.9		1.7				
Sulindac	7.2		18					2.0	
Suprofen		5	5		0.15			4.6	
Tometin.Na	1.3								
Zomepirac	0.7		0.6		3.2			1.2	
Paracetamol		216	216		> 100			216	
Dipyrone		50	50		> 400				
Codeine		21	21		5.6			23	

Abbreviations: PBQ, phenyl benzoquinone writhing assay; AA/flex, adjuvant arthritis flexion test; HAc, acetic acid writhing; ACh, Acetylcholine writhing.
[a] Drugs given 30 min p.o. before 0.03% phenylquinone i.p.
[b] Drugs given 2 min before s.c. injection of 5% formalin. ED_{50} R(–) > 270mg/kg p.o. S(+) 16(7–36)mg/kg p.o.
References: (**1**) Pong *et al.* (1985); (**2**) Griswold *et al.* (1991); (**3**) Otterness and Bliven (1985); (**4**) Amanuma *et al.* (1984); (**5**) Malmberg and Yaksh (1992a).

Essentially negative results have been obtained with ibuprofen and other NSAIDs in several other chronic models of arthritic disease. Thus no improvement has been found from ibuprofen treatment in antigen-induced arthritis in BALB/c mice (Cottney *et al.*, 1980; Hunneyball *et al.*, 1986; Crossley *et al.*, 1987), the adriamycin-induced paw inflammation in mice (Siegel *et al.*, 1980), the collagen II/Freund's Complete Adjuvant arthritis in mice (Griswold *et al.*, 1988), the Dumonde–Glynn chronic immune synovitis induced by local injections of albumin into the joints of rabbits (Goldlust and Rich (1981), the Arthus reaction in rats (Pflum and Greame, 1979), or the autoimmune lupus disease in NZB/W mice (Kelley *et al.*, 1982). Most DMARDs or immunosuppressant drugs are effective in these models (Pflum and Greame, 1979; Cottney *et al.*, 1980; Hunneyball *et al.*, 1986; Crossley *et al.*, 1987, 1989; Schuurs *et al.*, 1989). These results suggest that ibuprofen, like many other NSAIDs, does not exhibit disease-modifying activity such as would be evident with the agents (D-penicillamine, gold salts) used to treat autoimmune arthropathies.

Mice HAc ED$_{50}$ (mg/kg) (95% CL) (4)	Mice ACh ED$_{50}$ (mg/kg) (95% CL) (4)	Mice tail pressure ED$_{50}$ (mg/kg p.o.) (95% CL) (5)	Rat AgNO$_3$ arth. ED$_{50}$ (mg/kg p.o.) (95% CL) (5)	Rat formalin ED$_{50}$ (mg/kg p.o.) (95% CL)[b]	
				Intrathecal (5)	Intraperitoneal (5)
112 (79–190) 227 (121–425)	7.2 (4.3–12.1) 23 (11–45)	319 (184–547) > 400	115 (58–230) 440 (244–792)	18.9 (9–38)/ 27(18–41)	8 (514–12)
11.7 (5.3–26)	0.6 (0.3–1.3)	> 20	> 20	2.1 (1–4.3) 1.9 (1.2–4) 5.2 (3–8)	3.1 (2.3–4) 2.6 (1.3–5) 3.0 (2–4)
45 (18–112) 300 (174–519)	3.9 (2–8) 28 (14–57)	306 (184–509) > 300	343 (150–781) 115 (58–230)		
				5.9 (4–9) 257 (163–405)	5.5 (2–14) 6.0 (0.8–46)

5.1.3 Analgesic activity

Most frequently employed animal models for assaying analgesic activity of the NSAIDs include (a) abdominal writhing (induced by phenylquinone, acetic acid or acetylcholine) in mice; (b) the Randall–Selitto test in rats (in which pain is elicited by subplantar injection of ~20% yeast); or (c) the joint flexion of rats in whom adjuvant arthritis has been induced. The first two models are acute while the latter is a chronic model. Other acute models employ subplantar injection of pain-eliciting noxious agents (e.g. intra-articular silver nitrate in rats; Amanuma *et al.*, 1984).

NSAIDs and analgesics vary considerably in their pain inhibitory effects in these models (Table 5.4). The variation depends on (a) the pain elicited by the noxious agent and the peak of pain response compared with control (or the 'delta') produced by the pharmacological agent, (b) the rate of absorption and clearance of the drug in the animal species, and (c) experimental variables such as timing of the dose of drug in relation to that of the analgesic agent or pain-eliciting procedure. The effects of different classes of analgesic agents will depend on their respective sites and mechanisms of action in the peripheral compared with central or spinal nervous pathways of pain transmission.

The oral analgesic activities of 15 NSAIDs (including ibuprofen) in the phenylquinone visceral writhing test in mice have been shown to be linearly correlated with the recommended human analgesic or anti-inflammatory dosages (Pong et al., 1985). This suggests that it is possible to use the data from the phenylquinone visceral writhing assay to predict the human dosage of NSAIDs required for analgesia (Pong et al., 1985). This prediction does not take into account the varying clearances of the drugs in the two different species.

Current concepts of the mode of action of NSAIDs in controlling pain suggest that these drugs act at both peripheral and spinal/higher nervous centres (Urquhart, 1993; Bannwarth et al., 1995a: Björkman, 1995; Walker, 1995; Cashman, 1996; McCormack and Urquhart, 1995). The classical view that pain relief from NSAIDs is partly due to the anti-inflammatory activity of the drugs, has in recent years been modified by recognition that these drugs also have actions at different loci of the spino-thalamic pathways of nerve transmission and the modulation of painful stimuli (Urquhart, 1993; Bannwarth et al., 1995; Björkman, 1995; Walker, 1995; Cashman, 1996; McCormack, 1994; McCormack and Urquhart, 1995). A recent analysis by McCormack and Urquhart (1996) shows that the potency of NSAIDs as analgesics relative to their anti-inflammatory activity varies with clinical efficacy. This analysis implies that the analgesic effects can be dissociated from the anti-inflammatory activity of NSAIDs.

Mechanisms of NSAID analgesia involve prostaglandin-independent, as well as PG-dependent mechanisms. Musculoskeletal pain involves excitation of nerves that results in both peripheral and central sensitization (Woolf, 1989, 1991). Neural mediation of central sensitization involves (a) the excitatory amino acids glutamate and aspartate acting on N-methyl-D-aspartate (NMDA) receptors, and (b) substance P and related neurokinins acting on NK-1 receptors (Björkman, 1995; Walker, 1995; Cashman, 1996; McCormack, 1994; McCormack and Urquhart, 1995). Hyperalgesia leads to increased levels of immunoreactive PGE_2 and increased expression of the inducible cyclooxygenase, COX-2, in the dorsal horn concomitant with expression of *jun/fos* oncogene proteins (Malmberg and Yaksh, 1995; Buritova et al., 1996a). There is evidence that there are interactions between the spinal production of PGE_2 and NMDA-receptor mediated events during inflammatory nociceptive transmission (Buritova et al., 1996a,b). Furthermore, inhibition of PG production by NSAIDs alone or in combination with an NMDA-receptor agonist inhibits the expression of spinal c-Fos (Buritova et al., 1996a,b). There is also evidence for the participation of nitric oxide in nociceptive transmission and in the analgesic effects of NSAIDs (Björkman, 1995; Granados-Soto et al., 1995).

Effects of ibuprofen compared with other NSAIDs in analgesic models

In the mouse phenylbenzoquinone writhing model the ED_{50} for ibuprofen varies considerably between different studies, being 4.9–98 mg/kg (Table 5.4). To some extent this variability is attributable to variations in the time of dosage and other experimental factors. The 95% confidence limits (CL) reported for the ED_{50} values by one group (Amanuma *et al.*, 1984) reflect the high variability with this as well as other NSAIDs in this model. The data suggest that the responses obtained reflect high intra-animal variability, a feature that is well known to those experienced with this experimental model. The main factor accounting for this variability is the fact that the counting of the number of writhes following injection of the irritant has appreciable behavioural as well as observer error. If the averaged ED_{50} values for ibuprofen are compared with two other established standards, aspirin and indomethacin (Table 5.4), it is seen that ibuprofen is 4.3 times more potent than aspirin and 6.7 times less potent than indomethacin. More precise estimates of relative potency may be obtained by comparing the individual potencies of these drugs using data of Pong *et al.* (1985), Otterness and Bliven (1985) and Amanuma *et al.* (1984). This analysis reveals that ibuprofen is 10 times more potent than aspirin and 11 times less potent than indomethacin. Probably the best interpretation of the data overall in this model is that ibuprofen is about half way in between the potency extremes of aspirin (at the low end) and indomethacin (at the upper end) of ranges of analgesic activity. In comparison, paracetamol is about half the potency of aspirin, and thus ibuprofen has greater potency than paracetamol (Otterness and Bliven, 1985).

Similar variability in responses to NSAIDs is observed in the mouse writhing models where acetic acid or acetylcholine are employed (Table 5.4). However, the data on drug effects on acetylcholine from the same authors (Amanuma *et al.*, 1984) in studies of NSAIDs in the acetic acid and phenylbenzoquinone models appear to have smaller confidence intervals, reflecting lower experimental error. The relative potencies in the acetylcholine writhing model indicate that ibuprofen is 3.2 times more potent than aspirin and 12 times less potent than indomethacin. In contrast, in the acetic acid writhing model all these NSAIDs were consistently about 10–12 times less potent than in the acetylcholine model (Table 5.4). Ibuprofen is twice as potent as aspirin and 9.6 times less potent than indomethacin.

In the tail pressure assay in mice, NSAIDs (including ibuprofen) have such high ED_{50} values as to indicate lack of pharmacological selectivity. This model is probably more selective for opiates, so that the lack of effects of NSAIDs probably indicates their relative inactivity on CNS pathways involving mediation by opiates.

Studies on the various acute and chronic pain models in rats, as in mice mentioned above, also showed variations in drug potency between the models (Table 5.4). The data of Amanuma *et al.* (1984) show a consistently lower order of potency in the yeast paw pain or Randall–Selitto models compared with others (Table 5.4). The data from these authors indicate that ibuprofen is 2.8 times more potent than aspirin, which is 17.5 times less potent than indomethacin. In their review, Otterness and Bliven (1985) state that ibuprofen is 10 times more potent in this test than aspirin and 2.8 times less so than indomethacin.

Intrathecal ibuprofen has been shown to be 1.4 times more potent as an analgesic than aspirin and 10 times less so than indomethacin (Table 5.4). The relative doses for effects of the NSAIDs given intrathecally were comparable with their effects following intraperitoneal administration, with the exception of aspirin which was about 3.3 times less potent when given intrathecally. The relative effects of the other NSAIDs given by the two routes suggests that they have appreciable central effects, especially at the level of spinal nerves adjacent to where the NSAIDs were administered. Interestingly, paracetamol was 43 times less potent when given intrathecally than intraperitoneally, suggesting this drug has more pronounced peripheral than central analgesic effects. Discrimination of central analgesic effects of the two enantiomers of ibuprofen was seen in these studies. Thus, the PG synthesis-inhibitory (S)-(+) enantiomer was > 17 times more potent than (R)-(–)-ibuprofen (Table 5.4). This suggests that the component of central analgesia from ibuprofen (i.e. (R)-(–) vs (S)-(+)) is largely due to effects of the (S)-(+) enantiomer in inhibiting PG synthesis.

Another feature noted in these studies was that the rank order of potency of intrathecally administered NSAIDs in rats related to their inhibitory effects on *ex vivo* PG synthesis reported by others in mouse brain (Malmberg and Yaksh, 1992a). Unfortunately, the authors did not examine the effects of intraperitoneally administered racemate or the enantiomers of ibuprofen in this study, so it is not possible to conclude any peripheral versus central effects of the enantiomers of ibuprofen.

However, Wang and co-workers (1994) observed that intrathecally administered (S)-(+)-ibuprofen 0.25–1.5 mg produced a dose-related and time-dependent increase in tail-flick latency in rats. Interestingly, these authors also observed that there was no significant difference between the effects of 1.5 or 0.5 mg (S)-(+)-ibuprofen and 0.025 or 0.05 mg morphine. These results suggest that (S)-(+)-ibuprofen has direct spinal analgesic effects which, though not identical mechanistically, are comparable with that of morphine.

Among the convincing evidence of direct CNS/spinal analgesic activity of NSAIDs is that from the studies by Malmberg and Yaksh (1992a), in which they studied the analgesic response in rats after intrathecal compared with intraperitoneal administration of NSAIDs. It should be noted that the experimental protocol employed by these authors involved use of halothane anaesthesia prior to subcutaneous administration in the dorsal surface of the right hind paw with 50 μl 5% formalin. The anaesthetic may have caused some masking of the flinching response in the phase I period after administering formalin and the test drugs, which is why the authors may not have observed pronounced analgesic effects of the NSAIDs. The data obtained on the dose–response effects of NSAIDs (Table 5.4) was on the slope of the pain response elicited at 10–30 min after formalin injection at which there was, typically, most active response to NSAIDs.

In a later study using the same animal model, Malmberg and Yaksh (1995) showed that (S)-(+)- but not (R)-(–)-ibuprofen at 10 mg/kg, but not 1 mg/kg, given i.p. inhibited the release into the lumbar subarachnoid space (into which a dialysis probe was placed) of PGE_2, as well as the excitatory amino acids glutamate and aspartate. The results show that the active PG synthesis inhibitory (S)-(+)-ibuprofen is responsible for the release of the excitatory amino acids and that this is the analgesic component of *rac*-ibuprofen.

The effects of (S)-(+)-ibuprofen on NMDA receptor mediated scratching, biting and licking behaviour (SBL) in rats was investigated by Björkman (1995). The SBL behaviour may be considered a visceral-cutaneous nociceptive model reflecting noxious stimuli from Aδ- and C-fibres (Björkman, 1995). This author found that there was a dose-dependent decline in the behaviours and the total duration of responses induced by intrathecally administered NMDA 0.5 nmol with (S)-(+)-ibuprofen i.p., the ED_{50} being 5 μmol or 1.0 mg/kg. Diclofenac sodium and paracetamol both exhibited the same dose-related inhibition of behavioural response to NMDA with an ED_{50} of 1.0 μmol and 1.0 mmol, or 0.3 and 150 mg/kg, respectively. This shows that (S)-(+)-ibuprofen has potent inhibitory effects against the NMDA receptor activated pain signals in the nervous system.

The effects of (S)-(+)-ibuprofen on the nitric oxide-mediated NMDA activation in SBL was shown by the reversal of the effects of (S)-(+)-ibuprofen in this system by the metabolic precursor to nitric oxide, L-arginine, but not the inactive D-arginine (Björkman, 1995). Similar results were obtained with diclofenac sodium (Björkman, 1995). Thus, the analgesic effect of (S)-(+)-ibuprofen is mediated by inhibition of the NMDA-receptor activation by the excitatory amino acids glutamate and aspartate, and nitric oxide has an important role in mediating the effects of this and other NSAIDs. Similar actions of (S)-(+)- compared with (R)-(−)-ibuprofen as well as other NSAIDs appear to occur with spinal receptors for substance P and AMPA (α-amino-3-hydroxy-5-methyl-4-isoxalone) (Malmberg and Yaksh, 1992b). The inhibition of neural PG production clearly plays a central role in the effects of (S)-(+)-ibuprofen in mediating NMDA-receptor activation in analgesia.

The participation of synaptosomal adenosine transport in the analgesic actions of ibuprofen and other NSAIDs was investigated by Phillis and Wu (1981). These authors showed there was a marked inhibition of synaptosomal uptake of adenosine in rat brain synaptosomes *in vitro*, the IC_{50} being 0.14 μmol/l compared with that of indomethacin which was 0.15 μmol/l. This may represent another mechanism for the action of ibuprofen and other NSAIDs in the CNS.

In the adjuvant-induced chronic arthritis model in rats, ibuprofen has been shown in two separate studies to be 12–16 times more potent as an analgesic than aspirin and 6–11 times less so than indomethacin (Table 5.4). The potency of ibuprofen in this model is high relative to that of other NSAIDs and especially paracetamol (Table 5.4). Ibuprofen, like some other NSAIDs, is less potent in the intra-articular silver nitrate model of so-called 'arthritis' in rats (Malmberg and Yaksh, 1992a). The latter is probably more representative of acute joint inflammation than of a model of analgesia per se.

5.1.4   Antipyretic activity

NSAIDs, including ibuprofen, as well as non-narcotic analgesics, exhibit antipyretic activity that is generally considered to relate to their inhibitory activity on prostaglandin synthesis, especially of PGE_2, which is enhanced in the hypothalamic nuclei by pyrogens such as

CHAPTER 5

TABLE 5.5

Effects of ibuprofen compared with other NSAIDs on yeast-induced hyperthermia in rats

Drug	ED_{50} (mg/kg, p.o.) (95% CI)	
	(1)	(2)
Ibuprofen	0.43 (0.25–0.70)	5.53 (0.32–94.6)
Aspirin	36.7 (19.0–95.7)	78.3 (30.6–200)
Fenclofenac		54.3 (14.3–206)
Flufenamic acid	0.68 (0.21–1.34)	
Indomethacin	0.31 (0.06–1.80)	1.21 (0.41–3.53)
Phenylbutazone	9.13 (2.48–33.7)	12.4 (5.63–27.4)
Tolmetin. Na	7.16 (2.52–13.9)	

Fever induced by 15 ml/kg 15% baker's dry yeast s.c. 17 h before drug administration. Peak reduction of rectal temperature is at 2 h for ibuprofen and some other NSAIDs, but e.g. is 3 h for indomethacin and 2–4 h for tolmetin. *References*: (1) Shimizu *et al.* (1975); (2) Atkinson and Leach (1976).

interleukin-1 (IL-1) and endotoxin (Sobrado *et al.*, 1983; Dinarello *et al.*, 1984; Blatteis, 1988). IL-1 (formerly endogenous pyrogen) released by activated leukocytes during fever responses activates receptors at the blood–brain membrane loci adjacent to the hypothalamus, causing activation of phospholipase A_2 and consequent production of PGE_2 (Milton, 1982; Blatteis, 1988; Cao *et al.*, 1996). The antipyretic effect of ibuprofen is suggested as being localized at the hypothalamus since release of IL-1 from *Staphylococcus albus* activated human monocytes (Dinarello *et al.*, 1984). COX-2 is probably induced at these sites and vasculature and results in further amplification of the production of PGE_2 (Cao *et al.*, 1996). Ibuprofen has been shown to reduce the fever induced by IL-1 or endotoxin in guinea-pigs without affecting the systemic responses (serum zinc and iron, leukocytosis, and changes in amino acids), thus reflecting specific effects of ibuprofen on pyresis (Sobrado *et al.*, 1983).

Table 5.5 shows the relative antipyretic effects of ibuprofen compared with other NSAIDs in the yeast hyperthermia assay. It can be seen that ibuprofen is at least 16 times more potent than aspirin and is about comparable with indomethacin in this assay. The effects of NSAIDs in this assay are comparable with their potency as PG synthesis inhibitors.

5.1.5 General Toxicology

The acute and chronic toxicity of ibuprofen in most laboratory animal species is relatively low (Adams *et al.*, 1970). The acute toxicity (LD_{50}) for ibuprofen in rats has been reported to be 800 mg/kg p.o., which compares favourably with that of aspirin (1360 mg/kg), phenylbutazone (1280 mg/kg), naproxen (540 mg/kg) and indomethacin (25 mg/kg) (DiPasquale and Mellace, 1977). The usual cause of toxic reactions to this, as with other NSAIDs, is from gastrointestinal ulceration, bleeding and perforation (Adams *et al.*, 1970).

In rats, the therapeutic index (TI) of the ratio of acute toxicity/carrageenan paw oedema for ibuprofen is 68, which compares with aspirin 11, indomethacin 7, flufenamic acid 17, naproxen 190 and phenylbutazone 14 (Swingle *et al.*, 1976).

Gastrointestinal ulcerogenicity

Gastrointestinal ulcerogenicity is a major side-effect of the NSAIDs which can, in contrast to other adverse reactions from these drugs, be readily and reliably determined in laboratory animal models (Rainsford, 1989a,b, 1991). It was a major factor considered by Adams and co-workers in the choice of ibuprofen for clinical development (Chapter 1; Adams *et al.*, 1970).

Gastric mucosal lesions and ulcers with accompanying and focal hemorrhage develop with all NSAIDs when administered orally in single or multiple daily doses to fasted rodents and other small or large animals (Rainsford, 1989a). In rats or mice, typical hemorrhagic or craterous lesions which appear in the glandular stomach are generally visible either to the naked eye or with the aid of a dissecting or low-power microscope or lens (Rainsford, 1989a). Quantitation of the lesions varies with different authors employing various quantitative standards based on fixed points on the dose–response curves (Rainsford, 1989a,b).

Comparative ulcerogenicity of ibuprofen

The single dose levels of ibuprofen that are apparently non-irritant to the mucosa of mice, rats and dogs were found to be 200, 800 and 50 mg/kg (Adams *et al.*, 1970). The single doses of ibuprofen that were ulcerative were 400 mg/kg in mice, 1600 mg/kg in rats and 125 mg/kg in dogs. The relatively low dose of ibuprofen required to produce ulcers in dogs is typical for NSAIDs in this species.

The doses required for lesion development in these species following repeated long-term oral dosage of the drug were much lower in rats and dogs but less pronounced in mice than observed with the single dose of the drug in these species (Adams *et al.*, 1970). In the mouse given the drug for 13 weeks, the ulcer producing dose was 300 mg/kg and the non-irritant dose 75 mg/kg. In rats given ibuprofen for 26 weeks, the ulcerative dose was 180 mg/kg and the nonulcerative dose 60 mg/kg. However, in dogs the ulcerative dose was 16 mg/kg when given for 26 weeks and the non-irritant dose was 4 mg/kg over the same period. The drug was more ulcerogenic when given to pregnant rats or rabbits. The main site of ulceration in rats was the small intestine, while in dogs it was the gastric antrum and pylorus. In pregnant rats the main site of ulceration was the intestine.

The dose required for ulcer formation in mice given ibuprofen i.p. was the same as that when the drug was given orally, suggesting that the main effect of the drug is systemic and not from the local mucosal effects (Adams *et al.*, 1970).

The differences in species susceptibility for GI ulcerogenicity in dogs compared with rats appeared to relate to the plasma levels of the drug and metabolites when the

CHAPTER 5

radiolabelled drug was given orally for 2 weeks (Adams *et al.*, 1970). Much higher plasma levels of ibuprofen were found in dogs and in this species no metabolites are formed. In contrast, rats and humans metabolize the drug and, in both species, much lower plasma levels are obtained even after administration of a higher dose of the drug than was given to dogs, that species being only able to tolerate low doses of the drug (Adams *et al.*, 1970).

Comparing the ulcerogenicity of ibuprofen with other NSAIDs, the data in Table 5.6 show that in fasted normal or cold-treated rats given single oral doses of NSAIDs, ibuprofen has moderate mucosal irritancy compared with other NSAIDs, whether compared on a mass or molar basis (Rainsford, 1981). The cold treatment specifically sensitized the gastric mucosa to ulcerogenic effects of NSAIDs (Rainsford, 1975a, 1978, 1989a) and in this model ibuprofen has relatively low ulcerogenicity (Rainsford, 1977).

Repeated daily oral dosing of NSAIDs for 5–10 days produces in rats a different pattern of ulcerogenicity in the gastrointestinal tract from that observed after single doses of the drug (Rainsford, 1982b). Some drugs, e.g. diclofenac, ketoprofen, indomethacin or phenylbutazone, produce intestinal damage and this is related to the enterohepatic circulation of these drugs (Tsukada *et al.*, 1978; Rainsford, 1982c, 1983). Ibuprofen has a relatively low propensity to cause intestinal injury, especially in comparison to the potent intestinal ulcerogens noted above (Tsukada *et al.*, 1978; Ford and Houston, 1995), this being probably due to the lack of appreciable enterohepatic drug circulation in rats (Melarange *et al.*, 1992).

Adaptation of the gastric mucosa towards the ulcerogenic effects of NSAIDs has been described with some NSAIDs (Rainsford, 1984, 1992; Skeljo *et al.*, 1992). The evidence for adaptation comes from studies in which the drugs are given repeatedly for long periods (e.g. 2–4 weeks) and the mucosal damage after this is compared with that from single doses of the drugs. Skeljo *et al.* (1992) showed that adaptation of the gastric mucosa occurs in rats given repeated doses of ibuprofen. 'Short-acting' drugs like ibuprofen are claimed to exhibit mucosal adaptation, whereas others (e.g. indomethacin and naproxen) that are 'long-acting' do not exhibit this phenomenon. Cullen and co-workers (1995) have suggested that, based on endoscopic studies in humans, (S)-(+)-ibuprofen may exhibit greater adaptation than the racemic form of the drug.

The chronic gastro-ulcerogenic effects of nabumetone, diclofenac and ibuprofen were studied in rats given these drugs orally for 1 month at five times the ED_{25} dose for efficacy in the carrageenan oedema assay (Melarange *et al.*, 1994). Nabumetone 79 mg/kg/day was the least ulcerogenic followed by ibuprofen 88 mg/kg/day and diclofenac 11.5 mg/kg/day.

The blood loss in rats, measured with the ^{51}Cr-labelled red blood cell technique, from ibuprofen 100–400 mg/kg/day was found to exhibit a bimodal distribution with time (Suwa *et al.*, 1987). While this technique can be criticized on the grounds of lack of specificity, it is instructive to compare the GI bleeding with different NSAIDs. Thus, Suwa *et al.* (1987) related the second broad peak of blood loss from ibuprofen on days 8–18 to intestinal damage from the drug. This contrasts with the observations of Tsukada *et al.*

TABLE 5.6

Gastro-ulcerogenic activity of ibuprofen compared with other NSAIDs in rats

Drugs	Minimum ulcerogenic dose[a] (mg/kg, p.o.) at 3 h	24 h	UD$_{50}$ rats[b] (95% CI) 3.5 h	ED$_{10}$ cold treated rats[c] (mg/kg, p.o.)	(mmol/kg, p.o.)	Chronic (7 day)[d] ulcerogenicity in rats, score at dose (mg/kg/day)	mortality
	(1)		(2)	(3)		(1)	
Ibuprofen	6–13	6–13	148 (62.0–355)	14.4	0.07	3.1 @ 244	2/10
Alclofenac	30–60	60–120		9.5	0.042		
Aspirin	<15–30	<15–60	17.4 (8.7–34.8)	5.04	0.023	3.1 @ 215	0/10
Azapropazone				240	0.80		
Benoxaprofen				91	0.3		
Diclofenac.Na	4–8	4–8		1.0	0.003		
Fenclofenac	400–800	200–800		184	0.62	0.8 @ 180	0/10
Fenoprofen.Ca	30–60	30–60		20	0.04		
Flufenamic acid			174 (62.0–487)				
Indomethacin	1.3–2.5	2.5–5.0	6.6 (2.2–19.8)	2.5	0.0076	0.8 @ 5.7	0/10
Ketoprofen	0.6–1.3	5–10	6.8 (2.4–19.0)				
Mefenamic acid			548 (62.0–355)				
Naproxen	2–4	2–4		1.6	0.007		
Oxaprozin				851	2.9		
Phenylbutazone	40–80	38–75	96.0 (37.0–248)	25	0.081	1.1 @ 132	0/10
Piroxicam				0.01	0.0003		
Salicylic acid				60.7	0.44		

[a] In fasted female albino Sprague–Dawley normal rats given single oral dose of the drug. Mucosal damage was scored on a 0–4 scale of increasing severity and the minimum ulcerogenic dose determined as statistically significant.

[b] In fasted (24 h) male Donru rats.

[c] In fasted (24 h) male Sprague–Dawley rats exposed to –18°C for 35 min following single oral dose of drugs; lesions were determined at 2 h after dosing. ED$_{10}$ refers to the dose required to produce 10 lesions.

[d] Replete female rats dosed once daily for 6 days and lesions determined after last dose on day 7.

References: (1) Atkinson and Leach (1976); (2) Tsukada *et al.* (1978); (3) Rainsford (1987).

(1978) mentioned above. A similar second peak of blood loss occurred with indomethacin 4–16 mg/kg/day but not with aspirin 100–400 mg/kg/day.

Using the ^{51}Cr-EDTA technique, Ford et al. (1995) showed that (S)-(+)-ibuprofen was 10 times less potent in causing intestinal permeability than piroxicam. Using dosage procedures to achieve constant plasma concentrations of NSAIDs, Ford and Houston (1995) showed that the rank order of intestinal permeability using the ^{51}Cr-EDTA method was diclofenac>piroxicam>(S)-(+)-ibuprofen.

It is customary to relate the toxic effects of NSAIDs including the effects on specific organs (e.g. GI tract) to the doses required to produce therapeutic effects, in order to derive a therapeutic index (Rainsford, 1975b; Swingle et al., 1976; Gemmell et al., 1979; Suwa et al., 1987). The data obtained depend on the inflammatory/pain or other condition being assayed as well as on the species and treatment. Generally, there is a considerable scatter with the comparative data (Rainsford, 1981, 1987, 1989a). In most studies ibuprofen has relatively high values of therapeutic index (TI) of acute gastric irritancy in relation to acute inflammatory or pain conditions compared with other NSAIDs, although these vary according to the type of therapeutic parameter being compared (Rainsford, 1975a; Swingle et al., 1976; Gemmell et al., 1979). The relatively low intestinal ulcerogenicity with this drug gives a high TI in this region of the GI tract, which is in marked contrast to a number of other NSAIDs that are particularly ulcerogenic in this region (indomethacin, flurbiprofen, diclofenac, etc.) (Rainsford, 1982b).

Relatively little work has been published on the irritant effects of different formulations of ibuprofen on the gastrointestinal mucosa. Whitehouse and Rainsford (1987) found that the sodium salt of ibuprofen was about three times more irritant to the gastric mucosa of rats than was the parent acid. This enhancement of ulcerogenicity by solubilized salt formulations of acidic NSAIDs is a property of many of these drugs and probably relates to the enhancement of gastric mucosal absorption of the drug because it is more water-soluble. The lysine salt of ibuprofen has been found to have lower gastric irritancy than aspirin when observed by endoscopy in humans, but it does produce more damage than placebo (Müller and Simon, 1994).

The oral GI mucosal toxicity of aqueous suspensions of ibuprofen 17–44 mg/kg was compared with that of a wax microsphere-encapsulated drug in bethanechol chloride-stimulated rats (Adeyeye et al., 1996); the latter treatment stimulates acid and pepsin production in the stomach (Rainsford, 1987, 1989a,b). The in vitro release of the drug from the encapsulated drug was found to decline exponentially over 12 h, the half-time of release being approximately 2 h (Adeyeye et al., 1996). The disposition of ibuprofen was markedly different in the two formulations even though the total mass of drug absorbed reflected by the 12 h values of the area under the concentration curve (AUC_{12}) were the same with the two preparations. The maximum concentration with the encapsulated drug was about 1/3 that of the suspension and the time to reach peak concentrations was 3.6 h with the encapsulated drug compared with 0.32 h from the suspension. Both macroscopic

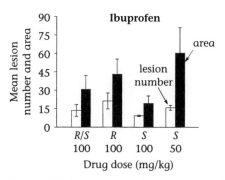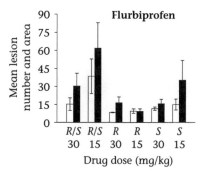

Figure 5.2: Gastric ulcerogenicity in mice of enantiomers (Rainsford, 1995)

and microscopic observations of mucosal damage at 7 h post treatment showed that the encapsulated drug produced much less mucosal injury than the suspensions of the drug, notably at the higher dose of 44 mg/kg ibuprofen. These studies are of particular interest for the potential of the wax-encapsulated formulation of ibuprofen being developed as a GI-safer formulation.

The gastric mucosal irritancy of the enantiomers of ibuprofen has been compared in mice with the racemate and with other enantiomeric NSAIDs (Rainsford, 1995; Figure 5.2). The relatively low ulcerogenicity of *rac*-ibuprofen in mice (Rainsford, 1987; Table 5.6) makes it difficult to determine ulcerogenicity of this drug compared with its enantiomers. However, in the cholinomimetic sensitized mouse model the (*R*)-(–) and (*S*)-(+) enantiomers of ibuprofen are about equally ulcerogenic with each other as well as with *rac*-ibuprofen at the upper dose of 100 mg/kg p.o. (Rainsford, 1995). Davies and co-workers (1996) have observed that both enantiomers of ibuprofen produce the same degree of increased intestinal permeability (determined by the ^{51}Cr-EDTA technique) in rats.

Studies of the effects of state of crystallization of (*S*)-(+)- and *rac*-ibuprofen on their plasma concentrations were performed in the rat by Walser *et al.* (1997) because it appeared that recrystallization of these forms led to better galenical or tableting properties. It was, however, found that there were no differences in the values for the AUCs from recrystallized compared with commercially available forms of these two drugs.

Mechanisms of ulcerogenicity

The role of endogenous microbial flora in the pathogenesis of mucosal injury has been investigated by several authors (Rainsford, 1983). Melarange and co-workers (1992) found that although gastric and intestinal mucosal injury and blood loss from ibuprofen in germ-free animals was the same as that in open-colony animals, indomethacin, as shown by others (Rainsford, 1983), produced more intestinal injury in conventional microbial-replete animals. These results suggest that although ibuprofen can produce intestinal damage, this does not depend on biliary excretion, and unlike that of indomethacin, which is excreted in the bile, this effect is not dependent on intestinal flora.

CHAPTER 5

TABLE 5.7

Effects of ibuprofen compared with other NSAIDs on the chopped tissue or *ex vivo* production of prostaglandins

Drug	Guinea-pig perfused lung ED$_{50}$ (μmol/l) PG[a] (1)	RCS[a] (1)	Guinea-pig chopped lung ID$_{50}$ (μmol/l) (2)	ST 3,24 h	DU 3,24 h	SI 3,24 h	LU 3,24 h	LI 3,24 h	KI 3,24 h	BR 3,24 h	Dose (mg/kg)
							(3)				
Ibuprofen (R/S)	1.5	1.5									
Aspirin	3.0	3.0	47.0[b]	× ○	× ○	○ ○	○ ○	○ ○	○ ○	× ○	16.4
Diclofenac,Na			8.4[a]	× ×	× ×	× ×	× ×	○ ×	○ ○	× ×	19.6
Flurbiprofen			5.1[a]								
Indomethacin	0.016	0.016	0.76[b]	× ×	× ×	× ×	× ×	× ○	× ×	× ×	28.8
Ketoprofen	0.002	0.0017									
Naproxen	0.035	0.025	3.9[a]								
Phenylbutazone	2.0	2.0		○ ○	○ ○	○ ○	○ ○	○ ×	○ ×	○ ○	12.0

Abbreviations and symbols: ST, stomach, DI, duodenum; SI, small intestine; LU, lungs; LI, liver; KI, kidney; BR, brain; × refers to inhibition of either PGF$_{2α}$ or PGE$_2$ or both; ○ refers to no inhibition.

[a] PG (prostaglandins) and RCS (rabbit aorta contracting substance) were determined by bioassay. RCS is the equivalent of thromboxane A$_2$.

[b] Doses of drugs given were based on achieving a body water concentration of 10 mmol/l, being sufficient to inhibit prostaglandin production based on IC$_{50}$ values in seminal vesicle assays. After excision, the tissues were autolyzed *in situ* for 30 min, weighed, spiked with [^{3}H]PGF$_{2α}$ homogenized and centrifuged, whereupon the supernatants were assayed for PGE$_2$ and PGF$_{2α}$ by RIA.

References: (1) Guyonnet and Julou (1976); (2) Vane (1971), Garcia-Rafanell and Forn (1979); (3) Fitzpatrick and Wynalda (1976).

Metabolism of (R)-(−)- to (S)-(+)-ibuprofen might be expected in the stomach or intestinal mucosa, and the production of the latter may reduce production of mucosal protective prostaglandins (Table 5.7). However, studies by Jeffrey *et al.* (1991) with rat intestinal tract sections perfused with enantiomers show that there is relatively little amount of (S)-(+) isomer formed after infusion of (R)-(−)-ibuprofen; the small amount of (S)-(+)-ibuprofen present could be accounted for by enantiomeric impurity. Thus, it is unlikely that (R)-(−)-ibuprofen is metabolized by the intestine during absorption.

While it is not possible to extrapolate these findings to the stomach, it is possible that no inversion of (R)-(−)- to (S)-(+)-ibuprofen occurs in this region as in the intestinal tract and that the major site of metabolic inversion is in the liver. The liver appeared to metabolize the (R)-(−) enantiomer almost exclusively (Jeffrey *et al.*, 1991). Hence the differences in the ulcerogenicity of ibuprofen enantiomers would be unlikely to be related to metabolism of (R)-(−)- to (S)-(+)-ibuprofen.

Recently, the relation of effects of ibuprofen enantiomers on the stomach to the effects on prostaglandin cyclooxygenase have been investigated by comparing the effects of (R)-(−)-, (S)-(+)- and *rac*-ibuprofen alone or in combination on prostaglandin production by pig mucosal explants in organ culture (Rainsford *et al.*, 1997b). These studies show that there is competitive interaction between the (R)-(−) and (S)-(+) forms in inhibiting production of PGE_2 and that this may reflect competition between these enantiomers on the active site of cyclooxygenase (Rainsford *et al.*, 1997b). The results show that *rac*-ibuprofen produces little if any inhibitory effects on prostaglandin production, whereas (S)-(+)-ibuprofen is a potent inhibitor. If these results are related to the situation *in vivo*, then the inhibition of production of mucosal protective prostaglandins may be less likely with *rac*-ibuprofen even at concentrations or doses double those in (S)-(+)-ibuprofen alone. This may reflect the competition between (R)-(−) and (S)-(+) for active sites on cyclooxygenases (Rainsford *et al.*, 1997b) (Figure 5.3).

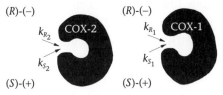

Figure 5.3: Postulated competition between the (R)-(−) and (S)-(+) enantiomers of ibuprofen and the cyclooxygenase (COX) isoenzymes that may be principally occurring in the upper gastrointestinal tract during contact with the mucosa and absorption. There is no intestinal metabolism of (R)-(−)-ibuprofen to its (S)-(+) antipode and this might also be absent in the stomach. Thus, at least half of the racemic form of the drug will be available for competing with the active sites on COX isoenzymes in the stomach and intestinal mucosal cells. It is suggested that the masking of the COX active sites by (R)-(−)-ibuprofen effectively prevents appreciable inhibition of prostaglandin production in the gastrointestinal mucosa, so accounting for the relatively low ulcerogenic activity and bleeding that is observed in clinico-epidemiological and experimental studies. (After Rainsford *et al.*, 1997b.)

While there is evidence that inhibition of gastric mucosal prostaglandin production by NSAIDs, such as ibuprofen, has a role in the development of mucosal injury, the exact relationship between inhibition of prostaglandin production and the development of mucosal damage has not been established (Rainsford, 1992; Wagner et al., 1995). This leads to postulates about other factors that may account for the development of mucosal damage (Rainsford, 1992). Among these are the influence of those cyclooxygenase inhibitors that are especially ulcerogenic in diverting the production of arachidonic acid to produce excess leukotrienes, which leads to vasoconstriction (from excess LTC_4 and metabolites) and leukocyte accumulation (from excess LTB_4) (Rainsford, 1992). Many dual inhibitors of both cyclooxygenase and lipoxygenase pathways are less gastro-ulcerogenic than corresponding and equipotent NSAIDs (with respect to anti-inflammatory activity) (Rainsford, 1992). Also, concurrent administration of 5-lipoxygenase inhibitors with cyclooxygenase inhibitory NSAIDs leads to reduction of the gastric mucosal injury from the latter (Rainsford, 1992). The fact that both enantiomers of ibuprofen have effects on leukocyte 5-lipoxygenase and reduce production of LTB_4 (see the later section on Effects on Leukotriene Production) may be a reason for the low ulcerogenicity of ibuprofen.

The somatostatin analogue octreotide was found by Scheiman and co-workers (1997) to prevent gastric mucosal lesions in rats from several NSAIDs including ibuprofen. These authors suggested that the effect of octreotide in preventing NSAID injury is to reduce adhesion of inflammatory leukocytes to gastric submucosal venules, an effect they showed in rats and humans with indomethacin. However, it is not clear whether ibuprofen enhances adherance of leukocytes to venules, so this NSAID-related mechanism of mucosal damage may not be apparent with ibuprofen.

Other factors that may account for the relatively low gastro-ulcerogenicity of ibuprofen may relate to the physicochemical properties of this drug in comparison with other NSAIDs. These factors are known to be especially important in determining the uptake of drugs into the mucosa and their interactions with the mucosal membranes and surface protective layer of phospholipids (McCormack and Brune, 1987, 1989; Kivinen et al., 1994; Lichtenberger et al., 1995; Lugea et al., 1997). The pK_a of ibuprofen (5.2) is relatively high compared with that of many other more ulcerogenic NSAIDs (e.g. aspirin and tolmetin, 3.5; naproxen, 4.2; indomethacin, 4.5; flurbiprofen, 4.6) (Barbito et al., 1997). Moreover, the partition and distribution coefficients of ibuprofen are also relatively high compared with those of other NSAIDs (Barbato et al., 1997). This, combined with the relatively high water-solubility of the drug (McCormack and Brune, 1990) and isothermal distribution in phospholipids, may be important in determining the effects of the drug on the interface between the stomach lumen and mucosal phospholipid/membrane layer such that relatively low disruption of this surface protective layer occurs.

Among the physicochemical characteristics of NSAIDs accounting for their gastrointestinal ulcerogenicity is the presence of a functional carboxyl moiety (Rainsford and Whitehouse, 1980; Rainsford, 1984; Whitehouse and Rainsford, 1980). Where the carboxyl moiety of acidic NSAIDs has been esterified with metabolizable groups that are readily hydrolyzed, this enables the mucosa to be masked against the irritant effects of the acidic groups of the drugs (Rainsford and Whitehouse, 1980; Whitehouse and Rainsford, 1980; Rainsford, 1984). Several such carboxyl-protected derivatives of ibuprofen that are effectively pro-drugs have been developed, among them various esters and amides (Möller *et al.*, 1989; Shanbhag *et al.*, 1992) and diethylcarbonates (Samara *et al.*, 1995), and most of these derivatives have shown low ulcerogenicity without appreciable effect on the anti-inflammatory activity inherent in ibuprofen. This shows that the carboxyl moiety of ibuprofen, as with other acidic NSAIDs, accounts for mucosal irritancy.

Among the ibuprofen derivatives that have been developed is the 5-aminosalicylic acid–ibuprofen amide conjugate (Möller *et al.*, 1989). This compound had acute anti-inflammatory activity in the carrageenan paw oedema model in rats that was about comparable with that of ibuprofen. It inhibited leukotriene production like 5-amino-salicylic acid itself, but was a somewhat less potent inhibitor of prostaglandin production in mouse macrophages *in vitro*. The ibuprofen derivative was less irritant to the gastric mucosa. This is a unique approach of developing a compound combining the anti-inflammatory properties of 5-aminosalicylic acid with those of ibuprofen.

The approach of developing these simple ester or amide derivatives of ibuprofen has potential utility as a means for reducing the propensity of ibuprofen to cause gastric mucosal irritancy. However, as with all these ester derivatives, it is essential to establish the kinetics of hydrolysis and the relationship of this to absorption as well as the contribution of systemic effects of the parent drug that is produced after gastric absorption in order to establish the potential therapeutic value of any such derivatives.

Bhattachacharya and co-workers (1991) observed that the gastric ulcerogenicity of ibuprofen 25 mg/kg/day given orally for 5 days with paracetamol 20 mg/kg/day caused much greater mucosal damage in rats subjected on the 6th day to pyloric ligation than did either of the drugs alone. Oral administration of many NSAIDs to pyloric ligated rats produces increased irritancy to the gastric mucosa compared with that in nonligated animals (Wagner *et al.*, 1995). However, this is less pronounced with ibuprofen (Wagner *et al.*, 1995). In their studies with paracetamol and ibuprofen, Bhattachacharya *et al.* (1991) showed that the free and total acidity as well as peptic activity was unaffected by any of these drug treatments compared with one another or with controls. The authors showed that the carbohydrate components of the mucus in these rats were significantly reduced by ibuprofen and the total content thereof more so by the combination of paracetamol and ibuprofen. This suggests that paracetamol may exacerbate the production of mucus when given in combination with ibuprofen and that this might, in part, account for the enhancement in ulcerogenic effects of ibuprofen by paracetamol. These results show that, far from being innocuous to the gastric mucosa, paracetamol can exacerbate injury when in combination with the NSAID ibuprofen.

Furthermore, Carryl and Spangler (1995) observed that combinations of diclofenac, naproxen and piroxicam, but not nabumetone, enhanced the gastric ulcerogenicity of ibuprofen in rats. This emphasizes the importance of drug combinations in the development of gastric mucosal injury and highlights the necessity of avoiding many combinations of NSAIDs with one another.

The studies by Bhattachacharya *et al.* (1991) showed that ibuprofen *in vivo* did not affect peptic activity in the rat. Wagner *et al.* (1995) observed that pepsinogen secretion was not increased in rats given ibuprofen. Furthermore, the secretion of pepsinogens I and II has been shown to be unaffected by (S)-(+)-ibuprofen in humans (Kullich *et al.*, 1994). However, 0.01–100 μmol/l ibuprofen, as with aspirin, has been found to stimulate histamine-induced pepsinogen secretion from isolated human peptic cells *in vitro* (Lanas *et al.*, 1995). These effects on the control of acid-pepsin secretion (Lanas *et al.*, 1995) may represent a non-prostaglandin-dependent mechanism for mucosal injury by ibuprofen where there is histamine stimulation. Basal secretion of pepsinogen was unaffected by these drugs and unrelated to effects on prostaglandin production. However, the effect of the two drugs on histamine-stimulated pepsinogen production was dependent on extracellular calcium. There may be an interaction of ibuprofen, as well as other NSAIDs, with the cyclic-AMP system controlling acid secretion (Silvola *et al.*, 1982a,b). Phosphodiesterase activity in the mucosa, which is responsible for the breakdown of cyclic-AMP, as well as adenylate cyclase have been shown to be competitively inhibited in the micromolar range by ulcerogenic NSAIDs (Silvola *et al.*, 1982a,b). However, ibuprofen did not exhibit any effects on these enzymes (Silvola *et al.*, 1982a,b), suggesting that it is unlikely to have appreciable effects on the cAMP regulation of acid secretion.

Hepatic toxicity

Following the observation that the progenitor to ibuprofen, ibufenac, exhibited liver toxicity in an appreciable proportion of rheumatic patients in the United Kingdom (Chapter 1), Adams and colleagues (1970) undertook detailed investigations in laboratory animals to establish whether ibuprofen had the liver toxicity observed with ibufenac. No significant biochemical changes were observed in the major liver function parameters in rats given ibuprofen 180 mg/kg/day for 16 weeks p.o., mice given 300 mg/kg/day of the drug in the diet for 13 weeks, or dogs given 16 mg/kg/day of the drug in gelatin capsules for 26 weeks (Adams *et al.*, 1970). No histological signs of damage were evident in the livers of these animals, although the liver weights of the rats and mice increased but returned to normal upon cessation of the drug. The authors noted that liver hypertrophy is a common reaction to high doses of drugs. They also observed that ibufenac caused significant elevation of plasma γ-glutamyl-transpepticlase (GTP), and in those rats given lethal doses of this drug focal hepatic necrosis was apparent at autopsy. These results show that ibuprofen was without the liver toxicity previously seen with ibufenac.

Interestingly, the body distribution of radiolabelled ibuprofen 20 mg/kg given for 4 weeks was markedy different in rats compared with that from the same dose of radio-labelled ibufenac given over the same period of time (Adams *et al.*, 1970). Thus, the concentrations of ibuprofen in the liver as well as in the plasma and kidney were some 10-fold less than those of ibufenac. There was also evidence of high accumulation of ibufenac in fat depots, where it was present in 20-fold greater amounts than observed with ibuprofen. In the ovary, the amount of ibufenac present was 10 times that of ibuprofen. Similar differences in body distribution were also observed in dogs given radiolabelled drugs twice daily for 2 weeks. These results show clearly that there is much greater body retention of ibufenac compared with that of ibuprofen in rats. The differences in distribution of these two drugs are particularly interesting in relation to their chemical structures. The only difference between the two drugs is that the α-carbon (or 2-carbon) attached to the carboxylic acid has a methyl substituent in ibuprofen whereas this is not present in ibufenac. Clearly, the lack of appreciable retention of ibuprofen is a major factor accounting for its relatively low overall toxicity in animals.

The clinical reports of idiosyncratic liver reactions from ibuprofen appear few, especially in comparison with drugs such as diclofenac, sulindac, naproxen, clometacine and phenylbutazone in which there have been a substantial number of cases of fulminant hepatitis and cholestasis (Prescott, 1992; Zimmerman, 1994; Boelsterli *et al.*, 1995). These cases usually comprise hepatocellular injury with some cholestasis (Zimmerman, 1994). A metabolic idiosyncrasy is usually ascribed to this adverse effect of ibuprofen (Zimmerman, 1994). The pathological mechanisms in the development of these liver reactions appear to be related to the metabolism of these drugs to their acyl glucuronides (Boelsterli *et al.*, 1995). It has been postulated that drug-glucuronides form covalent adducts with hepatic and plasma proteins and consequently become immunogenic (Boelsterli *et al.*, 1995). These long-life proteins then elicit either cytotoxic T cell-mediated or antibody-dependent cell-mediated toxicity involving participation of oxyradicals (Boelsterli *et al.*, 1995). It is unlikely that these mechanisms are involved with reactions involving ibuprofen. Indeed ibuprofen has been shown to reduce the Kupffer cell reaction during hemorrhage and increased production of pro-inflammatory cytokines (Chaudry *et al.*, 1995), so it is unlikely that the drug would enhance immunological responses in the liver. It has, however, been suggested that ibuprofen, like other propionic acid NSAIDs that are metabolized from their (*R*)-(−) enantiomeric forms via their acyl-CoA derivatives (Knights and Roberts, 1994), may lead either to potentially toxic 'hybrid' triglycerides in membranes or to effects related to the inhibition of β-oxidation of fatty acids (Boelsterli *et al.*, 1995). In the case of pirprofen it has been suggested that the latter effect may account for the development of microvesicular steatosis that has been observed in a few patients (Boelsterli *et al.*, 1995). There is no evidence for the development of idiosyncratic reactions from ibuprofen involving these proposed mechanisms.

CHAPTER 5

The direct effects of ibuprofen on liver cells *in vitro* were compared with those of two related propionic acids, flurbiprofen and butibufen, using cultured primary rat hepatocytes (Castell *et al.*, 1988). While none of these drugs affected acute toxicity (determined by Trypan blue exclusion), leakage of lactate dehydrogenase after 48 h in culture with normal therapeutic concentrations (about 0.1 mmol/l), at higher concentrations ibuprofen was the least cytotoxic of these NSAIDs. In rat liver tissue slices paracetamol produces extensive leakage of Trypan blue and this is not potentiated (nor indeed reversed) by ibuprofen (Beales and McLean, 1995). At supra-therapeutic concentrations ibuprofen and flurbiprofen were the least active in impairing albumin and urea synthesis, whereas at therapeutic concentrations ibuprofen and butibufen were the most potent in impairing gluconeogenesis from lactate. Brass and Garrity (1985) observed that ibuprofen caused a concentration-related increase in glycolysis, an effect that this drug shared with some other carboxylic acid NSAIDs (indomethacin, meclofenamic acid) but not piroxicam. Ibuprofen did not affect the rate of glycolysis in the presence of adrenaline or glucagon and neither did the drug affect hepatocyte adenylate cyclase activity alone or in the presence of glucagon. The inhibition of glycolysis by ibuprofen 80 μmol/l was inhibited by prostaglandin E_2. The authors suggested that ibuprofen might be affecting calcium uptake, thus indirectly affecting glucose non-hormonally-regulated metabolism.

Other effects of ibuprofen on liver functions involve the effects on the microsomal monooxygenase drug-metabolizing systems (Bélanger and Atitsé-Gbeassor, 1985). In rats, twice daily oral dosing with ibuprofen 10 mg/kg, as with indomethacin 10 mg/kg, ketoprofen 10 mg/kg and aspirin 100 mg/kg, for 3 days caused significant increases in liver microsomal cytochromes P450 and b_5, aminopyrene *N*-demethylase, *p*-anisole *O*-demethylase and aniline hydroxylase (Bélanger and Atitsé-Gbeassor, 1985). Naproxen 5 mg/kg only increased the activities of the latter three enzymes, while phenylbutazone 50 mg/kg and salicylic acid 100 mg/kg were without effect. All these drugs except aspirin and salicylic acid inhibited the aminopyrene *N*-demethylase, *p*-anisole *O*-demethylase and aniline hydroxylase activities *in vitro* (Bélanger and Atitsé-Gbeassor, 1985). Exceptionally high doses of ibuprofen (650 mg/kg s.c. or 400 mg/kg p.o.) inhibited aminopyrene *N*-demethylase *ex vivo* and reduced hexobarbital sleep times (Reinicke, 1977). In contrast to many NSAIDs (e.g. indomethacin, flurbiprofen) that decrease cytochrome P450 *in vitro*, ibuprofen does not appear to have this effect (Falzon *et al.*, 1986). It therefore appears that ibuprofen, like many NSAIDs, can induce liver microsomal drug-metabolizing enzymes *in vivo* as well as directly inhibiting the activities of these enzymes *in vitro*. However, ibuprofen does not affect cytochrome P450 stability *in vitro*. The exact significance of these effects of ibuprofen in relation to its metabolism or effects in the liver is not clear.

Renal injury

This aspect is discussed in Chapter 10. It is generally considered that renal effects occur with most NSAIDs to a varying degree (Reeves *et al.*, 1985; Whelton and Hamilton, 1994).

The major part of the mechanism of changes in renal function and the development of renal injury relates to the effects of these drugs in inhibiting prostaglandin production. The problem for many NSAIDs is exacerbated in the elderly, who have diminished renal function and therefore reduced ability to eliminate these drugs, especially in the case of those NSAIDs with long half-lives (Cusack, 1988; Schmitt and Guentert, 1989; Astbury and Bird, 1993; Ailabouni and Eknoyan, 1996). While the half-life of plasma ibuprofen is only slightly prolonged in the elderly, the clearance of the drug is reduced in this group (Schmitt and Guentert, 1989; Astbury and Bird, 1993). The clinical significance of this reduced clearance of ibuprofen is apparently relatively minor since the incidence of abnormalities of renal function is low compared with other NSAIDs (Committee on the Safety of Medicines/Medicines Control Agency, 1994).

Mutagenicity and carcinogenicity

Sister chromatid exchange is a sensitive technique for detecting alteration to DNA. Kullich and Klein (1986) did not observe any increase in sister chromatid exchange in the peripheral blood lymphocytes of nonsmoking patients with rheumatic diseases who had taken ibuprofen 1200 mg/day for 2 weeks; similar negative results were observed in patients who had received a range of other NSAIDs for the same period. An almost identical study published more recently by Ozkul *et al.* (1996) has confirmed these results. Phillpose and co-workers (1997) showed that ibuprofen, like the two other propionic acids ketoprofen and naproxen, was without any mutagenic activity in the Ames tests (in strains TA97a, TA100 and TA102) and only weakly genotoxic in the sister chromatid exchange test in mouse bone marrow cells *in vivo.*

Carcinogenicity studies did not reveal any potential for ibuprofen to affect the natural incidence of tumours that spontaneously develop in mice or rats of either sex given the drug continuously for 43 or 56 weeks, respectively (Adams *et al.*, 1970). Ibuprofen, like many other NSAIDs, has been shown to inhibit the oxidation of some proximate carcinogens, *trans*-dihydrodiol derivatives, by rat liver cytosolic dihydrodiol dehydrogenase (Smithgall and Penning, 1986). Again the exact significance of this effect of ibuprofen is not understood, though it implies that the drug, like other NSAIDs, may prevent the formation of the ultimate aromatic hydrocarbon carcinogen metabolites.

Reproductive toxicity

While ibuprofen is regarded as having low teratogenic potential (Adams *et al.*, 1970) it can, like other NSAIDs given in relatively high doses, cause some premature death of newborn rats (Powell and Cochrane, 1982). It does not appear that ibuprofen causes alterations in the length of gestation in rats (Powell and Cochrane, 1982).

Csapo (1977) studied the effects of ibuprofen on uterine contractility from pregnant and post-partum rabbits. The isometric contraction was found to be inhibited in a dose-dependent manner by 125–500 µg/ml ibuprofen in both preparations. However, greater inhibition was observed in tissues from post-partum animals.

To establish the relevance of these effects on myometrial activity *in vivo* Hahn and co-workers (1982) observed that pretreatment of guinea-pigs during the late oestrous cycle with ibuprofen and other NSAIDs i.v. before i.v. administration of arachidonic acid or prostaglandin $F_{2\alpha}$ reduced the myometrial hyperactivity from the latter in relationship to the potency of the NSAIDs as prostaglandin synthesis inhibitors. The authors also found that there was reduction in histologically observed catecholamine fluorescence in the myometrial nerves in tissues from animals given the NSAIDs and suggested that part of the effects of the drugs may be to reduce the sympathetic nerve activity. These authors suggested that, as the contraction of the myometrium is inhibited by NSAIDs in relation to their inhibitory activity on prostaglandin production, this *in vivo* system may be used as an *in vivo* assay for effects of NSAIDs on prostaglandin production. Lewis *et al.* (1975) previously showed that the contractile activity of the spontaneously active rat uterus was inhibited by NSAIDs in relationship to their potency as prostaglandin synthesis inhibitors. They also suggested that this assay could be employed for determining effects of NSAIDs on prostaglandin production in an intact tissue system *in vitro*.

5.1.6   Effects on prostaglandin production related to pharmacological activities

Inhibition of PG production is classically a major feature underlying the anti-inflammatory, analgesic and antipyretic activities of NSAIDs. However, the mechanisms of action of these drugs on the COX enzymes and other components of the prostaglandin synthesizing systems vary considerably from drug to drug. Table 5.7 summarizes the differing actions and potencies of ibuprofen compared with other NSAIDs on the components of the PG synthesizing systems. From Table 5.8 it can be seen that (S)-(+)-ibuprofen is an appreciably more potent inhibitor of COX-1 and COX-2 than the (R)-(–) enantiomer, but their relative potencies vary in different systems. It is possible that this variation depends on (a) variations in the bioconversion of (R)-(–)- to (S)-(+)-ibuprofen in different systems, (b) differences in the affinities of the two enantiomers for the active sites of the COXs, and (c) variations in the substrate (arachidonate) availability in different cell systems such that inhibitory effects of the drugs may be reversed when there is high concentration of arachidonate.

Effects of ibuprofen on production of prostaglandins and other eicosanoids

Following the pioneering studies by Vane (1971) showing that aspirin and indomethacin inhibit the synthesis of prostaglandins in chopped guinea-pig lung incubated with arachidonic acid, there quickly followed a considerable number of reports that other NSAIDs, including ibuprofen, also inhibit prostaglandin synthesis in various assay systems (Ham *et al.*, 1972; Tomlinson *et al.*, 1972; Flower *et al.*, 1972, 1973; Flower and Vane, 1972;

Flower 1974 and Vane; Table 5.8). These studies represented key findings in support of the general concept of Vane (1971) that inhibition of prostaglandin production could explain the anti-inflammatory, analgesic and antipyretic activities of NSAIDs (Ferreira, 1972; Flower et al., 1972; Tomlinson et al., 1972). Moreover, the analgesic and antipyretic activities of paracetamol, amidopyrene, dipyrone and other non-narcotic analgesics were accounted for by inhibition of prostaglandins (Flower and Vane, 1972; Flower, 1974). The weak anti-inflammatory activity of these analgesics related to their limited ability to accumulate in inflamed sites and little or no effects on prostaglandin production in inflamed tissues or inflammatory cells (Brune et al., 1981a; Rainsford et al., 1981). Hence, differentiation of the actions of NSAIDs from those of non-narcotic analgesics could be explained in both pharmacokinetic and pharmacodynamic terms.

The early studies showed that ibuprofen was a moderately potent inhibitor of prostaglandin biosynthesis in bovine or ovine seminal vesicle particulate or microsomal enzyme preparations, microsomes from other tissues, and cells from synovia, fibroblasts or macrophages (Table 5.8). The bovine or ovine microsomal (particulate) preparations would now be recognized as having the COX-1 isoform. The rheumatoid synovial ex-plants and mouse peritoneal macrophages stimulated with the phorbol ester TPA (tetrahydro-phorbol-13-acetate) (Table 5.8; Robinson et al., 1978; Brune et al., 1981b) would now be recognized as having appreciable *inducible* COX-2 activity. The production of COX-2 enzyme combined with the stimulated release of arachidonate by activation of phospholipases would account for the varying potency of ibuprofen compared with other anti-inflammatory and analgesic drugs in these tissue/cellular systems compared with microsomal preparations (Table 5.8). Also an important issue in comparing data of prostaglandin production from cellular systems having inducible COX-2 activity is that some drugs may affect induction of the COX-2 enzyme as well as its activity. Furthermore, the inhibitory effects of NSAIDs on COX-2 compared with COX-1 vary considerably from drug to drug (Rabasseda, 1996).

In the seminal vesicle and other microsomal preparations, the marked differences in inhibitory effects of ibuprofen compared with other NSAIDs can be explained by the varying assay conditions employed by different authors (Flower et al., 1973; Cushman and Cheung, 1976; Procaccini et al., 1977) as well as by chemical structure and reactivity towards cyclooxygenase(s) (Rome and Lands, 1975). The issue of differences in IC_{50} values of the NSAIDs being due to variations in substrate concentrations is illustrated by the data from Cushman and Cheung (1976) (Table 5.8). Thus, when bovine seminal vesicle microsomes are incubated with 1 mmol/l arachidonic acid, ibuprofen produces 100 times less inhibition of prostaglandin production than when incubated with 1000-fold less (1 μmol/l) substrate (indicative of the competitive inhibition of the enzyme). Similar, though even more marked, differences are observed with some NSAIDs. Thus, naproxen has some 460 times higher potency, indomethacin 60 times, phenylbutazone 12 times and aspirin equal potency when incubated with 1 μmol/l compared with 1 mmol/l arachidonic acid (Table 5.8; Cushman and Cheung, 1976). These differences can be explained in

TABLE 5.8

Comparative inhibitory effects on prostaglandin production of ibuprofen and other anti-inflammatory analgesic drugs in microsomal and cellular systms

Drug	Bovine seminal vesicle microsomes incubated with 1.0 mmol/l AA (IC_{50} mmol/l)				PGE_2 incubated with 1 μmol/l AA IC_{50} (mmol/l)	Bovine seminal vesicle IC_{50} (μmol/l)	Ovine vesicle preparation	
	PGF_2	$PGF_{2\alpha}$	PGD_2	MDA			Interference with substrate binding K_1 (μmol/l)	Time-dependent loss of enzyme activity (k_{app}/I) (μmol/l^{-1} min^{-1})
Ibuprofen *rac*	2.0[a], 0.65[b]	2.3[a], 0.5[b]	2.1[a], 0.6	1.8[a]	0.006	1.5	3.0	0
Ibuprofen R(−)								
Ibuprofen S(+)								
Aminopyrine	> 10[a]	> 10[a]	> 10[a]	> 10[a]				
Aspirin	9.0[a,b], 9.9[b]	> 10[a,b] > 10[b]	> 10[a].> 10[b]	> 10[a]	11.0	83	14 000	0.0003
Benzydamine	5.0[a,b] (by 150% @ 1 mmol/l)	1.1[a], 1.1[b]	1.5[a,e], 1.5[b]	0.7[a]	0.16			
Carprofen								
Diclofenac,Na								
Diflunisal								
Fenoprofen,Ca		> 10.0[a]	0.43[a]	0.38[a]	0.35			
Flazalone								
Flurbiprofen							1.0	1.1
Flufenamic acid	0.024[b]	0.037[b]	0.027[b]		0.0008[b]	2.7		
Indomethacin	0.04[a], 0.04[b]	0.03[a], 0.03[b]	0.03[a], 0.031[b]	0.02[a]	0.0006[b]	0.5	100	0.04
Ketoprofen *rac*								
Meclofenamic acid	0.01[a], 0.007[b]	0.02[a], 0.014[b]	0.02[a], 0.014[b]	0.01[a]	0.0006[b]	4.0	4.0	0.4
Mefenamic acid	0.017[b]	0.025[b]	0.021[b]		0.0007[b]		1.0	0
Naproxen	0.37[a], 0.37[b]	0.48[a], 0.48[b]	0.45[a], 0.48[b]	0.50[a]	0.0008[b]	6.1		
Niflumic acid	0.1[a]	0.15[b]	0.25[b]		0.0003[b]			
Paracetamol	5.5[b]	5.0[b]	5.5[b]		0.48[b]			
Phenylbutazone	1.4[a], 0.43[b]	1.2[a], 0.37[b]	> 10[a]	> 10[a]	0.037[b]			
Piroxicam								
Salicylate,Na								
Sulindac								
Sulindac Sulphide								
Tolmetin								
Author	(1)	(2)	(2)	(2)	(3)	(4)	(4)	

[a] Individual PG's assayed by radiometric-TLC method following incubation for 3–5 min at 37°C with ^{3}H-arachidonic acid (+1.0) mmol/l non-radioactive arachidonic acid), 5 mmol/l adrenaline and 5 mmol/l glutathione. $PGF_{2\alpha}$ was produced in greater amounts than PGE_2 or PGD_2 although at lower substrate concentrations PGE_2 was produced in greater amounts. MDA was determined spectrophotometrically by reaction with thiobarbituric acid.

[b] Assay methods same as in a except that PG production was measured with 1 μmol/l arachidonic acid (AA).

[c] As well as with 1.0 mmol/l AA as substrate.

[d] Enzyme preparation incubated for 8 min with ^{14}C-arachidonate in a similar system to that described by Tomlinson *et al.* (1972) and the PGE_2 concentration determined by radiometric-TLC assay.

[e] Microsomal enzyme preparation incubated for 5 min at 37°C with ^{3}H-arachidonate 0.33 mmol/l, 3 mmol/l adrenaline, 3.0 mmol/l glutathione and assayed by radiometric-TLC system.

[f] Microsomes were incubated with 0.33 mmol/l arachidonic acid, 2.3 mmol/l adrenaline and assayed spectrophotometrically.

Bovine seminal vesicle[d,e,f] IC$_{50}$ (µmol/l)	Bovine seminal vesicle microsomes[g] IC$_{50}$ (µmol/l)	Rabbit brain microsomes[g]	Rabbit kidney medulla microsomes[g] IC$_{50}$ (µmol/l)	Guinea-pig 'gut' microsomes IC$_{50}$ (µmol/l)	Human rheumatoid synovial explants[h] PGE$_2$ IC$_{50}$ (µmol/l)	Mouse fibroblast MC5-5 cells[i] PGE$_2$ IC$_{50}$ (µmol/l)	Mouse primary peritoneal macrophages[j] PGE$_2$ IC$_{50}$ IC$_{50}$ (µmol/l)
84[d], 120[e], 8600[d], 52	50.0	41.3	41.8	29	2.0	3.8	0.55
23 200	176	193	188	3300	20.0	110	6.6
4.6[e], 3.6[f]							0.0096
				0.3			1.4
62[e]	56.0	36.8	73.3			9.1	1.4
				0.6		1.4	0.0033
24.1[f]	15.1	2.3	3.88		0.2		0.016
6.0[d], 6.2[f]	0.07	0.61	0.15		0.005	0.6	0.00017
						0.9	0.022
6.0[d], 19.2[f]	1.45	1.08	0.485				
4.0[d], 5.8[f]	0.26	0.25	0.25	6.5			
	14.4	14.7	47.7		20.0	6.8	0.28
32.0[d], 96[f]				32			
	15.0	0.8	3.8		100		79.4
204[d]	142	22.0	87.7		10.0	12.0	5.5
						0.8	0.10
					> 1000		0.00058
						5.4	0.96
(5)	(6)	(7)	(8)	(9)	(10)	(11)	(12)

[g] Microsomes were incubated with 20 µg sodium arachidonate 100 µg glutathione and 10 µg hydroquinone for 20 min at 37°C following preincubation for 5 mins with the drugs alone.

[h] Organ culture explants were incubated in DMEM + 10% fetal calf serum at 37°C for 3 days and the PGE$_2$ concentration in the media measured by RIA.

[i] Cells preincubated in MEME medium for 2 h with drugs then fresh MEME media containing drugs + 5 µg arachidonic acid was added and incubated at 37°C for 1 h. The media was then removed and PGE$_2$ concentration determined by RIA.

[j] Resident mouse peritoneal macrophages were preincubated in *serum-free* DEMM at 37°C with drugs alone, followed 1 h later by 0.1 µmol/l phorbol ester, TPA; 2 h later the medium was collected and assayed for PGE$_2$ and 6-keto PGF$_{1\alpha}$ by RIA. *References*: (1) Flower et al. (1973); (2) Cushman and Cheung (1976); (3) Ham et al. (1972); (4) Rome and Lards (1975); (5) Adams et al. (1976); (6) Taylor and Salata (1976); (7) Garcia-Rafanell and Forn (1979); (8) Dembińska-Kiec et al. (1976); (9) Krupp et al. (1976); (10) Robinson et al. (1978); (11) Carty et al. (1980); (12) Brune et al. (1981).

CHAPTER 5

179

terms of varying affinity of the drug for the active site of the enzyme compared with that of the substrate and the time dependence of inhibitory effects of the drug (Rome and Lands, 1975; Taylor and Salata, 1976). This time-dependent inhibition of COX activity has been related to the presence of the carboxylate moiety; methyl esterification of the carboxyl groups virtually eliminates this time-dependence (estimated by the ratio of k_{app}/I value; Table 5.8) (Rome and Lands, 1975). Interference of substrate binding was observed with indomethacin and aspirin but not with ibuprofen, and the former two drugs were found to have lower K_I values upon methyl esterification of the carboxylic acid group but this was not evident with ibuprofen (Rome and Lands, 1975). These and other mechanistic studies (Flower, 1974; Kulmacz *et al.*, 1991) all suggest that there are marked differences in the mechanisms of inhibition of prostaglandin G/H synthases (PGHS) or Cyclo-oxygenases (COXs) by NSAIDs. Thus, the well-established covalent acetylation by aspirin of cyclo-oxygenases at the entrance to the substrate binding pocket near the active site of these enzymes leads to irreversible blockade of substrate binding that is maintained for the biological life of the enzyme protein (Smith *et al.*, 1996; Wennogle *et al.*, 1995; Vane and Botting, 1996).

Other NSAIDs may have high affinity for the active site and exhibit tight-binding or pseudoirreversibility by non-covalent reactions. Some such as ibuprofen have reversibility of binding to the active site of cyclooxygenases (Ku *et al.*, 1975; Taylor and Salata, 1976; Procaccini *et al.*, 1977). Thus, varying substrate (arachidonate) concentration causes marked changes in the IC_{50} values for reversible inhibitors of cyclooxygenase.

Recent reports suggest that exceptionally low concentrations of ibuprofen *stimulate* prostaglandin production in mouse peritoneal macrophages (Sergeeva *et al.*, 1997a,b). It is claimed that these cells, being non-stimulated, contain the constitutive cyclooxygenase, COX-1, which is stimulated by 1 nmol/l ibuprofen. The mechanism for this stimulatory effect was not apparent from these authors' work. However, it is possible that the self-destruction of the enzyme that occurs as a result of peroxy-fatty acid metabolism could be protected by ibuprofen transiently occupying a region near the peroxidative region of the enzyme. Thus, Wessels and Hempel (1996) showed that the inhibitory effect of hydrogen peroxide (H_2O_2) on PGH synthase could be prevented by ibuprofen. They showed that ibuprofen did not chelate Fe^{2+} (such as might be present in the enzyme active site) nor did the drug scavenge $OH^{\bullet}$. They concluded that ibuprofen displaces oxidant species from the COX site of PGH synthase, thereby preventing the oxidation of functional groups responsible for the activity of this enzyme.

Relevance of tissue concentrations to effects on eicosanoid production *in vitro*

Relevance of *in vitro* data on inhibition of cyclooxygenase activity depends on relating IC_{50} values *in vitro* to the expected concentration of drug expected at sites of action *in vitro* (Brune *et al.*, 1977; Brune *et al.*, 1981a; Urquhart, 1991). The dynamics of accumulation

TABLE 5.9

Pharmacological concentrations of ibuprofen and enantiomers in synovial joints and lumbar regions of human subjects after oral dosing of ibuprofen

Dose (mg)	Enantiomer	Compartment	Concentration (µmol/l)	Author(s)
400–1200	rac	Synovial fluid	4.0–63 [0.6–1.6][a]	Wallis and Simkin (1983)
		Synovial tissue	126–150	
800	rac	synovial fluid	11 (S)-(+) 6.4 (R)-(–)	Cox et al. (1991)
600	rac	Synovial fluid	9.7 (S)-(+)[b] 8.6 (R)-(–)	Geisslinger et al. (1993)
400	(S)-(+)	Synovial fluid	10.6 (S)-(+)[c]	
1200	rac	Synovial fluid	3.3–4.9 (S)-(+)	Seideman et al. (1994)
			2.4–4.4 (R)-(–)	
		Blister fluid	2.4–6.0 (S)-(+)	
			and (R)-(–)	
800	rac	Lumbar CSF	1.5	Bannworth et al. (1995b)

[a] Free concentrations from estimates of free fraction ~0.026.
[b] t_{max} ~2.4 h.
[c] t_{max} ~2.3 h.

and retention of NSAIDs in synovial tissues and fluids varies considerably from drug to drug, pathological state (Wallis and Simkin, 1983) and protein binding of synovial fluid and plasma (Wanwimolruk *et al.*, 1983). Synovial fluid concentrations are about half those in tissues (Wallis and Simkin, 1983) and data for free (non-protein-bound) ibuprofen are only available for synovial fluid (Table 5.9). The *total* concentrations of ibuprofen in the synovial fluid range from 2.4 to 63 µmol/l in synovial fluid and from 126 to 150 µmol/l in plasma following therapeutic doses of 400–1200 mg to arthritic patients (Table 5.9; Glass and Swannell, 1978; Wallis and Simkin, 1983; Mäkelä *et al.*, 1981; Wanwimolruk *et al.*, 1983; Gallo *et al.*, 1986). More relevant to the potential effects on cyclooxygenase activity in synovial tissues are the free concentrations, which are about 0.26 those of total concentrations (Urquhart, 1991), so that in synovial fluid the range would be about 0.6–1.6 µmol/l. With most of the reported data for inhibition of cyclooxygenase activity *in vitro*, this is probably within the range of concentrations that would be considered effective for inhibiting prostaglandin production *in vivo*; higher doses of 2400 mg/day used in treatment of rheumatic diseases would be expected to have greater potential inhibitory effects based on these calculations.

Accumulation of ibuprofen enantiomers in cerebrospinal fluid in patients who received 800 mg *rac*-ibuprofen with nerve-root compression (probably an indication of effective pain-relieving concentrations at sites where the drug is acting) has shown that concentrations of (S)-(+)-ibuprofen averaged 1.5 µmol/l (Bannwarth *et al.*, 1995b).

Effects of ibuprofen enantiomers on prostaglandin synthesis

The pioneering studies of Adams and co-workers (1976) have proved to be fundamental in showing that the (S)-(+) enantiomer of ibuprofen was appreciably more potent as an

CHAPTER 5

inhibitor of prostaglandin production than the (R)-(–) form. Furthermore, these authors gave evidence of the potential for the (R)-(–) enantiomer to be biologically converted to the (S)-(+) form. These pioneering observations were important also for the understanding of the anti-inflammatory and analgesic actions of all propionic acid NSAIDs in relationship to their inhibitory effects on prostaglandin synthesis. It is now well-established that an appreciable proportion of the anti-inflammatory activity of propionic acids is due to the effects of their (S)-(+) enantiomers in inhibiting prostaglandin production. Furthermore, the clinical efficacy of ibuprofen, like that of other propionic acid derivatives, has been shown to be related to the effects of the (S)-(+) enantiomer (Geisslinger et al., 1989; Evans et al., 1991) and its formation.

Understanding of the metabolic pathways of the (R)-(–)-ibuprofen to (S)-(+) enantiomeric conversions came from the pioneering studies of Wechter and colleagues (1974), who propose that the inversion of (R)-(–)-ibuprofen to the (S)-(+) enantiomer occurs via the formation of a coenzyme A thioester intermediate. These observations were later supported in studies by Nakamura et al. (1981), Hutt and Caldwell (1983), Williams and Day (1985, 1988), Williams et al. (1986), Caldwell et al. (1988), Mayer et al. (1988), Tracy et al. (1993) and Knights and Roberts (1994). Proof of the route of metabolic conversion of (R)-ibuprofen with accompanying epimerization and hydrolysis of the ibuprofenyl coenzyme A conjugate came from the studies of Tracy and co-workers (1993). These authors showed that rat and human liver homogenates and rat liver microsomes had highly potent activity capable of forming ibuprofenyl-coenzyme A. The V_{max}/K_m values were for the rat liver homogenate 0.022 µg/min/mg protein, for the human liver homogenate 0.005 µg/min/mg protein and for rat liver microsomes 0.047 µg/min/mg. Corresponding values for rat liver mitochondria were 0.027 ml/min/mg for the rate of formation of ibuprofenyl-coenzyme A. Interestingly, these authors showed that the (S)-(+) enantiomer of ibuprofen could inhibit formation of ibuprofenyl-coenzyme A; the exact significance of this is not as yet determined.

The exact contribution of the bioconversion of (R)-(–)-ibuprofen to the anti-inflammatory and prostaglandin synthesis inhibitory effects of racemic mixtures of ibuprofen that are conventionally used depends on the pharmacokinetics of this drug in different systems. In general there is estmated to be 30–60% bioconversion of (R)-(–)- to (S)-(+)-ibuprofen (Rudy et al., 1991; Bannwarth et al., 1995b; see also Chapter 4 in this book).

Effects of metabolic intermediates

While inhibition of prostaglandin production by ibuprofen occurs with the (S)-(+) but not the (R)-(–) enantiomer (Adams et al., 1976), recent studies have also implicated the (R)-(–)- and (S)-(+)-ibuprofenyl-coenzyme A intermediates formed during metabolism of (R)-(–)-ibuprofen to the (S)-(+) antipode (table 5.13). Thus, calculations of expected drug concentrations required for inhibition of cyclooxygenase based on in vitro data should take account of the concentration of (S)-(+)-ibuprofen and the two coenzyme A derivatives. In the absence of data on the latter two intermediates from rheumatic patients the

(S)-(+)-ibuprofen concentrations following 600–1200 mg of racemic ibuprofen range from 49 to 98 μmol/l (Cox *et al.*, 1991; Geisslinger *et al.*, 1993; Seideman *et al.*, 1994). The concentrations of (R)-(–)-ibuprofen achieved are usually about $^1/_3$–$^1/_2$ those of the (S)-(+) enantiomer, so accounting for conversion of (R)-(–)-ibuprofen to the coenzyme A derivatives probably would mean that the total concentrations of (S)-(+)-ibuprofenyl-CoA and (R)-(–)-ibuprofenyl-CoA would be accounted for by adding 50% to the above figures for (S)-(+)-ibuprofen to give a value of approximately 75–150 μmol/l. If the free fraction is the same for enantiomers as for the racemic drug, then this would give free concentrations of the order of 1.95–3.9 μmol/l. As with the calculations based on racemic concentrations, these values are within the range expected for cyclooxygenases to be inhibited.

Effects on cyclooxygenase isoforms

The recognition of the importance of the two cyclooxygenase isoenzymes for regulation of prostaglandin production and the actions of NSAIDs on the relative activities of these enzymes has recently attracted much interest (Vane and Botting, 1995). Concepts of the tissue selectivity of effects of different NSAIDs on the relative effects of NSAIDs and non-narcotic analgesics on the activities of the two cyclooxygenases that have been identified so far have formed the basis for recognizing that there may be varying effects of these drugs on prostaglandins derived physiologically compared with those under pathological conditions (Vane and Botting, 1995; Jouzeau *et al.*, 1997). The basis of this comes from the understanding that the non-inducible form of cyclooxygenase (COX-1) produces prostaglandins that are important for physiological regulation, e.g. control of blood flow, gastric acid secretion, mucus production, regulation of certain reproductive functions. The second form of cyclooxygenase (COX-2) has importance for inflammation in that the production of the enzyme protein is enhanced by inflammatory stimuli such as by cytokines following gene induction of the AP-1 gene-regulated sequence that is in the promoter region located up-stream from the gene responsible for transcribing the message sequence for COX-2. This *inducible form* of cyclooxygenase is subject to glucocorticoid inhibition by inhibition of the glucocorticoid reactive element (GRE) sequence in the promoter region. Micromolar concentrations of both aspirin and salicylate have been shown to inhibit the production of COX-2 enzyme protein, but the mechanism of this is as yet unclear. That inhibition of COX-2 induction is achieved by almost similar concentrations of aspirin and salicylate and at concentrations in relationship to aspirin that are much lower than the irreversible inhibition of the enzyme suggests that the almost equivalent anti-inflammatory activity of both aspirin and salicylate seen in some model animal systems and in humans being treated with high doses of both these drugs may be explained by inhibiting the production of the enzyme COX-2.

(S)-(+)-Ibuprofen differs from drugs such as indomethacin or aspirin that are irreversible or pseudoirreversible inhibitors respectively of COX-1 and COX-2 (Jouzeau *et al.*, 1997). Various studies have indicated that ibuprofen exhibits a degree of reversibility that can be

CHAPTER 5

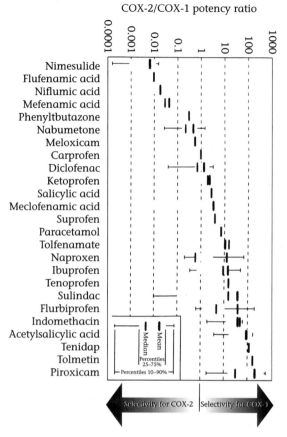

Figure 5.4: Relative potency against cyclooxygenase 1 (COX-1) and cyclooxygenase 2 (COX-2) of several NSAIDs currently available. (Reproduced with permission from Rabasseda (1996).)

seen by washing enzyme or cell preparations free of the drug as well as from kinetic analysis of pure enzyme systems.

Relative inhibitory effects of ibuprofen compared with other NSAIDs on cyclooxygenase isoenzymes

The potency of currently available NSAIDs in inhibiting COX-2 compared with COX-1 varies considerably with different drugs (Figure 5.4; Rabasseda, 1996). The data shown in Table 5.10 are a comparison of the effects of *rac*-ibuprofen with other NSAIDs on inhibition of the cyclooxygenases COX-1 and COX-2 in different cellular and enzymic systems. Considerable variation is evident in the respective molar potency ratios of COX-2 compared with COX-1 inhibition by *rac*-ibuprofen in different cellular systems; these ratios range from 0.018 to 15.0, although the data on phorbol ester-stimulated mouse macrophages (COX-2) compared with guinea-pig microsomes (COX-1) would seem the most extreme (Table 5.10). It may be that comparison of a cell-based system of macrophages with that of

TABLE 5.10

Comparison of the effects of ibuprofen with other NSAIDs and analgesics on cyclooxygenase isoenzymes. Data are IC_{50} (molar) potency rations of COX-2/COX-1 (with ratios relative to ibuprofen = 1)

Drug	Cultured LPS-stimulated J774.2 MΦ (COX-2)/bovine aortic endothelial cells (COX-1) (1)	Cultured human synovial (COX-2) gastric cells (COX-1) (2)	Transfected COX-2/COX-1 in murine enzymes COX-1 cells (3)	Human recombinant COX-2/COX-1 enzymes (4)	Transfected human COX-2/COX-1 enzymes into COX-1 cells (5)	Phorbol ester-stimulated mouse MΦ COX-2 (6) guinea-pig 'Gut' microsomes (COX-1) (7)
Ibuprofen (R/S)	15 (1)	1.3 (1)	0.7 (1)	0.6 (1)	3.1 (1)	0.018 (1)
Aspirin	166 (11)					0.0002 (0.011)
Carprofen (R/S)	1.0 (0.07)					
Diclofenac.Na	0.7 (0.047)	0.5 (0.39)		1.7 (2.8)	7.6 (2.5)	0.032 (1.7)
Etodolac(+/−)		0.1 (0.077)			0.8 (0.26)	
Flurbiprofen (R/S)	1.3 (0.087)		5.7 (8.1)	12.8 (21.3)	6.4 (2.1)	
Indomethacin	60 (4)	1.1 (0.85)	22.3 (31.9)	14.7 (24.5)	74.1 (23.9)	0.0002 (0.011)
Ketoprofen (R/S)				4.7 (7.8)		
Meclofenamic acid			6.9 (9.9)		6.5 (2.1)	
Mefenamic acid				0.03 (0.05)		
Meloxicam	0.8 (0.053)					
Nabumetone metabolite						
6-Methoxy-2-nqphthyl acetic acid						
Naproxen,Na	0.6 (0.04)	1.0 (0.77)	0.1 (0.14)	0.3 (0.5)	1.5 (0.48)	
Nimesulide	0.1 (0.0003)			3.3 (5.5)	5.9 (1.9)	0.043 (2.4)
Paracetamol	7.4 (0.49)					
Phenylbutazone						0.17 (0.94)
Piroxicam	250 (16.7)	0.2 (0.15)	9.5 (13.6)		6.3 (2.0)	
Salicylate,Na	2.8 (0.19)				28.2 (9.1)	
Sulindac	100 (6.7)					
Sulindac sulfide			30.9 (44.1)		39.0 (12.6)	
Tolfenamic acid	16.7 (1.1)					
Tolmetin.Na	175 (11.7)					

References: (1) Vane and Botting (1995); (2) Adams *et al.* (1990); (3) Meade *et al.* (1993); (4) Barnett *et al.* (1994); (5) Laneuville *et al.* (1994); (6) Brune *et al.* (1981); (7) Krupp *et al.*, 1976; Ku *et al.*, 1995 (mouse).

TABLE 5.11

Time-dependent changes in inhibitory effects of NSAIDs on COX-1 and COX-2 activities[a]

Drug (type of inhibition)	Microsomal enzymes			20-min pre-incubated microsomal enzymes			30-min pre-incubated HUVECs (COX-1) and A-549 (COX-2)*		
	COX-1	COX-2	Ratio COX-1/COX-2	COX-1	COX-2	Ratio COX-1/COX-2	COX-1	COX-2	Ratio COX-2/COX-1
Indomethacin (pseudo-irreversible time-dependent)	13.5	>1000	>74	0	0.35	3.5			
Ibuprofen *rac* (reversible, non-time-dependent)	4.0	12.5	3.1	14	80	5.7	0.5	0.4	0.9
Meloxicam (reversible)	–	–	–	36.6	0.49	0.013	0.15	0.05	0.3

From Vane and Botting (1996). *Data from William Harvey Research Institute, London.
[a] Values are IC$_{50}$ (μmol/l) or ratio of IC$_{50}$ values.

an isolated enzyme preparation of gut microsomes does not reflect the standard conditions, especially those employed in transfected cell systems where the cell environment for substrate (arachidonate) release would be expected to be similar in the two cell systems that have been transfected with human or murine recombinant prostaglandin H Synthase-1 (PGHS-1) or cyclo-oxygenase-1 (COX-1) and PGHS-2 (COX-2) isoenzymes. In the data on COS-1 transfected cells the ratios of COX-2/COX-1 inhibitory activity by *rac*-ibuprofen range from 0.6 to 3.1 which, considering the differences in assay methodology, is a reasonable range of variability.

The data from cultured cells is more variable, with the COX-2/COX-1 ratios being 1.3 and 15 (Table 5.10). These differences may reflect variations in intrinsic COX activity and availability of substrate. It may, however, also be argued that systems such as human synovial (COX-2) and gastric cells (COX-1) may reflect the expected drug effects on the two populations of cells wherein drug effects are manifest relative to their anti-inflammatory (COX-2) activity compared with mucosal irritancy (COX-1) related effects respectively.

Comparisons of the COX-2/COX-1 inhibitory ratios of different NSAIDs *relative* to ibuprofen (set at 1; Table 5.10) also show marked variability within each drug type. There is, however, a trend for the data from transfected cell lines to show similar ratios compared with those data from established cell lines. Again, as discussed above, the arguments for or against these two systems giving information about drug effects relative to their expected *in vivo* actions is debatable.

One source of variability of COX selectivity with different NSAIDs is the time-dependent and mechanistic influences on the respective cyclooxygenases (Table 5.11; Vane and Botting, 1996), this being an extension of the effects noted in microsomal systems noted previously. Time-dependent changes in the inhibitory effects of indomethacin (a pseudo-irreversible inhibitor) are particularly evident in the potent inhibitory effects of this drug on activity of both COXs following pre-incubation of the drug with the isolated microsomal enzyme compared with that where the drug has been added simultaneously with the substrate (Table 5.11; Vane and Botting, 1996).

The more pronounced inhibition of COX-2 and COX-1 with pre-incubated enzyme preparations is not evident with ibuprofen, a reversible enzyme inhibitor (Table 5.11). Indeed, there is a trend towards somewhat more potent effects of simultaneous incubation of drug with substrate compared with that where the enzyme was pre-incubated with drug (Table 5.11). As noted above, the relative inhibitory effects of drugs in isolated enzyme preparations differ considerably from those in cell lines (Table 5.11), making interpretation of the relative drug effects somewhat more difficult.

Differences in COX-selectivity of NSAIDs are evident in comparing the drug effects on isolated enzyme preparations, broken cells and whole cells (Table 5.12; Mitchell *et al.*, 1994; Kargman *et al.*, 1996; Vane and Botting, 1996). The potency of various drugs on purified enzymes is strikingly similar to that on broken cell preparations, but both are

TABLE 5.12

Comparison of the effects of ibuprofen and other NSAIDs on purified ovine prostaglandin G/H synthases (cyclooxygenases), with that in whole and disrupted J774.2 macrophages

| | COX-1/COX-2 ratios | | | Whole cell IC_{50} (nmol/l) | |
Drug	Purified enzymes	Broken cells[a]	Whole cells[a]	COX-1	COX-2
Ibuprofen	46	53.3	15	3.0	50
Aspirin	42	25	167	1.7	270
Indomethacin	50	40	60	0.0028	0.17
Salicylate. Na	Inactive	Inactive	2.9	219	625

From Vane and Botting (1996).
[a] J774.2 Macrophages were stimulated with *E. coli* lipopolysaccharide to serve as a source of COX-2 activity. Purified enzymes were ovine seminal vesicles (COX-1) and ovine placenta (COX-2).

markedly different from the inhibitory effects on COX-2 and COX-1 in isolated cells. This reflects availability of substrate, cofactors and influence on the environment in respective intracellular compartments where the cyclooxygenases are localized.

As noted previously, there are marked differences in the potencies of (R)-(−) and (S)-(+) enantiomers of ibuprofen compared with racemic ibuprofen on cyclooxygenase activities. Furthermore, the inhibitory effects of these isomers varies according to the cellular or enzymic system being considered (Table 5.13). The values of COX-2/COX-1 ratio in whole primary cell populations range from 1.3 to 7.2, whereas that in purified human enzyme preparations is 67 (Table 5.13). The same arguments regarding different experimental conditions noted above also apply here. Of particular interest in relation to the pharmacokinetics of *rac*-ibuprofen are the relative potencies of the metabolic intermediates of (R)-(−)- to (S)-(+)-ibuprofen bioconversion and their respective ratios (Table 5.13). COX-1 inhibition by (R)-(−)-ibuprofenyl-CoA and all these are appreciably less potent as inhibitors of COX-1 than (S)-(+)-ibuprofen (Table 5.13). However, (R)-(−)-ibuprofenyl-CoA and (S)-(+)-ibuprofenyl-CoA are relatively potent inhibitors of COX-2, even though they are not quite as potent as (S)-(+)-ibuprofen (Table 5.13). These data suggest that in respect of pharmacological actions at inflamed sites, both metabolic intermediates have the potential for inhibiting prostaglandin production together with that of (S)-(+)-ibuprofen. Thus, the inhibition of prostaglandin production at inflamed sites reflects that from the amount of conversion of (R)-(−)- to (S)-(+)-ibuprofen (with both intermediates present) as well as (S)-(+)-ibuprofen itself. The potential for both the CoA metabolites of ibuprofen to cause inhibition of COX-1 in the stomach mucosal or renal systems, where side-effects occur related to COX-1 inhibition, is, however, much lower (Table 5.13). This is because both coenzyme A (CoA) metabolites are appreciably less potent inhibitors of COX-1 (Table 5.13).

TABLE 5.13

Effects of racemic compared with the (R)-(−) and (S)-(+) enantiomers of ibuprofen and their thioester-CoA derivatives on prostaglandin G/H synthases (cyclooxygenases)

Drugs	Human purified isoenzymes[a] (1)			Human platelets (COX-1) Rat mesangial cells + IL-1 (COX-2) (1)			Human whole blood[b] (2)		
	COX-1	COX-2	Ratio COX-2/COX-1	COX-1	COX-2	Ratio COX-2/COX-1	COX-1	COX-2	Ratio COX-2/COX-1
rac-Ibuprofen	0.015	1.0	67	380	500	1.3	6.5	46.7	7.2
(S)-(+)-Ibuprofen	0.09	0.4	4.4	70	150	2.4	2.1	1.6	0.76
(S)-(+)-Ibuprofenyl-CoA							22.5	11.8	0.52
(R)-(−)-Ibuprofen	0.6	4.0	6.6	6500	2000	0.3	34.9	> 250	
(R)-(−)-Ibuprofenyl-CoA							219	5.6	0.026

Values are IC_{50} (μmol/l) or ratio of IC_{50} values.
[a] Values are approximate only, derived from published concentration-response.
[b] COX-2 determined in subjects who had previously consumed 500 mg aspirin at 2 days before withdrawal of blood to eliminate COX-1 activity, the whole blood being stimulated with E. coli lipopolysaccharide to induce COX-2.
References: (1) Boneberg et al. (1996); (2) Neupert et al. (1997).

Another factor that influences the potential of *rac*-ibuprofen to inhibit COX-1 production of physiologically important prostaglandins is the relative effects of the enantiomers in the diastereoisomeric mixture compared with the individual enantiomers. It is evident (Table 5.13) that *rac*-ibuprofen has inhibitory effects between those of (S)-(+)- and (R)-(–)-ibuprofen. However, these effects are not consistent in different cellular/enzymic systems, probably reflecting the influence of substrate availability and other experimental variables noted previously. The concentration–response curves are also non-identical (Boneberg *et al.*, 1996). However, the fact that inhibitory potency of *rac*-ibuprofen is between those of (S)-(+)- and (R)-(–)-ibuprofen combined, with these forms being reversible inhibitors of COXs, suggests that a model for inhibition of cyclooxygenase activity could be formulated to indicate that the individual enantiomers are competitive with one another for action at the active sites on cyclooxygenases (Figure 5.3). The relative affinity of the (R)-(–) enantiomer for the active site would be expected to be less than that of the (S)-(+) antipode, but similarity of their respective structures and relative sizes would allow for appreciable occupancy of cyclooxygenase active sites by (R)-(–) in the presence of (S)-(+); these effects being, of course, dependent on substrate concentration. As indicated previously, support for the concept of competitive interactions of the enantiomers of ibuprofen for the active site of cyclooxygenases has come from recent studies on prostaglandin in pig gastric mucosa in organ culture (Rainsford *et al.*, 1997b). These reversible interacting effects of *rac*-ibuprofen constituent enantiomers may have significance for sparing of the stomach, kidney and other organs wherein COX-1 is an important physiological regulator of prostaglandin production.

5.1.7 Effects on leukotriene production

In general ibuprofen has been regarded as being inactive as an inhibitor of the 5-lipoxygenase pathway. However, studies by Villlaneuva *et al.* (1993) have shown that the (R)-(–) and (S)-(+)enantiomers and the racemic form of ibuprofen inhibit production of leukotriene B_4 (LTB$_4$) in calcium ionophore-stimulated human neutrophils. The IC$_{50}$ for both isoforms was within the same potency range, being 0.14–0.36 µmol/l. Moreover, Vanderhoek and Bailey (1984) showed that 5-lipoxygenase activity was inhibited by *rac*-ibuprofen with an IC$_{50}$ of 0.42 µmol/l. This is within the range of inhibition of LTB$_4$ production observed by Villaneuva *et al.* (1993), suggesting that the mechanism of the reduction of LTB$_4$ production is by the inhibition of 5-lipoxygenase activity.

It is also possible that there could be a more generalized effect of ibuprofen on the release of phospholipids from membranes that underlies this apparent inhibition of leukotriene production. Thus, Vanderhoek and Bailey (1984) observed that 5 mmol/l ibuprofen inhibited the synthesis in neutrophils of di- and triglycerides and phospholipids from arachidonic acid.

The effects of ibuprofen on other pathways of arachidonic acid metabolism have also been found to be more complex. Vanderhoek and Bailey (1984) showed that ibuprofen 1.0 and 5.0 mmol/l *enhanced* the production of the 15-lipoxygenase enzyme protein. While the effects of ibuprofen on phospholipid and 15-lipoxygenase activity are apparent at higher concentrations than observed with the effects on 5-lipoxygenase, they illustrate more complex actions on eicosanoid and phospholipid metabolism than hitherto realized.

5.1.8   Smooth-muscle contractility

The above observations suggest that ibuprofen and other NSAIDs may, in general, have inhibitory effects on the contraction of smooth muscle. Famaey and co-workers (1977) showed that the contractions of the isolated guinea-pig ileum induced by prostaglandin E_2 alone or with acetylcholine, histamine or nicotine were inhibited by ibuprofen 40 µg/ml (194 µmole/l). (Where concentrations have been expressed in mass units, the value of their molar concentration is shown for comparison with other pharmacological effects and tissue/plasma concentrations during therapy (see table 5.9)). Other NSAIDs had similar effects on muscle contraction induced by these stimuli.

Ono *et al.* (1977) showed that ibuprofen and a range of other NSAIDs inhibited the resting tonus of the guinea-pig tracheal chain in a concentration-related manner. Furthermore, there was a linear correlation between the logarithm of the concentration required for inhibition of the resting tonus and the logarithm of the arachidonic acid-induced contraction of the rat fundus strip, implying that the inhibition of prostaglandin production by the NSAIDs relates to their inhibitory effects on smooth-muscle contractility (Ono *et al.*, 1977).

It therefore appears that ibuprofen has the property, like other NSAIDs, of inhibiting smooth-muscle contractility. The pharmacological consequences of these effects on intestinal muscle may be to promote side-effects on the gastrointestinal tract involving GI motility.

5.1.9   Effects on nitric oxide production

The production of nitric oxide (NO) and the subsequent combination with superoxide to form the very potent peroxynitrite ($HOONO^-$) anion appear to play a major role along with prostaglandins and other inflammatory mediators in the development of inflammation (Moncada *et al.*, 1991; Teixeira *et al.*, 1993; Pryor and Squadrito, 1995; Verissimo de Mello *et al.*, 1997). Moreover, there is considerable interrelation between NO and PG systems since (a) inducible nitric oxide synthase (iNOS) and COX-2 are co-expressed in inflammatory cells, (b) NO inhibits both COX-2 activity and induction, (c) inhibition of NO production stimulates PG production. In contrast, inhibition of PG synthesis by indomethacin has no effect on NO production in cultured macrophages (Swierkosz *et al.*, 1995).

TABLE 5.14

Effects of ibuprofen compared with other anti-inflammatory/analgesic drugs on inducible (inflammatory) nitric oxide synthase

Drug	System/treatment	Response(s)	Authors
Ibuprofen	Rat glial cells stimulated with LPS and IFN-γ	Enzyme activity unaffected. However, induction of iNOS inhibited @ IC_{50} 760 μmol/l; iNOS protein synthesis inhibited @ IC_{50} 890 μmol/l; iNOS. mRNA inhibited IC_{50} > 2 mmol/l	Stratman et al. (1997)
Ibuprofen Aspirin Indomethacin Salicylate.Na	Rat alveolar macrophages stimulated with LPS and IFN-γ	All drugs inhibited iNOS enzyme by pretranslational inhibition.	Aeberhard et al. (1995)
Aspirin Indomethacin Paracetamol Salicylate.Na	Mouse macrophages stimulated with LPS	Inhibition of iNOS (protein) synthesis by ibuprofen and aspirin IC_{50} = 3 mmol/l but no effect by other drugs.	Amin et al. (1995)
Ibuprofen	Human umbilical vein endothelial cells	Inhibition of cNOS but activation of iNOS.	Menzel and Kolarz (1997)

The summary of data from recent published reports of the effects of ibuprofen on nitric oxide synthase activity shown in Table 5.14 indicates that there are apparently differences in the effects of this drug, as well as other NSAIDs, on iNOS in macrophage compared with endothelial cells (Aeberhard *et al.*, 1995; Amin *et al.*, 1995; Menzel and Kolarz, 1997; Stratman *et al.*, 1997). While the NSAIDs do not appear to affect the NOS enzymic activity in macrophage cell lines or primary cells (Swierkosz *et al.*, 1995; Stratman *et al.*, 1997), ibuprofen and other NSAIDs seem to inhibit the induction of iNOS in mouse and rat primary macrophages and rat glial cells (Aeberhard *et al.*, 1995; Amin *et al.*, 1995; Stratman *et al.*, 1997). In endothelial cells, cNOS is inhibited but iNOS is increased (Menzel and Kolarz, 1997). There does not appear to be any reason for these differences in the response to ibuprofen on iNOS and cNOS in endothelial cells compared with macrophages.

5.1.10   Leukocytes and vascular permeability

Emigration of polymorphonuclear and mononuclear leukocytes into inflamed sites and their subsequent activation to produce inflammatory mediators (eicosanoids, oxyradicals, peroxynitrite, proteases/hydrolases) is well known to constitute a major component of the inflammatory process (Weissmann *et al.*, 1978; Abramson *et al.*, 1984; Eiserich *et al.*, 1998). The initial events involving adhesion and immigration of leukocytes to the endothelia adjacent to foci of inflammation are now well described and involve interactions of specific surface adhesion receptors on the respective cells (integrins, selectins) in a complex repertoire of events. NSAIDs have been known to affect initial stages of leukocyte adhesion to and migration through endothelia *in vitro* and *in vivo* (Meacock and Kitchen, 1976; Simchowitz *et al.*, 1979; Dawson, 1980; Abramson *et al.*, 1984; Kaplan *et al.*, 1984; Perianin *et al.*, 1984; Shimanuki *et al.*, 1985a,b; DiMartino *et al.*, 1989). Recent studies have shown that ibuprofen inhibits expression of vascular adhesion molecules (VCAM-1) (Kapiotis *et al.*, 1996; see also later section), so there may be regulation of the surface adhesion receptors related to these events by ibuprofen. These events may form a major part of the actions of ibuprofen in mediating the early stages of its anti-inflammatory activity.

Vascular changes and oedema

Inhibition of the development of oedema, as reflected by reduced protein and fluid accumulation, has been found with ibuprofen in several animal models (Meacock and Kitchen, 1976; Martin *et al.*, 1994). Discrimination of the effects of ibuprofen on vascular permeability from the accumulation and activation of leukocytes and their interaction with the microvasculature is an important issue in understanding the mode of action of this drug. Like many NSAIDs, ibuprofen has been found to have inhibitory effects on permeability to various agents and may also influence microvascular dynamics (Adams and Traber, 1982; Slater and House, 1993; Marzi *et al.*, 1993). Studies by Rampart and Williams (1986) in a rabbit skin model *in vivo* have shown differences in response to ibuprofen in inhibiting oedema formation measured by ^{125}I-albumin depending on the route of administration and inflammagen(s) employed. These authors found that the leakage of albumin following local or i.v. injection of C5a-des-arg or bradykinin, with arachidonic acid, was suppressed by ibuprofen, but when the latter fatty acid was replaced by PGE_2 local injection of ibuprofen had no effect while i.v. ibuprofen was inhibitory. Since the PGE_2 would have been extensively metabolized when given i.v., the local effect of the prostaglandin must have ameliorated the effects of ibuprofen. The authors concluded that the anti-oedemic effects of ibuprofen are independent of cyclooxygenase inhibition. However, the interpretation may be further complicated by the fact that the metabolism of the inflammatory peptides could also be inhibited by ibuprofen. It is possible that both a prostaglandin-dependent as well as an independent mechanism could be acting in the anti-oedemic effects of ibuprofen.

Endothelial cell–leukocyte interaction *in vitro*

Underlying the early stages of leukocyte adhesion and subsequent migration through the endothelial cells of the microvasculature are a series of complex events centring on the interactions of these various cells. The first aspect to be considered is the responses of various leukocyte populations to chemotactic substances *in vitro* and *ex vivo*.

In vitro chemotaxis and adhesion

In vitro migration of leukocytes can be inhibited by some NSAIDs although the effect depends on the nature of the chemoattractant and other experimental variables. Using mixed rat leukocyte populations comprising 40–50% monocytes and 20–30% polymorpho-nuclear neutrophil leukocytes (PMNs) derived from peritoneal fluids of carrageenan-treated rats, Meacock and Kitchen (1976) were unable to show inhibitory effects of ibuprofen 25–100 µg/ml (121–485 µmole/l)) or several other NSAIDs with the exception of 10 µg/ml (28 µmole/l) indomethacin or 50–100 µg/ml (162–324 µmole/l) phenylbutazone on migration of these cells in glass capillaries. However, prior *in vivo* treatment for 4 h with 50 mg/kg ibuprofen p.o. induced reduction of leukocyte migration *in vitro* in glycogen-activated rat peritoneal leukocytes (Dawson, 1980). Similar results were obtained in this model with other NSAIDs (Dawson, 1980) so it is assumed this is a generalized effect in this class of drugs.

Ibuprofen has been found to inhibit the chemotactic response of PMNs from humans or rodents to various stimuli (formyl-methiomyl-leucyl peptide (fMLP), complement C_{5a} (C5a), casein) at concentrations that are within or at the high end of those in plasma during therapy (Rivkin *et al.*, 1976; Brown and Collins, 1977; Spisani *et al.*, 1979; Tursi *et al.*, 1982; Flynn *et al.*, 1984; Goodwin, 1984; Skubitz and Hammerschmidt, 1986; Nielson and Webster, 1987; Maderazo *et al.*, 1984). Earlier studies showed variable effects of the drug on spontaneous migration, but more recent studies have clearly shown that ibuprofen has a more potent effect on chemotaxis than on chemokinesis, the latter being evident at relatively high concentrations (1 mg/ml) in the presence of fMLP (Nielson and Webster, 1987).

Inhibition by ibuprofen of adherence to plastic surfaces and bovine pulmonary artery endothelial cells has been shown when the PMNs are stimulated with fMLP or the phorbol ester TPA (PMA) (Nielson and Webster, 1987). Ibuprofen, like that of the other NSAIDs, indomethacin and piroxicam, inhibits fMLP-induced neutrophil aggregation (Abramson et al., 1984).

Part of the effect of ibuprofen on fMLP-induced migration and adherence appears to be due to inhibition of the binding of fMLP to its receptors on the surface of PMNs (Skubitz and Hammerschmidt, 1986).

Panerai, Locatelli and Sacerdote (1992, 1993) observed that NSAIDs including ibuprofen inhibited the chemotaxis of human neutrophils and monocytes induced by substance P. Since substance P is known to stimulate production of prostaglandins and pro-inflammatory cytokines (Parrish et al., 1994) it is not known whether part of the inhibitory actions of these drugs could be attributed to the effects of NSAIDs on the release of these mediators in response to substance P. The relevance of the in vitro effects of ibuprofen on PMN leukocyte aggregation to the situation in vivo has been investigated by Abramson et al. (1984). These authors showed that neutrophils from volunteers who had taken 2400 mg/day ibuprofen for 3 days had a 44% reduction in fMLP-induced aggregation; similar effects were observed with neutrophils from subjects who took indomethacin 100 mg/day or piroxicam 20 mg/day for the same period. As with all studies on drug effects of cell–cell interactions, particular note should be taken that many of these studies were performed on cells from normal subjects. It is known that leukocyte interactions in cells isolated from rheumatic patients have subnormal or abnormal chemoattractant functions (Spisani et al., 1982).

It appears that ibuprofen affects the dynamics of neutrophil–neutrophil and neutrophil–endothelial cell interactions. The other component leukocytes involved in the expression of the cellular kinetics of the inflammatory process are also affected by ibuprofen. Thus, Nielsen and Bennedsen (1983) observed that ibuprofen inhibited the zymosan-activated serum (ZAS)-induced chemotaxis of human blood monocytes at concentrations about 25 µg/ml (121 µmole/l), the IC_{50} being 70 µg/ml (340 µmole/l). While naproxen also inhibited ZAS-induced chemotaxis with an IC_{50} of 62 µg/ml (270 µmole/l), indomethacin, which also inhibited chemotaxis above 1 µg/ml (2.79 µmole/l), did not reach an IC_{50} value. The authors concluded that inhibition of monocyte chemotaxis is not a general property of all NSAIDs.

Chemotaxis of ZAS-activated rat peritoneal monocytes has also been shown to be inhibited by 100 µg/ml but not 30 µg/ml ibuprofen (Dawson, 1980). Of other NSAIDs investigated by Dawson (1980), only benoxaprofen (15–30 µg/ml (121 µmole/l)) was found to be inhibitory.

CHAPTER 5

Lymphocyte chemotaxis induced by phytohemagglutinin was found to be inhibited by high concentrations of ibuprofen (Panayi, 1975). In a similar system, ibuprofen at a concentration of 25 μg/ml (12 μmole/l) inhibited lymphocyte chemotaxis but did not affect blast-cell transformation except for weak effects at 150 μg/ml (0.73 μmole/l) (Tursi *et al.*, 1982).

These results suggest that ibuprofen has effects on chemotaxis of all main leukocyte populations but at concentrations that are probably within the higher range of plasma values encountered during therapy with this drug.

Leukocyte–endothelial interactions *in vitro*

As previously mentioned, leukocyte–endothelial interactions are inhibited by micromolar concentrations of ibuprofen (Slater and House, 1993). This effect is different from that of indomethacin which, paradoxically, increases these cell interactions in response to fMLP (Slater and House, 1993). There is one report showing that interactions between bovine endothelial cells and neutrophils are not affected by ibuprofen, indomethacin or aspirin (Dunn *et al.*, 1986). It is possible that the source of cells and the conditions may not have been suitable for demonstrating effects of ibuprofen in this system. In the systems where ibuprofen has been shown to be active, it is possible that the mechanisms involve drug effects on the expression of surface adhesion receptors on endothelial cells and/or leukocytes.

It has recently been found that ibuprofen inhibits endotoxin (pyrogen)-induced adhesion of human leukocytes to cultured human umbilical vein endothelial cells (HUVECs) (Kapiotis *et al.*, 1996). This effect was related to inhibition by ibuprofen of both interleukin 1α, (IL-1α)-induced and tumour necrosis factor-α (TNF-α)-induced expression of vascular cell adhesion molecule-1 (VCAM-1; CD106); an effect which was observed at relatively high IC_{50} values of 0.5 mmol/l with both cytokines (Kapiotis *et al.*, 1996). The drug was less potent as an inhibitor of pyrogen-induced intercellular adhesion molecule-1 (ICAM-1; CD54) and was inactive on E-selectin (CD62E) expression (Kapiotis *et al.*, 1996). These results suggest that ibuprofen may have effects at the earliest phase of vascular–leukocyte interactions during the development of inflammation by reducing the expression of VCAM-1.

The effects of ibuprofen on more complex cell–cell interactions were investigated by Smith, Mooney and Korn (1993). These authors found that the ability of PMNs to adhere to human fibroblast and endothelial cells was unaffected by prior intake by normal volunteers of 1800 mg/day ibuprofen for 4–5 days, although there were reduced amounts of the adhesion molecule Mac-1 on neutrophils. They also found that this drug treatment augmented adhesion of T-lymphocytes to fibroblast and endothelial cells but was without affect on expression of LFA-1 receptors.

Ottonello *et al.* (1992) found that the inhibition by ibuprofen of neutrophil chemotaxis induced by fMLP was unrelated to the surface expression of the glycoprotein,

CD11b-CD18, required for both aggregation and chemotaxis. Also, the drug did not affect the release of lactoferrin from the secondary granules that contain the CD11b-CD18 glycoprotein molecules, indicating that it did not affect the storage or release of these molecules.

Overall, these results suggest that the main effects of ibuprofen on leukocyte–endothelial interactions probably relate to inhibition of the expression of the vascular adhesion molecule VCAM-1. Since there are known to be more complex cell–cell interactions, it is obviously important to investigate the actions of this drug in comparison with that of other NSAIDs, especially in cells derived from patients with inflammatory diseases.

Migration and activation of leukocytes *in vivo*

NSAIDs vary considerably in their effects and specificity of *in vivo* actions on leukocytes (Meacock and Kitchen, 1976; Dawson, 1980; Klein *et al.*, 1982; Abramson *et al.*, 1984; Kankaanranta *et al.*, 1994; Kaplan *et al.*, 1984; Perianin *et al.*, 1984; Blackham *et al.*, 1985; Shimanuki *et al.*, 1985b; Martin *et al.*, 1994, 1995). The modes of action of NSAIDs on leukocyte migration and accumulation in inflamed sites *in vivo* can vary considerably according to the animal model employed and the nature of the inflammatory stimulus.

In the reverse passive Arthus reaction in rats, where the main infiltrating cell is the polymorphonuclear (PMN) leukocyte, myeloperoxidase activity attributed to the latter was significantly reduced in the skin sites at 4 h after oral dosing with 30 and 60 mg/kg ibuprofen but not with 15 mg/kg of the drug (Bailey and Sturm, 1983). This dose-related effect of ibuprofen was not related to the oedema since no significant changes were observed in the oedema (as wet weight of tissue) at the injected site (confirmed by accumulation of radioiodinated bovine serum albumin). These results are in contrast to the effects of dexamethasone 0.025–0.1 mg/kg p.o., which affected both oedema formation and myeloperoxidase activity (Bailey and Sturm, 1983). The lack of effects of ibuprofen on oedema formation could be related to the low doses of the drug employed since higher doses may be necessary to prevent the vascular damage induced in the Arthus reaction. In contrast to these observations, Myers *et al.* (1985) observed that PMN accumulation in the reverse passive Arthus reaction induced in the pleural cavity of rats was inhibited by doses > 150 mg/kg ibuprofen given for 4 h but oedema formation was inhibited by 30% with 35 mg/kg ibuprofen. A similar effect of the NSAIDs indomethacin and benoxaprofen was observed in this model in that anti-oedemic activity was obtained at much lower doses than required for inhibition of PMN accumulation (Myers *et al.*, 1985). More potent inhibition of PMN accumulation was observed with potent dual cyclooxygenase–lypoxygenase inhibitors (Myers *et al.*, 1985).

Using carrageenan as an inducer of hind-paw inflammation in rats and animals pretreated for 3 days with methotrexate to deplete them of circulating polymorphonuclear leukocytes, it was found that prior treatment (before injection of carrageenan) with

CHAPTER 5

ibuprofen 2×75 mg/kg p.o. at 3 and 0.5 h markedly inhibited the paw inflammation (Meacock and Kitchen, 1976). The effects of ibuprofen were more pronounced than those of indomethacin 2×1 mg/kg p.o., phenylbutazone 2×50 mg/kg p.o. or aspirin 2×75 mg/kg p.o. given under the same conditions. This shows that ibuprofen has direct effects on the development of oedema independent of leukocyte effects.

In the rat pleurisy model, Meacock and Kitchen (1976) found that both the same dose of ibuprofen (2×75 mg/kg p.o.) employed in the paw oedema studies and a single dose of 150 mg/kg of the drug significantly inhibited mononuclear cell emigration at 24 h and 6 h respectively. These authors were unable to show similar effects with several other NSAIDs (e.g. aspirin, fenoprofen, naproxen), although benoxaprofen and high doses of phenylbutazone and indomethacin were inhibitory; as expected, corticosteroids were also inhibitory in this model. Higgs *et al.* (1980) also showed that ibuprofen inhibited leuko-cyte accumulation in the rat carrageenan model but that some other NSAIDs were also inhibitory.

Using a 6-day air pouch model in rats, Martin and co-workers (1994) showed that ibuprofen 0.1–1.0 mg/kg p.o. reduced the leukocyte (principally PMN) accumulation induced by injection into the pouch of carrageenan. A higher dose of 1.0 mg/kg p.o. of the drug reduced oedema but had no effect on protein levels. These results suggest that the effects of ibuprofen on leukocytes (which are evident in the lower dose range) can be dif-ferentiated from the vascular permeability changes underlying oedema formation.

Rampart and Williams (1986) showed that the accumulation of ^{125}I-albumin in the skin of rabbits injected locally with various combinations of C5a-des-Arg, PGE_2 and bradykinin showed differing effects of ibuprofen depending on the route of administration and combinations of inflammagens employed. The authors concluded that part of the anti-oedemic effect of ibuprofen could be ascribed to effects on neutrophil accumulation. Other authors have reported varying effects of ibuprofen on PMN leukocyte accumulation in rats (Goto *et al.*, 1976; Higgs and Flower, 1981; Martin *et al.*, 1980; Satoh *et al.*, 1982), but overall the inhibitory response to ibuprofen in these carrageenan models is rela-tively consistent. In one study variable effects of ibuprofen were found on leukocyte accumulation induced by the leukoattractant fMLP injected into the rabbit anterior eye chamber (Shimanuki *et al.*, 1985). Thus, 10 mg/kg/day ibuprofen given s.c. twice daily for 3 days prior to fMLP inhibited leukocyte migration, whereas the higher dose of 100 mg/kg s.c., like lower doses of 0.1–1.0 mg/kg s.c. of the drug, were ineffective. High doses of 10 mg/kg/day indomethacin or flurbiprofen s.c. were inhibitory in this system, whereas lower doses of these drugs or aspirin up to 100 mg/kg were without effect. A later study by the same group (Shimanuki *et al.*, 1985) showed that ibuprofen inhibited leuko-cyte accumulation in this model in a dose-related manner with an ID_{50} of 8 mg/kg/day.

Using calcium pyrophosphate crystals or decomplemented isologous rat serum as inflammagens in the rat pleural inflammation model, Perianin *et al.* (1984) observed that ibuprofen 6 mg/kg p.o. inhibited leukocyte accumulation induced by the former but not the latter. Flurbiprofen 1.5 mg/kg p.o. and indomethacin 3.0 mg/kg, p.o. in contrast, reduced the accumulation of leukocytes induced by both inflammagens. Ibuprofen, like the other NSAIDs, reduced the fluid accumulation produced by both agents. It is regrettable that the authors did not explore the effects of higher doses of ibuprofen in their study as this would have given important dose–response information, especially as the dose of 5 mg/kg of ibuprofen is relatively low for inhibiting inflammation.

In the skin abrasion model in rabbits, Palder *et al.* (1986) found that oral pretreatment with ibuprofen reduced leukocyte accumulation in leukotriene B_4^- and zymosan-activated serum injected sites.

In the mouse ear oedema model, in which inflammation is induced by local application to the inner side of the ear of 2 mg arachidonic acid, the prior (0.5 h) oral administration of 1.0–10 mg ibuprofen failed to cause reduction in oedema and myeloperoxidase as indeed did other cyclooxygenase inhibitors; cyclooxygenase–lipoxygenase inhibitors and glucocorticoids were, however, inhibitory in this model (Kotyuk *et al.*, 1993). The low dose of ibuprofen may not have been sufficient for expression of anti-inflammatory activity in this model, especially as the rate of clearance of this as well as other NSAIDs from the body is usually high in mice.

Accumulation of leukocytes and platelets occurs during the early stages of acute myocardial infarction and this inflammatory response is considered to be important to the development of myocardial injury. In the canine model of acute myocardial injury induced by left circumflex coronary artery occlusion, ibuprofen 12.5 mg/kg i.v. every 4 h beginning 0.5 h before occlusion significantly reduced accumulation of ^{111}In-labelled leukocytes but not of ^{111}In-labelled platelets coincident with an approximate 50% reduction in infarct size (Romson *et al.*, 1982). In the canine occlusion/alternating reperfusion model of myocardial infarction, Allan *et al.* (1985) showed that prior treatment with ibuprofen 12.5 mg/kg i.v. did not alter the accumulation of PMNs (assayed by the myeloperoxidase method) and actually increased the infarct size. Clearly, the differences between this study and that of Romson *et al.* (1982) relate to methodology and the period of i.v. administration of ibuprofen and require resolution. Higher doses of ibuprofen should also be investigated.

Further complications are evident from another study in pigs where it was found by Ito *et al.* (1989) that ibuprofen had only a slight effect on neutrophil trapping induced by intracoronary administration of the complement component C5a.

Rinaldo and Dauber (1985) and Rinaldo and Pennock (1986) showed that ibuprofen exhibited a paradoxical effect on endotoxin-induced neutrophilic alveolitis in rats. An enhancement of neutrophils was observed at 3 mg/kg p.o. and no effect at 10–20 mg/kg p.o., but inhibition was evident at the higher dose of 30 mg/kg p.o. Ibuprofen pretreatment has been found to reduce the early phase (involving leukocyte accumulation, elevation of lymph and pulmonary pressure) of endotoxin-mediated lung injury in unanaesthetized sheep (Traber *et al.*, 1984).

CHAPTER 5

Balk *et al.* (1988) observed that single doses of 1–20 mg/kg ibuprofen given i.v. to dogs 15 min after endotoxin inhibited the accumulation of neutrophils in the aorta at 2 h while the higher dose of 20 mg/kg ibuprofen reduced adherence at 0.5 h. In contrast, the adherence of neutrophils to the pulmonary artery was unaffected by the drug and it did not affect the development of lung injury.

In a model of lung injury in rabbits induced by hyperoxia (exposure to 100% oxygen for 1–4 days), Das and co-workers (1988) were unable to show any effects of oral ibuprofen on ^{111}In-labelled PMN accumulation or pathological changes in the lungs. This is a particularly severe model of lung injury and the authors noted that there was a 50% mortality after 96 h of oxygen exposure. Clearly, more experiments are necessary to determine the effects of various doses of ibuprofen compared with oxyradical scavenging drugs and NSAIDs at lower oxygen concentrations in this model.

The overall conclusions that can be drawn from these investigations on the effects of ibuprofen on leukocyte accumulation are:

(1) Ibuprofen inhibits accumulation of PMNs and monocytes in response to carrageenan in rats.
(2) Variable effects have been reported in animal models of myocardial or lung injury. These effects of ibuprofen on the accumulation of PMNs depend on the site, the timing and dosage of the drug and the duration and severity of induced injury.

Clearly, further work is required to examine these aspects in detail. As indicated in the subsequent section, there appear to be more profound effects of the drug on leukocyte *activation* and this may be of greater significance than the effects of the drug on accumulation of leukocytes per se in these models.

5.1.11   Leukocyte functions

Phagocytosis

Smith (1977) studied the effects of ibuprofen and other NSAIDs on the phagocytosis by guinea-pig neutrophils of serum-treated (or activated) zymosan particles and concomitant release of the lysosomal enzyme β-glucuronidase. Ibuprofen 10–1000 μmol/l was inactive on both phagocytosis and enzyme release, as were the same concentrations of aspirin and fenoprofen. Indomethacin, naproxen and chloroquine phosphate at 100 and 1000 μmol/l were inhibitory on both responses. Of interest in relation to the mechanisms of action of NSAIDs on prostaglandin production was the observation that PGE_2, PGE_1 and $PGF_{2\alpha}$ inhibited both phagocytosis and enzyme release from neutrophils.

In contrast with these results obtained with guinea-pig neutrophils, Tursi *et al.* (1982) observed a concentration-related inhibition of the phagocytosis of yeast particles by human neutrophils. While the effect of ibuprofen was not particularly marked, being

27% inhibition at 50 µg/ml (242 µmole/l) and 29% at 75 µg/ml (363 µmole/l) compared with hydrocortisone and carprofen, there were some mild inhibitory effects.

In a carrageenan–zymosan-induced model of peritonitis in rats, Goto, Hisadome and Imamura (1979) observed that prior (–1 h or –2 h) oral administration of 30 or 100 mg/kg ibuprofen reduced the activity of the lysosomal enzyme arylsulphatase. Similar inhibitory effects were observed with other standard NSAIDs at pharmacologically relevant doses of drugs.

Intramammary injection of ibuprofen to dairy cows with bacterial infections may reduce udder inflammation (Nickerson *et al.*, 1986). With interest in examining the mechanism of these effects, Nickerson *et al.* (1986) found that ibuprofen decreased bacterial cell viability while increasing leukocyte degranulation, phagocytosis and bacterial killing.

It appears, therefore, that ibuprofen has slight inhibitory effects on phagocytosis and inhibits release of lysosomal enzymes.

Oxyradical production and enzyme release and myeloperoxidase activity

Among the responses that neutrophils manifest in inflammation are the production of oxyradicals and tissue-destructive enzymes. Simchowitz *et al.* (1979) observed that ibuprofen inhibited fMLP induced production of superoxide by human neutrophils with an IC_{50} of 0.9 mmol/l. Indomethacin and phenylbutazone also inhibited superoxide production with an IC_{50} of 0.1 and 0.01 mmol/l respectively, but aspirin was without effects. The concentrations of ibuprofen required for inhibition of superoxide productions were relatively high in this study and are high with respect to those encountered in the plasma during therapy with this drug. The authors did not find that ibuprofen affected the binding of fMLP to neutrophils.

In contrast to the above results, Abramson *et al.* (1984) were unable to show any effects of ibuprofen on fMLP–induced superoxide production *in vitro* even though as noted previously, ibuprofen inhibited aggregation induced by this stimulus. Furthermore, they observed that neutrophils from subjects who had ingested 2.4 g/day ibuprofen for 3 days also failed to inhibit fMLP-induced superoxide production although aggregation was inhibited. Similar lack of effect on superoxide production but with inhibition of aggregation was observed in neutrophils from subjects that had ingested 100 mg/day indomethacin for 3 days. However, they found that piroxicam 20 mg/day for 3 days inhibited both neutrophil superoxide production and aggregation. Piroxicam 50 mmol/l also inhibited both superoxide production and aggregation *in vitro*.

Studies in sheep neutrophils has shown that pharmacological concentrations of ibuprofen inhibit the release of free oxyradicals, while meclofenamic acid is an oxyradical scavenger (Tahamont and Gee, 1986). Both these previous results contrast with observations in human neutrophils, where Nielson and Webster (1987) showed that ibuprofen (≤ 5 mg/ml) did inhibit fMLP-induced superoxide production but not by an oxyradical scavenging mechanism involving xanthine oxidase. These drug effects were found when C5a

CHAPTER 5

was employed as a stimulus, but there was no apparent toxicity of the drug as determined by lactate dehydrogenase release. Furthermore, these authors observed that ibuprofen did not affect the phorbol ester-induced oxyradical production or enzyme release. The inhibitory effects of ibuprofen were not reversed by addition of PGE_1, or PGE_2 (0.3–300 μmol/l).

In a later study, Shelly and Hoff (1989) observed that ibuprofen inhibited superoxide release, but in contrast with the studies of Simchowitz, Mehta and Spilberg (1979) they did find that ibuprofen affected the binding of fMLP to neutrophils.

Villanueva *et al.* (1992, 1993) examined the effects of the two enantiomers of ibuprofen and the racemic form of the drug on neutrophil superoxide production, release of lysosomal β-glucuronidase and leukotriene B_4 formation. This study is interesting because the authors determined the concentrations of the enantiomers in the cells and compared these with those in the media. The results showed that the concentrations of (R)-(−)-, (S)-(+)- or *rac*-ibuprofen in the cells were identical to those in the media.

Of particular interest was that fMLP-induced superoxide production and release of β-glucuronidase and calcium ionophore (calimycin)-induced production of leukotriene B_4 were all inhibited *equally* by *all* the forms of ibuprofen. The concentration range for effect was 100–1000 μmol/l although slight inhibition was observed on superoxide production with *rac*- and (S)-(+)-ibuprofen at 30 μmol/l. The IC_{50} values for oxyradical production were 0.6 mmol/l for *rac*-ibuprofen, 0.5 μmol/l for (S)-(+)-ibuprofen and 0.43 mmol/l for (R)-(−)-ibuprofen. Similarly, the IC_{50} values for effects of ibuprofen release of β-glucuronidase (range 0.44–0.58 mmol/l) and leukotriene B_4 generation (range 0.14–0.36 mmol/l) were identical for all three forms of the drug.

Differences in the effects of *rac*-ibuprofen on superoxide production observed by Villanueva *et al.* (1993) and Simchowitz *et al.* (1979) with the apparently negative effects observed by Abramson *et al.* (1984) may be due to the concentrations of the stimulus, fMLP, employed by these authors. Thus, the positive (i.e. inhibitory) effects of ibuprofen observed by Villanueva *et al.* (1993) and Simchowitz *et al.* (1979) were obtained at lower concentrations of fMLP (30 and 40 mmol/l respectively) than those employed by Abramson *et al.* (1984), which were appreciably higher (100 mmol/l). The higher concentrations of the stimulus could not have been optimal for establishing the effects of the drug and could have been such as to overcome any inhibitory effects of the drug.

The similarity of IC_{50} values for release of superoxide, leukotriene B_4 and β-glucuronidase indicates that the effects of the various forms of the drug on these events are independent of the prostaglandin system. Of particular interest as well is the effect of all forms of the drug on production by stimulated cells of leukotriene B_4; the IC_{50} values for this effect are about one-half to one-third lower than those for the other two actions of the drug.

The direct effect of ibuprofen on xanthine oxidase, a source of superoxide, is considered unlikely from studies by Carlin *et al.* (1985), Nielson and Webster (1987) and Chatham *et al.* (1995). However, using the xanthine oxidase-induced depolymerization of hyaluronic acid as an assay of drug effects on superoxide functions (e.g. via scavenging of this anion), Carlin *et al.* (1985) observed that ibuprofen, like several other NSAIDs as well as paracetamol, inhibited this reaction; the IC_{50} for ibuprofen was 0.33 mmol/l, which was comparable with that of aspirin and some other NSAIDs but was appreciably higher than that of paracetamol, which was 0.05 mmol/l.

Ibuprofen 200 mg/kg p.o. was found to reduce the liver microsomal lipid oxidation induced by carbon tetrachloride in normal and carrageenan-inflamed rats (Parola *et al.*, 1984). This effect was not evident with phenylbutazone or indomethacin. Ibuprofen did not affect the production of glutathione in these rats.

Overall, these results suggest that ibuprofen has direct effects on the functions of oxyradicals, including lipid peroxidation, but the production of superoxide is not affected by the drug.

Cytokine production

Lang *et al.* (1995) observed that ibuprofen 100 µmol/l stimulated the production of TNF-α by zymosan-stimulated mouse peritoneal macrophages. Similar stimulatory effects were observed with flurbiprofen 10 µmol/l and indomethacin 20 µmol/l, but the corticosteroid dexamethasone 20 µmol/l inhibited TNF-α production in this system. Ibuprofen 100 µmol/l also stimulated TNF-α production in lipopolysaccharide-stimulated and thioglycollate-stimulated mouse macophages.

Recently, Jiang, Ting and Seed (1998) observed that phorbol ester (TPA/PMA)-stimulated human monocytes exhibited a concentration-dependent inhibition of TNF-α production. The IC_{50} value for ibuprofen was 485 µmol/l compared with that of indomethacin, which was 53 µmol/l, and fenoprofen, 265 µmol/l. A similar rank order of inhibition of TNF-α production was observed when okadaic acid was employed as an inducer; the IC_{50} for ibuprofen being 142 µmol/l. These inhibitory concentrations are at the high end of drug concentrations encountered in the plasma of patients during drug therapy.

Jiang, Ting and Seed (1998) showed that the production of the mRNA coding for TNF-α was inhibited by 1 mmol/l ibuprofen as well as the same concentration of indomethacin and fenoprofen, thus indicating that these drugs act as pretranslational modifiers of TNF-α production. Part of the mechanism may be mediated through the interruption by these NSAIDs of the amplifying effects of PGE_1 and 6-keto-$PGF_{1\alpha}$ on TNF-α production.

These results suggest that modulation of production of TNF-α by monocytes on NSAIDs, such as ibuprofen, may depend on the stimulus and/or state of priming of the monocytes to form macrophages as in the studies by Lang *et al.* (1995). Clearly, further investigations are necessary to clarify the meaning of these observations for the actions of drugs such as ibuprofen.

The proliferation of human peripheral T-lymphocytes by IL-2 has been found to be inhibited by ibuprofen 50–100 µg/ml (242–285 µmole/l) as well as by the same concentration

CHAPTER 5

of naproxen compared with that of tenidap 15–40 µg/ml (46.8–125 µmole/l) (Hall and Wolf, 1997). Similar effects have been observed with other NSAIDs (Goodwin and Ceuppens, 1983). Part of this effect may relate to the actions of these drugs in reducing production of prostaglandins which can affect T-cell proliferation (Goodwin and Ceuppens, 1983). However, it seems that a component of the actions of ibuprofen as well as of naproxen may be due to this drug inhibiting the binding of IL-2 to its receptor (Hall and Wolf, 1997). This effect is, apparently, not evident with tenidap (Hall and Wolf, 1997). These effects of ibuprofen may be of significance for its antirheumatic activity.

5.1.12   Immune functions

Of potential significance for NSAID effects on the immune system is an understanding of the distribution of the drugs within the compartments and cells of the immune system. Thus, Oelkers and co-workers (1996) observed that there was accumulation of ibuprofen enantiomers and metabolites in the lymph of rats given oral *rac*-ibuprofen. A total of 0.26% of the drug and metabolites was recovered in the thoracic duct after oral administration of 25 mg/kg of the drug. While not an appreciable amount, it is possible that this may have pharmacological consequences for the immune system, especially since the major component present was the prostaglandin synthesis inhibitory (S)-(+) enantiomer.

The above-mentioned effects of ibuprofen on cytokine production and actions have potential significance for drug effects on cell-mediated immune functions. NSAIDs have been shown to have effects on the proliferation and activation of lymphocytes that are probably largely due to the actions of these drugs in overcoming the suppressive effects of prostaglandin E_2 on lymphocyte proliferation (Ceuppens and Goodwyn, 1985). The inhibitory effects of ibuprofen on peripheral blood cells (Adkinson *et al.*, 1997) would be expected to result in sufficient reduction in prostaglandin E_2 to reduce its suppressive effects on lymphocyte proliferation.

Of the mononuclear and antibody responses that may be regulated by cytokines, that involving stimulation by viruses may be another target for the actions of ibuprofen. However, Graham and co-workers (1990) were unable to show any effects of ibuprofen in normal volunteers infected intranasally with rhinovirus type 2 on virus shedding and serum neutralizing antibody response, although aspirin and paracetamol did affect these reponses. These results suggest that immune responsiveness is not unduly affected by ibuprofen.

Gyte and Williams (1985) studied the effects of some NSAIDs on granulopoiesis in human bone marrow cells *in vitro*. The colony-forming unit (CFU-GM) was inhibited in 18 bone marrow samples by ibuprofen 24 µg/ml (117 µmole/l), although the range of inhibitory concentrations for this as well as the other NSAIDs was quite extensive. An analogue of ibuprofen, indoprofen, as well as phenylbutazone, both of which produce agranulocytosis, also inhibited CFU-GM activity *in vitro*.

Infection with *Listeria monocytogenes* leads to facultative localization of the organism in monocytes and macrophages (Hockertz *et al.*, 1995). Treatment with 4 mg/kg ibuprofen one day before led to a 10-fold reduction in the number of viable *L. monocytogenes* in the spleen (Hockertz *et al.*, 1995). These results suggest that ibuprofen may protect against infection by this organism by reinforcing the host response to the bacteria.

There have been several reports of NSAID-takers having Streptococcal Group A bacteraemia, featuring, in particular, necrotizing fasciitis and toxic shock (Bardham and Anderson, 1997). Serious infections initiated by other bacteria may also be precipitated, albeit rarely, by NSAIDs (Bardham, 1997). Recent reports in the lay press suggesting that non-prescription use of ibuprofen may be associated with the development of necrotizing fasciitis have been challenged on the grounds of accuracy of the reporting details (Melis, 1996). The association of streptococcal infection with NSAIDs in the development of necrotizing fasciitis suggests that NSAIDs may somehow predispose the individual with a particular susceptibility to the bacterial infection. However, a direct effect on the growth of the bacteria is unlikely. Elvers and Wright (1995) have shown that ibuprofen prevented growth of *Staphyloccocus areus*, the inhibitory effects being more pronounced at pH 6 than at pH 7.

5.1.13   Effects on articular joint integrity

It is clear from the above that ibuprofen has the potential to control a variety of local inflammatory reactions in diarthrodial arthritic joints. These multiple reactions involve not only the production of eicosanoids but also the components of inflammation derived from leukocyte accumulation and their activation to produce oxyradicals, nitric oxide, cytokines and the leukocyte-derived tissue destructive enzymes. The control of these inflammatory reactions is an important part of control of joint destruction in arthritis. The other components of joint destruction in arthritis involving cartilage and bone are also sites where ibuprofen may have important protective effects.

Cartilage proteoglycans

Inhibition of the synthesis of the structural components of cartilage comprising pro-teoglycans and collagens and the reactions involving intermediary metabolism and the mitochondrial production of adenosine triphosphate (ATP) were regarded around 30–40 years ago as an important property of NSAIDs, especially that of the salicylates, underlying their anti-inflammatory activity in joints (Whitehouse, 1965; Smith, 1966; Rainsford, 1984). The focus of attention then was the control of the proliferating pannus and other reactions leading to the abnormal growth of connective tissues in joints in patients with *rheumatoid arthritis* (RA). Today, however, this is considered in a different context, for much of the attention has been directed to the long-term effects of NSAIDs on the joint integrity in *osteoarthritis* (OA) (Brandt and Palmoski, 1984; Ghosh, 1988; Rainsford *et al.*, 1992; Rashad *et al.*, 1992; Rainsford, 1996). The joint destructive process, while involving a similar array of cellular enzymic reactions within the chondrocyte and bone (e.g. metallo-proteinases) in RA and OA, may differ appreciably when it comes to the extracellular processes that lead to the pattern of bone and joint destruction and reactions (e.g. pannus in RA and osteophytes in OA) (Fassbender, 1994). Thus, the biochemical influences of NSAIDs in OA may differ from those in RA. Whether or not inhibition of cartilage proteo-glycan and collagen synthesis is potentially undesirable in RA, as it appears to be in OA, is therefore debatable. Indeed, there are differences in the rate of glycosaminoglycan synthe-sis and turnover in cartilage from patients with OA compared with RA, these being greater in the former (Dingle, 1992).

McKenzie *et al.* (1976) observed that ibuprofen 0.02–0.2 mmol/l had no effect on the uptake of $^{35}SO_4$ into the papain digestible-resistent glycosaminoglycans (GAGs) of one specimen of human femoral neck cartilage surgically removed following subcapital frac-ture. However, in another sample, inhibition of radiosulfate uptake was observed at 0.02 mmol/l and to a lesser extent at 0.1 mmol/l, whereas at 0.2 mmol/l ibuprofen appeared to stimulate GAG synthesis. With some other NSAIDs there appeared to be more consistent results, with indomethacin and salicylate showing concentration-related reduction in the synthesis of GAGs in most specimens. Thus, it is not possible to conclude from the studies of these authors whether ibuprofen affects the synthesis of GAGs in human cartilage.

Karzel and Padberg (1977) showed that ibuprofen 0.01–1.0 mmol/l inhibited the biosynthesis of $^{35}SO_4$-GAGs in mouse embryonic fibroblasts in a concentration-dependent manner. Only the highest concentration of 1.0 mmol/l inhibited cell growth, so that inhibition of the synthesis of GAGs occurred within therapeutic concentrations but not at those likely to cause inhibition of cell growth. Other NSAIDs studies also inhibited the synthesis of GAGs in this system in concentrations that did not result in effects on cell numbers.

Dingle (1992) observed that ibuprofen 100 µg/l (485 µmol/l) but not 50 µg/l (243 µmol/l) inhibited the synthesis of $^{35}SO_4$-GAGs in cartilage from a 'young' human population. The former drug concentration is above that encountered therapeutically in plasma, so the significance of this finding is unclear. Moreover, the cartilage concentra-tion of ibuprofen is 3.0 µg/g (0.015 µmol/g) during therapy (Bannwarth and Dehais, 1991), so the effects described by Dingle are at concentrations far in excess of those likely to be encountered in cartilage *in situ*.

Dingle (1992) also showed that in the presence of hrIL-1α, which stimulates pro-teoglycan catabolism, ibuprofen 50 µg/l (243 µmol/l) caused a statistically significant reduction in $^{35}SO_4$-labelled GAGs at 2 and 4 days of culture, but not after 1 day. Again the concentration for this effect is far above that in synovial fluid and cartilage, although it may be encountered in plasma (Table 5.9). Aspirin 30 µg/ml (167 µmol/l) also caused a reduction in $^{35}SO_4$-GAG synthesis, but this probably reflects effects of salicylate formed by hydrolysis during culture. The concentration of the drug added is within the range encountered in plasma during therapy with this drug.

Brandt and Palmoski (1984) reported that ibuprofen 35 µg/ml (170 µmol/l) inhibited the $^{35}SO_4$-GAG synthesis in normal canine articular cartilage *in vitro*. This concentration for effect is within that encountered in plasma during therapy (Table 5.9) but higher than that in the cartilage (3.0 µg/ml) during therapy (Bannwarth and Dehais, 1991). Several other NSAIDs, including salicylate, inhibited the synthesis of $^{35}SO_4$-GAGs in this system.

Bjelle and Eronen (1991) observed that 20 µg/ml (97 µmol/l) but not the higher concentration of 100 µg/ml (485 µmol/l) of ibuprofen inhibited the synthesis of $^{35}SO_4$-GAGs in the matrix of articular chondrocytes. Less variable concentration-dependent reduction in $^{35}SO_4$-GAG synthesis occurred with diclofenac, indomethacin, naproxen and salicylate in the same system (Bjelle and Eronen, 1991).

Ibuprofen 40 µg/ml (194 µmol/ml), like that of many non-salicylate NSAIDs was not found to inhibit the synthesis of $^{35}SO_4$-GAGs in mouse patella *in vitro* (de Vries *et al.*, 1988). In this model (as well as in a modification of this in which trypsin digested cartilage is employed to mimic arthritic changes) salicylate is the most consistent inhibitor of GAG synthesis. It is also of interest that chronic paracetamol administration to rats reduces the GAG content of cartilage (van der Kraan *et al.*, 1990), even though the synthesis of GAGs is unaffected by the drug *in vitro* (de Vries *et al.*, 1988).

Overall, these studies suggest that relatively high concentrations of ibuprofen may reduce the synthesis of sulfated proteoglycans *in vitro*, but often the concentrations required for effect exceed those encountered in the joints during therapy. The relevance of this to the *in vivo* situation has not been determined. It should be noted that suppression of radiosulfate incorporation into GAGs has been suggested to be an artefact associated with *in vitro* studies (de Vries *et al.*, 1986). Thus, interpretation of these studies on the effects of ibuprofen on $^{35}SO_4$-GAGs synthesis may depend on the amount of non-radioactive sulfate in the medium affecting the specific activity of the $^{35}SO_4^{2-}$ as well as the effects of growth factors in serum (de Vries *et al.*, 1986).

Other metabolic precursors in the synthesis of GAGs have been studied as possible sites where NSAIDs, including ibuprofen, may exert inhibitory effects. David *et al.* (1992) showed that ibuprofen 15 µg/ml (73 µmol/l) did not exert any effects on the activity of glucuronyltransferases and xylyltransferases (assayed using exogenous acceptor molecules) present in articular cartilage from the femoral head of patients with OA, whereas indomethacin and salicylate had inhibitory activity. Hugenberg and co-workers (1993) also found that glucuronyltransferase from bovine liver was unaffected by 85 or 170 µmol/l *rac*-, (*R*)-(–)- or (*S*)-(+)-ibuprofen (i.e. within those concentrations found in synovial fluid). However, a higher concentration of 340 µmol/l (*S*)-(+)-ibuprofen, but not the (*R*)-(–)- or racemic forms of the drug, caused a statistically significant reduction in the activity of this enzyme. Moreover, aspirin and salicylate inhibited the activity of this enzyme at concentrations within those in synovial fluid during therapy. Furthermore, Hugenberg *et al.* (1993) found that bovine liver UDP-glucose dehydrogenase and glutamine-fructose-6-phosphate aminotransferase was unaffected by therapeutic

CHAPTER 5

concentrations of ibuprofen, aspirin or salicylate. It therefore appears that ibuprofen, unlike aspirin or salicylate, does not affect the biosynthesis of the oligosaccharide precursor required for chondroitin sulfate synthesis.

Protection against degradation of proteoglycans has been suggested as a potential effect of NSAIDs (Vignon *et al.*, 1991; Rainsford, 1996). Using the hide powder azure assay for human leukocyte elastase, Stephens *et al.* (1980) were unable to show any inhibitory effects of 1.0 mmol/l ibuprofen, whereas indomethacin, flurbiprofen and phenylbutazone exhibited inhibitory effects at 0.4 and 1.0 mmol/l. Blackburn *et al.* (1991) also found that ibuprofen at > 200 µmol/l did not affect neutrophil collagenase activity, although indomethacin, piroxican and tenidap inhibited this enzyme with IC_{50} values of 14, 69 and 19 µmol/l, respectively.

As indicated previously, ibuprofen inhibits hyaluronic acid degradation induced by oxyradicals (Carlin *et al.*, 1985). Studies by Salkie, Hannah and McNiel (1976) show that ibuprofen inhibits hyaluronidase activity in a concentration-dependent manner in the range of 20–100 mg/l (97–490 µmol/l) but only in the presence of heat-inactivated serum. This suggests that ibuprofen may interact with serum to release factors that prevent hyaluronic acid degradation. In contrast, betamethasone exerted inhibitory effects in the presence and absence of inactivated serum while flufenamic acid inhibited hyaluronic acid degradation without serum added. These results suggest there may be unique effects of ibuprofen in controlling hyaluronic acid degradation. These studies warrant further study to establish their relevance *in vivo*.

Joint integrity

Changes in the functions of joints and composition of bone and cartilage may have importance in the effects of NSAIDs on the progression of OA (Rashad *et al.*, 1992). To investigate the effects of ibuprofen on joint integrity and function, Michelsson (1980) treated rabbits that had the right knee immobilized by extension for 5 weeks with ibuprofen 100 mg/day p.o. (approximately 30 mg/kg/day). The thickening that accompanies the development of degenerative changes was significantly less and radiological changes were smaller in those rabbits that had received ibuprofen compared with untreated controls. The author concluded that ibuprofen has a prophylactic effect in preventing the underlying pathological changes during joint immobilization.

In contrast to these studies, Törnkvist and Lindholm (1980) observed that ibuprofen 16 mg/day (given p.o. to rats weighing 430–530 g; i.e. average 34 mg/kg/day) reduced bone mass and calcium in rats in whom fracture of callus had been induced in the tibia. However, they did observe that in the long term the effect is weakened and the changes in the bones become almost normal.

Byrick *et al.* (1992) observed that ibuprofen 20 mg/kg i.v. did not affect the hemodynamic changes or pulmonary fat or marrow embolism in dogs in whom bilateral cemented arthroplasty had been perfomed. This lack of effect occurred despite the reduction in plasma concentrations of 6-keto-prostaglandin $F_{1\alpha}$ or thromboxane B_2. While not demonstrating any effects on joint integrity, this study is important for showing the lack of effects on systemic body functions during arthroplasty.

Overall, it appears that ibuprofen exhibits variable effects on joint integrity depending on the model employed. The main effects of the drug may be confined to prevention of hyaluronic acid degradation and local effects on production of eicosanoids, TNF-α and leukocyte accumulation (as mentioned in the previous sections).

5.1.14 Miscellaneous biochemical and cellular actions

Hybrid triglyceride and lipid metabolism

The contribution of the bioconversion of (R)-(–)-ibuprofen to the pharmacological and toxicological effects of *rac*-ibuprofen depends on the rates of metabolism of this drug in different organs. With 30–60% bioconversion of (R)-(–) occurring to (S)-(+)-ibuprofen (Rudy *et al.*, 1991; Bannwarth *et al.*, 1995b; see also Chapter 4, there is appreciable 'metabolic load' required for the metabolism of (R)-(–)-ibuprofen. In this metabolic conversion (R)-(–)-ibuprofen forms a coenzyme A intermediate, which suggests that there may be substantial influences of (R)-(–)-ibuprofen on those steps involved in lipid metabolism involving coenzyme A (Evans, 1996; Mayer, 1996). Of particular interest is the propensity of ibuprofen to be incorporated into triglycerides as shown by Williams *et al.* (1986). In this pathway one of the fatty acids in the triglyceride chain is replaced to form so-called 'hybrid triglycerides'. Another propionic acid, flurbiprofen, which does not undergo chiral inversion via the formation of a coenzyme A thioester, does not lead to the formation of hybrid triglycerides. Other propionic acids such as ketoprofen and fenoprofen may also produce hybrid triglycerides as observed with ibuprofen (Mayer, 1996). Interestingly, these three propionic acids that are known to undergo metabolic inversion have also coincidentally been shown to reduce serum lipid levels and the rate of fatty acid synthesis (Mayer, 1996). This hypolipidemic action of these drugs is probably as a consequence of the inhibition of acetyl-coenzyme A carboxylase, a rate-limiting step in fatty acid biosynthesis (Mayer, 1996). Other metabolic consequences of this surrogate use of the acetyl-CoA pathway of fatty acid metabolism have not been identified, although there has been some speculation (Evans, 1996).

Mitochondrial β-oxidation of fatty acids has been shown to be inhibited by ibuprofen *in vitro*; there being an apparent selective effect of (R)-(–)-ibuprofen on the β-oxidation of palmitic acid (Frenaeux *et al.*, 1990). Zhao and co-workers (1992) have shown that (R)-(–)- and (S)-(+)-ibuprofen 0.25 and 0.5 mmol/kg i.p. inhibited the β-oxidation of palmitic acid in rats *in vivo*. There were no differences in the inhibitory effects of the enantiomers and the mechanism does not appear to involve effects on CoA.

Tvrzická and co-workers (1994) found that addition of 0.6 mg/day ibuprofen to the diet of male mice for 6 weeks resulted in increased levels of phospholipids and decreased

CHAPTER 5

neutral lipids in the kidneys. The effects on phospholipids were considered to be a consquence of the inhibition of prostaglandin metabolism by the drug. A novel component was observed in the heart and was identified by GC-MS to be isopropyl myristate. The isopropyl group was postulated to derive from the cleavage of the isobutyl group of ibuprofen. No obvious toxic effects were correlated with the changes in lipid composition, although there was increased body and liver mass.

Some interaction with lipid metabolism may be of benefit in choleretic states. Thus, Marks and co-workers (1996) observed that ibuprofen prevented the increase in saturation of bile with cholesterol and gallbladder contraction in obese subjects during weight loss. The authors suggested that ibuprofen may have benefit in preventing gallstones. Kaminski and co-workers (1985) performed a double-blind placebo-controlled trial to establish whether ibuprofen reduces the pain from gallbladder disease in relation to the histological signs of inflammation and the content of prostaglandins E and F in the gallbladder mucosal cells and muscle tissues. They found that ibuprofen was effective in reducing the pain from cholecystitis and reduced the PGE production by the gallbladder mucosa and muscle, but there was a poor correlation between pain relief and inhibition of prostaglandin production. In some respects this is not a surprising finding as the authors had studied prostaglandin production *ex vivo* and in homogenized tissues. Under these conditions prostaglandin production can be affected by the *in vitro* incubation, and with a drug that has reversible effects on cyclooxygenase activity the uncontrolled release of arachidonic acid will lead to reversal of the inhibition by ibuprofen. However, the findings that ibuprofen provided relief from the pain in cholecystitis and reduced the inflammation is an important therapeutic indication for the drug. This is especially important in relation to the relative gastrointestinal safety of ibuprofen.

Other metabolic or cellular effects

Several biochemical and cellular actions of ibuprofen have been described the exact significance of which for understanding of the therapeutic actions or side-effects of the drug is not yet clear. Thus, Penning and Talalay (1983) and Penning et al. (1985) have shown that ibuprofen and a number of other NSAIDs inhibit the activity of 3α-hydroxysteroid dehydrogenase, a NAD$^+$-linked enzyme involved in interconversion of steroid alcohols and ketones, in rat liver and brain respectively. Interestingly, the potency for inhibition of this enzyme is similar to that of the COX-1 activity in seminal vesicle preparation. The authors suggest that the effects on this enzyme may have significance for the anti-inflammatory effects of the NSAIDs. However, little evidence is available to support this interesting suggestion even though the rank order of inhibition of 3α-hydroxysteroid dehydrogenase relates to the acute anti-inflammatory activity of the NSAIDs.

Antimitotic activity has been observed in isoproteronol-treated parotid glands of rats dosed for 3 or 20 days with ibuprofen 80 mg/kg/day (Dorietto de Menezes and Catanzaro-Guimaraes, 1985). Inhibition of ornithine decarboxylase, a rate-limiting enzyme involved in nucleic acid biosynthesis, has been observed in rats *in vivo* given 12.5–50 mg/kg (R)-$(-)$- or (S)-$(+)$-ibuprofen i.p.; the (R)-$(-)$ enantiomer was somewhat the more potent of the two (Bruni *et al.*, 1990). Effects on membrane functions have been described for NSAIDs, including ibuprofen, as they influence lymphocyte and mitochondrial functions (Famaey and Whitehouse, 1975). These effects may have consequences for both anti-inflammatory and other actions of ibuprofen (Dorietto de Menezes and Catanzaro-Guimaraes, 1985).

5.2 EXPERIMENTAL THERAPEUTICS

In this section the potential application of ibuprofen in prevention or treatment of a variety of disease states is considered. These studies have been based on the understanding of the pharmacological actions of ibuprofen. Not only is the effect of the drug on prostaglandin production exploited but also its actions on leukocyte accumulation and activation, effects on oxyradical production and other anti-inflammatory and antipyretic effects of the drug. In some cases unique actions have been uncovered as the result of applying ibuprofen in some experimentally induced inflammatory or degenerative states.

5.2.1   Endotoxin shock

Experimentally induced endotoxinemia has been regarded as a model of septic shock, adult respiratory distress syndrome (ARDS) and other syndromes or conditions in humans where there has been an overriding bacterial infection.

During systemic endotoxin administration there is extensive arachidonic acid metabolism to its oxygenated products — prostaglandins, thromboxane, leukotrienes, lipoxins and other inflammatory products. To investigate the effects of administering a cyclooxygenase inhibitor to prevent the production of prostanoids during induction of endotoxinemia, and thus prevent the development of symptoms of shock and the mortality that occur during this state, Wise *et al.* (1980) pretreated rats at 30 min with ibuprofen 0.1–30 mg/kg i.v. before i.v. administration of 20 mg/kg *Salmonella enteritidis* endotoxin. They observed a dose-related improvement in survival of the rats with 0.1–30 mg/kg ibuprofen. At doses of 3.75 mg/kg and 30 mg/kg ibuprofen there was a reduction in plasma thromboxane and 6-keto-prostaglandin $F_{1\alpha}$, thrombin-induced platelet thromboxane B_2 production, and fibrin and lysosomal products. These results suggest that ibuprofen may act in preventing endotoxin-induced shock by reducing the pathogenic effects of arachidonic acid metabolites by cyclooxygenase inhibition. There may also be other actions of the drug in controlling the products of coagulopathy, e.g. fibrin degradation products (Ehrlich *et al.*, 1987).

Mansilla-Roselló and co-workers (1997) showed that the endotoxin-induced toxicity was reduced in CBA/H mice by two doses of ibuprofen 1 mg/kg 1 h before and 30 min after septic challenge. This was accompanied by an increase in the serum levels of IL-1α, TNF-α and IL-6 but reduced levels of PGE_2. This suggests that ibuprofen inhibits the

CHAPTER 5

production of PGE_2, while at the same time actually increasing the production of endotoxin-induced pro-inflammatory cytokines. Clearly the main effect in endotoxinemia is the inhibition of prostaglandin production.

In a model of streptococcal sepsis in newborn suckling rats by Short, Miller and Fletcher (1982), ibuprofen 4 mg/kg i.p. improved the survival time of animals given group B *Streptococcus* organisms (Type III) and its protective effects were more pronounced than those of indomethacin 3 mg/kg.

Sheep have often been employed for studies of the effects of endotoxin treatments because among other advantages they allow for monitoring of cardiovascular and other physiological effects of the endotoxin. To investigate the effects of ibuprofen on cardiopulmonary responses to the cyclooxygenase produced by endotoxin treatment, Adams and Traber (1982) gave this drug at a dose of 14 mg/kg 15 min before and 1 h 45 min after infusion of *Escherichia coli* endotoxin. They compared the responses (Pa_{O_2} neutrophil count, lymph/plasma ratio, mean arterial pressure, body temperature, hematocrit, lymph flow and total plasma protein concentrations) before and after treatments. Ibuprofen caused a statistically significant reduction in the changes elicited during the initial phases (phase I) of the endotoxin-mediated responses but not in the subsequent phases (II and III). The authors concluded that the effect of ibuprofen was to reduce the production of prostaglandins that mediate inflammatory reactions accompanying extravascular fluid movement and reduce the microvascular hydrostatic pressure-induced oedema and hypovolemia that occur in the early stages of endotoxin injury. Similar results were obtained by Traber *et al.* (1984) in a later study comparing the effects of ibuprofen with the antihistamine diphenhydramine.

Snapper *et al.* (1983) studied the effects of ibuprofen i.v. and meclofenamate sodium i.v. treatment on the alterations in lung mechanics induced by endotoxin (*E. coli*) treatment to unanaesthetized sheep. They observed that both drugs reduced the effects of endotoxin. Unfortunately, relatively little data was provided in this study on the effects of ibuprofen since the authors concentrated on those of meclofenamate sodium.

In dogs, ibuprofen was found to reduce the hypotension induced by endotoxin as well as to reverse the dimunition in platelet and leukocyte counts (Almqvist *et al.*, 1984; Yamanaka *et al.*, 1993). Ibuprofen has also been shown to reduce the pulmonary platelet trapping induced by endotoxin (Almqvist *et al.*, 1984; Ekstrom *et al.*, 1986). There appears to be a differential role of cyclooxygenase inhibition in controlling hypotensive responses including total peripheral resistance from that of the actions of platelet-activating factor (PAF) in reduced cardiac output and effective vascular compliance (Yamanaka *et al.*, 1993). Combination of ibuprofen with the PAF antagonist TCV-309 markedly attenuates the hypotensive effects in endotoxic shock more than the drugs alone (Yamanaka *et al.*, 1993).

Rinaldo and Dauber (1985) observed that prior treatment with 3.75 mg/kg ibuprofen prevented the *E. coli* endotoxin-induced bronchoalveolar inflammation in rats. They observed that here was a significant reduction in the total leukocytes in the bronchoalveolar lavage as well as the percentage and total of neutrophils recovered. Interestingly, methylprednisolone had no effects in this system.

The selective effects of ibuprofen given as a bolus dose of 12.5 mg/kg i.v. at the time of endotoxin administration and again 90 and 180 min later during the hypertensive (phase 1) and permeability (phase 2) components of endotoxin-induced pulmonary microvascular injury were also shown by Demling (1982). This author showed that indomethacin given as a bolus dose of 5 mg/kg i.v. and followed by an infusion of 3 mg/kg/h of this drug for 5 h had a similar effect to that of the ibuprofen treatment. These and other studies reported by Demling (1982) suggest that the hypertensive component of endotoxin-induced lung injury is due to thromboxane production with accompanying elevation of PGI_2 and $PGF_{2\alpha}$. The effects of ibuprofen are to reduce the production of these prostanoids concomitantly with reduction in hypertension and lymph flow but with no effect on the diminution of white cell counts that occurs during endotoxinemia. The early-stage hypoxia and increased respiratory rate were also decreased by the ibuprofen treatment (Demling, 1982). There is also reduced platelet trapping in the lung by ibuprofen as a consequence of this drug inhibiting thromboxane production (Ekstrom *et al.*, 1986).

Studies in rabbits have shown that ibuprofen can reduce influx of neutrophils into hyperoxic lungs (Das *et al.*, 1988) so there may be an added effect of the drug on leukocyte accumulation during lung injury independent of any lack of effects on circulating white cell counts as observed by Demling (1982). Ibuprofen 12.5 mg/kg i.v. at the same time as endotoxin followed by the same dose at 120 min reduced the neutrophil generation of superoxide in pigs (Carey *et al.*, 1992).

The production of TNF-α is also a major factor in the pathogenesis of endotoxin-induced lung injury in pigs (Wheeler *et al.*, 1992; Mullen *et al.*, 1993). Ibuprofen 14 mg/kg prevented the pulmonary arterial hypertension and changes in blood gases due to TNF-α in sheep (Wheeler *et al.*, 1992). Ibuprofen also appears to reduce TNF-α production in porcine sepsis (Carey *et al.*, 1991). Whether the reduction in superoxide production by neutrophils in this model (Carey *et al.*, 1991) is the mechanism for the action of ibuprofen in reducing the production of TNF-α or vice versa is not known. Ibuprofen has also been shown to reduce neutrophil hypochlorous acid production in pigs (Carey *et al.*, 1990). Studies by Leeper-Woodford and co-workers (1991) in a sepsis model in pigs induced by infusion of live *Pseudomonas aeruginosa* showed that ibuprofen 12.5 mg/kg i.v. reduced the induced production of TNF-α by about one-half that of the peak value concomitant with restoration of all hemodynamic and pulmonary parameters. Mullen and co-workers (1993) observed a reduction in TNF-α in the same type of model when the pigs were treated with ibuprofen 12.5 mg/kg i.v. with anti-TNF-α 5 mg/kg antibody, but this was not accompanied by reduction in the early-phase pulmonary vascular resistance, this only being evident at 60 min after initiation of the drug/antibody treatments. These results suggest that reduction of the activity of TNF-α by antibody treatment did not appreciably influence the effects of ibuprofen on respiratory functions.

CHAPTER 5

The shock-like condition involving hypotension, leukopenia and thrombocytopenia induced by a 2 h infusion of interleukin-1β in rabbits was shown by Okusawa *et al.* (1988) to be prevented by ibuprofen when given 15 min before the IL-1. However, when the drug was given 1 h after the infusion was initiated there was a reversal of hemodynamic changes but not the thrombocytopenia or leukopenia. Pretreatment with ibuprofen also reversed the shock-like effects of a low-dose combination of IL-1β and TNF-α. These results suggest that ibuprofen has benefits in preventing the symptoms of shock induced with either of the two cytokines given alone or together and that the effects of the drug are clearly temporal in nature.

Ibuprofen has been observed to inhibit the endotoxin-induced early rise in plasma TNF-α and the later increase in IL-6 and elastase in plasma in healthy human volunteers (Spinas *et al.*, 1991). Thus, the observations in animal model systems described above would appear to have relevance for potential human application of ibuprofen in treatment of sepsis. The main effect of the drug appears to be in attenuating the induced production of TNF-α during sepsis. It is, however, worth noting that septic shock is such a severe condition that it is unlikely that ibuprofen, or for that matter any other NSAID, would *alone* have a major outcome given in this condition. The effects of ibuprofen being confined to the early hypertensive/platelet neutrophil phase of endotoxin-mediated injury would be suggestive of limited utility of this drug given alone. Moreover, the later phase cytokine production (Spinas *et al.*, 1991) and involvement of platelet activating factor (Yamanaka *et al.*, 1993), which is also produced in abundance in septic shock, is indicative of the need for agents to control production of these potent inflammatory mediators to be given with ibuprofen in order to obtain significant therapeutic benefit in septic-shock injury.

5.2.2   Acute lung injury induced by exposure to chemicals

Induction of lung injury in dogs by aspiration of acid produces thrombocytopenia, platelet entrapment in the lung, elevated thromboxane production, sequestration of white blood cells and oedema in the lungs (Utsunomiya *et al.*, 1982). In some respects this model is similar to the early phases of endotoxin-induced pulmonary injury described above, but probably has fewer longer-term sequelae. A bolus infusion of 12.5 mg/kg ibuprofen to dogs at 1 h after acid aspiration inhibited TXB_2 production by platelets and white blood cells as well as the TXB_2 concentrations of white blood cells and the pulmonary oedema. However, this treatment did not reduce the entrapment of platelets, this being achieved, however, by infusion of the antiplatelet prostaglandin PGI_2 (Utsunomiya *et al.*, 1982). It is possible that if the dose of ibuprofen had been given at the same time as the acid aspiration the platelet entrapment could have been reduced as shown in the above-mentioned studies with endotoxin. However, the animal model of lung injury described by Utsunomiya *et al.* (1982) is of a therapeutic type and the authors did show that ibuprofen restored the lung morphology to normal appearance accompanying the reduction in thromboxane production and leukocyte accumulation.

The infamous wartime gas phosgene ($COCl_2$) produces a fulminant, noncardiogenic oedema when given to rodents that, depending on the dose applied, results in rapid death of the animals (Sciuto et al., 1996; Sciuto, 1997). It is suggested that as exposure of mice to phosgene results in extensive lung injury, this may be regarded a model of adult respiratory distress syndrome (Sciuto et al., 1996). Intraperitoneal administration of ibuprofen 15–300 mg/kg 30 min prior to, and 1 h after, exposure to phosgene (80 mg/m^3 for 20 min) resulted in a dose-related reduction in pulmonary oedema (Sciuto et al., 1996). This effect was potentiated by the phosphodiesterase inhibitor pentoxyfylline, which reduces leukocyte phagocytosis and superoxide production. These results suggest that there may be added benefits from control of leukocyte functions over those achieved by ibuprofen alone in the phosgene-induced lung injury.

In a test of lethality from phosgene-induced lung injury in mice exposed to 32 mg/m^3 of phosgene for 20 min, Sciuto (1997) observed a dose-related, and time-dependent, increase in survival from ibuprofen 1.5–7.5 mg/mouse i.p. (approximately 60–300 mg/kg), the survival being less after 24 h compared with 12 h. There was a reduction in pulmonary oedema and at high dose reduced malondialdehyde content (reflecting lipid peroxidation/ glutathione depletion) from ibuprofen.

In contrast to these results, ibuprofen 10 mg/kg/day for 14 days did not reduce the effects of intratracheal bleomycin, an inducer of oxyradical injury, and hypoxia in hamsters (Giri and Hollinger, 1996).

Amphotericin-β-induced elevation of pulmonary arterial pressure and lymph flow in sheep was found by Hardie et al. (1992) to be reduced by ibuprofen.

Ahn and co-workers (1994) observed that thrombin-induced oedema in rats was reduced to the same extent by 5 mg/kg (S)-(+)- or (R)-(–)-ibuprofen i.v.; (S)-(+)-ibuprofen also reduced the mean pulmonary artery pressure but had a somewhat lesser depressive effect on systemic arterial pressure. This drug also prevented the reduction in pH, Pa_{O_2} and Pa_{CO_2} induced by thrombin. While the reduction in oedema by (R)-(–)-ibuprofen might be ascribed, in part, to the metabolic chiral inversion of the drug, the fact that there appeared to be no significant difference between the anti-oedemic effects of both enantiomers is of interest in that this indicates a high degree of activity of the (R)-(–) enantiomer in this model. The effects of the (S)-(+) enantiomer on blood gases, pH and pulmonary pressure are further evidence of a cyclooxygenase-dependent mechanism for ibuprofen in alleviating lung injury. The authors also showed that ibuprofen did not have any direct antithrombotic activity in vitro, thus ruling out any masking of the actions of thrombin by ibuprofen in this model.

5.2.3   Acute myocardial injury and coronary functions

A substantial number of investigations have been performed suggesting that ibuprofen has some beneficial effects in acute myocardial injury and blood flow. The mechanisms of the protective effects of ibuprofen are probably similar to those involved in other organ injury such as discussed above. Additionally, there is a component involving inhibition of platelet aggregation and the mechanism of this is discussed in the later section on this topic linked to effects on thrombogenesis. Here the physiological, molecular and cellular effects of ibuprofen on myocardial injury and blood flow are considered.

In acute myocardial injury induced in baboons by coronary artery ligation, ibuprofen 12.5 mg/kg i.v. given 30 min after occlusion caused a reduction in neutrophil accumulation and loss of plasma creatinine phosphokinase activity, the latter representing a reduction in infarct area in the myocardium (Crawford *et al.*, 1981). There was, however, no accompanying reduction by ibuprofen in the accumulated complement components, C3, C4 and C5 localized at infarct sites. The components were reduced in the same study by cobra venom, another myocardial protectant (Crawford *et al.*, 1981).

Myocardial infarction induced by left coronary artery occlusion is a well-established model in dogs and has been used extensively to investigate the effects of potential myocardial protective agents. In this model Romson *et al.* (1982) showed that treatment with ibuprofen 12.5 mg/kg i.v. every 4 h beginning 30 min before occlusion reduced the infarct size by 40% compared with that in control animals with accompanying 67% reduction in the accumulation of ^{111}In-labelled leukocytes. However, the authors did not observe any reduction in the accumulation of ^{111}In-labelled platelets, suggesting that the mechanism of this protective effect is due to the reduction by ibuprofen in the leukocyte-mediated inflammatory responses. These processes contribute to the pathogenesis of early myocardial injury probably by leukocytes producing hydroxyl radicals and hydrogen peroxide (Rowe *et al.*, 1983; Hess *et al.*, 1985). The activated neutrophils in producing these oxyradicals disrupt the transport of calcium ions by the cardiac sarcoplasmic reticulum (Hess *et al.*, 1985). This process has been shown to be rectified by ibuprofen and indomethacin as well as by combinations of superoxide dismutase and catalase *in vitro* (Hess *et al.*, 1985; Werns *et al.*, 1985), implying from the latter that oxyradicals from stimulated leukocytes play a major role in damage to the calcium transport system in the sarcoplasmic reticulum.

The importance of the effects of ibuprofen on the release of oxyradicals, as well as the release of leukocyte lysosomal enzymes, has been shown by Flynn *et al.* (1984) in their feline model of acute myocardial injury induced by ligation of the anterior descending coronary artery. They observed that ibuprofen 2.5–20 mg/kg given i.v. immediately before and 2 h after ligation caused a reduction by about one-half to two-thirds in the infarct size, which was not evident in cats given aspirin 5–150 mg/kg in the same treatment protocol. These authors showed that superoxide production and release of the lysosomal enzymes β-glucuronidase and lysozyme from human leukocytes was inhibited *in vitro* in a concentration-related manner by 0.4 mmol/l ibuprofen but not by aspirin. Ibuprofen 0.5 mmol/l, but not aspirin 1.1 mmol/l, reduced the granulocyte-mediated endothelial injury *in vitro*. Unfortunately, Flynn *et al.* (1984) did not provide evidence of the effects of ibuprofen compared with aspirin on leukocyte oxyradical production and lysosomal enzyme release in their feline myocardial injury model *in vivo.*

Another mechanism of the action of ibuprofen in myocardial injury relates to possible effects on coronary vessels. Apstein and Vogel (1982) showed that ibuprofen produced coronary arterial vasodilation in the isolated perfused rabbit heart, the IC_{50} for this effect being 50 µg/ml (242 µmole/l). The change in vascular resistance by ibuprofen did not result from physiological changes in coronary tone as oxygen demand and metabolism by the myocardium were unaffected by the drug treatment. This was confirmed in a similar study by Grover and Weiss (1985).

Using the isolated perfused rat heart (Langendorff) technique, in which arachidonic acid (0.5–2.0 µg) induced a vasoconstrictor effect initially followed about half a minute later by a prolonged coronary vasodilatation (extending over the subsequent 4–5 min), it was found that ibuprofen 14.5 µmol/l reduced both the vasoconstriction and dilatation of the coronary vessel in a reversible manner. These results imply that cyclooxygenase inhibition affects production of both vasoconstrictor and vasodilator prostaglandins when there is release of arachidonic acid. Clearly, the nature of the vasoactive stimulus determines response to ibuprofen. Reconciling these responses to the earlier study by Apstein and Vogel (1982) suggests that, aside from the possibility of variations with different animal models, in situations where there is release of arachidonate there could be blockade of vasoactivity by ibuprofen but not when there is no evident physiological stimulus as provided in the studies by Apstein and Vogel (1982).

It is possible that part of the blockade of vasoactive effects of ibuprofen arise from drug-related effects on nitric oxide (NO)/endothelium-dependent relaxation factor (EDRF) produced by the coronary artery (Kleha *et al.*, 1995) through drug effects on the production of the nitric oxide synthases (see section 5.1.9, Effects on Nitric Oxide Production).

In contrast to the reported cardioprotective effects of ibuprofen in models discussed above, Allan and co-workers (1985) were unable to demostrate reduction of accumulated neutrophils in the alternating occlusion/reperfusion of the left anterior descending coronary artery model in dogs. Furthermore, they observed an apparent increase in myocardial injury by ibuprofen pre-treatment (12.5 mg/kg i.v.) in this model. These results are difficult to interpret in relation to the previous studies except inasmuch as the pathology of the injury or, perhaps more significantly, the extent and severity of injury to the myocardium are somehow different in the myocardium following coronary occlusion and subsequent perfusion. Clearly, this aspect requires more detailed investigation before it can be resolved.

In another study Ito and co-workers (1989) were unable to show that blockade of thromboxane production by NSAIDs did not prevent the myocardial ischemia, coronary flow or neutrophil trapping induced by infusion of complement $C5_a$ in pigs.

Overall, these studies suggest that although ibuprofen may have some protective effects involving accumulation and activation of leukocyte and possibly thromboxane

CHAPTER 5

production effects in some systems the results of other studies clearly need to be reconciled before it can be claimed that the drug has any potential benefit in myocardial injury. Furthermore, it should be noted that these studies have all been performed in acute models which may not be representative of the more complex pathology in human coronary/myocardial disease where cardiac arrhythmias and artheriosclerosis present confounding pathology.

5.2.4　Cerebral injury

The potential protective effects of ibuprofen against injury induced in the brain of rats have been investigated using two models. Thus, Patel and co-workers (1993) found that ibuprofen 15 mg/kg given i.v. into the external jugular vein prevented the histologically-observed injury in the CA3 region of the dorsal hippocampus induced after 3 days by 10 mins of bilateral carotid artery occlusion and simultaneous hypotension in rats. The authors also observed that the same dose of ibuprofen in this model reduced the concentrations of thromboxane B_2 and 6-keto-prostaglandin $F_{1\alpha}$ in the caudate nucleus and 6-keto $PGF_{1\alpha}$ in the hippocampus at various time intervals up to 5.5 h post-ischemia. These results suggest that ibuprofen may protect against the ischemia-induced damage in some regions of the brain and that the mechanism involves reduction in the elevated levels of prostanoids. Unfortunately, with lack of information on the regional changes of blood supply in the brain it is not possible to relate the specific changes in blood supply to those regions of the brain where injury was observed and the limited effects of ibuprofen in the hippocampus.

In a model of cortical injury in which the dura of rats is exposed to a frozen ($-50°C$) probe for 5 s, Pappius and Wolfe (1983) investigated the effects of ibuprofen 36 mg/kg/day compared with indomethacin as a single dose of 7.5 mg/kg on glucose uptake, blood flow and prostaglandin concentration in the area of the lesion. The local utilization of the nonmetabolizable sugar, [^{14}C]deoxyglucose observed by autoradiography was markedly reduced in many areas of the focally-traumatized brain. The effects of the trauma were significantly reversed after 3 days' treatment with both ibuprofen and indomethacin. Local cerebral blood flow, measured by the [^{14}C]iodoantipyrine autoradiographic technique, was markedly altered by the trauma and showed evidence of extensive hyperemia, especially in the cerebral hemisphere wherin the lesion had developed. Ibuprofen did not produce any significant change in lesioned animals and neither did the treatment with indomethacin. The concentrations of prostaglandin E_2, $F_{2\alpha}$ and D_2 as well as arachidonic acid were markedly elevated within 1 min of injury to the brain. By 24 h after indomethacin treatment, the concentration of $PGF_{2\alpha}$ (the only prostaglandin measured) and arachidonic acid was significantly inhibited. Unfortunately, the authors did not study the effects of ibuprofen on prostaglandin concentrations in this model, so it can only be assumed that this drug had reduced prostaglandin metabolism. It is also unfortunate that the effects of ibuprofen were not investigated at time intervals other than at 3 days and also at other higher doses of the drug. This is especially important since changes in local blood flow may have been observed at earlier time intervals following treatment with ibuprofen, concomitant with effects on prostaglandin metabolism. None the less, the results suggest that ibuprofen treatment does markedly reverse the decline in glucose uptake induced by trauma in the brain.

Cerebral blood flow in the rat was found by Phillis *et al.* (1986) to be increased from the resting state in otherwise untreated (but anesthetized) rats following intraperitoneal administration of a single dose of either 0.1 mg/kg and 0.01 mg/kg ibuprofen as well as by the same dose of indomethacin and following 24 s of anoxia treatment.

While the models employed by Phillis *et al.* (1986) and Pappius and Wolfe (1983) differ, it is possible to interpret these results by postulating that short-term treatment with ibuprofen may result in exacerbation of the reactive hyperemia but not after prolonged cerebral injury and ibuprofen treatment.

Overall, the results of these studies suggest that ibuprofen probably has only limited beneficial effects in models of cerebral injury. It should be stressed, however, that the lack of adequate dose- and time-dependent studies and some methodological limitations of the reported studies do not allow for definitive statements to be made about the potential for ibuprofen to be considered as a therapeutic agent in treating cerebral injury.

5.2.5 Tourniquet-shock ischemia

Further evidence that ibuprofen may have anti-ischemic activity has been provided from the studies by Ward *et al.* (1995) in a rat model of tourniquet injury. In this model rats suffer a severe form of circulatory shock with oxidative stress, leading finally to multiple organ system failure and death within 24 h. Ward and co-workers (1995) investigated the effects of treatment with ibuprofen 12.5 mg/kg given i.p. at 24 and 2 h prior to application of tourniquets. They found the drug increased liver thiol concentrations and reduced thiobarbituric acid-reactive substances (TBARS; a measure of oxyradical attack on biomolecules) in the livers of rats at 5 h after tourniquet application and 2 h after hind-limb perfusion concomitant with reduced plasma levels of the aspartate and alanine aminotransferases compared with in control animals. Furthermore, the elevated numbers of activated neutrophils in the circulation following hind-limb perfusion were reduced by ibuprofen treatment.

While these studies, like many others performed to examine the protective effects of ibuprofen on oxyradical-medicated organ/tissue injury, were performed at a single dose level of the drug, the results do indicate that ibuprofen has protective effects in these systems. Part of the protective activity of ibuprofen seems to involve reducing the activity, numbers or organ accumulation of neutrophils, though the effect of the drug on neutrophil dynamics varies from model to model. Finally, it should be noted that there do not appear to have been clear indications from the studies performed to date whether the

CHAPTER 5

protection observed by ibuprofen could be exploited in post-treatment organ injury. This would be indicative of the potential of ibuprofen for therapeutic, as distinct from prophylactic, activity after organ injury.

5.2.6 Transcutaneous hypoxia

Another model of organ injury in skin in which leukocytes and reactive oxygen species play a role that is affected by ibuprofen has been studied by Maderazo *et al.* (1986). They found that transcutaneous hypoxia induced by i.v. infusion of fMLP 1 nmol/kg was reversed by ibuprofen with an ID_{50} of 4.6 mg/kg. This corresponded to a plasma concentration of 11 µg/ml, which is within the plasma concentration of the drug encountered during therapy. The results compared favourably with the effects of methylprednisolone, which had an ID_{50} of 2.7 mg/kg.

5.2.7 Cytokines and surgical stress

Surgical stress induces a range of hormonal changes, as well as production of pro-inflammatory cytokines and oxyradicals. Chambrier *et al.* (1996) showed that prior treatment at 12 and 2 h and postoperative administration of 500 mg ibuprofen suppositories every 8 h up to the 3rd day after cholecystectomy reduced the elevated plasma levels of ACTH and cortisol as well as glucose, accompanied by a marked reduction in circulating levels of interleukin (IL)-6 and total leukocytes. There was a small transient reduction in circulating levels of IL-1 and TNF-α in the 1–4 h postoperative period, but these changes did not reach statistical significance. Surprisingly, the late postoperative elevation in levels of C-reactive protein were unaffected by the ibuprofen treatments despite the reduction in IL-6.

Generally, production of pro-inflammatory cytokines by activated leukocytes *in vitro* is unaffected or possibly slightly increased by ibuprofen in common with that of many cyclooxygenase inhibitors (Hartman *et al.*, 1993). However, it is apparent that ibuprofen can modulate the responses to induce changes from production *in vivo* of cytokines or subsequent stimulation of pro-inflammatory cytokines (e.g. IL-6) by 'primary' pro-inflammatory cytokines (e.g. IL-1) (Sobrado *et al.*, 1983; Chambrier *et al.*, 1996). Alternatively ibuprofen could reduce the production of prostaglandins induced by inflammatory mediators (e.g. endotoxin) that induced cytokines or IL-1 itself (Dinarello and Bernheim, 1991; Sobrado *et al.*, 1983).

Some of these effects of ibuprofen on cytokine production may be evident when the drug has been given with cimetidine in restoring the helper/suppressor T-lymphocyte ratio in mice that have undergone severe trauma (e.g. from 20% burn injury, 40% hepatectomy or crush amputation of a hind limb) (Zapata-Sirvent *et al.*, 1986).

5.2.8 Pleurisy from delayed hypersensitivity reaction

The well-established anti-inflammatory effects of ibuprofen in models of pleural inflammation (e.g. induced by carrageenan) have served as a basis for investigating the potential for using ibuprofen and other NSAIDs to prevent delayed-type hypersensitivity reactions (DTH). While ibuprofen, like other NSAIDs given orally, significantly reduced the carrageenan-induced pleural inflammation, these drugs did not appear to markedly inhibit either the volume of pleural effusions or leukocyte infiltration induced by intrapleural triple antigen (containing pertussis organisms as well as diphtheria and tetanus toxoid) with Freund's complete antigen in a DHT protocol (Satoh *et al.*, 1982). In contrast, steroidal anti-inflammatory drugs and auranofin were relatively potent inhibitors of both these parameters of the pleural inflammation in this DHT model. However, only two doses of the NSAIDs were given, at 1 h and 24 h after challenge with the triple antigen, and the pleural inflammation was determined 48 h after challenge. It is, therefore, possible that the poor response to treatment with the NSAIDs was related to the lack of adequate drug concentrations in the animals at 48 h because of rapid renal clearance of these drugs in rats. Steroids and auranofin might be expected to have had a longer residence time and hence their effects would have been related, in part, to their longer retention in the rat. It would probably have been more appropriate to have given the NSAIDs twice or three times daily in divided doses for two days of treatment in the DHT model employed by Satoh *et al.* (1982). Thus, it is not possible to conclude unequivocally about the utility of ibuprofen or other NSAIDs in controlling manifestations of the DHT reaction.

5.2.9 Abdominal adhesions

Two conflicting reports have appeared from studies with the same model of peritoneal adhesions induced in White New Zealand rabbits by abrading and crushing the uterine horns (Holtz, 1982; Bateman, Nunley and Kitchen, 1982). In the study by Holtz (1982) ibuprofen 12.54 mg/kg intramuscularly at 15 mins before surgery and thereafter twice daily for 3 days failed to affect the initial lesion score or number of reformed lesions. However, Bateman *et al.* (1982) observed that intravenous administration of 10 mg/kg ibuprofen 30 min prior to surgery and then 3 times daily for 4 days significantly reduced the scores for adhesions. The differences between these two studies that could account for the opposite results are the route of administration (i.m. by Holtz and i.v. by Bateman *et al.*) as well as the cumulative dose (75 mg/kg in the study by Holtz compared with 120 mg/kg in the study by Bateman *et al.*). While the former author terminated the study at 2 weeks and the latter at 3 weeks this difference in timing is unlikely to have influenced the outcome since the pathological consequences of this procedure would have been established and are due effects fully manifest at either of these time intervals. The most likely factor accounting

CHAPTER 5

for these differences in response to the drug treatment are the cumulative dose. It is, therefore, likely that ibuprofen does prevent the development of abdominal adhesions.

O'Brien *et al.* (1982) observed that ibuprofen 5 mg/kg i.m. reduced the histologically-observed indices of wound healing in left oophorectomized and right salpingo-oophorectomized ewes that involved reduced vascular ingrowth, fibroblast proliferation and mesothelial regeneration. There were no differences in the overall formation of adhesions in ibuprofen or control animals.

Overall, therefore, the potential of ibuprofen on adhesion formation and wound healing deserve further investigations especially in the clinical setting.

5.2.10   Uveitis

Inflammatory conditions in the eye are commonly treated with glucocorticoids, though their prolonged use is controversial (Szary, 1979). In a model of experimental iridocyclitis induced in rabbits, Szary (1979) observed that 250 mg/kg ibuprofen given p.o. twice daily for varying periods up to 72 h postoperatively resulted in marked reduction in the protein content, sialic acid, seromucoid, proteolytic activity and prostaglandin concentration in the aqueous humor at 8–48 h following induction of iridocyclitis. The effects of indomethacin 50 mg/kg intravenously administered were similar to or more pronounced than those of ibuprofen. Unfortunately, the lack of statistical analyses of the data did not allow for quantitative comparisons of the results. These studies suggest that ibuprofen given orally may be useful for treatment of inflammatory conditions of the eye and may be useful as an adjuct or alternative to corticosteroids.

5.3   CLINICAL PHARMACOLOGY AND TOXICOLOGY

This section addresses the effects of ibuprofen in various experimentally induced and clinically occurring conditions. Not included in this section are studies concerning the pharmacokinetics of ibuprofen, which can be found in Chapter 4, and other relevant clinical studies in Chapters 6 and 8.

5.3.1   Experimental inflammation

Following the earlier studies by Adams and co-workers (1969) in which they discovered the anti-inflammatory activity of ibuprofen in the ultraviolet-induced erythema, Edwards and co-workers (1982) studied the effects of ibuprofen 400 mg every 4 h for a total of 4 doses, aspirin 1.2 g every 4 h for a total of 3 doses, and indomethacin 25 mg every 4 h for a total of 4 doses in 15 healthy volunteers who were exposed to UV-B from fluorescent sun lamps; the exposure to UV radiation took place 2 h after the initial dose of the drugs. The minimal dose of light to produce erythema (MED) was determined for each subject with and without the drugs. Ibuprofen caused an increase in the MED of 250% compared with aspirin 230% and indomethacin 250%. These results clearly showed that ibuprofen was like aspirin and indomethacin in being a potent inhibitor of the erythema response in humans. Thus these results provided clinical confirmation of the studies that had been done in guinea-pigs by Adams and co-workers (1969).

An important clinical aspect that results from the potential protective effects of ibuprofen against UV erythema arises from the studies of Bayerl *et al.* (1996) in which they observed that prior administration of 200 mg of ibuprofen 4 times daily for a total of 3 days prevented the formation of sunburn cells in the epidermis of patients with sun reactive skin (types 1 or 2) that had not been undergoing tanning before these studies. The skin area examined was that around the hips: an area of skin not normally exposed to sunlight. The effects of ibuprofen were pronounced in the group that had basal cell carcinoma or squamous cell carcinoma and the authors suggested that the reduced formation of sunburn cells after ibuprofen treatment may reflect reduction in DNA damage and in reactions during photocarcinogenesis.

Walker, Nguyen and Day (1994) examined the effects of ibuprofen 800 mg 4 times over 36 h or a matched placebo in a double-blind crossover design in volunteers who had received an intradermal injection of urate crystals (heat sterilized to remove endotoxin) into the skin of the forearm. The peak inflammatory response in the forearm appeared at 32 h and had dissipated by 56 h post urate injection. The logarithmic mean area of the wheal was significantly reduced after ibuprofen treatment by about 20%. This relatively weak response to ibuprofen was offset by marked intra- and inter-subject variability over the 4 treatment periods. Intra-subject variability was found to be appreciable with ibuprofen, being approximately 50% in both ibuprofen- and placebo-treated subjects. As the authors had not determined plasma concentrations of the drug, it was not possible to establish whether the variability observed related in any way to pharmacokinetic variations. Moreover, it would have been useful to have dose–response data in this study since it might have been possible to determine the component of variability with respect to dosage.

5.3.2   Experimental pain

Nielsen and co-workers (1990) observed that ibuprofen 400 or 800 mg was superior to placebo in analgesic effects in a double-blind, crossover design study in normal healthy volunteers in whom pain was induced by application of low-energy (50 mW) argon laser beam to the dorsal region of the right hand. While the peak plasma levels observed after intake of 800 mg ibuprofen were greater than those after 400 mg, there were no differences in the pain relief obtained with these two dosages of the drug. These results suggest that there is a limit to the dose-related efficacy of ibuprofen in this pain model.

Forster and co-workers (1992) compared the effects of ibuprofen 800 mg with those of paracetamol 1000 mg or dipyrone 1000 mg and with placebo on the pain elicited by repeated pinching at 2 min intervals of the interdigital web skin between the first and second and the second and third fingers. To examine the potentially confounding effects of the reflex diminution of blood flow in the stimulated hand, the authors applied a laser Doppler flow meter on the surface of the thumb and a plethysgmograph around the thumb to measure the local vasoconstriction and pyresis. The drugs were administered 30 min prior to the initial stimulus. It was found that ibuprofen and dipyrone both showed statistically significant analgesic effects, but paracetamol was ineffective in this model. The reduction in pain was not accompanied by sympathetic reflex vasoconstriction but there was a reduction by ibuprofen in the flow reaction around the pinched skin sites.

In a similar study, Petersen *et al.* (1997) determined the effects of ibuprofen 600 mg compared with placebo for up to 120 min during application of pain across the interdigital web between the second and third finger as well as the primary and secondary hyperalgesia induced by 7 min burn injury to the calf. In this double-blind, randomized, two-way crossover study, it was found that ibuprofen reduced the pain induced by static mechanical pressure in the interdigital web as well as that induced by motor brush stimulation of the area of secondary hyperalgesia following burn injury. However, ibuprofen did not reduce the area of secondary hyperalgesia following pin prick or stroke after the burn injury.

In another model of physical pain, Korbal and co-workers (1994) studied the effects of 400 and 800 mg of ibuprofen on experimentally induced tonic and phasic pain. Phasic pain was induced by application of a stream of dry carbon dioxide to the right nostril. The left nostril was stimulated with a constant stream of dry air which produced a tonic painful sensation described as dull and burning. Subjects recorded the pain intensity by means of a visual analogue scale displayed on a computer monitor. In addition, the electrophysical response to pain was recorded using EEG recorded at three positions Fz, Cz and Pz, thus enabling measurement of the chemosomatosensory event-related potentials (CSSERP). The authors observed that there was no significant difference in the pain responses observed before the drug treatments and 90 min after the drugs with both the tonic and phasic pain stimuli. They did, however, claim that the nonsignificant effect was dose-related in terms of a decrease in stimulus. However, there was a statistically dose-related decrease in the CSSERP amplitudes. These results suggest that measurement of the electrophysiological responses to pain by EEG is more sensitive than the use of visual analogue scales. A potential problem with this study design is that the exposure to CO_2 and dry air can be decidedly unpleasant and it is possible that the objectionable nature of the pain response could mask psychologically the expected analgesic response to the drugs.

Kilo and co-workers (1995) observed that ibuprofen 3×400 mg or 800 mg over a 2 h period one day following freezing of a small area of skin produced significant inhibition of hyperalgesia in comparison to placebo in a double-blind crossover study. A similar analgesic effect was observed in response to pinching of the interdigital web of the skin. Interestingly, there was no effect of ibuprofen on the flare and allodynia induced by capsaicin. This suggests that ibuprofen has different effects on substance P-mediated pain as compared with local pain induced by mechanical noxious stimulation.

In the earlier section on studies performed in animal and *in vitro* systems, the effects of ibuprofen on pain mechanisms were shown to be mediated not only by peripheral mechanisms but also by central mechanisms. Thus, intrathecally administered (*S*)-(+)-ibuprofen has been shown to have direct spinal analgesic effects in rats which, though not identical mechanistically, are comparable with that of morphine (Wang *et al.*, 1994). One of the central mechanisms that is known to be important in modulating pain is that involving the opiate system. On the hypothesis that prostaglandin E inhibits the release of the endogenous opiate β-endorphin from pituitary cells, Troullos and co-workers (1997) examined the effects of inhibiting prostaglandin production with ibuprofen before surgical stress in human subjects undergoing dental surgery (under outpatient conditions). These authors showed that plasma immunoreactive β-endorphin was increased during surgical stress but that, in comparison with placebo, prior oral administration (at 1 h) of ibuprofen 600 mg resulted in a doubling of the plasma levels of the opioid compared with placebo. Likewise, methylprednisolone 125 mg given under the same conditions caused a marked suppression of the release of β-endorphin. These results are interesting not only for the potential that β-endorphin has in mediating the pain-relieving effects of ibuprofen but also in terms of the actions of steroids versus the nonsteroidal drugs presumably mediated by regulation of prostaglandin synthesis.

5.3.3   Effects on platelet aggregation and thrombosis

The first studies of the effects of ibuprofen on platelet aggregation *ex vivo* were performed by Baele, Deweerdt and Barbier (1970). They undertook a study in hospitalized subjects who took either 400 mg ibuprofen, 1 g aspirin or two tablets of placebo. Blood was collected 1 h later and platelet-rich plasma was obtained by conventional centrifugation. Platelet aggregation was measured using the turbidimetric method; the platelet-rich plasma was incubated with (a) adenosine diphosphate, (b) adrenaline, or (c) collagen. The data obtained by these workers was highly scattered. It was, therefore, difficult to determine with accuracy whether positive inhibitory effects had been obtained by aspirin. However, ibuprofen prior treatment did impair the aggregation induced by collagen but not by the other treatments. Part of the problem in this experimental design was that the platelet-rich plasma obtained by centrifugation would have had a relatively low drug concentration. Since additional medium is required to be added to the platelet-rich plasma containing the various stimulants, it is not surprising that a high degree of scatter was obtained in the results. Furthermore, as ibuprofen is a reversible inhibitor of cyclooxygenase, the platelet production of thromboxane could be partially or completely reversed by endogenous substrate produced by stimulation of the platelets. In contrast, the effects of aspirin would be expected to be irreversible since this drug irreversibly acetylates the platelet cyclooxygenase

■ CHAPTER 5 ■

■ 225

(Rainsford, 1984). Thus, it is difficult to understand why aspirin did not produce consistent results, although the authors believed that the lower dose (*sic.*) of aspirin employed may have accounted for the lack of effects observed with some of the stimuli.

Following these initial studies there have been a number of reports showing that ibuprofen inhibits platelet aggregation induced by adrenaline, arachidonic acid, collagen and thrombin (O'Brien, 1968; Brooks *et al.*, 1973; Ikeda, 1977; McIntyre *et al.*, 1978; Parks *et al.*, 1981; Adesuyi and Ellis, 1982; Cronberg *et al.*, 1984; Longenecker *et al.*, 1985; Cox *et al.*, 1987; Evans *et al.*, 1991; Villaneuva *et al.*, 1993). The mechanism of this inhibition of platelet aggregation is thought to be due to the reduced synthesis of thromboxane A_2. Despite the consensus that the mechanism of ibuprofen inhibition of platelet aggregation is related to the inhibition of thromboxane synthesis, the recent studies by Stichtenoth *et al.* (1996), were unable to demonstrate significant reduction in thromboxane B_2 production in subjects who had ingested ibuprofen 3×400 mg/day or 3×200 mg/day for 5 days prior to isolation of the platelets. However, the authors did observe reduction in platelet aggregation in subjects who had ingested 3×25 mg/day or 3×50 mg/day of ketoprofen, a very potent cyclooxygenase inhibitor. Again, the reasons for this may be similar to those identified from the study by Baele *et al.* (1970) mentioned above. In addition to the extensive studies showing effects of ibuprofen on platelet aggregation and thromboxane production in platelets derived from humans (Brooks *et al.*, 1973; Cox *et al.*, 1987; Ikeda, 1977; Longenecker *et al.*, 1985; McIntyre *et al.*, 1978; O'Brien, 1968; Parks *et al.*, 1981; Evans *et al.*, 1991; Villaneuva *et al.*, 1993) studies have shown that ibuprofen like aspirin, inhibits platelet aggregation *ex vivo* in rabbits (Adesuyi and Ellis, 1982). Thus, doses of 6–24 mg/kg ibuprofen i.v. for 30 min significantly inhibited aggregation *ex vivo* in the presence of arachidonic acid. The authors also found that prostacyclin (PGI_2) production was inhibited by ibuprofen 12 and 24 mg/kg i.v. (Adesuyi and Ellis, 1982).

Fujiyoshi *et al.* (1987) observed that ibuprofen, like indomethacin, phenylbutazone and aspirin, inhibited the platelet aggregation induced by collagen and arachidonic acid but not that by adenosine diphosphate (ADP) in rabbit platelets *in vitro*. The IC_{50} value for ibuprofen against collagen-induced aggregation was 176 µmol/l compared with that of aspirin 118 µmol/l. The corresponding IC_{50} values when arachidonic acid was employed were 65 µmol/l for ibuprofen compared with 71 µmol/l for aspirin. Thus, *in vitro* ibuprofen is equipotent as an inhibitor of rabbit platelet aggregation when the platelets are stimulated by collagen and arachidonic acid. Indomethacin by comparison is approximately 10-fold more potent as an inhibitor of collagen-induced aggregation and 20-fold more potent as an inhibitor of arachidonic acid-induced aggregation.

In a more extensive study, Fujiyoshi *et al.* (1987) observed a dose-dependent inhibition of the aggregation of rat platelets *ex vivo* following oral administration of ibuprofen 25–100 mg/kg compared with indomethacin 5–25 mg/kg, phenylbutazone 50–250 mg/kg and aspirin 50–200 mg/kg. The respective ED_{50} values were for ibuprofen 37.2 mg/kg, for indomethacin 6.6 mg/kg, for phenylbutazone 134.9 mg/kg and for aspirin 147.9 mg/kg.

In a model of antithrombotic activity, DiPasquale and Mellace (1977) have shown that the mortality induced by i.v. injection of high doses of arachidonic acid to rabbits is reduced by ibuprofen; the protective activity, PD_{50}, being 31.4 mg/kg/ml i.p. The potency of ibuprofen is lower than with many other NSAIDs (cf. aspirin PD_{50} 0.98 mg/kg/ml i.p.; naproxen PD_{50} 7.0 mg/kg/ml i.p.; indomethacin PD_{50} 0.07 mg/kg/ml i.p.) (DiPasquale and Mellace, 1977). These results suggest that the antithrombotic acivity of ibuprofen is relatively weak *in vivo*.

To examine the relationship between inhibition of platelet thromboxane production and the plasma concentrations of the active form of ibuprofen, i.e. the (S)-(+) enantiomer, Evans *et al.* (1991) studied the effects of oral dosage of *rac*-ibuprofen 200–1200 mg as a single dose, with blood samples collected up to 48 h afterwards. The plasma concentrations of (S)-(+) ibuprofen were determined and also the plasma bound drug concentration. Platelet thromboxane production was stimulated by thrombin. The authors showed that all doses of the drug inhibited thromboxane production to the extent of > 90%. They observed that the inhibition of platelet thromboxane production was directly related to the unbound (i.e. non-plasma-protein-bound) concentration of (S)-(+)-ibuprofen in the plasma. These results show that the effects of *rac*-ibuprofen-induced inhibition of platelet thromboxane production is directly related to the active form of the drug. Unfortunately, the authors did not measure the platelet aggregation induced by thrombin or other stimuli to relate these to the effects on thromboxane production. This would have been a useful observation since it would enable the thromboxane effect of ibuprofen to be discriminated from that of other stimuli. This is of particular significance in view of the studies by Villanueva *et al.* (1993), who observed differences between the effects of *rac*-ibuprofen and the individual enantiomers of the drug on platelet aggregation induced by collagen in platelet-rich plasma as well as in washed platelets compared with those of thromboxane production in the same system. Thus the IC_{50} value for inhibition of platelet aggregation with (S)-(+)-ibuprofen was 88 mmol/l compared with thromboxane production, which was 26 mmol/l. This contrasts with the effects of the inactive enantiomer of ibuprofen, that is (R)-(–)-ibuprofen which had an IC_{50} value of 1260 mmol/l compared with thromboxane production, which was 380 mmol/l in platelet-rich plasma. Curiously, *rac*-ibuprofen showed inhibition of thromboxane production and platelet aggregation at IC_{50} values that were much closer to those of the (S)-(+)-ibuprofen than of (R)-(–)-ibuprofen, suggesting that *rac*-ibuprofen has appreciably greater inhibitory effects on both these processes than would be expected if the effect were half-way between the inhibitory concentrations for the two enantiomers. In washed platelets the effects of *rac*-ibuprofen and the enantiomers was appreciably greater than in the platelet-rich plasma, a reflection of the effects of the added plasma proteins that are present in the platelet-rich plasma preparations. The inhibitory effects of *rac*-ibuprofen were about the same as those of (S)-(+)-ibuprofen, but again the inhibitory effects of (R)-(–)-ibuprofen were much less than those of either of the other two forms.

CHAPTER 5

Inhibition of cyclooxygenase may not be the only mechanism of drug action on platelets due to the inhibition resulting from arachidonic acid metabolism. Thus, Siegel and co-workers (1980) showed that aspirin and several other NSAIDs inhibit the conversion of 12L-hydroperoxy-5,8,10,14-eicosatetraenoic acid (12-HPETE) to the corresponding hydroxy acid via the 12-lipoxygenase in platelets. The IC_{50} for inhibition of the conversion of 12-HPETE to 12-HETE for ibuprofen was 200 mmol/l compared with those of aspirin 500 mmol/l, indomethacin 25 mmol/l, and phenylbutazone 50 mmol/l (Siegel *et al.*, 1979, 1980). Paracetamol, which does not inhibit platelet aggregation, also was found by these authors to be inactive. The significance of the inhibitory effects of ibuprofen and the other NSAIDs on 12-HPETE peroxidase activity in platelets in relationship to their inhibitory effects on platelet aggregation is not known. However, hydroxyl radicals generated from the conversion of 12-HPETE to 12-HETE might be expected to contribute to the manifestations of intracellular activation reactions.

Overall, although ibuprofen has some modest antiplatelet effects, these relate to the effects of the (S)-(+) enantiomer and possibly effects on 12-lipoxygenase activity. In contrast to aspirin, ibuprofen does not have long lasting antiplatelet effects, i.e. effective through the half-life of the platelet *in vivo*.

5.3.4 Gastrointestinal injury and bleeding

Clinico-epidemiological data on the gastrointestinal (GI) ulcerogenicity and bleeding from ibuprofen in comparison with other NSAIDs are discussed at length in Chapter 9. The evidence from these studies is that ibuprofen is among the NSAIDs that have the lowest GI risk. Moreover, ibuprofen has a relatively low degree of gastric intolerance in rheumatoid patients with prior history of peptic ulcer disease (Cardoe, 1975).

Some clinico-experimental data are reviewed to highlight further the reactions of ibuprofen compared with other NSAIDs on the human GI tract. Experimental studies in laboratory animals have been reviewed in section 5.1.5 of this chapter. These studies show that ibuprofen has moderately low GI ulcerogenicity in most animal models relative to therapeutic activity in comparison with other NSAIDs.

Thompson and Anderson (1970) were the first to investigate the gastrointestinal blood loss from ibuprofen 800–1800 mg/day compared with that from aspirin (calcium salt) 4.8 g/day, paracetamol 4 g/day, phenylbutazone 300 mg/day and placebo. The studies were performed in unspecified patients, using the radiochromium ^{51}Cr red cell technique. The treatment periods varied over a considerable range, from 13 to 56 days on ibuprofen and similarly from 19 to 72 days on the other drugs. No detailed statistical comparisons were perfomed on the data. However, the average blood loss observed was 1.4, 1.75 and 1.5 ml/day with ibuprofen 800, 1200 and 1800 mg/day respectively. This was not different from that from placebo, which was 1.3 ml/day, but was appreciably lower than that from aspirin, which averaged 3.3 ml/day.

Schmid and Culic (1976) performed a double-blind crossover comparison of the gastrointestinal blood loss from ibuprofen 900–1350 mg/day with that from aspirin 2.7–5.1 g/day and the preparations were taken for 2 weeks at the outset or (with a few exceptions) for 1 year in an open-label parallel group study. Blood loss from the gastrointestinal tract was studied over a 4-day period at five times during the treatment period using the ^{51}Cr technique. In the 2-week group blood loss from ibuprofen was 3.0 ± 2.0 (SD) ml in 4 days from ibuprofen and 6.7 ± 1.7 ml/4 days on aspirin. After 1 year the blood loss in 7 patients was 6.2 (± 2.7) ml/4 days on ibuprofen and 4.2 (± 1.2) ml/4 days in 9 others. This compared with 18.2 (± 16.6) and 20.6 (± 7.0) ml/4 days in the two aspirin groups, the difference being statistically significant.

Similar observations showing that ibuprofen caused less blood loss than aspirin have been reported by others using the ^{51}Cr blood loss technique, and ibuprofen is often used as a basis for comparing blood loss with other NSAIDs or analgesics since it consistently shows low gastrointestinal bleeding (Bianchi Porro et al., 1977; Warrington et al., 1982; Bidlingmaier et al., 1995). Being a 'bench standard' as a low-blood-loss drug is recognition of the relatively low propensity for this drug to produce damage in the gastrointestinal tract. The low gastrointestinal blood loss with ibuprofen can, in part, be related to the short-lived and relatively limited effects on platelets (McIntyre et al., 1978), thus limiting the degree of blood loss from damaged mucosa. Even in hemophiliac patients, platelet functions and bleeding are not affected more than in control subjects (McIntyre et al., 1978), reflecting the low potential for ibuprofen to contribute to bleeding from damaged sites such as from the GI mucosa. Moreover, the low biliary elimination of ibuprofen (0.82%) observed by Schneider et al. (1990) in patients with cholangiodrainage compared with that of indomethacin (6.4%) and diclofenac (4.6%) may also account for the relatively low blood loss with ibuprofen arising from intestinal injury.

A considerable number of upper GI endoscopic investigations have been performed comparing the mucosal irritancy of ibuprofen in therapeutic doses with that of aspirin and other NSAIDs (Vasconcelos Tiexeira et al., 1977; Lanza et al., 1976a, 1981, 1987; Bergmann et al., 1992; Müller and Simon, 1994). Ibuprofen consistently produced relatively low damage to the gastroduodenal mucosa compared with aspirin and some other ulcerogenic NSAIDs (Lanza et al., 1979, 1981, 1987; Bergmann et al., 1992; Müller and Simon, 1994; see also Chapter 9). Again, as with GI blood loss studies, ibuprofen has been used as a low-GI-irritant standard for comparison in investigations, especially of new NSAIDs. Conventional tablets of ibuprofen (Motrin™) produced superior bioavailability yet comparable or slightly lower gastroduodenal injury observed endoscopically than did disintegrated tablets taken with water or orange juice (Friedman et al., 1990).

The relatively benign character of ibuprofen on the GI tract of rheumatic patients has been illustrated by the study of Vasconcelos Tiexeira et al. (1977), who found that daily oral intake of ibuprofen 1200 mg for 1–6 weeks did not result in any changes in pentagastrin-stimulated acid secretion compared with that in the same subjects before

CHAPTER 5

treatment with the drug. Moreover, they observed that, although many of the subjects had pre-existent gastroduodenal pathology (e.g. gastritis, duodenal ulcers), neither endoscopic nor microscopic observations revealed any effects on this pathology from treatment with ibuprofen.

Miscellaneous observations on GI effects

The monoamine oxidase inhibitor moclobemide was not found to increase blood loss from ibuprofen (Guentert *et al.*, 1992). This suggests that amine oxidase activity does not influence the mucosal absorption, gastric emptying or other processes underlying its effects on the gastrointestinal tract, and that these two drugs may be given safely together.

Ibuprofen, like other NSAIDs, has infrequently been associated with exacerbation of the symptoms of colitis (Gibson *et al.*, 1992). Roediger and Millard (1995) have shown that ibuprofen 2.0–7.5 mmol/l but not the anticolitis drug 5-aminosalicylic acid inhibited the fatty acid metabolism of butyrate in isolated rat colonocytes and those cells isolated from the proximal and distal colon from human subjects. The highest concentration of both these drugs inhibited lactate formation from glucose. These authors suggested that the inhibition of fatty acid biosynthesis by ibuprofen may be important in the exacerbation of colitis seen with ibuprofen as well as being of benefit in prevention of colon cancer (see later section).

5.3.5   Hypersensitivity and other immunological reactions

As a class, NSAIDs are associated with the development of asthma and bronchospasm, urticaria, erythematous rash, angioneurotic oedema and other hypersensitivity reactions (Assem, 1976; Settipane, 1983; Fowler, 1987; Arnaud, 1995; Biscarini, 1996). Such class-related effects belie the considerable variablity that exists in the propensity of different NSAIDs to cause these reactions and the type they elicit (Settipane, 1983; Fowler, 1987; Arnaud, 1995; Biscarini, 1996). There is a high degree of variability in reports of these conditions, e.g. aspirin-sensitive bronchospasm or asthma (Fowler, 1987). Subjects with aspirin-sensitive asthma and urticaria/angioneurotic oedema are often sensitive to indomethacin and some other NSAIDs, but not the fenamates or non-narcotic analgesics (Fowler, 1987). It has been suggested that the lack of reactivity of these subjects to the fenamates may be related to the effect these drugs have in antagonizing the bronchoconstrictor effects of prostaglandin $F_{2\alpha}$ (Fowler, 1987). There are indications that some individuals are sensitive to certain classes of drugs, for example aspririn-sensitive asthma being evident in middle-aged females and those with food or other allergies (Fowler, 1987). There is considerable controversy over whether aspirin-sensitive asthma and related hypersensitivity reactions are immunological in character (Settipane, 1983; Fowler, 1987). Ibuprofen has a low association with asthma though it can provoke bronchospasm in certain asthmatics (Biscarini, 1996). In aspirin-intolerant individuals the extent of cross reaction with challenge has been reported to be 5% with ibuprofen, benzoate and tartrazine, in contrast to that from indomethacin, which is 100% (Settipane, 1983).

It is also worth noting that some NSAIDs or non-narcotic analgesics can be used in individuals with non-aspirin-sensitive asthma and may even relieve the symptoms of this condition (Assem, 1976; Rainsford, 1984).

Reports of hypersensitivity reactions to ibuprofen are infrequent (Biscarini, 1996). In analyses of adverse reactions from non-prescription use of the drug there appear to be no serious hypersensitive reactions recorded (Furey *et al.*, 1992; Rainsford *et al.*, 1997a). Mostly these involve urticaria and other mild skin reactions (Furey *et al.*, 1992; Rainsford *et al.*, 1997a). Higher prescription use of the drug can lead to the development of skin rashes (Biscarini, 1996). These comprise urticarial, purpuric and erythematous changes, while two cases of bullous pemphigoid lesions have been reported (Biscarini, 1996). Photosensitization has been reported with ibuprofen, though to a lower extent than with drugs such as benoxaprofen (Biscarini, 1996). Phototoxic reactions with red blood cells exposed *in vitro* to visible light limited to 5% UV-A and added NSAIDs did not lead to any photohemolysis with ibuprofen, although several other NSAIDs that produce phototoxic effects did cause an effect in this system (Becker *et al.*, 1996). This suggests that the relative phototoxic activity of ibuprofen may be low relative to that of NSAIDs with greater potential to produce this reaction *in vivo*.

In Sweden, where reporting of adverse reactions is compulsory, there was, in the period 1975–84, only one report of Stevens–Johnson's syndrome from prescription use of ibuprofen, whereas during 1970–84 there were 24 reports with the butazones (oxyphenbutazone and phenylbutazone), the most frequently reported drugs associated with this side-effect (Wiholm *et al.*, 1987).

A patient who developed Coombs'-positive hemolytic anemia associated with ingestion of a formulation of ibuprofen (Mortin-400™) was later found to have reacted to the orange dye coating on the tablet (Law *et al.*, 1979). This underlines the importance of considering the excipients in formulations of NSAIDs before ascribing hypersensitivity or other actions to the drug itself.

The mechanisms of NSAID-associated allergic reactions are considered, in part, to involve the pharmacological properties of the drugs as cyclooxygenase inhibitors (Arnaud, 1995). In intolerant patients there is upregulation of the 5-lipoxygenase pathway, and with inhibition of the cyclooxygenase pathway there is diversion of arachidonate through the lipoxygenase pathway to produce excess bronchoconstrictor leukotrienes (Arnaud, 1995). There is also evidence for IgE-dependent allergic reactions (Arnaud, 1995). Histamine release has been shown to be enhanced by some NSAIDs in ragweed-treated leukocytes from individuals allergic to household dusts or ragweed (Wijnar *et al.*, 1980). However, a few drugs such as fenbufen, ibufenac and paracetamol inhibited this reaction, ibuprofen being inactive in this assay. These results suggest that in contrast to other

CHAPTER 5

NSAIDs ibuprofen has no effect on *in vitro* reactions thought to underlie immediate-type hypersensitivity reactions.

Recent studies suggest that the immune reactivity of some NSAIDs (e.g. tolmetin, zomepirac) that are known to induce hypersensitivity reactions may be due to the reaction of the drug–glucuronide conjugates with endogenous proteins, e.g. human serum albumin (Zia-Amirhosseini *et al.*, 1995). This hypothesis presupposes that the reactivity of the respective NSAID-glucuronides will depend on their stability and reactivity *in vivo*. Clearly, further studies are required to establish whether ibuprofenyl-glucuronides have similar reactivity to those of other reactive drugs such as zomepirac-glucuronide. It would be suspected, however, that the stability/reactivity of ibuprofenyl-glucuronide would be relatively low in view of the relatively low number of reports of hypersensitivity with ibuprofen.

5.3.6   Gynaecological and obstetric uses

Ibuprofen is used extensively for the treatment of dysmenorrhoea and other painful gynaecological conditions (see Chapter 7); this therapeutic activity is related to effects on prostaglandin production. The beneficial effects on menstrual pain may be related to the effects of the drug on contraction of the myometrium induced by arachidonic acid metabolites. Thus, Smith and co-workers (1975) found that ibuprofen, in common with a range of other NSAIDs, inhibited the contraction *in vitro* of human myometrial strips from pregnant individuals induced by prostaglandin $F_{2\alpha}$. In most experiments the NSAIDs reduced the amplitude of contractions as well as their rate. Similar inhibitory effects were observed in uterine tissues derived from non-pregnant rabbits.

The reduction in mononuclear phagocytic activity observed during menstruation is not affected by ibuprofen (Stratton *et al.*, 1984).

The endometrial inflammation induced by intrauterine contraceptive devices (IUDs) has been shown experimentally in rats to be reduced by ibuprofen as well as by other NSAIDs (Srivastava *et al.*, 1989). This finding indicates that ibuprofen may have an added benefit in those women with IUDs apart from effects on menstrual pain.

Recurrent vaginal candida infection in women leads to impairment of proliferative capacity of lymphocytes stimulated with mitogens or the presence of macrophages (Witkin *et al.*, 1986). Addition of ibuprofen or indomethacin reduced the inhibitory effects of macrophages on lymphocyte proliferation (Witkin *et al.*, 1986). This suggests that there may be benefits in employing ibuprofen in control of the immunoinflammatory reactions in candidiasis.

Therapeutic use of ibuprofen as a tocolytic agent has not been associated with congenital malformations (Østensen, 1994). Mild constriction of the ductus arteriosus has been reported in a few subjects (Østensen, 1994). Coceani *et al.* (1979) showed that ibuprofen induces premature closure of the ductus arteriosus in the lamb. This effect has the benefit of preventing patent ductus arteriosus development in premature infants (Varvarigou *et al.*, 1996).

Alterations of photopic and scotopic electroretinography have, however, been observed in the newborn piglet (Hanna *et al.*, 1995). The latter effect appears to be a property of propionic acids and in newborn piglets is accompanied by reduction in retinal concentrations of the principal prostaglandins (Hanna *et al.*, 1995). The effect is unlikely to be due to changes by ibuprofen in chloride-sensitive channels of retinal epithelia, although other NSAIDs (e.g. niflumic acid) cause these changes (Bialek *et al.*, 1996).

Intake of NSAIDs including ibuprofen with a decongestant in the first trimester may lead to gastroschisis (Werler *et al.*, 1992). The mechanism of this effect is not known but probably relates only to the inhibition of prostaglandin production by the drug since there are a wide range of other pharmacological agents that do not affect prostaglandin production but that produce this effect (Werler *et al.*, 1992).

Oral intake of ibuprofen is unlikely to lead to substantial excretion in milk (Weibert *et al.*, 1982). However, when the drug was given in multiple doses of 400 mg to a patient undergoing maxillary surgery it was found to be excreted into the milk (Walter and Dilger, 1997). This suggests that caution should be used when the drug is taken during lactation where there has been surgery, but otherwise it should be relatively safe to take.

5.3.7 Effects on lung inflammation in cystic fibrosis

The anti-inflammatory properties of ibuprofen have been the basis for establishing its utility in ameliorating the lung inflammation in patients with cystic fibrosis (Konstan *et al.*, 1995; Konstan, 1996). Konstan (1996) has pointed out that the use of prednisone (1 mg/kg) to control airway inflammation in cystic fibrosis, while possibly beneficial, results in an unacceptably high incidence and severity of side-effects. The case is made by this author for using ibuprofen – probably the safest among the NSAIDs – given at high dose, in preference to corticosteroids. Support for the use of ibuprofen comes from a study by Konstan and co-workers (1995) in which they compared the effects of high-dose ibuprofen in a double-blind, placebo-controlled study in 85 patients with cystic fibrosis aged 5–39 years in two cystic fibrosis centres in Cleveland, Ohio (USA) and having mild lung disease (forced expiratory volume in one second (FEV_1) ≥ 60% of predicted value). Doses of ibuprofen were individually adjusted to give plasma concentrations of 50–100 µg/ml (240–490 µmol/l). The authors found that ibuprofen treatment had a significantly lower rate of annual decline in FEV_1, body weight and chest inflammation radiographic score over 4 years. There were no differences between the groups in the frequency of hospitalization. Only one patient withdrew from the study because of conjunctivitis and one other because of epistaxis related to ibuprofen. Clearly, these results attest to the benefits of high-dose ibuprofen in ameliorating the lung symptoms without side-effects as observed with corticosteroids. Further larger scale investigations are warranted to quantify the

CHAPTER 5

benefits of long-term high-dose ibuprofen in subsets of patients with cystic fibrosis. One important aspect worth considering is whether ibuprofen given to young children at early stages of the disease would confer particular benefit. Also, combinations of ibuprofen with other agents such as pentoxyfylline and fish oils (Konstan, 1996) to control other components of the inflammatory process mediated by cytokines and lipoxygenase products would have added benefit in control of airway inflammation and the decline in lung functions.

5.3.8   Colo-rectal, mammary and other cancers

In addition to providing effective pain relief (Ventafridda *et al.*, 1990) long-term intake of a number of NSAIDs has been found to be associated with reduction in the risk of developing colon and other cancers (Muscat *et al.*, 1994; Berkel *et al.*, 1996; Morgan, 1996; Peleg *et al.*, 1996). Also, acute-phase proteins (C-reactive protein and IL-6) have been shown to be reduced by ibuprofen 1200 mg/day for 8–11 days in colorectal cancer patients. This suggests that ibuprofen may reduce the systemic inflammatory components in cancer.

Extensive studies in experimental animal models and in cancer cells *in vitro* have given support to the concept that NSAIDs may control some of the components of cancer cell growth and proliferation (Levy, 1997). Results suggest that though there may be some component related to the inhibition of COX-2-derived prostaglandins (Reddy *et al.*, 1996; Reich and Martin, 1996; Levy, 1997) there is also clear evidence of a prostaglandin-independent pathway involving the induction of apoptosis by NSAIDs (Hanif *et al.*, 1996; Levy, 1997). The latter has been highlighted by the effects of sulindac sulfone (the non-prostaglandin synthesis inhibitory metabolite of sulindac) in reducing the development of adenomas and carcinomas induced in rats by azoxymethane (Piazza *et al.*, 1997). Sulindac has been shown to induce apoptosis in cancer cell populations and has been shown to reduce the risk of colorectal proliferation in patients with familial adenomatous polyposis (Pasricha *et al.*, 1995).

The evidence in epidemiological studies for individual NSAIDs showing reduction in risk of colorectal and other cancers has not been focused on any one drug, with the exception of aspirin (Muscat *et al.*, 1994; Berkel *et al.*, 1996; Morgan, 1996; Peleg *et al.*, 1996). In many of the studies it is possible that ibuprofen, being a frequently ingested NSAID, might have been taken, and so the data may reflect the intake of this drug as well as of aspirin and other NSAIDs.

More specific associations have come from the studies of Harris, Namboodiri and Farrar (1996), who observed that ibuprofen intake had a slightly better odds ratio (OR = 0.57) than aspirin (OR = 0.69) or any NSAID (OR = 0.66) in risk of breast cancer, although these differences did not approach statistical significance. None the less, ibuprofen intake appears to be potentially capable of reducing the risk of breast cancer.

Stimulation by dietary supplementation with ibuprofen 400 ppm, and several other NSAIDs, of rat mucosal glutathione *S*-transferase (GST) μ and π levels and GST activity was observed by van Leishout and co-workers (1997). The authors suggested that enhanced activity of these GST isoforms may play a role in detoxification during chemical carcinogenesis and may partly explain the potential anticarcinogenic activity of NSAIDs.

McMillan and co-workers (1977) reported that combination of megestrol acetate and ibuprofen increased body weight and reduced levels of the acute-phase reactant, C-reactive protein, in patients with advanced gastrointestinal cancer. This suggests that control of cachexia may be achieved by combination of the steroid with ibuprofen.

In animal studies, McCarthy and Daun (1993) showed that ibuprofen, like indomethacin, reduced tumour growth by 30–40% and lowered body temperature in anorexic rats implanted with the Walker 256 tumour. However, these drugs had no effect on food intake and body weight of tumour-bearing animals. The authors suggested that prostaglandin synthesis inhibition has no relation to tumour-mediated anorexia. Clearly, further studies are warranted to establish the efficacy and mechanism of the control of cachexia in cancer patients given ibuprofen and other drugs that may enhance anabolic activity.

Further studies are clearly warranted on the mechanisms of ibuprofen in preventing the growth, proliferation and induction of apoptosis of cancer cells, as well as clinico-epidemiological investigations of the potential of ibuprofen in comparison with other NSAIDs to prevent cancers in various body sites.

5.3.9   Alzheimer's and related dementias

As with the above-mentioned investigations on NSAIDs in cancer, there have been a substantial number of investigations indicating from epidemiological data that there is reduction in the onset of and reduced risk of developing Alzheimer's disease in subjects taking NSAIDs (Andersen et al., 1995; Breitner et al., 1995; Breitner, 1996; McGeer and McGeer, 1996; Stewart et al., 1997). Stewart and co-workers (1997) in their longitudinal study showed that ibuprofen was one of the NSAIDs that was associated with reduced risk of developing Alzheimer's disease and the decline in cognitive function. Interestingly, intake of paracetamol was not associated with any reduction in risk of developing this disease.

There is substantial evidence supporting the development of an immunoinflammatory basis for Alzheimer's in the region where senile plaques develop in this disease (Chen et al., 1996; Griffin et al., 1996; Sheng et al., 1996). Production of inflammatory cytokines occurs in this region. There is a major role of IL-1, IL-6 and complement C3 in the inflammatory reactions in this disease (Chen et al., 1996; Griffin et al., 1996; Sheng et al., 1996). Curiously, COX-2 mRNA expression appears to be decreased 3-fold in the neocortex of Alzheimer's disease patients (Chang et al., 1996). This observation makes it difficult to reconcile the beneficial effects of the COX-2 inhibition by NSAIDs in preventing the onset of symptoms or the decline in cognitive state in this disease. It may be that these drugs act to control manifestations of oxyradical damage in the regions of the brain where

CHAPTER 5

degenerative changes occur (McGeer and McGeer, 1996). Other non-prostaglandin effects of these drugs as well as their actions on vascular prostaglandin production may also be important in their apparent protective effects.

5.3.10 Prevention of cataract

Epidemiological studies suggest that intake of ibuprofen or aspirin and paracetamol may prevent cataract formation in susceptible individuals, e.g. those with diabetes mellitus or rheumatoid arthritis (Cotlier and Sharma, 1981; Harding and van Heyningen, 1988). Several non-prostaglandin mechanisms may be involved in this preventative activity of ibuprofen. Among these, evidence indicates that the non-enzymic modification of lens proteins as well as albumin by glucose and fructose is prevented *in vitro* by relatively high concentrations of ibuprofen (10–20 mmol/l) (Raza and Harding, 1991). The modification of proteins by sugars such as glucose involves formation of Schiff's bases that then undergo Amadori rearrangement to form ketoamine derivatives of predominantly cyclic Maillard compounds. Glycation of crystallins increases with age and conditions such as diabetes mellitus. Ibuprofen has been shown to reduce the rate of binding of glucosamine, fructose, galactose and cyanate to crystallin (Ajiboye and Harding, 1989; Roberts and Harding, 1990; Raza and Harding, 1991).

Recent studies by Plater *et al*. (1997) have shown that ibuprofen prevented the post-translational modification of α-crystallin to the γ-form, so protecting the chaperone-like activity of the former. The authors suggested that ibuprofen exerted its protective effects by binding of ibuprofen breakdown products to lysine groups of α-crystallin, so preventing post-translational modification that accounts for loss of chaperone-like activity of this protein.

5.4 CONCLUSIONS

Ibuprofen is a moderately potent anti-inflammatory/analgesic/antipyretic drug with a relatively low systemic toxicity and gastrointestinal irritancy. Its mode of action involves the inhibition by the (S)-(+) enantiomer and the CoA intermediates of COX-1- and COX-2-derived prostanoids. There is evidence that both enantiomers of the drug inhibit production of leukocyte-derived lipoxygenase products. Ibuprofen may also affect the production of oxyradicals and nitric oxide via inhibition of iNOS induction. The production and actions of certain pro-inflammatory cytokines may also be affected by this drug.

Recent studies have shown that there is considerable potential for ibuprofen to have beneficial effects in a number of chronic inflammatory and degenerative diseases as well as in some cancers. More extensive investigations should be undertaken to determine the relative efficacy of ibuprofen in these states and its mechanisms of action.

REFERENCES

ABRAMSON, S., EDELSON, H., KAPLAN, H., GIVEN, W. and WEISSMANN, G. (1984) The inactivation of the polymorphonuclear leukocyte by nonsteroidal anti-inflammatory drugs. *Inflammation* 8, S103–S108.

ADAMS, L., NEUMAN, R.G., SACHS, J. and BARLOW, S.P. (1990) Efficacy and gastric safety of etodolac as determined by cultured human gastric and synovial cells. *Gastroenterology* 98(Suppl.), A14 (abstract).

ADAMS, S.S. and COBB, R. (1963) The effect of salicylates and related compounds on erythema in the guinea-pig and man. In: DIXON, A.ST.J., MARTIN, B.K., SMITH, M.J.H. and WOOD, P.H.N. (eds), *Salicylates. An International Symposium*. London, J and A Churchill, 127–134.

ADAMS, T. JR and TRABER, D.L. (1982) The effects of a prostaglandin synthetase inhibitor, ibuprofen, on the cardiopulmonary response to endotoxin in sheep. *Circulatory Shock* 9, 481–489.

ADAMS, S.S., McCULLOUGH, K.F. and NICHOLSON, J.S. (1969) The pharmacological properties of ibuprofen, an anti-inflammatory, analgesic and antipyretic agent. *Archives Internationale Pharmacodynamie et de Thérapie* 178, 115–129.

ADAMS, S.S., BOUGH, R.G., CLIFFE, E.E. *et al.* (1970) Some aspects of the pharmacology, metabolism, and toxicology of ibuprofen. *Rheumatology and Physical Medicine* 11(Suppl.), 9–22.

ADAMS, S.S., BRESLOFT, P. and MASON, C.G. (1976) Pharmacological differences between the optical isomers of ibuprofen: evidence for metabolic inversion of the (–)-isomer. *Journal of Pharmacy and Pharmacology* 28, 256–257.

ADESUYI, S.A. and ELLIS, E.F. (1982) The effect of ibuprofen dose on rabbit platelet aggregation and aortic PGI_2 synthesis. *Thrombosis Research* 28, 581–585.

ADEYEYE, C.M., BRICKER, J.D., VILIVALAM, V.D. and SMITH, W.I. (1996) Acute gastrointestinal toxic effects of suspensions of unencapsulated and encapsulated ibuprofen in rats. *Pharmaceutical Research* 13, 784–793.

ADKINSON, N.F., BARRON, T., POWELL, S. and COHEN, S. (1977) Prostaglandin production by human peripheral blood cells *in vitro*. *Journal of Laboratory and Clinical Medicine* 90, 1043–1053.

AEBERHARD, E.E., HENDERSON, S.A., ARABOLOS, N.S. *et al.* (1995) Nonsteroidal anti-inflammatory drugs inhibit the expression of the inducible nitric oxide gene. *Biochemical and Biophysical Research Comunications* 208, 1053–1059.

AHN, C.M., SANDLER, H., WEGENER, T. and SALDEEN, T. (1994) Effect of ibuprofen on thrombin-induced pulmonary oedema in the rat. *Pulmonary Pharmacology* 7, 393–399.

CHAPTER 5

AILABOUNI, W. and EKNOYAN (1996) Nonsteroidal anti-inflammatory drugs and acute renal failure in the elderly. *Drugs and Aging* **9**, 341–351.

AJIBOYE, R. and HARDING, J.J. (1989) The non-enzymic glycosylation of bovine lens proteins by glucosamine and its inhibition by aspirin, ibuprofen and glutathione. *Experimental Eye Research* **49**, 31–41.

ALLAN, G., NHATTACHERJEE, P., BROOK, C.D., READ, N.G. and PARKE, A.J. (1985) Myeloperoxidase activity as a quantitative marker of polymorphonuclear leukocyte accumulation into an experimental myocardial infarct — the effect of ibuprofen on infarct size and polymorphonuclear leukocyte accumulation. *Journal of Cardiovascular Pharmacology* **7**, 1154–1160.

ALMQVIST, P.M., KUENZIG, M. and SCHWARTZ, S.I. (1984) Treatment of experimental canine endotoxin shock with ibuprofen, a cyclooxygenase inhibitor. *Circulatory Shock* **13**, 227–232.

AMANUMA, F., OKUYAMA, S., ORIKASA, S. *et al.* (1984) The analgesic and antipyretic effects of a nonsteroidal anti-inflammatory drug, oxaprozin, in experimental animals. *Folia Pharmacologia Japonica* **83**, 345–354.

AMIN, A.R., VYAS, P., ATTUR, M. *et al.* (1995) The mode of action of aspirin-like drugs: effect on inducible nitric oxide synthase. *Proceedings of the National Academy of Sciences of the USA* **92**, 7926–7930.

ANDERSEN, K., LAUNER, L.J., OTT, A., HOES, A.W., BRETELER, M.M.B. and HOFMAN, A. (1995) Do nonsteroidal anti-inflammatory drugs decrease the risk for Alzheimer's disease? The Rotterdam Study. *Neurology* **45**, 1441–1445.

APSTEIN, C.S. and VOGEL, W.M. (1982) Coronary arterial vasodilator effect of ibuprofen. *Journal of Clinical Pharmacology* **220**, 167–171.

ARNAUD, A. (1995) Allergy and intolerance to nonsteroidal anti-inflammatory agents. *Clinical Reviews in Allergy and Immunology* **13**, 245–251.

ASSEM, E.S.K. (1976) Immunological and non-immunological mechanisms of some of the desirable and undesirable effects of anti-inflammatory and analgesic drugs. *Agents and Actions* **6**, 212–218.

ASTBURY, C. and BIRD, H.A. (1993) Nonsteroidal anti-inflammatory drugs and their metabolic pathways in the elderly. *Journal of Drug Development* **6**, 57–61.

ATKINSON, D.C. and LEACH, E.C. (1976) Anti-inflammatory and related properties of 2-(2,4-dichlorophenoxy)phenylacetic acid (fenclofenac). *Agents and Actions* **6**, 657–666.

BAELE, G., DE WEERDT, G.A. and BARBIER, F. (1970) Preliminary results of platelet aggregation before and after administration of ibuprofen. *Rheumatology and Physical Medicine* **11**(Symposium), 9–26.

BAILEY, P.J. and STURM, A. (1983) Immune complexes and inflammation. A study of the activity of anti-inflammatory drugs in the reverse passive arthus reaction in the rat. *Biochemical Pharmacology* **32**, 475–481.

BALK, R.A., JACOBS, R.F., TRYKA, A.F., TOWNSEND, J.W., WALLS, R.C. and BONE, R.C. (1988) Effects on ibuprofen on neutrophil function and acute lung injury in canine endotoxin shock. *Critical Care in Medicine* **16**, 1121–1127.

BANNWARTH, B. and DEHAIS, J. (1991) Concentration des anti-inflammatories non-stéroïdiens dans le cartilage articulaire chez l'Homme. *Revue du Rhumatisme* **58**, 879–882.

BANNWARTH, B., DEMONTES-MAINARD, F., SCHAEVERBEKE, T., LABAT, L. and DEHAIS, J. (1995a) Central analgesic effects of aspirin-like drugs. *Fundamentals of Clinical Pharmacology* **9**, 1–7.

BANNWARTH, B., LAPICQUE, F., PEHOURCQ, F. *et al.* (1995b) Stereoselective disposition of ibuprofen enantiomers in human cerebrospinal fluid. *British Journal of Clinical Pharmacology* **40**, 266–269.

BARBITO, F., ROTONDA, M.I. and QUAGLIA, F. (1997) Interactions of nonsteroidal anti-inflammatory drugs with phospholipids: comparison between octanol/buffer partition coefficients and chromatographic indices on immobilized artificial membranes. *Journal of Pharmaceutical Sciences* **86**, 225–229.

BARDHAM, M. (1997) Nonsteroidal anti-inflammatory drugs: concurrent or causative drugs in serious infection. *Clinics in Infectious Diseases* **25**, 1272–1273.

BARDHAM, M. and ANDERSON, A.W. (1997) Nonsteroidal anti-inflammatory drugs (NSAIDs). A predisposing factor for streptococcal bacteraemia? In: HORAUD, T., SICARD, M., BOUVET, A. and DE MONTCLOS, H. (eds), *Streptococci and The Host*. New York, Plenum Press, 145–147.

BARNETT, J., CHOW, J., IVES, D. *et al.* (1994) Purification, characterization and selective inhibition of human prostaglandin G/H synthase 1 and 2 expressed in baculovirus system. *Biochimica et Biophysica Acta* **1209**, 130–139.

BATEMAN, B.G., NUNLEY, W.C. and KITHIN, J.D. (1982) Prevention of postoperative peritoneal adhesions with ibuprofen. *Fertility and Sterility* **38**, 107–108.

BAYERL, C., BOHNET, E., MOLL, I. and JUNG, E.G. (1996) Quantification of sunburn cells *in vivo* after exposure to UV and ibuprofen. *European Journal of Dermatology* **6**, 362–364.

BEALES, D. and McLEAN, A.E. (1995) Cell injury and protection in long-term incubation of liver slices after *in vivo* initiation with paracetamol: cell injury after *in vivo* initiation with paracetamol. *Toxicology* **103**, 113–119.

BECKER, L., EBERLEIN KONIG, B. and PRZYBILLA, B. (1996) Phototoxicity of nonsteroidal anti-inflammatory drugs: *in vitro* studies with visible light. *Acta Dermato-Venereologica* **76**, 337–340.

CHAPTER 5

BÉLANGER, P.M. and ATTISÉ-GBEASSOR (1985) Effect of nonsteroidal anti-inflammatory drugs on the microsomal monooxygenase system of rat liver. *Canadian Journal of Physiology and Pharmacology* **63**, 798–803.

BENSLAY, D.N. and NICKANDER, R. (1982) Comparative effects of benoxaprofen and other anti-inflammatory drugs on bone damage in the adjuvant arthritic rat. *Agents and Actions* **12**, 313–319.

BERGMANN, J.F., CHASSANY, O., GENÈVE, J., ABITEBOUL, M., CAULIN, C. and SEGRESTAA, J.M. (1992) Endoscopic evaluation of the effect of ketoprofen, ibuprofen and aspirin on the gastroduodenal mucosa. *European Journal of Clinical Pharmacology* **42**, 685–688.

BERKEL, H.J., HOLCOMBE, R.F., MIDDLEBROOKS, M. and KANNAN, K. (1996) Nonsteroidal anti-inflammatory drugs and colorectal cancer. *Epidemiologic Reviews* **18**, 205–217.

BERTELLI, A. and SOLDANI, G. (1979) Polymyxin B-induced oedema in the hind paw of the rat as an assay for anti-inflammatory drugs. *Arzneimittel-Forschung* **29**, 777–778.

BHATTACHARYA, S.K. and DAS, N. (1984) Effect of central prostaglandins on carrageenan-induced pedal oedema in rats. *Journal of Pharmacy and Pharmacology* **36**, 766–767.

BHATTACHARYA, S.K., GOEL, R.K., BHATTACHARYA, S.K. and TANDON, R. (1991) Potentiation of gastric toxicity of ibuprofen by paracetamol in the rat. *Journal of Pharmacy and Pharmacology* **43**, 520–521.

BIALEK, S., QUONG, J.N., YU, K. and MILLER, S.S. (1996) Nonsteroidal anti-inflammatory drugs alter chloride and fluid transport in bovine retinal epithelium. *American Journal of Physiology* **270**, C1175–C1189.

BIANCHI PORRO, G., CORVI, G., FUCCELLA, L.M., GOLDANIGA, G.C. and VALZELLI, G. (1977) Gastro-intestinal blood loss during administration of indoprofen, aspirin and ibuprofen. *Journal of International Medical Research* **5**, 155–160.

BIDLINGMAIER, A., HAMERMAIER, A., NAGYIVANAYI, P., PABST, G. and WAITZINGER, J. (1995) Gastrointestinal blood loss induced by three different nonsteriodal anti-inflammatory drugs. *Arzneimmitel-Forschung* **45**, 491–493.

BISCARINI, L. (1996) Anti-inflammatory analgesics and drugs used in gout. In: Dukes, M.N.G. (ed.), *Meyer's Side Effects of Drugs*, 13th edn. Amsterdam, Elsevier, 204–264.

BJELLE, A. and ERONEN, I. (1991) The *in vitro* effect of six NSAIDs on the glycosaminoglycan metabolism of rabbit chondrocytes. *Clinical and Experimental Rheumatology* **9**, 369–374.

BJÖRKMAN, R. (1995) Central antinociceptive effects of nonsteroidal anti-inflammatory drugs and paracetamol. *Acta Anaesthesiologica Scandavica* **39**(Suppl. 103), 9–44.

BLACKBURN, W.D., LOOSE, L.D., HECK, L.W. and CHATHAM, W.W. (1991) Tenidap, in contrast to several available nonsteroidal anti-inflammatory drugs, potently inhibits the release of activated neutrophil collagenase. *Arthritis and Rheumatism* **34**, 211–216.

BLACKHAM, A., NORRIS, A.A. and WOODS, F.A.M. (1985) Models for evaluating the anti-inflammatory effects of inhibitors of arachidonic acid metabolism. *Journal of Pharmacy and Pharmacology* 37, 787–793.

BLATTEIS, C.M. (1988) Neural mechanisms in the pyrogenic and acute-phase responses to interleukin-1. *International Journal of Neuroscience* 38, 223–232.

BOELSTERLI, U.A., ZIMMERMAN, H.J. and KRETZ-ROMMEL, A. (1995) Idiosyncratic liver toxicity of nonsteroidal anti-inflammatory drugs: molecular mechanisms and pathology. *Critical Reviews in Toxicology* 25, 207–235.

BOLAM, J.P., ELLIOTT, P.N.C., FORD-HUTCHINSON, A.W. and SMITH, M.J.H. (1974) Histamine, 5-hydroxytryptamine, kinins and the anti-inflammatory activity of human plasma fraction in carrageenan-induced paw oedema in the rat. *Journal of Pharmacy and Pharmacology* 26, 434–440.

BONEBERG, E.M., ZOU, M.-H. and ULLRICH, V. (1996) Inhibition of cyclooxygenase-1 and -2 by (R)-(−)- and (S)-(+)-ibuprofen. *Journal of Clinical Pharmacology* 36, 16S–19S.

BRANDT, K.D. and PALMOSKI, M.J. (1984) Effects of salicylates and other nonsteroidal anti-inflammatory drugs on articular cartilage. *American Journal of Medicine* 77(1A), 65–69.

BRASS, E.P. and GARRITY, M.J. (1985) Effect of nonsteroidal anti-inflammatory drugs on glycogenolysis in isolated hepatocytes. *British Journal of Pharmacology* 86, 491–496.

BREITNER, J.C.S. (1996) The role of anti-inflammatory drugs in the prevention and treatment of Alzheimer's disease. *Annual Review of Medicine* 47, 401–411.

BREITNER, J.C.S., WELSH, K.A., HELMS, M.J., GASKELL, P.C., GAU, B.A., ROSES, A.D., PERICAKVANCE, M.A., and SAUNDERS, A.M. (1995) Delayed onset of Alzheimer's disease with nonsteroidal anti-inflammatory and histamine H2 blocking drugs. *Neurobiology of Aging* 16, 523–530.

BROOKS, C.D., SCHLAGEL, C.A., SEKHAR, N.C. and SOBOTA, J.T. (1973) Tolerance and pharmacology of ibuprofen. *Current Therapeutic Research* 15, 180–189.

BROWN, K.A. and COLLINS, A.J. (1977) Action of nonsteroidal, anti-inflammatory drugs on human and rat peripheral leukocyte migration *in vitro*. *Annals of the Rheumatic Diseases* 36, 239–243.

BROWN, K.A. and COLLINS, A.J. (1978) *In vitro* effects of nonsteroidal anti-inflammatory drugs on human polymorphonuclear cells and lymphocyte migration. *British Journal of Pharmacology* 64, 347–352.

BRUNE, K., GRAF, P. and RAINSFORD, K.D. (1977) Biodistribution of acidic anti-inflammatory drugs: a clue to the understanding of their effects and side-effects. *Drugs under Experimental and Clinical Research* 2, 155–168.

BRUNE, K., RAINSFORD, K.D. and SCHWEITZER, A. (1981a) Biodistribution of mild analgesics, *British Journal of Clinical Pharmacology* 10, 279S–284S.

CHAPTER 5

■ 241

BRUNE, K., RAINSFORD, K.D., WAGNER, K. and PESKAR, B.A. (1981b) Inhibition by anti-inflammatory drugs of prostaglandin production in cultured macrophages. Factors influencing the apparent drug effects. *Naunyn-Schmiedeberg's Archives of Pharmacology* **315**, 269–278.

BRUNI, G., RUNCI, F.M., FIASCHI, A.I. and SEGRE, G. (1990) Inhibition of ornithine-decarboxylase produced by (*S*)-(+)- and (*R*)-(–)-ibuprofen in rats. *Pharmacological Research* **22**, 97–102.

BURITOVA, J., CHAPMAN, V., HONORÉ, P. and BESSON, J.-M. (1996a) Selective cyclooxygenase-2 inhibition reduces carrageenan oedema and associated spinal c-Fos expression in the rat. *Brain Research* **715**, 217–220.

BURITOVA, J., CHAPMAN, V., HONORÉ, P. and BESSON, J.-M. (1996b) Interactions between NMDA- and prostaglandin receptor-mediated events in a model of inflammatory nociception. *European Journal of Pharmacology* **303**, 91–100.

BYRICK, R.J., WONG, P.Y., MULLEN, J.B. and WIGGLESWORTH, D.F. (1992) Ibuprofen pretreatment does not prevent hemodynamic instability after cemented arthroplasty in dogs. *Anesthesia and Analgesia* **75**, 515–522.

CALDWELL, J., HUTT, A.J. and FOURNEL-GIGLEUX, S. (1988) The metabolic chiral inversion and dispositional enantioselectivity of the 2-arylpropionic acids and their biological consequences. *Biochemical Pharmacology* **37**, 105–114.

CAO, C., MATSUMURA, K., YAMAGATA, K. and WANTANABE, Y. (1996) Endothelial cells of the rat brain vasculature express cyclooxygenase-2 mRNA in response to systemic interleukin-1β: a possible site of prostaglandin synthesis responsible for fever. *Brain Research* **733**, 263–272.

CARDOE, N. (1975) 'Brufen' in the treatment of rheumatoid disease in patients with gastric intolerance. *Current Medical Research and Opinion* **3**, 518–521.

CAREY, P.D., BYRNE, K., JENKINS, J.K. et al. (1990) Ibuprofen attenuates hypochlorous acid production from neutrophils in porcine acute lung injury. *Journal of Surgical Research* **49**, 262–270.

CAREY, P.D., LEEPER-WOODFORD, S.K., WALSH, C.J., BYRNE, K., FOWLER, A.A. and SUGERMAN, H.J. (1991) Delayed cyclooxygenase blockade reduces the neutrophil respiratory burst and plasma tumor necrosis factor levels in sepsis-induced acute lung injury. *Journal of Trauma* **31**, 733–740.

CAREY, P.D., JENKINS, J.K., BYRNE, K., WALSH, C.J., FOWLER, A.A. and SUGERMAN, H.J. (1992) The neutrophil respiratory burst and tissue injury in septic acute lung injury: the effect of cyclooxygenase inhibition in swine. *Surgery* **112**, 45–55.

CARLIN, G., DJURSÄTER, R., SMEDGARD, G. and GERDIN, B. (1985) Effect of anti-inflammatory drugs on xanthine oxidase and xanthine oxidase induced dipolymerization of hyaluronic acid. *Agents and Actions* **16**, 377–384.

CARRYL, O.R. and SPANGLER, R.S. (1995) Comparative effects of nabumetone, naproxen, piroxicam and diclofenac on rat gastric irritancy following exposure to OTC non-steroidal anti-inflammatory agents and their gastric irritants. *Scandavian Journal of Rheumatology* **24**, 336–341.

CARTY, T.J., ESKRA, J.D., LOMBARDINO, J.G. and HOFFMAN, W.W. (1980) Piroxicam, a potent inhibitor of prostaglandin production in cell culture, structure-activity study. *Prostaglandins* **19**, 51–59.

CASHMAN, J.N. (1996) The mechanisms of action of NSAIDs in analgesia. *Drugs* **52**(Suppl. 5), 13–23.

CASTELL, J.V., LARRAURI, A. and GOMEZ-LECHON, M.J. (1988) A study of the relative hepato-toxicity *in vitro* of the nonsteroidal anti-inflammatory drugs ibuprofen, flurbiprofen and butibufen. *Xenobiotica* **18**, 737–745.

CEUPPENS, J.L. and GOODWYN, J.S. (1985) Immunological responses in treatment with non-steroidal anti-inflammatory drugs, with particular reference to the role of prostaglandins. In: RAINSFORD, K.D. (ed.), *Anti-Inflammatory and Antirheumatic Drugs. Volume I: Inflamma-tion Mechanisms and Actions of Traditional Drugs.* Boca Raton FL, CRC Press, 89–105.

CHAMBRIER, C., CHASSARD, D., BIENVENU, J. *et al.* (1996) Cytokine and hormonal changes after cholecystectomy. Effect of ibuprofen pretreatment. *Annals of Surgery* **224**, 178–182.

CHANG, J.W., COLEMAN, P.D. and O'BANION, M.K. (1996) Prostaglandin G/H synthase-2 (cyclooxygenase-2) mRNA expression is decreased in Alzheimer's disease. *Neurobiology of Aging* **17**, 801–808.

CHATHAM, W.W., BAGGOTT, J.E., LOOSE, L.D. and BLACKBURN, W.D. JR (1995) Effects of tenidap on superoxide-generating enzymes. Non-competitive inhibition of xanthine oxidase. *Biochemical Pharmacology* **50**, 811–814.

CHAUDRY, I.H., ZELLWEGER, R. and AYALA, A. (1995) The role of bacterial translocation on Kuppfer cell immune function following hemorrhage. *Progress in Clinical and Biological Research* **392**, 209–218.

CHEN, S., FREDRICKSON, R.C.A. and BRUNDEN, K.R. (1996) Neuroglial-mediated im-munoinflammatory responses in Alzheimer's disease: complement activation and therapeutic approaches. *Neurobiology of Aging* **17**, 781–787.

COCEANI, F., WHITE, E., BODACH, E. and OLLEY, P.M. (1979) Age-dependent changes in the response of the lamb ductus arteriosus to oxygen and ibuprofen. *Canadian Journal of Physiology and Pharmacology* **57**, 825–831.

COMMITTEE ON THE SAFETY OF MEDICINES/MEDICINES CONTROL AGENCY (1994) Relative safety of oral non-aspirin NSAIDs. *Current Problems in Pharmacovigilance* **20**, 9–11.

CONNOLLY, K.M., STECHER, V.J., SPEIGHT, P.T., BECKER, R. and RATHMAN, J. (1989) Differential effects of antiarthritic agents on subnormal plasma iron levels in adjuvant arthritic rats. *Agents and Actions* **27**, 328–331.

CHAPTER 5

COTLIER, E. and SHARMA, Y.G. (1981) Aspirin and senile cataracts in rheumatoid arthritis. *Lancet* **i**, 338–339.

COTTNEY, J., BRUIN, J. and LEWIS, A.J. (1980) Modulation of the immune system in the mouse. 2. Drug administration following antigen sensitization. *Agents and Actions* **10**, 48–56.

COX, S.R., VAN DER LUGT, J.T., GUMBLETON, T.J. and SMITH, R.B. (1987) Relationships between thromboxane production, platelet aggregability, and serum concentrations of ibuprofen and flurbiprofen. *Clinical Pharmacology and Therapeutics* **41**, 510–521.

COX, S.R., GALL, E.P., FORBES, K.K., GRESHAM, M. and GORIS, G. (1991) Pharmacokinetics of the (*R*)-(–) and (*S*)-(+) enantiomers of ibuprofen in the serum and synovial fluid of arthritic patients. *Journal of Clinical Pharmacology* **31**, 88–94.

CRAWFORD, M.H., MCMANUS, L.M., GROVER, F.L., WEBSTER, S.A., PINKARD, R.N. and O'ROURKE, R.A. (1981) Myocardial preservation by ibuprofen or Cobra Venom Factor (CVF) given after experimental infarction in the baboon. *Clinical Research* **29**, 184A.

CRONBERG, S., WALLMARK, E. and SODERBERG, I. (1984) Effect on platelet aggregation of oral administration of 10 nonsteroidal analgesics to humans. *Scandinavian Journal of Haematology* **33**, 155–159.

CROSSLEY, M.J., SPOWAGE, M. and HUNNEYBALL, I.M. (1987) Studies on the effects of pharmacological agents on antigen-induced arthritis in BALB/c mice. *Drugs under Experimental and Clinical Research* **13**, 273–277.

CROSSLEY, M.J., HOLLAND, T., SPOWAGE, M. and HUNNEYBALL, I.M. (1989) Monoarticular antigen-induced arthritis in rabbits and mice. In: CHANG, J.Y. and LEWIS, A.J. (eds), *Pharmacological Methods in the Control of Inflammation*. New York, Alan R. Liss, 415–439.

CSAPO, A.I. (1977) Inhibition of prostaglandin synthesis and contractility in the rabbit and rat uterus by ibuprofen. *Prostaglandins* **13**, 735–743.

CULLEN, D.J., HUDSON, N., ATHERTON, J.C., FILIPOWICZ, B. and HAWKEY, C.J. (1995) Acute gastric tolerability of (*S*)-(+)-ibuprofen compared to racemic ibuprofen. *Gut* **36**(Suppl. 1): abstract F234.

CUSACK, B.J. (1988) Drug metabolism in the elderly. *Journal of Clinical Pharmacology* **28**, 571–576.

CUSHMAN, D.W. and CHEUNG, H.S. (1976) Effect of substrate concentration on inhibition of prostaglandin synthetase of bull seminal vesicles by anti-inflammatory drugs and fenamic acid analogs. *Biochimica et Biophysica Acta* **424**, 449–459.

DAS, D.K., BANDYOPADHYAY, D., HOORY, S. and STEINBERG, H. (1988) Role of polymorphonuclear leukocytes in hyperoxic lung injury. Prevention of neutrophil influx into the lung endothelium during oxygen exposure by ibuprofen. *Biomedica Biochimica Acta* **47**, 1023–1036.

DAS, G., COLLINS, J. and WEISSLER, A.M. (1981) Natural history of electrical interventricular septal force in the course of left ventricular hypertrophy in man. *Clinical Research* **29**, 184A.

DAVID, M.G., VIGNON, E., PESCHARD, M.J., BROQUET, P., LOUISOT, P. and RICHARD, M. (1992) Effect of nonsteroidal anti-inflammatory drugs (NSAIDS) on glycosyltransferase activity from human osteoarthritic cartilage. *British Journal of Rheumatology* **31**(Suppl. 1), 13–17.

DAVIES, N.M., WRIGHT, M.R., RUSSELL, A.S. and JAMALI, F. (1996) Effect of the enantiomers of flurbiprofen, ibuprofen, and ketoprofen on intestinal permeability. *Journal of Pharmaceutical Sciences* **85**, 1170–1173.

DE VRIES, B.J., VAN DEN BERG, W.B., VITTERS, E. and VAN DE PUTTE, L.B.A. (1986) The effect of salicylate on anatomically intact articular cartilage is influenced by sulfate and serum in the culture medium. *Journal of Rheumatology* **13**, 686–693.

DAWSON, W. (1980) The comparative pharmacology of benoxaprofen. *Journal of Rheumatology* **7**(Suppl. 6), 5–11.

DEMBINSKA-KIEC, A., ZMUDA, A. and KRUPINSKA, A. (1976) Inhibition of prostaglandin synthetase by aspirin-like drugs in different microsomal preparations. In: SAMUELSON, B. and PAOLETTI, R. (eds), *Advances in Prostaglandin and Thromboxane Research*, vol. 1. New York, Raven Press, 99–103.

DEMLING, R.H. (1982) Role of prostaglandins in acute pulmonary microvascular injury. *Annals of the New York Academy of Sciences* **384**, 517–534.

DE VRIES, B.J., VAN DEN BERG, W.B., VITTERS, E. and VAN DE PUTTE, L.B.A. (1988) Effects of NSAIDs on the metabolism of sulfated glycosaminoglycans in healthy and (post) arthritic murine cartilage. *Drugs* **35**(Suppl. 1), 24–32.

DIMARTINO, M.J., WOLFF, C.E., CAMPBELL, G.K. and HANNA, N. (1989) The pharmacology of arachidonic acid-induced rat PMN leukocyte infiltration. *Agents and Actions* **27**, 325–327.

DINARELLO, C.A. and BERNHEIM, H.A. (1981) Ability of human leukocytic pyrogen to stimulate brain prostaglandin synthesis *in vitro*. *Journal of Neurochemistry* **37**, 702–708.

DINARELLO, C.A., BISHAI, I., ROSENWASSER, L.J. and COCEANI, F. (1984) The influence of lipoxygenase inhibitors on the *in vitro* production of human leukocytic pyrogen and lymphocyte activating factor (interleukin-1). *International Journal of Immunopharmacology* **6**, 43–50.

DINGLE, J.T. (1992) NSAIDs and human cartilage metabolism. In: RAINSFORD, K.D. and VELO, G.-P. (eds), *Side-effects of Anti-inflammatory Drugs 3*. Lancaster, Kluwer Academic Publishers, 261–268.

DIPASQUALE, G. and MELLACE, D. (1977) Inhibition of arachidonic acid induced mortality in rabbits with several nonsteroidal anti-inflammatory drugs. *Agents and Actions* **7**, 481–485.

CHAPTER 5

DI ROSA, M., GIROUD, J.P. and WILLOUGHBY, D.A. (1971) Studies of the mediators of the acute inflammatory response induced in rats in different sites by carrageenan and turpentine. *Journal of Pathology* **104**, 15–29.

DOLLERY, C. (ed.) (1991) Ibuprofen. In: *Therapeutic Drugs*, vol. 2. Edinburgh, Churchill-Livingstone, 11–16.

DORIETTO DE MENEZES, M.R. and CATANZARO-GUIMARAES, S.A. (1985) Determination of the anti-inflammatory and antimitotic activities on nonsteroidal anti-inflammatory drugs ibuprofen, diclofenac and fentiazic. *Cellular and Molecular Biology* **31**, 455–461.

DUNN, C.J. (1991) Cytokines as mediators of chronic inflammatory disease. In: KIMBALL, E.S. (ed.), *Cytokines and Inflammation*. Boca Raton FL, CRC Press, 1–33.

DUNN, C.J., FLEMING, W.E., McGUIRE, J.C., OHLMANN, G.M. and GRAY, G.D. (1986) The role of cyclooxygenase and lipoxygenase pathways in the adhesive interaction between bovine polymorphonuclear leukocytes and bovine endothelial cells. *Prostaglandins and Leukotrienes in Medicine* **21**, 221–230.

EDWARDS, E.K., HORWITZ, S.N. and FROST, P. (1982) Reduction of the erythema response to ultraviolet light by nonsteroidal anti-inflammatory agents. *Archives of Dermatological Research* **272**, 263–267.

EHRLICH, H.P., MacGARVEY, U., McGRANE, W.L. and WHITE, M.E. (1987) Ibuprofen as an antagonist of inhibitors of fibrinolysis in wound fluid. *Thrombosis Research* **45**, 17–28.

EISERICH, J.P., HISTORA, M., CROSS, C.E. *et al.* (1998) Formulation of nitric oxide-derived inflammatory oxidants by myeloperoxidase in neutrophils. *Nature* **391**, 393–397.

EKSTROM, B.F., KUENZIG, M. and SCHWARTZ, S.I. (1986) Pulmonary platelet trapping in *Escherichia coli* endotoxin-injected dogs treated with methylprednisolone, ibuprofen and naloxone. *Acta Chirologica Scandinavica* **152**, 181–185.

ELVERS, K.T. and WRIGHT, S.J.L. (1995) Antibacterial activity of the anti-inflammatory compound ibuprofen. *Letters in Applied Microbiology* **20**, 82–92.

EVANS, A.M. (1996) Pharmacodynamics and pharmacokinetics of the profens: enantioselectivity, clinical implications, and special reference to (S)-(+)-ibuprofen. *The Journal of Clinical Pharmacology* **36**, 7S–15S.

EVANS, A.M., NATION, R.L., SANSOM, L.N., BOCHNER, F. and SOMOGYI, A.A. (1991) Effect of racemic ibuprofen dose on the magnitude and duration of platelet cyclooxygenase inhibition: relationship between inhibition of thromboxane production and the plasma unbound concentration of (S)-(+)-ibuprofen. *British Journal of Clinical Pharmacology* **31**, 131–138.

FALZON, M., NIELSCH, A., BURKE, M.D. (1986) Denaturation of cytochrome P-450 by indomethacin and other nonsteroidal anti-inflammatory drugs: evidence for a surfactant mechanism and a selective effect of a *p*-chlorophenyl moiety. *Biochemical Pharmacology* **35**, 4019–4024.

FAMAEY, J.-P. and WHITEHOUSE, M.W. (1975) Interaction between nonsteroidal anti-inflammatory drugs and biological membranes — IV. Effects of nonsteroidal anti-inflammatory drugs and of various ions on the availability of sulphydryl groups on lymphoid and mitochondrial membranes. *Biochemical Pharmacology* 24, 1609–1615.

FAMAEY, J.P., FONTAINE, J. and REUSE, J. (1977) The effects of nonsteroidal anti-inflammatory drugs on cholinergic and histamine-induced contractions of guinea-pig isolated ileum. *British Journal of Pharmacology* 60, 165–171.

FASSBENDER, H.-G. (1994) Inflammatory reactions in arthritis. In: DAVIES, M.E. and DINGLE, J.T. (eds), *Immunopharmacology of Joints and Connective Tissue*. London, Academic Press, 165–198.

FERREIRA, S.H. (1972) Prostaglandins, aspirin-like drugs. *Nature New Biology* 240, 200–203.

FERREIRA, S.H. and VANE, J.R. (1974) New aspects of the mode of action of nonsteroid anti-inflammatory drugs. *Annual Reviews of Pharmacology* 14, 57–73.

FITZPATRICK, F.A. and WYNALDA, M.A. (1976) *In vivo* suppression of prostaglandin bio-synthesis by nonsteroidal anti-inflammatory agents. *Prostaglandins* 12, 1037–1051.

FLOWER, R.J. (1974) Drugs which inhibit prostaglandin synthesis. *Pharmacological Reviews* 26, 33–67.

FLOWER, R.J. and VANE, J.R. (1972) Inhibition of prostaglandin synthesis in brain explains the antipyretic activity of paracetamol (4-acetamido-phenol). *Nature* 240, 410–411.

FLOWER, R.J. and VANE, J.R. (1974) Inhibition of prostaglandin biosynthesis. *Biochemical Pharmacology* 23, 1439–1450.

FLOWER, R.J., GRYGLEWSKI, R., HERBACZYNSKACEDRO, K. and VANE, J.R. (1972) The effect of anti-inflammatory drugs on prostaglandin synthesis. *Nature New Biology* 238, 104–106.

FLOWER, R.J., CHEUNG, H.S. and CUSHMAN, D.W. (1973) Quantitative determination of prostaglandins and malondialdehyde formed by the arachidonate oxygenase (prostaglandin synthetase) system of bovine seminal vesicle. *Prostaglandins* 4, 325–341.

FLYNN, P.J., BECKER, W.K., VERCELLOTTI, G.M. *et al.* (1984) Ibuprofen inhibits granulocyte responses to inflammatory mediators. A proposed mechanism for reduction of experimental myocardial infarct size. *Inflammation* 8, 33–38.

FORD, J. and HOUSTON, J.B. (1995) Concentration–response relationships for three non-steroidal anti-inflammatory drugs in the rat intestine. *Human Experimental Toxicology* 14, 573–579.

FORD, J., MARTIN, S.W. and HOUSTON, J.B. (1995) Assessment of intestinal permeability changes induced by nonsteroidal anti-inflammatory drugs in the rat. *Journal of Pharmacological and Toxicological Methods* 34, 9–16.

FORSTER, C., MAGERL, W., BECK, A. *et al.* (1992) Differential effects of dipyrone, ibuprofen, and paracetamol on experimentally induced pain in man. *Agents and Actions* 35, 112–121.

CHAPTER 5

FOWLER, P.D. (1987) Aspirin, paracetamol and nonsteroidal anti-inflammatory drugs. A comparative review of side-effects. *Medical Toxicology* **2**, 338–366.

FRENAEUX, E., FROMENTY, B., BERSON, A. *et al.* (1990) Stereoselective and non-stereoselective effects of ibuprofen enantiomers on mitochondrial β-oxidation of fatty acids. *Journal of Pharmacology and Experimental Therapeutics* **255**, 529–535.

FRIEDMAN, H., SECKMAN, C., LANZA, F., ROYER, G., PERRY, K. and FRANCOM, S. (1990) Clinical pharmacology of predisintegrated ibuprofen 800 mg tablets: an endoscopic and pharmacokinetic study. *Journal of Clinical Pharmacology* **30**, 57–63.

FUJIYOSHI, T., IIDA, H., MURAKAMI, M. and UEMATSU, T. (1987) Inhibitory effect of EB-382, a nonsteroidal anti-inflammatory agent, on platelet aggregation. *Yakugaku Zasshi* **107**, 76–81.

FUREY, S.A., WAKSMAN, J.A. and DASH, B.H. (1992) Nonprescription ibuprofen: side-effect profile. *Pharmacotherapy* **12**, 403–407.

FURST, D.E. (1994) Are there differences among nonsteroidal anti-inflammatory drugs? Comparing acetylated salicylates, nonacetylated salicylates, and nonacetylated nonsteroidal anti-inflammatory drugs. *Arthritis and Rheumatism* **37**, 1–9.

GALLO, J.M., GALL, E.P., GILLESPIE, W.R., ALBERT, K.S. and PERRIER, D. (1986) Ibuprofen kinetics in plasma and synovial fluid of arthritic patients. *Journal of Clinical Pharmacology* **26**, 65–70.

GARCIA-RAFANELL, J. and FORN, J. (1979) Correlation between anti-inflammatory activity and inhibition of prostaglandin biosynthesis induced by various nonsteroidal anti-inflammatory agents. *Arzneimittel-Forschung* **29**, 630–633.

GEISSLINGER, G., STOCK, K.-P., BACH, G.L., LOEW, D. and BRUNE, K. (1989) Pharmacological differences between (R)-(–)- and (S)-(+)-ibuprofen. *Agents and Actions* **27**, 455–457.

GEISSLINGER, G., STOCK, K.P., LOEW, D., BACH, G.L. and BRUNE, K. (1993) Variability in the stereoselective disposition of ibuprefen in patients with rheumatoid arthritis. *British Journal of Clinical Pharmacology* **35**, 603–607.

GEMMELL, D.K., COTTNEY, J. and LEWIS, A.J. (1979) Comparative effects of drugs on four paw oedema models. *Agents and Actions* **9**, 107–116.

GHOSH, P. (1988) Antirheumatic drugs and cartilage. *Baillière's Clinical Rheumatology* **2**, 309–338.

GIBSON, G.R., WHITACRE, E.B. and RICOTTI, C.A. (1992) Colitis induced by nonsteroidal anti-inflammatory drugs. *Archives of Internal Medicine* **152**, 625–632.

GIRI, S.N. and HOLLINGER, M.A. (1996) Effect of nordihydroguaiaretic acid and ibuprofen on bleomycin and hyperoxia-induced changes in lung superoxide dismutase, prostaglandins and lethality. *Archives of Toxicology* **70**, 271–276.

GLASS, R.C. and SWANNELL, A.J. (1978) Concentrations of ibuprofen in serum and synovial fluid from patients with arthritis. *British Journal of Clinical Pharmacology* **6**, 453P–454P.

GOLDLUST, M.B. and RICH, L.C. (1981) Chronic immune synovitis in rabbits, II. Modulation by anti-inflammatory and antirheumatic agents. *Agents and Actions* **11**, 729–735.

GOODWIN, J.S. (1984) Mechanism of action of nonsteroidal anti-inflammatory agents. *American Journal of Medicine* **77**, 57–64.

GOODWIN, J.S. and CEUPPENS, J.L. (1983) Effects of nonsteroidal anti-inflammatory drugs on immune function. *Seminars in Arthritis and Rheumatism* **13**(Suppl. 1), 134–143.

GOTO, K., HISADOME, M. and IMAMURA, H. (1976) Studies on anti-inflammatory agents XXXIX: Effects of 2(5H-[1]benzopyrano-[2,3] pyridin-7-yl) propionic acid (Y-8004) on leukocyte emigration and enzyme release from emigrated leukocytes *in vivo*. *Journal of the Pharmaceutical Society of Japan* **96**, 1013–1021.

GOTO, K., HISADOME, M. and IMANURA, H. (1979) Effects of 2-{4-(2-imidazo[1,2-a]-pyridyl)phenyl} propionic acid (Y-9213) on *in vivo* release of lysosomal enzymes from rat polymorphonuclear leukocytes during phagocytosis of particles. *Japanese Journal of Pharmacology* **29**, 67–75.

GRAHAM, N.M., BURRELL, C.J., DOUGLAS, R.M., DEBELLE, P. and DAVIES, L. (1990) Adverse effects of aspirin, acetaminophen, and ibuprofen on immune function, viral shedding, and clinical status in rhinovirus-infected volunteers. *Journal of Infectious Diseases* **162**, 1277–1282.

GRANADOS-SOTO, V., FLORES-MURRIETA, F.J., CASTAÑEDA-HERNÁNDEZ, G. and LÓPEZ-MUÑOZ, F.J. (1995) Evidence for the involvement of nitric oxide in the antinociceptive effect of ketorolac. *European Journal of Pharmacology* **277**, 281–284.

GRIFFIN, W.S.T., SHENG, J.G. and MRAK, R.E. (1996) Inflammatory pathways. Implications in Alzheimer's disease. In: WASCO, W. and TANZI, R.E. (eds), *Molecular Mechanisms of Dementia*. Totowa NJ, Humana Press, 169–176.

GRISWOLD, D.E., HILLEGASS, L.M., MEUNIER, P.C., DiMARTINO, M.J. and HANNA, N. (1988) Effects of inhibitors of eicosanoid metabolism in murine collagen-induced arthritis. *Arthritis and Rheumatism* **31**, 1406–1412.

GROVER, G.J. and WEISS, H.R. (1985) Effect of ibuprofen and indomethacin on the O_2 supply/consumption balance in ischemic rabbit myocardium. *Proceedings of the Society for Experimental Biology and Medicine* **180**, 270–276.

GUENTERT, T.W., SCHMITT, M., DINGEMANSE, J., BANKEN, L., JONKMAN, J.H. and OOSTERHUIS, B. (1992) Unaltered ibuprofen-induced faecal blood loss upon co-administration of moclobemide. *Drug Metabolism and Drug Interactions* **10**, 307–322.

GUYONNET, J.C. and JULOU, L. (1976) Relationship between the inhibitory activity on 'RCS' and prostaglandin synthesis and the anti-inflammatory activity of ketoprofen and several other nonsteroidal anti-inflammatory agents. *Rheumatology and Rehabilitation* **17**(Suppl.), 11–14.

GYTE, G.M.L. and WILLIAMS, J.R.B. (1985) The effects of some nonsteroidal anti-inflammatory drugs on human granulopoiesis *in vitro*. *Alternatives for Testing in Laboratory Animals* **13**, 38–47.

HAHN, D.W., CARRHER, R. and McGUIRE, J.L. (1982) Effects of suprofen and other pro-staglandin synthetase inhibitors in a new animal model for myometrial hyperactivity. *Prostaglandins* **23**, 1–16.

HALL, V.C. and WOLF, R.E. (1997) Effects of tenidap and nonsteroidal anti-inflammatory drugs on the response of cultured human T cells to interleukin 2 in rheumatoid arthritis. *Journal of Rheumatology* **24**, 1467–1470.

HAM, E.A., CIRIELLO, K.J., ZANETTI, M., SHEN, T.Y. and KUEHL, F.A. JR (1972) Studies on the mode of action of nonsteroidal anti-inflammatory drugs. In: RANWELL, P.W. and PHARRISS, B.R. (eds), *Prostaglandins in Cellular Biology*. New York, Plenum Press, 345–352.

HANIF, R., PITTAS, A., FENG, Y. *et al.* (1996) Effects of nonsteroidal anti-inflammatory drugs on proliferation and on induction of apoptosis in colon cancer cells by a prostaglandin-independent pathway. *Biochemical Pharmacology* **52**, 237–245.

HANNA, N., LaCHAPELLE, P., ROY, M.S., ORQUIN, J., VARMA, D.R. and CHEMTOB, S. (1995) Alterations in the electroretinogram of newborn piglets by propionic acid-derivative nonsteroidal anti-inflammatory drugs but not by indomethacin and diclofenac. *Pediatric Research* **37**, 81–85.

HANSBROUGH, J.F., ZAPATA-SIRVENT, R.L. and BENDER, E.M. (1986) Prevention of alterations in postoperative lymphocyte subpopulations by cimetidine and ibuprofen. *American Journal of Surgery* **151**, 249–255.

HARADA, Y., HATANAKA, K., KAWAMURA, M. *et al.* (1996) Role of prostaglandin H synthase-2 in prostaglandin E_2 formation in rat carrageenin-induced pleurisy. *Prostaglandins* **51**, 19–33.

HARDIE, W.D., WHEELER, A.P., WRIGHT, P.W., SWINDELL, B.B. and BERNARD, G.R. (1992) Effects of cyclooxygenase inhibition on amphotericin B-induced lung injury in awake sheep. *Journal of Infectious Diseases* **166**, 134–138.

HARDING, J.J. and VAN HEYNINGEN, R. (1988) Drugs, including alcohol, that act as risk factors for cataract. *British Journal of Opthalmology* **72**, 809–814.

HARRIS, R.E., NAMBOODIRI, K.K. and FARRAR, W.B. (1996) Nonsteroidal anti-inflammatory drugs and breast cancer. *Epidemiology* **7**, 203–205.

HARTMAN, D.A., OCHALSKI, S.J. and CARLSON, R.P. (1993) The effects of anti-inflammatory and antiallergic drugs on the release of IL-1β and TNT-α in the human whole blood assay. *Agents and Actions* **39**(Special Conference Issue), C70–C72.

HECHTMAN, H.B. (1982) Modification of inflammatory response to aspiration with ibuprofen. *American Journal of Physiology* **12**, H903–H910.

HESS, M.L., ROWE, G.T., CAPLAN, M., ROMSON, J.L. and LUCCHESI, B. (1985) Identification of hydrogen peroxide and hydroxyl radicals as mediators of leukocyte-induced myocardial dysfunction. Limitation of infarct size with neutrophil inhibition and depletion. *Advances in Myocardiology* **5**, 159–175.

HIGGS, G.A. (1989) Use of implanted sponges to study the acute inflammatory response. In: CHANG, J.Y. and LEWIS, A.J. (eds), *Pharmacological Methods in the Control of Inflammation*. New York, Alan R. Liss, 151–171.

HIGGS, G.A. and FLOWER, R.J. (1981) Anti-inflammatory drugs and the inhibition of arachidonate lipoxygenase. In: PIPER, P.J. (ed.), *SRS-A and Leukotrienes. Proceedings of the Royal College of Surgeons*. Chichester, Research Studies Press, 197–207.

HIGGS, G.A., EAKINS, K.E., MUGRIDGE, K.G., MONCADA, S. and VANE, J.R. (1980) The effects of nonsteroid anti-inflammatory drugs on leukocyte migration in carrageenin-induced inflammation. *European Journal of Pharmacology* **66**, 81–86.

HIROSE, K., KOJIMA, Y., EIGYO, M. *et al.* (1980) Pharmacological studies of benoxaprofen, a new anti-inflammatory drug (1). Anti-inflammatory and analgesic activities. *Pharmacometrics (Tokyo)* **19**, 569–580.

HOCKERTZ, S., HECKENBERGER, R., EMMENDORFFER, A. and MULLER, M. (1995) Influence of ibuprofen on the infection with *Listeria monocytogenes*. *Arzneimittel-Forschung* **45**, 104–107.

HOLTZ, G. (1982) Failure of a nonsteroidal anti-inflammatory agent (ibuprofen) to inhibit peritoneal adhesion reformation after lysis. *Fertility and Sterility* **37**, 582–583.

HORAKOVA, Z., BAYER, B.M., ALMEIDA, A.P. and BEAVEN, M.A. (1980) Evidence that histamine does not participate in histamine-induced pleurisy in rat. *European Journal of Pharmacology* **62**, 17–25.

HUGENBERG, S.T., BRANDT, K.D. and COLE, C.A. (1993) Effect of sodium salicylate, aspirin, and ibuprofen on enzymes required by the chondrocyte for synthesis of chondroitin sulfate. *Journal of Rheumatology* **20**, 2128–2133.

HUNNEYBALL, I.M., CROSSLEY, M.J. and SPOWAGE, M. (1986) Pharmacological studies of antigen-induced arthritis in BALB/c mice I. Characterization of the arthritis and the effects of steroidal and nonsteroidal anti-inflammatory agents. *Agents and Actions* **18**, 384–393.

HUTT, A.J. and CALDWELL, J. (1983) The metabolic chiral inversion of 2-arylpropionic acids. A novel route with pharmacological consequences. *Journal of Pharmacy and Pharmacology* **35**, 693–704.

IKEDA, Y. (1977) The effect of ibuprofen on platelet function *in vivo*. *Keio Journal of Medicine* **26**, 213–222.

ITO, B.R., ROTH, D.M., CHENOWETH, D.E., LEFER, A.M. and ENGLER, R.L. (1989) Thromboxane is produced in response to intracoronary infusions of complement C5a in pigs.

CHAPTER 5

Cyclooxygenase blockade does not reduce the myocardial ischemia and leukocyte accumulation. *Circulatory Research* **65**, 1220–1232.

JANAS-BORATYNSKA, M. and SCEWCZYK, Z. (1979) The effect of imminosuppressive and anti-inflammatory drugs on lymphocyte population and MIF in glomerulonephritis. *Archivum Immunologiae et Therapiae Experimentalis* **27**, 833–845.

JEFFREY, P., TUCKER, G.T., BYE, A., CREWE, H.K. and WRIGHT, P.A. (1991) The site of inversion of (R)-(–)-ibuprofen: studies using rat in-site perfused intestines/liver preparations. *Journal of Pharmacy and Pharmacology* **43**, 715–720.

JESMOK, G.J., FOWLER, A.A. 3D and SUGERMAN, H.J. (1993) Combined ibuprofen and monoclonal antibody to tumor necrosis factor-alpha attenuate hemodynamic dysfunction and sepsis-induced acute lung injury. *Journal of Trauma* **34**, 612–620.

JIANG, C., TING, A.T. and SEED, B. (1998) PPAR-γ agonists inhibit production of monokine inflammatory cytokines. *Nature* **391**, 82–86.

JOUZEAU, J.-Y., TERLAIN, B., ABID, A., NÉDÉLEC, E. and NETTER, P. (1997) Cyclooxygenase isoenzymes. How recent findings affect thinking about nonsteroidal anti-inflammatory drugs. *Drugs* **53**, 563–582.

KAISER, D.G. and GLENN, E.M. (1974) Aspirin–ibuprofen interaction in the adjuvant-induced polyarthritic rat. *Research Communications in Chemical Pathology and Pharmacology* **9**, 583–586.

KAMINSKI, D.L., DESHPANDE, Y., THOMAS, L., QUALY, J. and BLANKS, W. (1985) Effect of oral ibuprofen on formation of prostaglandins E and F by human gallbladder muscle and mucosa. *Digestive Diseases and Sciences* **30**, 933–940.

KANKAANRANTA, H., MOILANEN, E. and VAPAATALO, H. (1994) Effects of nonsteroidal anti-inflammatory drugs on polymorphonuclear leukocyte functions *in vitro*: focus on fenamates. *Naunyn-Schmiedeberg's Achives of Pharmacology* **350**, 685–691.

KAPIOTIS, S., SENGOELGE, G., SPERR, W.R. *et al.* (1996) Ibuprofen inhibits pyrogen-dependent expression of VCAM-1 and ICAM-1 on human endothelial cells. *Life Sciences* **58**, 2167–2181.

KAPLAN, H.B., EDELSON, H.S., KORCHAK, H.M., GIVEN, W.P., ABRAMSON, S. and WEISSMANN, G. (1984) Effects of nonsteroidal anti-inflammatory agents on human neutrophil functions *in vitro* and *in vivo*. *Biochemical Pharmacology* **33**, 371–378.

KARGMAN, S., WONG, E., GRIEG, G.M. *et al.* (1996) Mechanism of selective inhibition of human prostaglandin G/H synthase-1 and -2 in intact cells. *Biochemical Pharmacology* **52**, 1113–1125.

KARZELL, K. and PADBERG, D.-W. (1977) Untersuchungen über den Einfluß antirheumatisch aktiver Phenylessigsäuerderivate auf den Glykosaminoglykanstoffwechsel von Fibroblastenkulturen. *Arzneimittel-Forschung* **27**, 533–538.

KELLEY, V.E., IZUI, S. and HALUSHKA, P.V. (1982) Effect of ibuprofen, a fatty acid cyclo-oxygenase inhibitor, on murine lupus. *Clinical Immunology and Immunopathology* **25**, 223–231.

KILO, S., FORSTER, C., GEISSLINGER, G., BRUNE, K. and HANDWERKER, H.O. (1995) Inflammatory models of cutaneous hyperalgesia are sensitive to effects of ibuprofen in man. *Pain* **62**, 187–193.

KIVINEN, A., VIKHOLM, I. and TARPILA, S. (1994) A film balance study of the monolayer-forming properties of dietary phospholipids and the interaction with NSAIDs on the monolayers. *International Journal of Pharmaceutics* **108**, 109–115.

KLEHA, J.F., DEVELSY, P. and JOHNS, A. (1995) Endothelium derived relaxing factor release from canine coronary artery by leukocytes. *Canadian Journal of Physiology and Pharmacology* **73**, 404–408.

KLEIN, B., TIOMNY, A., GLOBERSON, A., ELAIN, I., NOTTI, I. and DJALDETTI, M. (1982) Effect of anti-inflammatory drugs on the phagocytic activity of peripheral blood monocytes. *Prostaglandins, Leukotrienes and Medicine* **9**, 321–330.

KNIGHTS, K.M. and ROBERTS, B.J. (1994) Xenobiotic acyl-CoA formation: evidence for kinetically distinct hepatic microsomal long-chain fatty acid and nafenopin-CoA ligases. *Chemical and Biological Interactions* **90**, 215–223.

KONSTAN, M.W. (1996) Treatment of airway inflammation in cystic fibrosis. *Current Opinion in Pulmonary Medicine* **2**, 452–456.

KONSTAN, M.W., BYARD, P.J., HOPPEL, C.L. and DAVIS, P.B. (1995) Effect of high dose ibuprofen in patients with cystic fibrosis. *New England Journal of Medicine* **332**, 848–854.

KORBAL, G., HUMMEL, C., GRUBER, M., GEISSLINGER, G. and HUMMEL, T. (1994) Dose-related effects of ibuprofen on pain-related potentials. *British Journal of Clinical Pharmacology* **37**, 445–452.

KOTYUK, B., RAYCHAUDHURI, A. and DIPASQUALE, G. (1993) Effect of anti-inflammatory compounds on oedema formation and myeloperoxidase activity in the arachidonic acid-induced ear model in the mouse. *Agents and Actions* **39** (Special Conference Issue), C46–C48.

KRUPP, P., MENASSÉ, R., RIESTERER, L. and ZIEL, R. (1976) The biological significance of inhibition of prostaglandin synthesis. In: LEWIS, G.P. (ed.), *The Role of Prostaglandin in Inflammation*. Berne, Hans Huber, 106–115.

KRUPP, P., MENESSÉ, R. and ZIEL, R. (1976) Chemistry and pharmacology of diclofenac. In: WAGENHÄUSER, R.J. (ed.), ®Voltaren. A new nonsteroid antirheumatic agent (diclofenac). Proceedings of a Symposium held during the VIIIth European Rheumatology Congress, Helsinki, 1975. Hans Huber, Bern, 13–18.

KU, E.C., WASVARY, J.M. and CASH, W.D. (1975) Diclofenac sodium (GP 45841, Voltaren), a potent inhibitor of prostaglandin synthetase. *Biochemical Pharmacology* **24**, 641–650.

CHAPTER 5

KULLICH, W. and KLEIN, G. (1986) Investigations of the influence of nonsteroidal anti-rheumatic drugs on the rates of sister-chromatid exchange. *Mutation Research* **174**, 131–134.

KULLICH, W., WALLNER, H. and KLEIN, G. (1994) Die Bestimmung von Serumpepsinogen I and II zur Beurteilung der gastroduodenalen Vertraglichkeit von (S)-(+)-ibuprofen. *Wiener Klinische Wochenschrift* **106**, 208–211.

KULMACZ, R., PALMER, G. and TSAI, A.-L. (1991) Prostaglandin H synthase: perturbation of the tyrosyl radical as a probe of anticyclooxygenase agents. *Molecular Pharmacology* **40**, 833–837.

LANAS, A.I., NERIN, J., ESTEVA, F. snd SÁINZ, R. (1995) Nonsteroidal anti-inflammatory drugs and prostaglandin effects on pepsinogen secretion by dispersed human peptic cells. *Gut* **36**, 657–663.

LANEUVILLE, O., BREUER, D.I.C., DEWITT, D.L., HLA, J., FUNK, C.D. and SMITH, W.L. (1994) Differential inhibition of human prostaglandin endoperoxide H synthase-1 and -2 by nonsteroidal anti-inflammatory drugs. *Journal of Pharmacology and Experimental Therapeutics* **271**, 927–934.

LANG, F., ROBERT, J.-M., BOUCROT, P., WELIN, L. and PETIT, J.-Y. (1995) New anti-inflammatory compounds that inhibit tumour necrosis factor production: probably interaction with protein kinase C activation. *Journal of Pharmacology and Experimental Therapeutics* **275**, 171–176.

LANZA, F.L., ROYER, G.L., NELSON, R.S., CHEN, T.T., SECKMAN, C.E. and RACK, M.F. (1979) The effects of ibuprofen, indomethacin, aspirin, naproxen, and placebo on the gastric mucosa of normal volunteers. A gastroscopic and photographic study. *Digestive Diseases and Sciences* **24**, 823–828.

LANZA, F.L., ROYER, G.L., NELSON, R.S., CHEN, T.T., SECKMAN, C.E. and RACK, M.F. (1981) A comparative endoscopic evaluation of the damaging effects of nonsteroidal anti-inflammatory agents on the gastric and duodenal mucosa. *American Journal of Gastroenterology* **75**, 17–21.

LANZA, F., RACK, M.F., LYNN, M., WOLF, J. and SANDA, M. (1987) An endoscopic comparison of the effects of etodolac, indomethacin, ibuprofen, naproxen, and placebo on the gastrointestinal mucosa. *Journal of Rheumatology* **14**, 338–341.

LAW, E. and LEWIS, A.J. (1977) The effect of systemically and topically applied drugs on the ultraviolet-induced erythema in the rat. *British Journal of Pharmacology* **59**, 591–597.

LAW, I.P., WICKMAN, C.J. and HARRISON, B.R. (1979) Coombs'-positive hemolytic anemia and ibuprofen. *Southern Medical Journal* **72**, 707–710.

LEEPER-WOODFORD, S.K., CAREY, P.D., BYRNE, K. *et al.* (1991) Ibuprofen attenuates plasma tumor necrosis factor activity during sepsis-induced acute lung injury. *Journal of Applied Physiology* **71**, 915–923.

LESKO, S.M. and MITCHELL, A.A. (1996) Paediatric ibuprofen and leukopenia. *Journal of the American Medical Association* **275**, 986.

LEVY, G.N. (1997) Prostaglandin H synthases, nonsteroidal anti-inflammatory drugs, and colon cancer. *FASEB Journal* **11**, 234–247.

LEWIS, A.J., COTTNEY, J. and SUGRUE, M.F. (1975) The spontaneously contracting pregnant rat uterus as a model for anti-inflammatory drug activity. *Journal of Pharmacy and Pharmacology* **27**, 375–376.

LICHTENBERGER, L.M., WANG, Z.M., ROMERO, J.J. *et al.* (1995) Nonsteroidal anti-inflammatory drugs (NSAIDs) associate with zwitterionic phospholipids: insight into the mechanism and reversal of NSAID-induced gastrointestinal injury. *Nature Medicine* **1**, 154–158.

LONGENECKER, G.L., SWIFT, I.A., BOWEN, R.J., BEYERS, B.J. and SHAH, A.K. (1985) Kinetics of ibuprofen effect on platelet and endothelial prostanoid release. *Clinical Pharmacology and Therapeutics* **37**, 343–348.

LUGEA, A., ANTOLÍN, M., MOURELLE, M., GUARNER, F. and MALAGELADA, J.-R. (1997) Deranged hydrophobic barrier of the rat gastroduodenal mucosa after parenteral nonsteroidal anti-inflammatory drugs. *Gastroenterology* **112**, 1931–1939.

MADERAZO, E.G., BREAUX, S.P. and WORONICK, C.L. (1984) Inhibition of human polymorphonuclear leukocyte cell responses by ibuprofen. *Journal of Pharmaceutical Sciences* **73**, 1403–1406.

MADARAZO, E.G., BREAUX, S.P. and WORONICK, C.L. (1986) Protective effects of ibuprofen and methylprednisolone on chemotactic factor-induced transcutaneous hypoxia. *Journal of Pharmacology and Experimental Therapeutics* **238**, 453–456.

MÄKELÄ, A.-L., LEMPIAEINEN, M. and YLIJOKI, H. (1981) Ibuprofen levels in serum and synovial fluid. *Scandinavian Journal of Rheumatology* **39**(Suppl.), 15–17.

MALMBERG, A.B. and YAKSH, T.L. (1992a) Antinociceptive actions of spinal nonsteroidal anti-inflammatory agents in the formalin test in the rat. *Journal of Pharmacology and Experimental Therapeutics* **263**, 136–146.

MALMBERG, A.B. and YAKSH, T.L. (1992b) Hyperalgesia mediated by spinal glutamate or substance P receptor blocked by spinal cyclooxygenase inhibition. *Science* **257**, 1276–1279.

MALMBERG, A.B. and YAKSH, T.L. (1995) Cyclooxygenase inhibition and the spinal release of prostaglandin E_2 and amino acids evoked by paw formalin injection: a microdialysis study in unanesthetized rats. *Journal of Neuroscience* **15**, 2768–2776.

MANSILLA-ROSELLÓ, A., FERRÓN-ORIHUELA, J.A., RUTZ-CABELLO, F., GARROTE-LARA, D., FERNÁNDEZ-MONDÉJAT, E. and DELGADO-CARRASCO, M.L. (1997) Differential effects of IL-1β and ibuprofen after endotoxin challenge in mice. *Journal of Surgical Research* **67**, 199–204.

CHAPTER 5

MARKS, J.W., BONORRIS, G.G. and SCHOENFIELD, L.J. (1996) Effects of ursodiol or ibuprofen on contraction of gallbladder and bile among obese patients during weight loss. *Digestive Diseases and Sciences* **41**, 242–249.

MARTIN, M.K., CARTER, G.W. and YOUNG, P.R. (1980) Comparative anti-inflammatory activity of cyclooxygenase and lipoxygenase inhibitors. *Pharmacologist* **22**, 255, Abstract no. 526.

MARTIN, S.W., STEVENS, A.J., BRENNAN, B.S., DAVIES, D., ROWLAND, M. and HOUSTON, J.B. (1994) The six-day-old rat air pouch model of inflammation: characterization of the inflammatory response to carrageenan. *Journal of Pharmacological and Toxicological Methods* **32**, 139–147.

MARTIN, S.W., STEVENS, A.J., BRENNAN, B.S., ROWLAND, M. and HOUSTON, J.B. (1995) Pharmacodynamic comparison of regional drug delivery for nonsteroidal anti-inflammatory drugs, using the rat air-pouch model of inflammation. *Journal of Pharmacy and Pharmacology* **47**, 458–461.

MARUYAMA, Y., IMAYOSHI, T., GOTO, K. and KADOBE, Y. (1977) Pharmacological studies of 2-(5*H*-[1] benzopyrano (2,3*b*) pyridin-7-yl) propionic acid (Y-8004) (III). Interactions of Y-8004 with anti-inflammatory agents. *Folia Pharmacologica Japonica* **73**, 113–122.

MARZI, I., BAUER, C., HOWER, R. and BUHREN, V. (1993) Leukocyte–endothelial cell interactions in the liver after hemorrhagic shock in the rat. *Circulatory Shock* **40**, 105–114.

MAYER, J.M. (1996) Ibuprofen enantiomers and lipid metabolism. *Journal of Clinical Pharmacology* **36**, 27S–32S.

MAYER, J.M., BARTOLUCCI, C., MAÎTRE, J.-M. and TESTA, B. (1988) Metabolic chiral inversion of anti-inflammatory 2-arylpropionates: lack of reaction in liver homogenates, and study of methine proton acidity. *Xenobiotica* **18**, 533–543.

McCARTHY, D.O. and DAUN, J.M. (1993) The effects of cyclooxygenase inhibitors on tumor-induced anorexia in rats. *Cancer* **71**, 486–492.

McCORMACK, K. (1994) The spinal actions of nonsteroidal anti-inflammatory drugs and the dissociation between their anti-inflammatory and analgesic actions. *Drugs* **47**(Suppl. 5), 28–45.

McCORMACK, K. and BRUNE, K. (1987) Classical absorption theory and the development of gastric mucosal damage associated with the nonsteroidal anti-inflammatory drugs. *Archives of Toxicology* **60**, 261–269.

McCORMACK, K. and BRUNE, K. (1989) The amphiprotic character of azapropazone and its relevance to the gastric mucosa. *Archives of Toxicology* **64**, 1–6.

McCORMACK, K. and URQUHART, E. (1995) Correlation between nonsteroidal anti-inflammatory drug efficacy in a clinical pain model and the dissociation of their anti-inflammatory and analgesic properties in animal models. *Clinical Drug Investigation* **9**, 88–97.

MCGEER, P.L. and MCGEER, E.G. (1996) Anti-inflammatory drugs in the fight against Alzheimer's disease. *Annals of the New York Academy of Sciences* **777**, 213–220.

MCINTYRE, B.A., PHILP, R.B. and INWOOD, M.J. (1978) Effect of ibuprofen on platelet function in normal subjects and hemophiliac patients. *Clinical Pharmacology and Therapeutics* **24**, 616–621.

MCKENZIE, L.S., HORSBURGH, B.A., GHOSH, P. and TAYLOR, T.K.F. (1976) Effect of anti-inflammatory drugs and sulfated drugs on sulfated glycosaminoglycan synthesis in aged human articular cartilage. *Annals of the Rheumatic Diseases* **35**, 487–497.

MCMILLAN, D.C., LEEN, E., SMITH, J. *et al.* (1995) Effect of extended ibuprofen administration on the acute phase protein response in colorectal cancer patients. *European Journal of Surgical Oncology* **21**, 531–534.

MCMILLAN, D.C., O'GORMAN, P., FEARON, K.C.H. and MCARDLE, C.S. (1997) A pilot study of megestrol acetate and ibuprofen in the treatment of cachexia in gastrointestinal cancer patients. *British Journal of Cancer* **76**, 788–790.

MEACOCK, S.C.R. and KITCHEN, E.A. (1976) Some effects of nonsteroidal anti-inflammatory drugs on leukocyte migration. *Agents and Actions* **6**, 320–325.

MEADE, E.A., SMITH, W.L. and DEWITT, D.L. (1993) Differential inhibition of prostaglandin endoperoxide synthase (cyclooxygenase) isoenzymes by aspirin and other non-steroidal anti-inflammatory drugs. *Journal of Biological Chemistry* **268**, 6610–6614.

MELIS, R. (1996) No basis for associating non-prescription ibuprofen and similar agents with necrotizing fasciitis. *American Journal of Health Systems Pharmacy* **53**, 2218.

MELARANGE, R., MOORE, G., BLOWER, P.R., COATES, M.E., WARD, F.W. and RONAASEN, V. (1992) A comparison of indomethacin with ibuprofen on gastrointestinal mucosal integrity in conventional and germ-free rats. *Alimentary Pharmacology and Therapeutics* **6**, 67–77.

MELARANGE, R., BLOWER, P. and SPANGLER, R. (1994) Comparison of the anti-inflammatory activity and gastrointestinal irritancy of nabumetone, ibuprofen and diclofenac in rats following chronic administration. *European Journal of Rheumatology and Inflammation* **14**, 23–27.

MENZEL, J.E. and KOLARZ, G. (1997) Modulation of nitric oxide synthase activity by ibuprofen. *Inflammation* **21**, 451–461.

MICHELSSON, J.E. (1980) The effect of ibuprofen on the thickening, stiffening and development of degenerative changes in the rabbit knee following immobilization. *Scandanavian Journal of Rheumatology* **9**, 141–144.

MIKAMI, T. and MIYASAKA, K. (1983) Effects of several anti-inflammatory drugs on the various parameters involved in the inflammatory response in rat carrageenin-induced pleurisy. *European Journal of Pharmacology* **95**, 1–12.

MILTON, A.S. (1982) Prostaglandins in fever and the mode of action of antipyretic drugs. In: MILTON, A.S. (ed.), *Pyretics and Antipyretics*. Berlin, Springer-Verlag, 257–303.

CHAPTER 5

MITCHELL, J.A., AKARASEREENONT, P., THIEMERMANN, C., FLOWER, R.J. and VANE, J.R. (1994) Selectivity of nonsteroidal anti-inflammatory drugs as inhibitors of constitutive and inducible cyclooxygenase. *Proceedings of the National Academy of Sciences of the USA* **90**, 11693–11697.

MÖLLER, N.L., DIETZEL, K.E., SCHNEIDER, H.T. and BRUNE, K. (1989) Novel 5-aminosalicylic acid conjugates: synthesis, pharmacological and toxicological properties. *European Journal of Medicinal Chemistry* **24**, 463–469.

MONCADA, S., PALMER, R.M.J. and HIGGS, E.A. (1991) Nitric oxide: physiology, pathophysiology, and pharmacology. *Pharmacological Reviews* **43**, 109–142.

MORGAN, G. (1996) Nonsteroidal inflammatory drugs and the chemoprevention of colorectal and oesophageal cancers. *Gut* **38**, 646–648.

MULLEN, P.G., WINDSOR, A.C., WALSH, C.J. *et al.* (1993) Combined ibuprofen and monoclonal antibody to tumor necrosis factor-alpha attenuate hemodynamic dysfunction and sepsis-induced acute lung injury. *Journal of Trauma* **34**, 612–620.

MÜLLER, P. and SIMON, B. (1994) Effects of ibuprofen lysine and acetylsalicylic acid on gastric and duodenal mucosa. Randomized single-blind placebo-controlled endoscopic study in healthy volunteers. *Arzneimttel-Forschung* **44**, 840–843.

MUSCAT, J.E., STELLMAN, S.D. and WYNDER, E.L. (1994) Nonsteroidal anti-inflammatory drugs and colorectal cancer. *Cancer* **74**, 1847–1854.

MYERS, R.F., ANTHES, J.C., CASMER, C.J. and SIEGEL, M.I. (1985) *Ex vivo* effects of nonsteroidal anti-inflammatory drugs on arachidonic acid metabolism in neutrophils from a reverse passive Arthus reaction. *Inflammation* **9**, 91–98.

NAKAMURA, Y., YAMAGUCHI, T., TAKAHASHI, S., HASHIMOTO, S., IWATANI, K. and NAKAGAWA, Y. (1981) Optical isomerization of $R(-)$-hydratropic acid derivatives. *Journal of Pharmacobio-Dynamics* **4**, S1.

NEUPERT, W., BRUGGER, R., EUCHENHOFER, C., BRUNE, K. and GEISSLINGER, G. (1997) Effects of ibuprofen enantiomers and its coenzyme A thioesters on human prostaglandin endoperoxide synthases. *British Journal of Pharmacology* **122**, 487–492.

NICKERSON, S.C., PAAPE, M.J., HARMON, R.J. and ZIV, G. (1986) Mammary leukocyte response to drug therapy. *Journal of Dairy Science* **69**, 1733–1742.

NIELSON, H. and BENNEDSEN, J. (1983) Effect of nonsteroidal anti-inflammatory drugs on human monocyte chemotaxis *in vitro*. *Immunopharmacology* **5**, 259–265.

NIELSEN, J.C., BJERRING, P., ARENDT-NIELSEN, L. and PETTERSON, K.-J. (1990) A double-blind, placebo controlled, cross-over comparison of the analgesic effect of ibuprofen 400 mg and 800 mg on laser-induced pain. *British Journal of Clinical Pharmacology* **30**, 711–715.

NIELSEN, V.G. and WEBSTER, R.O. (1987) Inhibition of human polymorphonuclear leukocyte functions by ibuprofen. *Immunopharmacology* **13**, 61–71.

NUSS, G.W., SMYTH, R.D., BREDER, C.D., HITCHINGS, M.J., MIR, G.N. and REAVEY-CANTWELL, N.H. (1976) The antiphlogistic, antinociceptive and antipyretic properties of fenclorac (α, m-dichloro-p-cyclohexylphenyl acetic acid, diethylammonium salt). *Agents and Actions* 6, 735–747.

O'BRIEN, J.R. (1968) Effect of anti-inflammatory agents on platelets. *Lancet* i, 894–895.

O'BRIEN, W.F., DRAKE, T.S. and BIBRO, M.C. (1982) The use of ibuprofen and dexamethasone in the prevention of postoperative adhesion formation. *Obstetrics and Gynecology* 60, 373–378.

OELKERS, R., IONAC, M., ERB, K., BRUNE, K. and GEISSLINGER, G. (1996) Transfer of different nonsteroidal anti-inflammatory drugs *via* the lymphatic system in the rat. *Drug Metabolism and Disposition* 24, 1107–1110.

OHNISHI, H., CHICHIRO, C., SUZUKI, K. *et al.* (1982) Effects of protizinic acid on the prostaglandins system and the production of oxygen radicals. *Folio Pharmacologia Japonica* 79, 561–569.

OKUSAWA, S., GELFAND, J.A., IKEJIMA, T., CONNOLLY, R.J. and DINARELLO, C.A. (1988) Interleukin 1 induces a shock-like state in rabbits. Synergism with tumor necrosis factor and the effect of cyclooxygenase inhibition. *Journal of Clinical Investigation* 81, 1162–1172.

ONO, T., OHTSUKA, M., SAKAI, S., OHNO, S. and KUMADA, S. (1977) Relaxant effect of aspirin-like drugs on isolated guinea-pig tracheal chain. *Japanese Journal of Pharmacology* 27, 889–898.

ØSTENSEN, M. (1994) Optimisation of antirheumatic drug treatment during pregnancy. *Clinical Pharmacokinetics* 27, 484–503.

OTTERNESS, I.G. and BLIVEN, M.L. (1985) Laboratory models for testing nonsteroidal anti-inflammatory drugs. In: LOMBARDINO, J.G. (ed.), *Nonsteroidal Anti-inflammatory Drugs*. New York, Wiley, 113–251.

OTTERNESS, I.G., WISEMAN, E.H. and GANS, D.J. (1979) A comparison of the carrageenan oedema test and ultraviolet light-induced erythema test as predictors of the clinical dose in rheumatoid arthritis. *Agents and Actions* 9, 177–183.

OTTONELLO, L., PASTORINO, G., DAPINO, P., BERETTA, A. and DALLEGRI, F. (1992) Ibuprofen inhibits adhesion-dependent neutrophil response by a glycoprotein-unrelated mechanism. *Drugs under Experimental and Clinical Research* 18, 23–27.

OZKUL, Y., ERENMEMISOGLU, A., EKECIK, A., SAATCI, C., OZDAMAR, S. and DEMIRTAS, H. (1996) Do nonsteroidal anti-inflammatory drugs induce sister chromatid exchanges in T lymphocytes. *Journal of International Medical Research* 24, 84–87.

PALDER, S.B., HUVAL, W., LELCUK, S. *et al.* (1986) Reduction of polymorphonuclear leukocyte accumulations by inhibition of cyclooxygenase and thromboxane synthase in the rabbit. *Surgery* 99, 72–81.

CHAPTER 5

PANAYI, G.S. (1975) The effect of ibuprofen on lymphocyte stimulation by phytohemag-glutinin *in vitro. Current Medical Research and Opinion* **3**, 513–515.

PANERAI, A.E., LOCATELLI, L. and SACERDOTE, P. (1992) Effects of piroxicam and ibuprofen on substance P induced chemotaxis of human monocytes and polymorphonuclear cells. *Pharmacological Research* **26**, 30–31.

PANERAI, A.E., LOCATELLI, L. and SACERDOTE, P. (1993) Inhibitory effect of NSAIDs on the chemotaxis induced by substance P on human monocytes and polymorphonuclear cells. *Annali dell Istituto Superiore di Sanita* **29**, 375–377.

PAPPIUS, H.M. and WOLFE, L.S. (1983) Effects of indomethacin and ibuprofen on cerebral metabolism and blood flow in traumatized brain. *Journal of Cerebral Blood Flow and Metabolism* **3**, 448–459.

PARKS, W.M., HOAK, J.C. and CZERVIONKE, R.L. (1981) Comparative effects of ibuprofen on endothelial and platelet prostaglandin synthesis. *Journal of Pharmacology and Experimental Therapeutics* **219**, 415–419.

PAROLA, M., PARADISI, L. and TORRIELLI, M.V. (1984) Nonsteroidal anti-inflammatory agents and hepatic lipid peroxidation in normal and carrageenin-treated rats. *Research Communications in Chemical Pathology and Pharmacology* **45**, 37–53.

PARRISH, M.B., RAINSFORD, K.D., JOHNSON, D.M. and DANIEL, E.E. (1994) NK_1 receptors mediated release of 6-keto-$PGF_{1\alpha}$ from the *ex vivo* perfused canine ileum. *Journal of Pharmacology and Experimental Therapeutics* **271**, 39–47.

PARTSCH, G., SCHWARZER, C. and EBERL, R. (1990) The effects of ibuprofen and diclofenac on the chemotaxis and adenosine triphosphate level of polymorphonuclear cells *in vitro. Journal of Rheumatology* **17**, 583–588.

PASRICHA, P.J., BEDI, A., O'CONNOR, K. *et al.* (1995) The effects of sulindac on colorectal proliferation and apoptosis in familial adenomatous polyposis. *Gastroenterology* **109**, 994–998.

PATEL, P.M., DRUMMOND, J.C., SANO, T., COLE, D.J., KALKMAN, C.J. and YAKSH, T.L. (1993) Effect of ibuprofen on regional eicosanoid production and neuronal injury after fore-brain ischemia in rats. *Brain Research* **614**, 315–324.

PAVELKA, K., SUSTA, A., VOJTISEK, O. *et al.* (1973) Double-blind comparison of ibuprofen and phenylbutazone in the short-term treatment of rheumatoid arthritis. *Rheumatology and Rehabilitation* **12**, 68–73.

PEARSON, C.M. and WOOD, F.D. (1959) Studies of polyarthritis and other lesions induced in rats by injection of mycobacterial adjuvant. I. General clinical and pathologic charac-teristics and some modifying factors. *Arthritis and Rheumatism* **2**, 440–459.

PELEG, I.I., LUBIN, M.F., COTSONIS, G.A., CLARK, W.S. and WILCOX, C.M. (1996) Long-term use of nonsteroidal anti-inflammatory drugs and other chemopreventors and risk of subsequent colorectal neoplasia. *Digestive Diseases and Sciences* **41**, 1319–1326.

PENNING, T.M. and TALALAY, P. (1983) Inhibition of a major NAD(P)-linked oxidoreductase from rat liver cytosol by steroidal and nonsteroidal anti-inflammatory agents and by prostaglandins. *Proceedings of the National Academy of Sciences of the USA* **80**, 4504–4508.

PENNING, T.M., SHARP, R.B. and KRIEGER, N.R. (1985) Purification and properties of a 3α-hydroxysteroid dehydrogenase from rat brain cytosol. Inhibition by nonsteroidal anti-inflammatory drugs and progestins. *Journal of Biological Chemistry* **260**, 15266–15272.

PERIANIN, A., ROCH-ARVEILLER, M., GIROUD, J.P. and HAKIM, J. (1984) *In vivo* interaction of nonsteroidal anti-inflammatory drugs on the locomotion of neutrophils elicited by acute nonspecific inflammations in the rat — effect of indomethacin, ibuprofen and flurbiprofen. *Biochemical Pharmacology* **33**, 2239–2243.

PERIANIN, A., GIROUD, J.P. and HAKIM, J. (1988) Differential *in vivo* effects of indomethacin, ibuprofen, and flurbiprofen on oxygen-dependent killing activities of neutrophils elicited by acute nonimmune inflammation in the rat. *Inflammation* **12**, 181–189.

PETERSEN, K.L., BRENNUM, J. and DAHL, J.B. (1997) Experimental evaluation of the analgesic effect of ibuprofen on primary and secondary hyperalgesia. *Pain* **70**, 167–174.

PFLUM, L.R. and GRAEME, M.L. (1979) The Arthus reaction in rats, a possible test for anti-inflammatory and antirheumatic drugs. *Agents and Actions* **9**, 184–189.

PHILLIS, J.W. and WU, P.H. (1981) Indomethacin, ibuprofen and meclofenamate inhibit adenosine uptake by rat microsomes. *European Journal of Pharmacology* **72**, 139–140.

PHILLIS, J.W., DELONG, R.E. and TOWNER, J.K. (1986) Indomethacin and ibuprofen enhance anoxia-enduced hyperemia in rat brain. *European Journal of Pharmacology* **124**, 85–91.

PHILLPOSE, B., SINGH, R., KHAN, K.A. and GIRI, A.K. (1997) Comparative mutagenic and genotoxic effects of three propionic acid derivatives ibuprofen, ketoprofen and naproxen. *Mutation Research — Genetic Toxicology and Environmental Mutagenesis* **393**, 123–131.

PIAZZA, G.A., ALBERTS, D.S., HIXSON, L.J. *et al.* (1997) Sulindac sulfone inhibits azoxymethane-induced colon carcinogenesis in rats without reducing prostaglandin levels. *Cancer Research* **57**, 2909–2915.

PLATER, M.L., GOODE, D. and CRABBE, M.J.C. (1997) Ibuprofen protects alpha-crystallin against posttranslation modification by preventing cross-linking. *Opthalmic Research* **29**, 421–428.

PONG, S.F., DEMUTH, S.M., KINEEY, C.M. and DEEGAN, P. (1985) Prediction of human analgesic dosage of nonsteroidal anti-inflammatory drugs (NSAIDs) from analgesic ED_{50} values in mice. *Archives Internationales de Pharmacodynamie et de Thérapie* **273**, 212–220.

POWELL, J.G. and COCHRANE, R.L. (1982) The effects of a number of nonsteroidal anti-inflammatory compounds on parturition in the rat. *Prostaglandins* **23**, 469–488.

PRESCOTT, L.F. (1992) The hepatotoxicity of nonsteroidal anti-inflammatory drugs. In: RAINSFORD, K.D. and VELO, G.P. (eds), *Side-effects of Anti-inflammatory Drugs 3*. Dordrecht, Kluwer Academic Publishers, 176–187.

CHAPTER 5

PRYOR, W.A. and SQUADRITO, G.L. (1995) The chemistry of peroxynitrite: a product from the reaction of nitric oxide with superoxide. *American Journal of Physiology* **268**, L699–L722.

PROCACCINI, R.L., SMYTH, R.D. and REAVEY-CANTWELL, N.H. (1977) Studies on the *in vitro* inhibition of prostaglandin synthetase by fenclorac (α, *m*-dichloro-*p*-cyclohexylphenylacetic acid) and indomethacin. *Biochemical Pharmacology* **26**, 1051–1057.

RABASSEDA, X. (1996) Nimesulide: a selective cyclooxygenase 2 inhibitor anti-inflammatory drug. *Drugs of Today* **32**(Suppl. D), 1–23.

RAINSFORD, K.D. (1975a) A synergistic interaction between aspirin, or other nonsteroidal anti-inflammatory drugs, and stress which produces severe gastric mucosal damage in rats and pigs. *Agents and Actions* **5**, 553–558.

RAINSFORD, K.D. (1975b) The biochemical pathology of aspirin-induced gastric damage. *Agents and Actions* **5**, 326–344.

RAINSFORD, K.D. (1977) The comparative gastric ulcerogenic activities of nonsteroidal anti-inflammatory drugs. *Agents and Actions* **7**, 573–577.

RAINSFORD, K.D. (1978) The role of aspirin in gastric ulceration. Some factors involved in the development of gastric mucosal damage induced by aspirin in rats exposed to various stress conditions. *American Journal of Digestive Diseases* **23**, 521–530.

RAINSFORD, K.D. (1981) Comparison of the gastric ulcerogenic activity of new-nonsteroidal anti-inflammatory drugs in stressed rats. *British Journal of Pharmacology* **73**, 79c–80c.

RAINSFORD, K.D. (1982a) Adjuvant polyarthritis in rats: is this a satisfactory model for screening antiarthritic drugs? *Agents and Actions* **12**, 452–458.

RAINSFORD, K.D. (1982b) A comparison of the gastric ulcerogenic activity of benoxaprofen with other nonsteroidal anti-inflammatory drugs in rats and pigs. *European Journal of Rheumatology and Inflammation* **5**, 148–164.

RAINSFORD, K.D. (1982c) An analysis of the gastrointestinal side-effects of nonsteroidal anti-inflammatory drugs, with particular reference to comparative studies in man and laboratory species. *Rheumatology International* **2**, 1–10.

RAINSFORD, K.D. (1983) Mechanisms of intestinal mucosal damage by nonsteroidal anti-inflammatory drugs. In: PHILLIPS, S.F., BARBARA, L. and PAOLETTI, R. (eds), *Gastroenterology: New Trends in Pathophysiology and Therapy of the Large Bowel*. Amsterdam, Elsevier/North Holland, 207–220.

RAINSFORD, K.D. (1984) *Aspirin and the Salicylates*. London, Butterworths.

RAINSFORD, K.D. (1987) Gastric ulcerogenicity of nonsteroidal anti-inflammatory drugs in mice with mucosa sensitized by cholinomimetic treatment. *Journal of Pharmacy and Pharmacology* **39**, 669–672.

RAINSFORD, K.D. (1989a) Gastrointestinal side-effects. In: CHANG, J.Y. and LEWIS, A.J. (eds), *Pharmacological Methods in the Control of Inflammation*. New York, Alan R. Liss, 343–362.

RAINSFORD, K.D. (1989b) Quantitation by computerized visual image analysis of gastric mucosal lesions induced in mice and rats by nonsteroidal anti-inflammatory drugs. *Acta Physiologica Hungarica* **72**, 371–378.

RAINSFORD, K.D. (1991) Uncoupling the toxicological morass in the development of new antirheumatic drugs — is there any hope? *British Journal of Pharmacology* **30**, 161–166.

RAINSFORD, K.D. (1992) Mechanisms of gastrointestinal ulceration from nonsteroidal anti-inflammatory drugs: a basis for use and development of protective agents. In: RAINSFORD, K.D. and VELO, G.P. (eds), *Side-Effects of Anti-inflammatory Drugs 3*. Lancaster, Kluwer Academic Publishers, 97–114.

RAINSFORD, K.D. (1995) Gastric ulcerogenicity in mice of enantiomers of nonsteroidal anti-inflammatory drugs having differing potency as prostaglandin synthesis inhibitors. *Pharmaceutical Sciences* **1**, 169–171.

RAINSFORD, K.D. (1996) Mode of action, uses, and side-effects of anti-inflammatory drugs. In: RAINSFORD, K.D. (ed.), *Advances in Anti-Rheumatic Therapy*. Boca Raton FL, CRC Press, 59–111.

RAINSFORD, K.D. and WHITEHOUSE, M.W. (1980) Anti-inflammatory/antipyretic salicylic acid esters with low gastric ulcerogenic activity. *Agents and Actions* **10**, 451–456.

RAINSFORD, K.D., SCHWEITZER, A. and BRUNE, K. (1981) Autoradiographic and biochemical observations on the distribution of nonsteroidal anti-inflammatory drugs. *Archives Internationale Pharmacodyamie et de Thérapie* **250**, 180–194.

RAINSFORD, K.D., RASHAD, S.Y., REVELL, P.A. *et al.* (1992) Effects of NSAIDs on cartilage proteoglycan and synovial prostaglandin metabolism in relation to progression of joint destruction in osteoarthritis. In: BÁLINT, G., GÖMÖR, B. and HODINKA, L. (eds), *Rheumatology, State of the Art*. Amsterdam, Excerpta Medica, 177–183.

RAINSFORD, K.D., ROBERTS, S.C. and BROWN, S. (1997a) Ibuprofen and paracetamol: relative safety in non-prescription doses. *Journal of Pharmacy and Pharmacology* **49**, 345–376.

RAINSFORD, K.D., FOX, J., MILNE, G.W.A. and HONG, H. (1997b) Gastro-ulcerogenicity of enantiomeric NSAIDs: relation to cyclooxygenases, 1996. *Rheumatology in Europe (EULAR '97 Meeting, Vienna Nov. 19–22, 1997)* **26**(Suppl.) 72, Abstract no. 290.

RAMPART, M. and WILLIAMS, T.J. (1986) Suppression of inflammation oedema by ibuprofen involving a mechanism independent of cyclooxygenase inhibition. *Biochemical Pharmacology* **35**, 581–586.

RANE, L.H. and LANDS, W.E.M. (1975) Structural requirements for time-dependent inhibition of prostaglandin production by anti-inflammatory drugs. *Proceedings of the National Academy of Sciences of the USA* **72**, 4863–4865.

CHAPTER 5

RASHAD, S., RAINSFORD, K., REVELL, P., LOW, F., HEMIGWAY, A. and WALKER, F. (1992) The effects of NSAIDs on the course of osteoarthritis. In: BÁLINT, G., GÖMÖR, B. and HODINKA, L. (eds), *Rheumatology, State of the Art*. Amsterdam, Excerpta Medica, 184–188.

RAZA, K. and HARDING, J.J. (1991) Non-enzymic modification of lens proteins by glucose and fructose: effects of ibuprofen. *Experimental Eye Research* 52, 205–212.

REDDY, B.S., RAO, C.V. and SIEBERT, K. (1996) Evaluation of cyclooxygenase-2 inhibitor for potential chemopreventive properties in colon carcinogenesis. *Cancer Research* 56, 4566–4569.

REEVES, W.B., FOLEY, R.J. and WEINMAN, E.J. (1985) Nephrotoxity from nonsteroidal anti-inflammatory drugs. *Southern Medical Journal* 78, 318–322.

REICH, R. and MARTIN, G.R. (1996) Identification of arachidonic acid pathways required for the invasive and metastatic activity of malignant tumor cells. *Prostaglandins* 51, 1–17.

REINICKE, C. (1977) Influence of nonsteroid anti-inflammatory drugs (NSAIDs) on liver enzymes. *Drugs under Experimental and Clinical Research* 2, 139–153.

RINALDO, J.E. and DAUBER, J.H. (1985) Effect of methylprednisolone and of ibuprofen, a nonsteroidal anti-inflammatory agent, on bronchalveolar inflammation following endotoxemia. *Circulatory Shock* 16, 195–203.

RINALDO, J.E. and PENNOCK, B. (1986) Effects of ibuprofen on endotoxin-induced alveolitis: biphasic dose response and dissociation between inflammation and hypoxemia. *American Journal of Medical Science* 291, 29–38.

RIVKIN, U., FOSCHI, G.V. and ROSEN, C.G. (1976) Inhibition of the *in vitro* neutrophil chemotaxis and spontaneous motility by anti-inflammatory agents. *Proceedings of the Society for Experimental Biology and Medicine* 153, 236–240.

ROBERTS, K.A. and HARDING, J.J. (1990) Ibuprofen, a putative anti-cataract drug. *Experimental Eye Research* 50, 157–164.

ROBINSON, D.R., McGUIRE, M.B., BASTIAN, D., KANTROWITZ, F. and LEVINE, L. (1978) The effects of anti-inflammatory drugs on prostaglandin production by rheumatoid synovial tissue. *Prostaglandins and Medicine* 1, 461–477.

ROEDIGER, W.E.W. and MILLARD, S. (1995) Selective inhibition of fatty acid oxidation in colonocytes by ibuprofen: a cause of colitis? *Gut* 36, 55–59.

ROME, L.H. and LANDS, W.E.M. (1975) Structural requirements for time-dependent inhibition of prostaglandin biosynthesis by anti-inflammatory drugs. *Proceedings of the National Academy of Sciences of the USA* 72, 4863–4865.

ROMSON, J.L., HOOK, B.G., RIGOT, V.H., SCHORK, M.A., SWANSON, D.P. and LUCCHESI, B.R. (1982) The effect of ibuprofen on accumulation of indium-111-labelled platelets and leukocytes in experimental myocardial infarction. *Circulation* 66, 1002–1011.

Rowe, G.T., Manson, N.H., Caplan, M. and Hess, M.L. (1983) Hydrogen peroxide and hydroxyl radical depression of cardiac sarcoplasmic reticulum. Participation of the cyclooxygenase pathway. *Circulation Research* **53**, 584–591.

Royer, G.L., Seckman, C.E., Schwartz, J.H. and Bennett, K.P. (1985) Effects of ibuprofen on normal subjects: clinical and routine and special laboratory assessments. *Current Therapeutic Research* **37**, 412–426.

Rudy, A.C., Knight, P.M., Brater, D.C. and Hall, S.D. (1991) Stereoselective metabolism of ibuprofen in humans: administration of *R-, S-* and racemic ibuprofen. *Journal of Pharmacology and Experimental Therapeutics* **259**, 1133–1139.

Salkie, M.L., Hannah, C.L. and McNeil, E.M. (1976) The effects of antirheumatoid drugs on the *in vitro* activity of human serum hyaluronidase. *Clinical Biochemistry* **9**, 184–187.

Samara, E., Avnir, D., Ladkani, D. and Bialer, M. (1995) Pharmacokinetic analysis of diethylcarbonate prodrugs of ibuprofen and naproxen. *Biopharmaceutics and Drug Disposition* **16**, 201–210.

Sasaki, S. (1970) Clinical trials of ibuprofen in Japan. Report from the Drug Evaluation Committee, the official organ of the Japan Rheumatism Association. *Rheumatology and Physical Medicine* **11**(Symposium), 32–39.

Satoh, H., Shimomura, K., Mukumoto, S., Ohara, K. and Mori, J. (1982) Effects of anti-inflammatory drugs on triple vaccine-induced pleurisy in rats. *Japanese Journal of Pharmacology* **32**, 909–919.

Scheiman, J.M., Tillner, A., Pohl, T. *et al.* (1997) Reduction of nonsteroidal anti-inflammatory drug induced gastric injury and leukocyte endothelial adhesion by octreotide. *Gut* **40**, 720–725.

Schmid, F.R. and Culic, D.D. (1976) Anti-inflammatory drugs and gastrointestinal bleeding: a comparison of aspirin and ibuprofen. *Journal of Clinical Pharmacology* **16**, 418–425.

Schmitt, M. and Guentert, T.W. (1989) Effect of age on the pharmacokinetics of tenoxicam in comparison to other nonsteroidal anti-inflammatory drugs (NSAIDs). *Scandinavian Journal of Rheumatology* (Suppl. 80), 86–89.

Schneider, H.T., Nuernberg, B., Dietzel, K. and Brune, K. (1990) Biliary elimination of nonsteroidal anti-inflammatory drugs. *British Journal of Clinical Pharmacology* **29**, 127–131.

Schuurs, A.H.W.M., Verheul, H.A.M. and Wick, G. (1989) Spontaneous autoimmune models. In: Chang, J.Y. and Lewis, A.J. (eds), *Pharmacological Methods in the Control of Inflammation*. New York, Alan R. Liss, 449–485.

Sciuto, A.M. (1997) Ibuprofen treatment enhances the survival of mice following exposure to phosgene. *Inhalation Toxicology* **9**, 989–403.

CHAPTER 5

SCIUTO, A.M., STOTTS, R.R. and HURT, H.H. (1996) Efficacy of ibuprofen and pentoxifylline in the treatment of phosgene-induced acute lung injury. *Journal of Applied Toxicology* **16**, 381–384.

SEIDEMAN, P., LOHRER, F., GRAHAM, G.G., DUNCAN, M.W., WILLIAMS, K.M. and DAY, R.O. (1994) The stereoselective disposition of the enantiomers of ibuprofen in blood, blister fluid and synovial fluid. *British Journal of Clinical Pharmacology* **38**, 221–227.

SELPH, J.L., BONCEK, V.M., SOROKO, F.E., HARRIS, T.M. and COCHRAN, F.R. (1993) The pharmacological evaluation of locomotor activity versus the inflammatory parameters in rat adjuvant arthritis. *Agents and Actions* **39**, C201–C203.

SERGEEVA, M.G., GONCHAR, M.V., CHISTYAKOV, V.V. and MEVKH, A.T. (1997a) Ultralow concentrations of ibuprofen activate cell prostaglandin synthesis. *Applied Biochemistry and Biotechnology* **61**, 167–171.

SERGEEVA, M.G., GONCHAR, M.V., NAMGALADZE, D.A., MEVKH, A.T. and VARFOLOMEYEV, S.D. (1997b) Prostaglandin H synthase of mouse macrophages: inhibiting and activating action of ibuprofen. *Biochemistry — Moscow* **62**, 269–274.

SETTIPANE, G.A. (1983) Aspirin and allergic diseases. *American Journal of Medicine* **74**(6A), 102–109.

SHARMA, J.N. and SHARMA, J.N. (1977) Comparison of the anti-inflammatory activity of Commiphora mukul (an indigenous drug) with those of phenylbutazone and ibuprofen in experimental arthritis induced by mycobacterial adjuvant. *Arzneimittel-Forschung* **27**, 1455–1457.

SHANBHAG, V.R., CRIDER, A.M., GOKHALE, R., HARPALANI, A. and DICK, R.M. (1992) Ester and amide prodrugs of ibuprofen: synthesis, anti-inflammatory activity, and gastrointestinal toxicity. *Journal of Pharmaceutical Sciences* **81**, 149–154.

SHELLY, J. and HOFF, S.F. (1989) Effects of nonsteroidal anti-inflammatory drugs on isolated human polymorphonuclear leukocytes (PMN): chemotaxis, superoxide production, degranulation and N-formyl-L-methionyl-L-leucyl-L-phenylalanine (FMLP) receptor binding. *General Pharmacology* **20**, 329–334.

SHENG, J.G., ITO, K., SKINNER, R.D., MRAK, R.E., ROVNAGHI, C.R., VANELOIK, L.J. and GRIFFIN, W.S.T. (1996) *In vivo* and *in vitro* evidence supporting a role for the inflammatory cytokine interleukin-1 as a driving force in Alzheimer's pathogenesis. *Neurobiology of Aging* **17**, 761–766.

SHIMANUKI, T., NAKAMURA, R.M. and DIZEREGA, G.S. (1985a) *In vivo* modulation of leukotaxis by nonsteroidal anti-inflammatory drugs. *Agents and Actions* **17**, 80–83.

SHIMANUKI, T., NAKAMURA, R.M. and DIZEREGA, G.S. (1985b) Modulation of leukotaxis by ibuprofen. A quantative determination *in vivo*. *Inflammation* **9**, 285–295.

SHIMIZU, M., NAKAMURA, H., MOTOYOSHI, S. and YOKOYAMA, Y. (1975) Pharmacological studies on 1-methyl-5-p-toluoylpyrrole-2-acetic acid (tolmetin), a new anti-inflammatory agent, in experimental animals I. Anti-inflammatory, analgesic and antipyretic activity. *Pharmacometrics* **10**, 293–310.

SHORT, B.L., MILLER, M.K. and FLETCHER, J.R. (1982) Improved survival in the suckling rat model of Group B Streptococcal sepsis after treatment with nonsteroidal anti-inflammatory drugs. *Paediatrics* **70**, 343–347.

SIEGEL, D.M., GIRI, S.N., SCHEINHOLTZ, R.M. and SCHWARTZ, L.W. (1980) Characteristics and effect of anti-inflammatory drugs on adriamycin-induced inflammation in the mouse paw. *Inflammation* **4**, 233–248.

SIEGEL, M.I., McCONNELL, R.T. and CUATRECASAS, P. (1979) Aspirin-like drugs interfere with arachidonate metabolism by inhibition of the 12-hydroperoxy-5,8,10,14-icosatetraenoic acid peroxidase activity of the lipoxygenase pathway. *Proceedings of the National Academy of Sciences of the USA* **76**, 3774–3778.

SIEGEL, M.I., McCONNELL, R.T., PORTER, N.A. and CUATRECASAS, P. (1980) Arachidonate metabolism via lipoxygenase and 12 L-hydroperoxy-5,8,10,14-icosatetraenoic acid peroxidase sensitive to anti-inflammatory drugs. *Proceedings of the National Academy of Sciences of the USA* **77**, 308–312.

SILVOLA, J., KANGASAHO, M., TOKOLA, O. and VAPAATALO, H. (1982a) Effects of nonsteroidal anti-inflammatory drugs (NSAIDs) on cyclic AMP phosphodiesterase (PDE) and adenylate cyclase (AC) activities. *Acta Physiologica Scandavica* (Suppl. 508), 40, Abstract 83.

SILVOLA, J., KANGASAHO, M., TOKOLA, O. and VAPAATALO, H. (1982b) Effects of nonsteroidal anti-inflammatory drugs on rat gastric mucosal phosphodiesterase activity. *Agents and Actions* **12**, 516–520.

SIMCHOWITZ, L., MEHTA, J. and SPILBERG, I. (1979) Chemotactic factor-induced generation of superoxide radicals by human neutrophils: effect of metabolic inhibitors and anti-inflammatory drugs. *Arthritis and Rheumatism* **22**, 755–763.

SIMON, B., KOCH, E.M., JACKISCH, P. and MÜLLER, P. (1993) Tageszeitliche Abhängigkeit der Ibuprofen-Gastropathie und der Schutzwirkung von Ranitidin. Eine endoskopische, kontrollierte Doppelblind-Pilostudie. *Arzneimmitel-Forschung* **43**, 989–991.

SKELJO, M.V., GIRAUD, A.S. and YEOMANS, N.D. (1992) Adaptation of rat gastric mucosa to repeated doses of non-salicylate nonsteroidal anti-inflammatory drugs. *Journal of Hepatology and Gastroenterology* **7**, 586–590.

SKUBITZ, K.M. and HAMMERSCHMIDT, D.E. (1986) Effects of ibuprofen on the chemotactic peptide-receptor binding and granulocyte response. *Biochemical Pharmacology* **35**, 3349–3354.

SLATER, C. and HOUSE, S.D. (1993) Effects of nonsteroidal anti-inflammatory drugs on microvascular dynamics. *Microvascular Research* **45**, 166–179.

CHAPTER 5

SMITH, I.D., TEMPLE, D.M. and SHEARMAN, R.P. (1975) The antagonism by anti-inflammatory analgesics of prostaglandin F_{2a}-induced contractions of human and rabbit myometrium *in vitro*. *Prostaglandins* **10**, 41–49.

SMITH, M.J.H. (1966) Anti-inflammatory activity of salicylates. In: SMITH, M.J.H. and SMITH, P.K. (eds), *The Salicylates. A Critical Bibliographic Review*. New York, Wiley-Interscience, 203–232.

SMITH, R.J. (1977) Modulation of phagocytosis by and lysosomal enzyme secretion from guinea-pig neutrophils: effect of nonsteroidal anti-inflammatory agents and prostaglandins. *Journal of Pharmacology and Experimental Therapeutics* **200**, 647–657.

SMITH, R.J. and BOWMAN, B.J. (1982) Stimulation of human neutrophil degranulation with 1-*O*-octadecyl-2-*O*-acetyl-*sn*-glycerol-3-phosphorylcholine: modulation by inhibitors of arachidonic acid metabolism. *Biochemical and Biophysical Research Communications* **104**, 1495–1501.

SMITH, T.H., MOONEY, J. and KORN, J.H. (1993) Modulation of cellular adhesion by anti-inflammatory drugs. *Arthritis and Rheumatism* **36**(Suppl. S2), Abstract D105.

SMITH, W.L., GARAVITO, R.M. and DEWITT, D.L. (1996) Prostaglandin endoperoxide H synthases (cyclooxygenases)-1 and -2. *Journal of Biological Chemistry* **271**, 33157–33160.

SMITHGALL, T.E. and PENNING, T.M. (1986) Inhibition of *trans*-dihydrodiol oxidation by the nonsteroidal anti-inflammatory drugs. *Carcinogenesis* **7**, 583–588.

SNAPPER, J.R., HUTCHISON, A.A., OGLETREE, M.L. and BRIGHAM, K.L. (1983) Effects of cyclooxygenase inhibitors on the alterations in lung mechanics caused by endotoxemia in the unanesthetized sheep. *Journal of Clinical Investigation* **72**, 63–76.

SOBRADO, J., MOLDAWER, L.L., BISTRAN, B.R., DINARELLO, C.A. and BLACKBURN, G.L. (1983) Effect of ibuprofen on fever and metabolic changes induced by continuous infusion of leukocyte pyrogen (interleukin 1) or endotoxin. *Infection and Immunity* **42**, 997–1005.

SPINAS, G.A., BLOESCH, D., KELLER, U., ZIMMERLI, W. and CAMMISULI, S. (1991) Pretreatment with ibuprofen augments circulating tumor necrosis factor-alpha, interleukin-6, and elastase during acute endotoxinemia. *Journal of Infectious Diseases* **163**, 89–95.

SPISANI, S., VANZINI, G. and TRANIELLO, S. (1979) Inhibition of human leukocytes locomotion by anti-inflammatory drugs. *Experientia* **35**, 803–804.

SPISANI, S., DOVIGO, L., CARLETTI, R. and TRANIELLO, S. (1982) Defective responsiveness to natural and pharmacological molecules of neutrophil locomotion in rheumatoid arthritis disease. *Scandanavian Journal of Rheumatology* **11**, 246–250.

SRIVASTAVA, K., DASGUPTA, P.K., SRIVASTAVA, A.K. and MURTHY, P.S. (1989) Role of plasminogen activators and leukocytes in IUD-induced inflammation: effect of some anti-inflammatory agents. *Advances in Contraception* **5**, 173–178.

STEPHENS, R.W., WALTON, E.A., GHOSH, P., TAYLOR, T.K.F., GRAMSE, M. and HAVEMANN, K. (1980) A radioassay for proteolytic cleavage of isolated cartilage proteoglycan 2.

Inhibition of human leukocyte elastase and cathepsin G by anti-inflammatory drugs. *Arzneimittel-Forschung* **30**, 2108–2112.

STEWART, W.F., KAWAS, C., CORRADA, M. and METTER, E.J. (1997) Risk of Alzheimer's disease and duration of NSAID use. *Neurology* **48**, 626–632.

STICHTENOTH, D.O., TSIKAS, D., GUTZKI, F.-M. and FRÖLICH, J.C. (1996) Effects of ketoprofen and ibuprofen on platelet aggregation and prostanoid formation in man. *European Journal of Clinical Pharmacology* **51**, 231–234.

STRATMAN, N.C., CARTER, D.B. and SETHY, V.H. (1997) Ibuprofen: effect on inducible nitric oxide synthase. *Molecular Brain Research* **50**, 107–112.

STRATTON, J.A., MILLER, R.D., KENT, D.R., THRUPP, L.D., RICHARDS, C. and DISAIA, P.J. (1984) Depressed mononuclear cell phagocytic activity associated with menstruation. *Journal of Clinical Immunology* **15**, 127–131.

SUWA, T., URANO, H., KOHNO, Y., SUZUKI, A. and AMANO, T. (1987) Comparative studies on the gastrointestinal lesions caused by several nonsteroidal anti-inflammatory agents in rats. *Agents and Actions* **21**, 167–172.

SWIERKOSZ, T.A., MITCHELL, J.A., WARNER, T.D., BOTTING, R.M. and VANE, J.R. (1995) Co-induction of nitric oxide and cyclooxygenase: interactions between nitric oxide and prostanoids. *British Journal of Pharmacology* **114**, 1335–1342.

SWINGLE, K.F., MOORE, G.G.I. and GRANT, T.J. (1976) 4-Nitro-2-phenoxymethanesulfonanilide (R-805): a chemically novel anti-inflammatory agent. *Archives Internationales de Pharmacodynamie et de Thérapie* **221**, 132–139.

SZARY, A. (1979) Studies on the experimental therapy of iridocyclitis. *Archivum Immunologiae et Therapiae Experientalis* **27**, 899–910.

TAHAMONT, M.V. and GEE, M.H. (1986) The effects of cyclooxygenase inhibition on chemiluminescence and aggregation in sheep neutrophils. *Prostaglandins and Leukotrienes in Medicine* **24**, 139–149.

TAKEUCHI, K., ITO, K., IWAMA, M. *et al.* (1985) Anti-inflammatory activity of the dry distillation tar of delipidated soybean (Glyteer) (1). *Folio Pharmacologica Japonica* **85**, 397–406.

TALESNIK, J. and HSIA, J.C. (1982) Coronary flow reactions to arachidonic acid are inhibited by docosahexaenoic acid. *European Journal of Pharmacology* **80**, 255–258.

TAYLOR, R.J. and SALATA, J.J. (1976) Inhibition of prostaglandin synthetase by tolmetin (Tolectin, McN-2559), a new nonsteroidal anti-inflammatory drug. *Biochemical Pharmacology* **25**, 2479–2484.

TEIXERA, M.M., WILLIAMS, T.J. and HELLEWELL, P.G. (1993) Role of prostaglandins and nitric oxide in acute inflammatory reactions in guinea-pig skin. *British Journal of Pharmacology* **110**, 1515–1521.

CHAPTER 5

THILO, D., NYMAN, D. and DUCKERT, F. (1974) A study of the effects of the antirheumatic drug ibuprofen (Brufen®) on patients being treated with the oral anti-coagulant phenprocoumon (Marcoumar®). *Journal of International Medical Research* **2**, 276–278.

THOMAS, P., HEPBURN, B., KIM, H.C. and SAIDI, P. (1982) Nonsteroidal anti-inflammatory drugs in the treatment of hemophilic arthropathy. *American Journal of Hematology* **12**, 131–137.

THOMPSON, M. and ANDERSON, M. (1970) Studies of gastrointestinal blood loss during ibuprofen therapy. *Rheumatology and Physical Medicine* **11**(Suppl.), 104–107.

TOMLINSON, R.V., RINGOLD, H.J., QUERSHI, M.C. and FORCHIELLI, E. (1972) Relationship between inhibition of prostaglandin synthesis and drug efficacy: support for the current theory on mode of action of aspirin-like drugs. *Biochemical and Biophysical Research Communications* **46**, 552–559.

TÖRNKVIST, H. and LINDHOLM, T.S. (1980) Effect of ibuprofen on mass and composition of fracture callus and bone. *Scandinavian Journal of Rheumatology* **9**, 167–171.

TRABER, D.L., ADAMS, T. JR, HENRIKSEN, N. and TRABER, L.D. (1984) Ibuprofen and diphenhydramine reduce the lung lesion of endotoxemia in sheep. *Journal of Trauma* **24**, 835–840.

TRACY, T.S., WIRTHWEIN, D.P. and HALL, S.H. (1993) Metabolic inversion of (*R*)-ibuprofen. Formation of ibuprofenyl-coenzyme A. *Drug Metabolism and Disposition* **21**, 114–120.

TROULLOS, E., HARGREAVES, K.M., TVRZICKÁ, A. and DIONNE, R.A. (1997) Ibuprofen elevates immunoreactive β-endorphin levels in humans during surgical stress. *Clinical Pharmacology and Therapeutics* **62**, 74–81.

TSUKADA, W., TSUBOKAWA, M., MASUKAWA, T., KOJIMA, H. and KASAHARA, A. (1978) Pharmacological study of 6,11-dihydro-11-oxodibenz[*b,e*]oxepin-3-acetic acid (oxepinac): a new anti-inflammatory drug. *Arzneimittel-Forschung* **28**, 428–438.

TURSI, A., LORIA, M.P., SPECCHIA, G. and CASAMESSIMA, D. (1982) *In vitro* studies of anti-inflammatory activity of carprofen. *European Journal of Rheumatology and Inflammation* **5**, 488–491.

TVRZICKÁ, E., CVRČKOVÁ, E., MÁCA, B. and JIRÁSKOVA, M. (1994) Changes in the liver, kidney and heart fatty acid composition following administration of ibuprofen to mice. *Journal of Chromatography B* **656**, 51–57.

URQUHART, E. (1991) A comparison of synovial fluid concentrations of nonsteroidal anti-inflammatory drugs with their *in vitro* activity. *Agents and Actions* **32**, 261–265.

URQUHART, E. (1993) Central analgesic activity of nonsteroidal anti-inflammatory drugs in animal and human pain models. *Seminars in Arthritis and Rheumatism* **23**, 198–205.

UTSUNOMIYA, T., KRAUSZ, M.M., DUNHAM, B. *et al.* (1982) Modification of inflammatory response to aspiration with ibuprofen. *Americal Journal of Physiology* **243**, H903–H910.

Van Arman, C.G., Begany, A.J., Miller, L.M. and Pless, H.H. (1965) Some details on the inflammations caused by yeast and carrageenin (with appendix on kinetics of the reaction). *Journal of Pharmacology and Experimental Therapeutics* **150**, 328–334.

Vanderhoek, J.Y. and Bailey, J.M. (1984) Activation of a 15-lipoxygenase/leukotriene pathway in human polymorphonuclear leukocytes by the anti-inflammatory agent ibuprofen. *Journal of Biological Chemistry* **259**, 6752–6756.

Vanderhoek, J.Y., Eckborg, S.L. and Bailey, J.M. (1984) Nonsteroidal anti-inflammatory drugs stimulate 15-lipoxygenase/leukotriene pathway in human polymorphonuclear leukocytes. *Journal of Allergy and Clinical Immunology* **74**, 412–417.

Van der Kraan, P.M., Vitters, E.L., de Vries, B.J., van den Berg, W.B. and van de Putte, L.B.A. (1990) The effect of chronic paracetamol administration to rats on the glycaminoglycan content of patellar cartilage. *Agents and Actions* **29**, 218–223.

Vane, J.R. (1971) Inhibition of prostaglandin synthesis as a mechanism of action for aspirin-like drugs. *Nature New Biology* **231**, 232–239.

Vane, J.R. and Botting, R.M. (1995) New insights into the mode of action of anti-inflammatory drugs. *Inflammation Research* **44**, 1–10.

Vane, J.R. and Botting, R.M. (1996) Overview — mechanisms of action of anti-inflammatory drugs. In: Vane, J., Botting, J. and Botting, R. (eds), *Improved Non-Steroid Anti-Inflammatory Drugs. COX-2 Enzyme Inhibitors*. Lancaster, Kluwer Academic Publishers, and London, William Harvey Press, 1–27.

van Leishout, E.M.M., Tiemesssen, D.M., Peters, W.H.M. and Jansen, J.B.M.J. (1997) Effects of nonsteroidal anti-inflammatory drugs on glutathione *S*-transferases of the rat digestive tract. *Carcinogenesis* **18**, 485–490.

Varvarigou, A., Bardin, C.L., Beharry, K., Chemtob, S., Papageorgiou, A. and Aranda, J.V. (1996) Early ibuprofen administration to prevent patent ductus arteriosus in premature newborn infants. *Journal of the American Medical Association* **275**, 539–544.

Vasconcelos Tiexeira, A., Abrunhosa, R. and Poças, L. (1977) Observations on the gastric mucosa of rheumatic patients before and after ibuprofen administration as studied by pentagastrin test, endoscopy, and light and electonmicroscopy. *Journal of International Medical Research* **5**, 243–252.

Ventafridda, V., De Conno, F., Panerai, A.E., Maresca, V., Monza, G.C. and Ripamonti, C. (1990) Nonsteroidal anti-inflammatory drugs as first step in cancer pain therapy: double-blind within-patient study comparing nine drugs. *Journal of International Medical Research* **18**, 21–29.

Verissimo de Mello, S.B., Novaes, G.S., Laurindo, I.M.M., Muscará, de Barros Maciel, F.M. and Cossermelli, W. (1997) Nitric oxide synthase inhibitor influences prostaglandin and interleukin-1 production in experimental arthritic joints. *Inflammation Research* **46**, 72–77.

■
CHAPTER 5
■

VIGNON, E., MATHIEU, P., LOUISOT, P. and RICHARD, M. (1991) *In vitro* effect of nonsteroidal anti-inflammatory drugs on proteoglycanase and collagenase activity in human osteoarthritic cartilage. *Arthritis and Rheumatism* **34**, 1332–1335.

VILLANUEVA, M., HECKENBERGER, R., PALMER, M. and SCHRÖR, K. (1992) Stereospecific and non-stereospecific effects of ibuprofen on human platelet and polymorphonuclear leukocyte functions. *Agents and Actions* **37**(Suppl.), 162–170.

VILLANUEVA, M., HECKENBERGER, H., PALMER, S.M. and SCHRÖR, K. (1993) Equipotent inhibition by (R)-(–)-, (S)-(+)- and racemic ibuprofen of human polymorphonuclear cell function *in vitro*. *British Journal of Clinical Pharmacology* **35**, 235–242.

VINEGAR, R., SCHREIBER, W. and HUGO, R. (1969) Biphasic development of carrageenin oedema in rats. *Journal of Pharmacology and Experimental Therapeutics* **166**, 96–103.

VINEGAR, R., TRAUX, J.F. and SELPH, J.L. (1976) Quantitative studies on the pathway to acute carrageenan inflammation. *Federation Proceedings* **35**, 2447–2456.

VINEGAR, R., TRAUX, J.F., SELPH, J.L. and VOELKER, F.A. (1982) Pathway of onset, development, and decay of carrageenan pleurisy in the rat. *Federation Proceedings* **41**, 2588–2595.

WAGNER, K.A., NANDI, J., KING, R.L. and LEVINE, R.A. (1995) Effects of nonsteroidal anti-inflammatory drugs on ulcerogenesis and gastric secretion in pyloris ligated rat. *Digestive Diseases and Sciences* **40**, 134–140.

WALKER, J.S. (1995) NSAID: an update on their analgesic effects. *Clinical and Experimental Pharmacology and Physiology* **22**, 855–860.

WALKER, J.S., NGUYEN, T.V. and DAY, R.O. (1994) Clinical response to nonsteroidal anti-inflammatory drugs in urate-crystal induced inflammation: a simultaneous study of intersubject and intrasubject variability. *British Journal of Pharmacology* **38**, 341–347.

WALLIS, W.J. and SIMKIN, P.A. (1983) Antirheumatic drug concentrations in human synovial fluid and synovial tissue. Observations on extra-vascular pharmacokinetics. *Clinical Pharmacokinetics* **8**, 496–522.

WALSER, S., HRUBY, R., HESSE, E., HEINZL, H. and MASCHER, H. (1997) Preliminary toxicokinetic study with different crystal forms of (S)-(+)-ibuprofen (dexibuprofen) and R,S-ibuprofen in rats. *Arzneimittel-Forschung* **47**, 750–754.

WALTER, K. and DILGER, C. (1997) Ibuprofen in human milk. *British Journal of Clinical Pharmacology* **44**, 211–212.

WALTON, E.A., GHOSH, P., TAYLOR, T.K.F., GRAMSE, M. and HAVEMANN, K. (1978) A radioassay for proteolytic cleavage of isolated cartilage proteoglycan. *Analytical Biochemisty* **90**, 726–736.

WANG, B.C., BUDZILOVICH, G., HILLER, J.M., ROSENBERG, C., HILLMAN, D.E. and TURNDORF, H. (1994) Antinociception with motor blockade after subarachnoid administration of S-(+)-ibuprofen in rats. *Life Sciences* **54**, 715–720.

WANWIMOLRUK, S., BROOKS, P.M. and BIRKETT, D.J. (1983) Protein binding of nonsteroidal anti-inflammatory drugs in plasma and synovial fluid of arthritic patients. *British Journal of Clinical Pharmacology* **15**, 91–94.

WARD, P.H., MALDONADO, M., ROA, J., MANRIQUEZ, V. and VIVALDI, E. (1995) Ibuprofen protects rat livers from oxygen-derived free radical-mediated injury after tourniquet shock. *Free Radical Research* **22**, 561–569.

WARRINGTON, S.J., HALSEY, A. and O'DONNELL, L. (1982) A comparison of gastrointestinal bleeding in healthy volunteers treated with tiaprofenic acid, aspirin or ibuprofen. *Rheumatology* **7**, 107–110.

WECHTER, W.J., LOUGHEAD, D.G., REISCHER, R.J., VAN GIESSEN, G.J. and KAISER, D.G. (1974) Enzymatic inversion of saturated carbon: nature and mechanism of the inversion of (R)-(–) p-iso-butyl hydratropic acid. *Biochemical and Biophysical Research Communications* **61**, 833–837.

WEIBERT, R.T., TOWNSEND, R.J., KAISER, D.G. and NAYLOR, A.J. (1982) Lack of ibuprofen excretion into human milk. *Clinical Pharmacy* **1**, 457–458.

WEISSMANN, G., SMOLEN, J.E. and HOFFSTEIN, S. (1978) Polymorphonuclear leukocytes as secretory organs of inflammation. *Journal of Investigative Dermatology* **71**, 95–99.

WENNOGLE, L.P., LIANG, H., QUINTAVALLA, J.C. *et al.* (1995) Comparison of recombinant cyclooxygenase-2 to native isoforms: aspirin labelling of the active site. *FEBS Letters* **371**, 315–320.

WERLER, M.M., MITCHELL, A.A. and SHAPIRO, S. (1992) First trimester maternal use in relation to gastroschisis. *Teratology* **45**, 361–367.

WERNS, S.W., SHEA, M.J. and LUCCHESI, B.R. (1985) Free radicals in ischemic myocardial injury. *Journal of Free Radicals in Biology and Medicine* **1**, 103–110.

WESSELS, D.A. and HEMPEL, S.L. (1996) Ibuprofen protects human endothelial cells prostaglandin H synthase from hydrogen peroxide. *American Journal of Physiology* **271**, C1879–C1886.

WHEELER, A.P., HARDIE, W.D. and BERNARD, G.R. (1992) The role of cyclooxygenase products in lung injury induced by tumor necrosis factor in sheep. *American Review of Respiratory Diseases* **145**, 632–639.

WHELTON, A. and HAMILTON, C.W. (1994) Renal toxicity of nonsteroidal anti-inflammatory drugs. In: LEWIS, A.J. and FURST, D.E. (eds), *Nonsteroidal Anti-Inflammatory Drugs. Mechanisms and Clinical Uses.* New York, Marcel Dekker, 195–205.

WHITEHOUSE, M.W. (1965) Some biochemical and pharmacological properties of anti-inflammatory drugs. *Progress in Drug Research* **8**, 321–429.

WHITEHOUSE, M.W. and RAINSFORD, K.D. (1980) Esterfication of acidic anti-inflammatory drugs suppresses their gastro-toxicity without adversely affecting their anti-inflammatory activity in rats. *Journal of Pharmacy and Pharmacology* **32**, 795–796.

CHAPTER 5

WHITEHOUSE, M.W. and RAINSFORD, K.D. (1987) Why are nonsteroidal anti-inflammatory drugs so gastrotoxic, even when given orally as solubilized salt formulations or parenterally? In: RAINSFORD, K.D. and VELO, G.P. (eds), *Side-effects of Anti-inflammatory Drugs. Part 2. Studies in Major Organ Systems.* Lancaster, MTP Press, 55–65.

WIHOLM, B.E., MYRHED, M. and EKMAN, E. (1987) Trends and patterns in adverse drug reactions to nonsteriodal anti-inflammatory drugs reported in Sweden. In: RAINSFORD, K.D. and VELO, G.P. (eds), *Side-effects of Anti-inflammatory Drugs. Part 1. Clinical and Epidemiological Aspects.* Lancaster, MTP Press, 55–70.

WIJNAR, R.J., HEARN, T. and STARKWEATHER, S. (1980) Augmentation of allergic histamine release from human leukocytes by nonsteroidal anti-inflammatory — analgesic agents. *Journal of Allergy and Clinical Immunology* 66, 37–45.

WILHELMI, G. (1949) Ueber die pharmakologischen Eigenschaften von Irgapyrin, einem neuen Präparat aus der Pyrazolreihe. *Schweizer Medizinische Wochenschrift* 79, 577.

WILLIAMS, K.M. and DAY, R.O. (1985) Stereoselective disposition — basis for variability in response to NSAIDs. In: BROOKS, P.M. and DAY, R.O. (eds), *Basis for Variability in Response.* Basel, Birkhäuser, 119–127.

WILLIAMS, K.M. and DAY, R.O. (1988) The contribution of enantiomers to variability in response to anti-inflammatory drugs. In: BROOKS, P.M., DAY, R.O., WILLIAMS, K. and GRAHAM, G. (eds), *Basis for Variability of Response to Anti-Rheumatic Drugs,* Proceedings of a Satellite Meeting of the Xth International Congress of Pharmacology. Basel, Birkhäuser, 76–84.

WILLIAMS, K., DAY, R., KNIHINICKI, R. and DUFFIELD, A. (1986) The stereoselective uptake of ibuprofen enantiomers into adipose tissue. *Biochemical Pharmacology* 35, 3405–3409.

WILLIS, A.L. (1970) Identification of prostaglandin E_2 in rat inflammatory exudate. *Pharmacological Research Communications* 2, 297–304.

WINDER, C.V., WAX, J., BURR, V., BEEN, M. and ROSIERE, C.E. (1958) A study of pharmacological influences on ultraviolet erythema in guinea-pigs. *Archives Internationale Pharmacodynamamie et de Thérapie* 116, 261–292.

WINTER, C.A., RISLEY, E.A. and NUSS, G.W. (1962) Carrageenin-induced oedema in the hind paw of the rat as an assay for anti-inflammatory drugs. *Proceedings of the Society of Experimental Biology and Medicine* 111, 544–547.

WISE, W.C., COOK, J.A., ELLER, T. and HALUSHKA, P.V. (1980) Ibuprofen impoves survival from endotoxic shock in the rat. *Journal of Pharmacology and Experimental Therapeutics* 215, 160–164.

WITKIN, S.S., HIRSCH, J. and LEDGER, W.J. (1986) A macrophage defect in women with recurrent Candida vaginitis and its reversal *in vitro* by prostaglandin inhibitors. *American Journal of Obstetrics and Gynecology* 155, 790–795.

PHARMACOLOGY AND TOXICOLOGY OF IBUPROFEN

WOOLF, C.J. (1989) Recent advances in the pathophysiology of acute pain. *British Journal of Anaesthesia* **63**, 139–146.

WOOLF, C.J. (1991) Generation of acute pain: central mechanisms. *British Medical Bulletin* **47**, 523–533.

YAMANAKA, S., IWAO, H., YUKIMURA, T., KIM, S. and MIURA, K. (1993) Effect of the platelet activating factor antagonist, TCV-309, and the cyclooxygenase inhibitor, ibuprofen, on the hemodynamic changes in canine experimental endotoxic shock. *British Journal of Pharmacology* **110**, 1501–1509.

ZAPATA-SIRVENT, R., HANSBROUGH, J.F. and BARTLE, E.J. (1986) Prevention of posttraumatic alterations in lymphocyte subpopulations in mice by immunomodulating drugs. *Archives of Surgery* **121**, 116–122.

ZHAO, B., GEISSLINGER, G., HALL, I., DAY, R.O. and WILLIAMS, K.M. (1992) The effect of the enantiomers of ibuprofen and flurbiprofen on the β-oxidation of palmitate in the rat. *Chirality* **4**, 137–141.

ZIA-AMIRHOSSEINI, P., HARRIS, R.Z., BRODSKY, F.M. and BENET, L.Z. (1995) Hypersensitivity to nonsteroidal anti-inflammatory drugs. *Nature Medicine* **1**, 2–4.

ZIMMERMANN, H.J. (1994) Hepatic injury associated with nonsteroidal anti-inflammatory drugs. In: LEWIS, A.J. and FURST, D.E. (eds), *Nonsteroidal Anti-Inflammatory Drugs. Mechanisms and Clinical Uses*. New York, Marcel Dekker, 171–194.

CHAPTER 5

Therapeutics of Ibuprofen in Rheumatic and Other Chronic and Painful Diseases

W F KEAN[1]**, W W BUCHANAN**[2] **AND K D RAINSFORD**[3]

[1]McMaster University Faculty of Health Sciences, Hamilton, Ontario,
Canada; [2]Sir William Osler Health Institute, Hamilton, Ontario, Canada;
[3]Division of Biomedical Sciences, Sheffield Hallam University, Sheffield, UK

Contents

6.1 INTRODUCTION

Ibuprofen (2-(4-isobutylphenyl)propionic acid), was the first of the phenylalkanoic acid class of therapeutic value to be introduced into most countries for clinical use (Adams, 1987; see also Chapter 1). Several phenylalkanoic acids were discovered over a 15-year period at The Boots Pure Drug Company, and four of the analogues were brought to clinical trials (Adams, 1987). Among the first of these analogues, BTS-10335 at 2–4 g/day was effective in rheumatoid arthritis, but skin rash occurred in many patients (Bower *et al.*, 1979; Adams, 1987). The next clinical candidate, ibufenac, 2–2.4 g/day was active in clinical studies but necessitated withdrawal because of increased incidence of hepatotoxicity (Adams *et al.*, 1963; Thompson *et al.*, 1964; Adams, 1987). Another analogue, BTS 10499, was more potent than the others but caused skin rash in approximately 20% of patients (Adams, 1987).

6.2 OVERVIEW OF CLINICAL PHARMACOLOGY

Aspects of the pharmacology and toxicology of ibuprofen relevant to its use in rheumatic diseases and various pain states are briefly reviewed.

The original reports by Adams and colleagues (1967, 1970) identified that ibuprofen was 4–8 times as active as ibufenac in the ultraviolet erythema model in guinea-pigs; 4 times as active as ibufenac in the acetylcholine-induced mouse writhing test; and 5 times more active in the yeast-induced fever in rats.

The initial studies indicated that there was no difference in biological activity between the two optically active enantiomers of ibuprofen. The inversion of (*R*)-(−)-ibuprofen to the (*S*)-(+) enantiomer occurs in the liver, the intestine and in adipose tissue through an acyl co-enzyme A intermediate which can proceed to the formation of a triglyceride species (Williams and Day, 1985; Williams *et al.*, 1986; Mayer *et al.*, 1988, 1996; Menzel-Soglowek *et al.*, 1993; Tracey *et al.*, 1993; Shirley *et al.*, 1994).

Ibuprofen has analgesic and anti-inflammatory properties and was initially identified to be equivalent to aspirin (Davies and Avery, 1971; Huskinsson *et al.*, 1976). The drug is available worldwide in a wide range of tablet forms, 200, 400, 600, 800 mg and as an oral suspension, 100 mg/5 ml (American Medical Association, 1995; Reynolds, 1996). The lowest dose of 200 mg is available in most countries for over-the-counter (OTC) use (American Medical Association, 1995; Reynolds, 1996).

The absorption of ibuprofen is rapid and complete (greater than 80%) after oral ingestion (Davies and Avery, 1971; Kantor, 1979; Dollery, 1991). Plasma levels appear in 0.5 to 1.5 h but absorption is delayed by food (Davies and Avery, 1971; Kantor, 1979; Dollery, 1991). Ibuprofen is transferred slowly into the synovial space and remains within the synovial cavity in high concentration after plasma concentrations have decreased (Glass

CHAPTER 6

and Swannell, 1978; Whitlam *et al.*, 1981). Ibuprofen is 90% bound to plasma protein at concentrations of 200 µg/ml (Whitlam *et al.*, 1981). The drug is not excreted in measurable quantities in breast milk. Ibuprofen is eliminated by biotransformation through the cytochrome P450 2C isoform to the 2-[4-{2-hydroxy-2-methylpropyl}phenyl]propionic acid and 2-[4-{carboxypropyl}phenyl] propionic acid (Adams *et al.*, 1970; Dollery, 1991; Rudy *et al.*, 1991; Fracasso *et al.*, 1992). These metabolites are glucuronidated and all metabolites are pharmacologically inactive (Dollery, 1991; Rudy *et al.*, 1991). A taurine conjugate of ibuprofen, formed through ibuprofenyl-coenzyme A thioester is only a minor metabolite; 1.5% formed after ingestion of 400 mg of ibuprofen (Shirley *et al.*, 1994). The hepatic metabolism of ibuprofen does not result in impaired aminopyrine clearance (Abernathy and Greenblatt, 1983) and the elimination half-life of ibuprofen is in the range of 2–2.5 h.

Concurrent administration of aspirin with ibuprofen results in a reduction of serum concentrations but does not affect the elimination half-life of ibuprofen (Grennan *et al.*, 1979). Patients with rheumatoid arthritis demonstrated a weak increased clinical benefit with moderate doses of soluble aspirin and ibuprofen (Grennan *et al.*, 1979). Interactions might occur between warfarin and ibuprofen (Penner and Albrecht, 1975; Hansen, 1979; Gabb, 1996), but the effect is probably low grade compared with that of aspirin, azapropazone and phenylbutazone (Browers and de Smet, 1994). In a study of 36 males receiving ibuprofen 1200–1600 mg/day and warfarin 7.5 mg/day for 14 days, no effect was noted on warfarin binding to albumin and there was no effect on prothrombin, partial thromboplastin times, and the levels of coagulation factors II, V, VII, IX (Penner and Albrecht, 1975). The lack of direct interaction of ibuprofen with warfarin is most likely related to the fact that ibuprofen and warfarin compete for different sites of albumin binding (Sudlow 1975, 1976; Birkett, 1980). However, a slightly increased bleeding time may be related to the moderate effect of ibuprofen on platelet aggregation (Browers and de Smet, 1994; see also Chapter 5).

In patients with alcoholic liver disease, ibuprofen kinetics have been shown to be within normal limits (Albert and Gernaat, 1984). The pharmacokinetics of ibuprofen in children resemble those in adults (Nahata *et al.*, 1991). Normal ibuprofen pharmacokinetics are not appreciably changed in patients with renal insufficiency (Dollery, 1991), febrile children (Nahata *et al.*, 1991) and patients with rheumatoid arthritis (Albert and Gernaat, 1984).

In the majority of studies, ibuprofen pharmacokinetics indicate a potentially wide safety profile in inflammatory diseases, and in conditions of compromised hepatic and renal function (see Chapters 4 and 10).

Magnesium hydroxide enhances the oral absorption of ibuprofen (Neuvonen, 1991). Ibuprofen has been shown to displace the binding of phenytoin to albumin (Bachmann *et al.*, 1986; Johnson *et al.*, 1994). Ibuprofen 600 mg t.i.d. has no effect on plasma digoxin levels (Jorgensen *et al.*, 1991) or the antihypertensive activity of hydrochlorothiazide or enalapril, although plasma renin activity was decreased by ibuprofen (Koopmans *et al.*, 1987; Velo *et al.*, 1987). Cardiovascular functions including blood pressure are unaffected by ibuprofen in normal individuals (Bradley, 1991) or in hypertensive subjects taking verapamil (Houston *et al.*, 1995). However, blood pressure can be affected by ibuprofen in elderly subjects with renal insufficiency (Murray *et al.*, 1997) and in hypertensive subjects taking antihypertensive drugs (Koopmans *et al.*, 1987; Radack *et al.*, 1987; Davies *et al.*, 1988; Camu *et al.*, 1992) and in diabetic patients (Bakris *et al.*, 1995). Interaction with antihypertensive agents is relatively low irrespective of whether diuretics or combinations of these with other antihypertensive agents are considered (Johnson *et al.*, 1994a,b). Ibuprofen 400 mg and 800 mg doses in normal subjects inhibit furosemide-induced diuresis but not natriuresis (Passmore *et al.*, 1990). Ibuprofen 800 mg in patients with diabetes mellitus does not affect natriuresis although glomerular filtration rate is reduced (Bakris *et al.*, 1995). Ibuprofen 1200 mg t.i.d. did not affect the control of fasting blood sugar with chlorpropamide (Shah *et al.*, 1984). These studies suggest that the pharmacokinetic and pharmacodynamic activity of ibuprofen demonstrates relatively few significant drug–drug or drug–disease interactions (Browers and de Smet, 1994).

Animal toxicity studies with ibuprofen have demonstrated that the principal toxicological effects are on the gastrointestinal tract, commonly in the form of gastric ulcers (Adams *et al.*, 1969; Rainsford, 1977; Whitehouse and Rainsford 1987; Suwa *et al.*, 1987; Wiseman and Noguchi, 1987; Dollery, 1991). Dogs appear to be more prone than rats to gastric ulcers during ibuprofen treatment and this is probably related to the longer elimination half-life of ibuprofen in this species (Adams *et al.*, 1969; Adams, 1987). There is no evidence of significant intestinal damage with ibuprofen except at very high doses for long periods (Adams *et al.*, 1969). In contrast, some NSAIDs (e.g. diclofenac, indomethacin, sulindac) can produce intestinal perforation, diaphragm-like strictures and adhesions in patients with rheumatic diseases (Cohen, 1976; Bjarnason, 1988; Rainsford, 1994; Rainsford and Quadir, 1995). The major site of adverse reactions to nonsteroidal analgesics, including ibuprofen, occurs in the upper gastrointestinal tract. Elderly patients with chronic oesophageal-gastric reflux have been reported to develop oesophageal injury (Semble *et al.*, 1989). The commonest problem, however, with ibuprofen and other nonsteroidal anti-inflammatory analgesics is dyspepsia. The most serious problem with this class of drug is gastrointestinal hemorrhage (Willett *et al.*, 1994). This can occur with ibuprofen therapy, especially in the elderly (Griffin *et al.*, 1988, 1991; Gabriel *et al.*, 1991), although the risk appears to be much less with ibuprofen than with other nonsteroidal anti-inflammatory analgesics (Table 6.1; Griffin *et al.*, 1991; Langman *et al.*, 1994; Garcia Rodriguez and Jick, 1994; Rainsford and Quadir, 1995; see also Chapter 9). Colitis has been described patients on ibuprofen (Tanner and Raghunath, 1988; Reynolds, 1996).

The evidence that women are more prone to gastrointestinal complications is conflicting (Matthewson *et al.*, 1988). Misoprostol has been shown to heal ibuprofen-induced gastric ulcers (Jaszewski *et al.*, 1992). Hepatic injury appears least likely from ibuprofen

CHAPTER 6

TABLE 6.1

Risks of upper gastrointestinal bleeding ulcers derived from case-controlled studies and meta-analysis

	CSM ranking	Garcia Rodriguez and Jick (1994)			Langman et al. (1994)			Griffin et al. (1991)			Laporte et al. (1989)			Carson et al. (1991)			Gabriel et al. (1991)		
		RR	Pos	95% CI	RR	Pos	95% CI	RR	Pos	95% CI	RR	Pos	95% CI	RR	Pos	95% CI	RR	Pos	95% CI
Ibuprofen	1	2.9	1	1.78–5.0	2.0	1	1.4–2.6	2.3	1	1.8–3.0				1.0	1	Ref.	2.27	1	1.85–2.80
Diclofenac	2	3.9	3	2.3–6.5	4.2	2	2.6–8.8	4.3	3	3.4–5.4	7.9	3	4.3–14.6	1.5	3	0.7–2.9	2.84	2	1.68–4.82
Naproxen	5	3.1	2	1.7–5.9	9.1	3	5.5–15.1				6.5	2	2.2–19.6						
Ketoprofen	6	5.4	4	2.6–11.3	23.7	6	7.8–74.2												
Indomethacin	9	6.3	5	3.3–12.2	11.3	4	5.3–20.3	3.8	2	2.4–6.0	4.9	1	2.0–12.2	1.1	2	0.5–2.2	4.69	3	2.97–7.41
Piroxicam	11	18.0	6	8.2–39.5	13.7	5	7.1–26.3	6.4	4	4.8–8.4	19.1	4	8.2–44.3				11.12	4	6.19–20.23
Azapropazone	12	23.4	7	6.9–79.3	31.5	7	10.3–96.9												
Aspirin																	3.38		2.26–5.01
Overall	N/A	4.7		3.8–5.7	4.5		3.6–5.8										8.0		6.37–10.06
Overlap in groups rating		1–5			1–6			1,2			1–4			1–3			1–3		

RR denotes relative risk from calculated odds ratios.

Pos = position in ranking.

CSM ranking is the ranking by the UK Committee on the Safety of Medicines based on yellow card reports.

The overlap in groups is the estimate of overlap of risks based on overlap of the confidence intervals. It should be noted that the assessment of risk with azapropazone is subject to very high error since there were relatively few cases recorded. These data are only included because of the mention of this in the original cited texts.

From Rainsford and Quadir (1995), reproduced with the permission of the publishers of *Inflammopharmacology*, Kluwer Academic Publishers.

compared to aspirin and other nonsteroidal anti-inflammatory analgesics (Rodriguez *et al.*, 1994). It has been proposed that the lack of appreciable difference of gastric mucosal ulceration in mice between (*R*)-(−) and (*S*)-(+) enantiomers of ibuprofen may be due to the low intrinsic ulcerogenicity of the drug combined with the metabolic inversion of ibuprofen in the mouse (Rainsford, 1995). The (*S*)-(+) isomer of ibuprofen is more active than the relatively inactive (*R*)-(−) isomer, for inhibition of cyclooxygenase-2 (Boneberg *et al.*, 1996). Racemic (*rac*-)ibuprofen is almost equipotent as an inhibitor of COX-1 and COX-2 (O'Neill *et al.*, 1993; Smith *et al.*, 1994; Laneuville *et al.*, 1994; Vane and Botting, 1995). The low ulcerogenic activity of ibuprofen is most likely related to its pro-drug like character of the (*R*)-(−) enantiomer present in half of the racemate, as well as other pharmacokinetic features (see Chapter 5). While the efficacy of (*S*)-(+)-ibuprofen has been demonstated in patients with lumbar pain, rheumatoid arthritis, ankle sprains, ankylosing spondylitis and osteoarthritis (Rahlfs and Stat, 1996), at present the evidence for the advantages of pure preparations of the (*S*)-(+) enantiomer (Kean *et al.*, 1991; Evans, 1996) must remain largely theoretical until proper studies are carried out comparing its efficacy and tolerability to those of the racemic preparation.

Paracetamol (acetaminophen) may enhance the ulcerogenicity of ibuprofen (Bhattacharya *et al.*, 1991) but this drug has not been shown to produce mucosal injury in endoscopic studies on volunteers (Lanza *et al.*, 1986).

Less common and rare side-effects of ibuprofen include thrombocytopenia (Jain, 1994), an acute thrombocytopenia from an antibody-mediated mechanism in a patient with ankylosing spondylitis (Meyer *et al.*, 1993), and ulcerative proctitis in juvenile systemic lupus (Khoury, 1989). There is a report of a mild constriction of the ductus arteriosus and reversible oliguria (Østensen, 1994). Hemolytic anaemia has been described, but the relationship to glucose-6-phosphate dehydrogenase deficiency is undefined (Sanford-Driscoll and Knodell, 1986). Central nervous system toxicity occurs, including visual disturbance in the form of reduced contrast sensitivity (Ridder and Tomlison, 1992). Ocular side-effects with ibuprofen were noted by Collum and Bowen (1971), but some of the patients were on Plaquenil™ (hydroxychloroquine), which is well known to cause ocular side-effects. A later study of 247 patients with rheumatoid arthritis showed that no macular lesions were discoved when they were examined on two separate occasions (Williamson and Sturrock, 1976). Generally, ibuprofen is not asociated with any effect on visual fields, acuity, and colour sensitivity (Ridder and Tomlison, 1992). Ibuprofen, like other NSAIDs and paracetamol, has been reported to have some moderately disruptive effects on normal sleep patterns, and ibuprofen delays the onset of the deeper stages of sleep (Murphy *et al.*, 1994). Other adverse events recorded, including hypersensitivity reactions, are typical of NSAIDs (Reynolds, 1996; Rainsford and Velo, 1992).

Although ibuprofen can be used to treat mild musculoskeletal symptoms in patients with systemic lupus erythematosus (Karsh *et al.*, 1980), its use requires special caution, especially as it has been reported to cause an aseptic lymphocytic or eosinophilic

CHAPTER 6

meningitis (Giansiracusa *et al.*, 1980; Quinn *et al.*, 1984; Day *et al.*, 1987). This complication has also been reported in patients with no clinical evidence of rheumatic disease but with a positive anti-nuclear antibody (Ewert, 1989). The meningitis respond quickly to discontinuation of therapy, and there are no sequelae. The cause is unknown, and the complication has been reported with the use of other nonsteroidal anti-inflammatory analgesics, including tolmetin (Ruppert and Barth, 1981) and sulindac (Ballas and Donta, 1983), and the antibiotic cotrimazole (Kremer *et al.*, 1983). Aseptic meningitis in patients with systemic lupus erythematosus has also been reported with over-the-counter doses of ibuprofen (Katona *et al.*, 1988). It has also been reported in NZBZ/NZW mice (Berliner *et al.*, 1985).

Ibuprofen may also have beneficial side-effects (see aso Chapter 5). Of potential clinical significance is that the drug has been reported to induce protection against brain trauma in mice (Hall, 1985) and experimentally induced myocardial damage (Evans *et al.*, 1985), including that from cytotoxic therapy (Inchiosa and Smith, 1990). It may also reduce the onset and development of Alzheimer's disease and related dementias (Stewart *et al.*, 1997) and reduce the incidence of breast cancer (Harris *et al.*, 1996). Ibuprofen inhibits glucose modification of lens protein in the eye and may therefore be of benefit in the prevention of cataract formation (Raza and Harding, 1991). Ibuprofen has beneficial effects on alcohol-induced behaviour and cognitive effects (Naranjo and Bremner, 1993a,b) and can inhibit alcohol-induced teratogenic activity (Randall *et al.*, 1991). Ibuprofen has been shown to relieve muscle soreness in exercise (Hasson *et al.*, 1993).

Acute renal failure can be precipitated in patients with chronic kidney damage (Whelton *et al.*, 1986; Cummings *et al.*, 1988). No NSAID, however, is free of renal complications (Schlondorff, 1993). Interstitial nephritis and nephrotic syndrome have been reported with ibuprofen (Pierucci and Patrono, 1992) and the drug has been recorded to cause polyuria and nocturia (Novak, 1975). Heaton and Bourke (1976) reported papillary necrosis as a result of vasculitis due to ibuprofen and hypersensitivity reactions such as abdominal pain, nausea, vomiting and elevated liver enzymes have been recorded (Soneblick and Abraham, 1978; Shoenfeld *et al.*, 1980). These reactions are extremely rare, and patients who have developed the syndrome have mostly suffered from systemic lupus erythematosus or mixed connective-tissue disease (Soneblick and Abraham, 1978; Shoenfeld *et al.*, 1980). Only one rheumatic patient has died (Lee *et al.*, 1983), but ibuprofen has been reported to exacerbate systemic lupus erythematosus (Stratton, 1985), and lupus-like syndromes (Bar-Sela *et al.*, 1980) with positive anti-nuclear tests have been reported following use of ibuprofen.

Since its introduction into clinical use in the late 1960s, the therapeutic benefits of ibuprofen have been established in literature reports that have identified clinical efficacy, patient preference, acceptable incidence of adverse reactions, and a high patient tolerance in clinical trials of rheumatoid arthritis, osteoarthritis, ankylosing spondylitis, the reactive arthritides, gout, soft-tissue rheumatism, and clinical pain models.

6.3   RHEUMATOID ARTHRITIS

6.3.1   Early studies

The first clinical trials of ibuprofen in the treatment of arthritic conditions were performed in 1966 in patients probably with active rheumatoid disease (see Chapter 1). These initial studies indicated that the drug was active at doses as low as 300–600 mg daily (Chalmers, 1969; Adams, 1987). Later Boardman, Nuki and Hart (1967) compared 900 mg/day ibuprofen for 7 days with placebo in the first double-blind trial in 20 patients with classical or definite rheumatoid arthritis as judged by criteria of the American Rheumatism Association. The period of treatment was probably inadequate and numbers of patients were of insufficient power to discern a statistically significant effect for such a low dose and period. Thus, in retrospect it is not surprising that despite the patients being well selected the trial showed that ibuprofen did not confer benefit over placebo. This type of study would probably rank today as an initial dose-finding Phase I type study where safety would be a primary outcome measure. In this respect ibuprofen produced mild side-effects that were no different from placebo. Two patients had dyspepsia with ibuprofen and three on placebo also reported this side-effect. The expected gastrointestinal side-effects of ibuprofen were obviously no different from placebo at the dose of 900 mg/day.

Later, Thompson, Fox and Newell (1968) compared the effects of 600 mg/day ibuprofen with 3 g/day paracetamol for 2 weeks in 44 patients with rheumatoid arthritis (diagnostic criteria not specified) in a double-blind 4-way crossover study (by today's criteria this might be considered an N of 1 study). The statistical analysis by trends showed that ibuprofen was significantly preferred by patients compared with paracetamol. Thus, at the low dose of ibuprofen employed, this study with sufficient numbers of patients to give reasonable statistical power showed that the drug was an effective treatment even in comparison with paracetamol. In an open-label type study following this, the same authors compared ibuprofen in 55 patients, of whom 51 had rheumatoid arthritis, 3 had psoriatic arthritis and 1 had ankylosing spondylitis, in a study in which ibuprofen was given for 4–94 weeks at doses of 300–1000 mg daily (Thompson *et al.*, 1968). This study showed that ibuprofen treatment was associated with improvement or unchanged physical symptoms (morning stiffness, grip strength, joint tenderness, functional capacity) in the majority of patients, about half of whom showed improvement in their parameters.

Some of the early studies contained small numbers of patients and were without evidence of responsive disease in the pre-trial washout period (Dick-Smith, 1969; Dick *et al.*, 1970; Hingorani, 1970; Huskisson *et al.*, 1970; Sasaki, 1970; Brooks *et al.*, 1970; Mills *et al.*, 1973; Dornan and Reynolds, 1974; McArthur *et al.*, 1979), but most importantly the ibuprofen dose was too low (Boardman *et al.*, 1967; Jasani *et al.*, 1968; Chalmers, 1969; Dick-Smith, 1969). These studies used dosages in the order of 600–900 mg/day. Although efficacy of the drug was not pronounced, good tolerance was observed.

CHAPTER 6

285

Among these earlier studies were two large double-blind, multicentre trials, one in the United States involving two studies of 127 and 122 rheumatoid arthritis patients respectively (Brooks *et al.*, 1970). In the first they received 600 mg/day ibuprofen and in the second the higher dose of 900 mg/day in a parallel randomized study in comparison with 3.6 g/day aspirin for a total of 4 weeks following 2 weeks' prior treatment (standardization) with aspirin (Brooks *et al.*, 1970). Both doses of ibuprofen were comparable with aspirin in efficacy. While a similar pattern of side-effects was evident (all mild), with the exception of tinnitus with aspirin, the gastrointestinal symptoms were more pronounced in the first trial with 600 mg ibuprofen than in the second study with 900 mg ibuprofen, where the incidence and number of gastrointestinal as well as non-gastrointestinal symptoms was appreciably lower with ibuprofen than aspirin. The gastrointestinal symptoms may have been a carryover from the initial aspirin pre-treatment. This may also have explained the relatively high incidence of guaiac-positive stools that were reported with patients in both studies who received ibuprofen; these were again higher for both ibuprofen and aspirin in the first study than in the second. The clinical chemistry and blood parameters were unaffected by ibuprofen or aspirin treatments.

The other multicentre trial was performed in Japan under the auspices of the Drug Evaluation Committee of the Japan Rheumatism Association (Sasaki, 1970). Again, as with the above study (Brooks *et al.*, 1970), a placebo was not employed for comparison but aspirin was employed as the comparator drug, on the grounds that the action of ibuprofen resembles that of aspirin and the latter is established as a standard treatment in rheumatoid arthritis. One wonders what the regulatory agencies such as the US Food and Drug Administration would make of the first judgement today. In this study the lower dosage of both ibuprofen 600 mg/day and aspirin 2 g/day was employed because 'in our experience of Japanese patients, their tolerance of drug is usually quite low. Genetic factors, dietary habits, and their slender build may be responsible for this low tolerance' (Sasaki, 1970). Certainly, their body weight was strikingly low by Western standards: 83% of patients were of less than 60 kg body weight and 14 of 97 patients in the trial were up to 30 kg! A total of 5 of the original 102 cases withdrew from treatment; 3 on ibuprofen because of 'epigastralgia' (2) and flare-up (1) and 2 on aspirin because of flare-up (1) and skin rash (1). Pain improvement at 56 days was noted in 23% of patients receiving ibuprofen and 28% on aspirin, with the difference being non-significant; the improvement being observed in the majority (about half the patients). Interestingly, there was a significant reduction in erythrocyte sedimentation rate with both drugs. Two subjects who had take ibuprofen had increased liver enzymes; one involved marked increase in SGPT (serum glutamate-pyruvate transaminases) and the other a slight elevation of this enzyme and increase alkaline phosphatase. No ibuprofen patients had occult blood in their stools, but two patients on aspirin had evidence of faecal blood. There was no recording of adverse reactions in this study.

Another trial was performed by Cremoncini (1970) in Milan, Italy, in 76 patients — 74 with osteoarthritis and 2 others non-defined — who participated in five studies. These comprised a double-blind comparison of ibuprofen 600 mg/day with mefenamic acid 760 mg/day for 15 days; two open studies with 600–1000 mg/day ibuprofen; an open trial of 600 mg ibuprofen sodium given as suppositories; and a single-dose study of the latter where blood levels were determined. In the double-blind study, ibuprofen was comparable with mefenamic acid in relief of symptoms; improvement being noted in about half the subjects. In the open study with ibuprofen given as suppositories, efficacy was similar to that following oral treatment, with the suppositories being well tolerated although the blood levels of the drug were variable. Side-effects were minor and comprised a rash in 3 subjects with a rise in SGPT in 3 others.

Thus these initial reports from several centres in the United Kingdom, Italy, Japan and the United States, presented at the first published Symposium on Ibuprofen (1970) held at the Royal College of Physicians in London on 13 March 1970, showed the efficacy of ibuprofen in treating rheumatic diseases. From there on, the use of ibuprofen became well established for treatment of rheumatoid arthritis as well as other arthritides.

6.3.2   Later higher dose studies

The clinical concept of rheumatoid arthritis has been refined over the last 30 years by a better understanding of the immune pathogenesis of the disorder. It is most likely that clinical trials of rheumatoid arthritis in the late 1960s and early 1970s contained some patients who were seronegative for rheumatoid factor and thus would better fit the current definition of the reactive arthritides. However, with appropriate randomization, it would be expected that equal numbers of these 'contaminant patients', if indeed they were included, would be distributed between the placebo and the ibuprofen group or the comparative drug group. Since ibuprofen has been shown to be of benefit in the reactive arthritides, it is most likely that the outcome of these early trials would not have been different if today's clinical definition of rheumatoid arthritis had been applied.

The original clinical studies of ibuprofen in rheumatoid arthritis were with dosages of 600–900 mg/day (see Chapter 1). It has been argued that the efficacy of ibuprofen in those dosages was not as great as has subsequently been shown with higher doses. Some authors stated that the 600–900 mg dosage displayed only analgesic effect but not an anti-inflammatory effect. Bloomfield and colleagues (1974) demonstrated that in low doses (300–900 mg/day) ibuprofen produced analgesic activity similar to that of aspirin. The study by P M Brooks and colleagues (1973) with doses of 1200–2400 mg showed superior efficacy at the higher dose although adverse reactions also increased in frequency (Godfrey and De la Cruz, 1975). One should be cautious in attempting to make such distinctions between analgesic and anti-inflammatory effects based solely on dose range for control of pain compared with soft-tissue swelling. The known pathophysiology of inflammation and pain transmission suggests that a distinction between analgesia and inflammation is probably a vague one between two ends of a continuous spectrum.

Hence, dose ranges for analgesic compared with anti-inflammatory effects inevitably overlap. Also, pharmacological dogma states that with NSAIDS much of their action in controlling pain derives from control of inflammation. Since the dose range for control of pain is lower than that for control of inflammation, this raises questions about the logic of the premise of separating analgesic from anti-inflammatory doses of NSAIDS such as ibuprofen in treating arthritic states. Thus, notwithstanding that NSAIDs express multiple individual activities on the different aspects of inflammation and pain transmission, the differences observed at low dose (600–900 mg) compared with a high dose (3200 mg) of ibuprofen in a clinical setting may merely display the responses at the extremes of the two ends of a continuum of the complex integrated process we refer to as chronic inflammation. Finally, it would be worth noting that it is very difficult to demonstrate anti-inflammatory effect in humans since measurement of, for example, digital joint circumference (having components of soft-tissue and joint swelling) is relatively crude.

Differences in response to ibuprofen are related to the dosage of the drug (Grennan et al., 1983). The study by Godfrey and De la Cruz (1975) showed a decrease in joint swelling with ibuprofen 2400 mg/day but not with 1200 mg/day. It is of interest that no significant difference was identified for these two doses in other measures of pain and inflammation, such as number of painful joints, grip strength, and morning stiffness. The evaluation of morning stiffness and grip strength is fraught with the dangers of interpretation biases for both, and with problems of reproducibility for grip strength. Mena and colleagues (1977) conducted a 6-week parallel double-blind study on 83 patients with rheumatoid arthritis using ibuprofen 3200 mg versus aspirin 4 g/day. Ibuprofen demonstrated similar analgesic activity to the aspirin, but aspirin was superior with respect to measures of joint swelling. The frequency of gastrointestinal tract adverse effects was less for ibuprofen but possibly not as advantageous as has been demonstrated in studies of ibuprofen using lower doses. In a 24-week multicentre double-blind controlled trial, Di Perri and colleagues (1987a) studied oral ibuprofen 600 mg t.i.d. versus oral imidazole salicylate 750 mg t.i.d. in 60 patients with classical or definite rheumatoid arthritis who were randomly assigned to one of the two treatments groups. Equal clinical benefit was identified for morning stiffness, grip strength, Ritchie's articular index and severity of joint pain. Systemic tolerability as assessed by hematological, liver, and kidney tests was normal in both groups. There was an overall low incidence of side-effects: 23% for imidazole salicylate and 33% for ibuprofen.

There are numerous studies that outline the clinical efficacy and good safety record of ibuprofen. The reviews by Adams and Buckler (1979), Kantor (1979) and Nicholson (1982), provide expert summaries of the first 10–12 years of the development and clinical use of ibuprofen. Ibuprofen has been demonstrated to be superior to placebo throughout a range of dosages (Jasani et al., 1968; Dick-Smith, 1969; Dick et al., 1970; Huskisson et al., 1970; Deodhar et al., 1973; Lee et al., 1976; Brugueras et al., 1978; Huskisson and Scott, 1979; Balogh et al., 1979; Australian Multi-Centre Trial Group 1980; Palmer et al., 1981).

Ibuprofen is of clinical value in the management of inflammatory rheumatoid arthritis in its early stages, in acute flare-up, and even in advanced disease. Overall, in nearly all the trials it has been demonstrated to be of equal efficacy to the majority of the currently available NSAIDs as shown in Table 6.2. The majority of clinical trials with ibuprofen have been of short duration (Deodhar *et al.*, 1973; Lee *et al.*, 1976; but see Wagenhauser, 1973, Neustadt, 1997, and later discussion).

An impressive array of studies have employed ibuprofen as a standard for comparison of all main parameters of efficacy and the range of tolerance with other NSAIDs in the treatment of rheumatoid arthritis (Table 6.2). Among the drugs that have been compared with ibuprofen are aspirin (Hadidi *et al.*, 1972; Hill *et al.*, 1990), benoxaprofen (now discontinued; Gum, 1980; Table 6.2), benorylate (Darlington and Coomes, 1975), choline magnesium trisalicylate (Ehrlich *et al.*, 1980), diclofenac (Garcia Rubio, 1976; Cardoe and Fowler, 1979; Brooks *et al.*, 1980; Meinicke and Danneskiold-Samsøe, 1980; Caldwell, 1986; Zuchner, 1986), diflunisal (Palmer *et al.*, 1981; Fasching, 1983; Bennett *et al.*, 1986), etodolac (Zwaifler, 1989; Neustadt, 1997), felbinac (topical ointment; Hosie and Bird, 1994), fenclofenac (now discontinued; Godfrey and Swain, 1985), fenoprofen (Reynolds and Whorwell, 1974; Gall *et al.*, 1982), flurbiprofen (Mena *et al.*, 1977; Buchanan and Kassam, 1986), ketoprofen (Mills *et al.*, 1973; Anderson *et al.*, 1974; Saxena and Saxena, 1978; Calin *et al.*, 1976; Montrone *et al.*, 1979; Kantor, 1986), mefenamic acid (Stockman *et al.*, 1976; Leslie, 1977), nabumetone (Friedel *et al.*, 1993; Morgan *et al.*, 1993), naproxen (Arendt-Racine *et al.*, 1978; Australian Multicentre Trial Group, 1980; Castles and Skosey, 1980; Gall *et al.*, 1982; Mungavin and Clarke, 1983; Taborn *et al.*, 1985; Todd and Clissold, 1990), oxaprozin (Hubsher and Walker, 1983; Appelrouth *et al.*, 1986; Poiley *et al.*, 1986), phenylbutazone (Pavelka *et al.*, 1973), piroxicam (Makisara and Nuotio, 1978; Balogh *et al.*, 1979; Turner *et al.*, 1982; Mungavin and Clarke, 1983; McLaughlin, 1985), pirprofen (Josef *et al.*, 1981; Todd and Beresford, 1986), sulindac (Burry and Witherington, 1979; Australian Multicentre Trial Group, 1980), proquazone (Ruotsi and Skrifvars, 1978), suprofen (now discontinued; Todd and Heel, 1985), tiaprofenic acid (Daymond *et al.*, 1979; Katona and Burgos-Vargas, 1981; Eastmond *et al.*, 1982; Bird *et al.*, 1984; Bird, 1985; Famaey and Huskisson, 1988; Todd and Clissold, 1991) and tolmetin (Gall *et al.*, 1982; McMillan, 1977, 1982). A variety of controlled and open-label studies have been performed showing the efficacy of ibuprofen in rheumatoid arthritis, and indeed in other rheumatic conditions (Symposium on Ibuprofen ('Brufen'), 1975).

Of the 50 trials in which ibuprofen was compared with other NSAIDs summarized in Table 6.2, the majority showed that ibuprofen was equipotent with other NSAIDs in the overall assessment of pain relief. It should be noted that in the assessment of these trials joint symptoms did not always relate to pain relief, and with some NSAIDs there were differences in these two overall parameters in the responses of ibuprofen compared with other NSAIDs.

CHAPTER 6

TABLE 6.2

Summary of comparative studies of ibuprofen with other NSAIDs in rheumatoid arthritis

Study	Sample size	Design[a]	Duration (days)	Outcome (drug, daily dose)[b]
Boardman et al. (1967)	20	DBC	14	IBU 900 mg = PLA
Jasani et al. (1968)	9	DBC	28	IBU 750 mg = ASA 5000 mg < PRED 15 mg
Chalmers (1969)	6	DBC	42	IBU 300–900 mg = ASA 3600 mg
Dick-Smith (1969)	30	DBC	42	IBU 1200 mg = ASA 2400–3600 mg > PLA
Dick et al. (1970)	9	DBC	28	IBU 400–800 mg = ASA 2400–3600 mg > PLA
Hingorani (1970)	38	DBC	14	IBU 600 mg = FLU 450 mg
Huskisson et al. (1970)	18	DBC	28	IBU 1200 mg = ASA 3600 mg > PLA
Sasaki (1970)	97	DBC	56	IBU 600 mg = ASA 2000 mg
Brooks et al. (1973)	127	DBP	28	IBU 600 mg = ASA 3600 mg
Deodhar et al. (1973)	37	DBC	35	IBU 1200 mg = IND 100 mg = NaS 400 mg > PLA
Hingorani (1973)	27	DBC	42	IBU 1200 mg = BEN 8000 mg
Mills et al. (1973)	35	DBC	28	IBU 1200 mg = KET 150 mg
Anderson et al. (1974)	150	SBP	14	IBU 1200 mg = KET 100–200 mg
Brooks (1974)	122	DBP	28	IBU 900 mg = ASA 3600 mg
Dornan and Reynolds (1974)	27	DBC	56	IBU 1200 mg = ASA 3600 mg
Reynolds and Whorwell (1974)	25	SBC	42	IBU 2400 mg = FEN 2400 mg = NAP 75 mg. AEs IBU = FEN > NAP
Blechman et al. (1975)	885	DBP/MCT	365	IBU 800–1000 mg = ASA 3600–6000 mg
Darlington and Coomes (1975)	43	DBC	42	IBU 600 mg = BEN 8000 mg
Godfrey and De La Cruz (1975)	41	DBP	28	IBU 2400 mg > IBU 1200 mg
	20	DBC	70	IBU 1600 mg = IND 100 mg
Huskisson et al. (1976)	90	DBC	56	IBU 1200 mg = FEN 2400 mg = KET 150 mg = NAP 500 mg. AEs IBU = NAP < FEN = KET
Lee et al. (1976)	684	SBC	14	IBU 1200 mg = ASA 319 mg = IND 100 mg = KET 100–200 mg = FLU 75 mg = MEF 1500 mg = ALC 3 g = BEN 4 g < PRED 15 mg > ACE 4 g and PLA
Stockman et al. (1976)	16	DBC	70	IBU 1200 mg = MEF 1500 mg > PLA
Calin et al. (1977)	102	DBP	90	IBU 1200 mg = KET 150 mg > PLA
McMillen (1977)	104	DBC	168	IBU 1600–2400 mg = TOL 1200–1800 mg for dropouts
Mena and Willkens (1977)	83	DBP	56	IBU 3200 mg = ASA 4000 mg
Mena et al. (1977)	208	DBP	42	IBU 2400 mg = FLU 1200 mg

Arendt-Racine et al. (1978)	64	DBP	112	IBU 1200 mg = NAP 500 mg = ASA 3600 mg. AEs IBU = NAP
Balogh et al. (1979)	20	SBC	28	IBU 1200 mg = PIR 20 mg. AEs IBU > PIR
Makisara and Nuotio (1978)	24	DBP	28	IBU 600–1200 mg = PIR 20 mg
Cardoe and Fowler (1979)	60	DBP	14	IBU 1600 mg = DCL 100 mg
Daymond et al. (1979)	41	DBC	28	IBU 1200 mg = TIA 600 mg
Huskisson and Scott (1979)	18	SBP	21	IBU 1200 mg = IDP 800 mg > PLA
Australian MTG (1980)	400	DBC	21 + 14	IBU 1200 mg = ASA 3900 mg = NAP 250–500 mg = SUL 200–400 mg > PLA
Brooks et al. (1980)	26	DBC	21 + 14	IBU 1200–1600 mg = DCL 75–100 mg
Gum (1980)		DBC	196	BEN 400–600 mg; ASA 4–6 g; IBU 1600–2400 mg all equal in efficacy but side-effects increased with ASA
Palmer et al. (1981)	20	DBC	42	IBU 1600 mg = DIF 750 mg > PLA
Scalie and Rivelis (1981)	30	DBP	30	IBU 1200 mg < IND 800 mg > PLA. AEs IBU = IND
Gall et al. (1982)	89	DBC	112	IBU 2400 mg = NAP 750 mg = FEN 3150 mg = TOL 1500 mg = ASA 4800 mg. AEs all IBU, NAP, FEN, TOL < ASA 3200 mg pretrial
Turner et al. (1982)	68	DBP/MCT	180	IBU 2400 mg = PIR 20 mg. AEs IBU > PIR
Mungavin and Clarke (1983)	373	DB	14	TIA 600 mg = IBU 1200 mg = IND 75 mg = NAP 500 mg = PIR 20 mg, BEN 600 mg
Bird et al. (1984)	30	DB	28	TEN 20–40 mg = IBU 2400 g
McLaughlin (1985)	21	DB	98	PIR 20 mg = IBU 2400 mg
Taborn et al. (1985)	75	DB	14	1600 mg IBU < NAP 750 mg in terms of morning stiffness/duration but not severity
Appelrouth et al. (1986)	152	MCT	52	IBU 1200–1800 mg = OXA 1200 mg AEs IBU = OXA
Poiley et al. (1986)	197	MCT	52	IBU 1200–1800 mg = OXA 1200 mg. AEs IBU = OXA
Bennett (1986)	210	DB	72	DIF/500–750 mg = IBU 1600–2400 mg
Caldwell (1986)	75	DB	70	DCL 150 mg > PLA = IBU 2400 mg
DiPerri et al. (1987a,b)	60	DB	168	IMS 75 mg = IBU 600 mg
Josef et al. (1981)	46	DB	6	IBU 1200 mg ≤ PPN 600 mg. AEs IBU < PPN
Neustadt (1997)	1446	DB/MCT	52	IBU 600 mg = 150 mg ETO < 600 mg ETO. AEs IBU = ETO

a DB, double blind; DBC, double blind crossover; DBP, double blind parallel; MCT, multicentre trial; SBP, single blind parallel; SBC, single blind crossover.

b >, greater than; <, less than; ACE, acetaminophen/paracetamol; ALC, alcofenac; ASA, aspirin; FEN, fenoprofen; BEN, benorylate; DCL, diclofenac; DIF, diflunisal; ETO, etodolac; FLU, flufenamic acid; IBU, ibuprofen; IMS, Imidazole salicylate; IND, indomethacin; IDP, indoprofen; KET, ketoprofen; MEF, mefenamic acid; OXA, oxaprozin; NAP, naproxen; NaS, sodium salicylate; PLA, placebo; PIR, piroxicam; PPN, pirprofen; PRED, prednisone; SUL, sulindac; TIA, tiaprofenic acid; TOL, tolmetin.

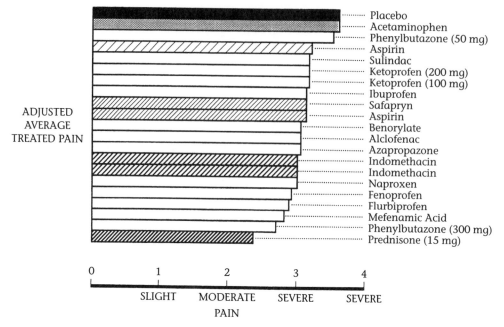

Figure 6.1: Comparison of the pain relief observed in rheumatoid arthritis patients receiving ibuprofen with that from other NSAIDs, steroids acetaminophen and placebo (Lee *et al.*, 1976)

The ranking of NSAIDs for their adjusted pain relief and mean satisfaction scores during therapy of rheumatoid arthritis where the drugs were given under standard dosage conditions has been reported by Buchanan and Kassam (1986) (Figure 6.1). While most scores were close to one another for all the NSAIDs, there was an appreciably lower score with prednisone 5 mg t.i.d. (Buchanan and Kassam, 1986). Paracetamol ranked with placebo, while mefenamic acid, flurbiprofen and indomethacin had the highest rating (Buchanan and Kassam, 1986). Next was aspirin, ibuprofen being equal with ketoprofen (Buchanan and Kassam, 1986). Mean satisfaction scores were similar to the pain relief scores (Buchanan and Kassam, 1986). These data suggest that most NSAIDs are similar to one another in pain relief and satisfaction although there are small differences between them; they are clearly less effective than corticosteroids and more effective than paracetamol.

6.3.3 Adverse events

In some of the studies summarized in Table 6.2 the adverse events reported with ibuprofen are less than with some NSAIDs, with others showing that the pattern and incidence are at least no worse than with comparator drugs. The incidence of adverse events appears to be dose-related.

The early studies with low dosage (300–900 mg) showed a low profile of side-effects for ibuprofen (Chalmers, 1969; Dick-Smith, 1969; Hingorani, 1970; Sasaki, 1970) and in some studies of higher dose, ibuprofen was shown to have a lower side-effect profile than aspirin (Dornan and Reynolds, 1974; Blechman *et al.*, 1975). However, the group studied by Blechman and colleagues (1975) had a lower hemoglobin level for pre-treatment values compared to the aspirin group at 1 year. In the high-dose study of ibuprofen 3200 mg/day versus aspirin 4000 mg/day by Mena *et al.* (1977), side-effects were more common in the aspirin group. The standard upper dose of ibuprofen, 2400 mg/day, versus high-dose flurbiprofen 120 mg/day (Mena *et al.*, 1977) showed a relatively low incidence of adverse effects for ibuprofen. In the studies by Huskisson and colleagues (1976) and Arendt-Racine (1978), the side-effect profile for ibuprofen was lower than that for ketoprofen and fenoprofen in the former study, and lower than for aspirin in the latter study. Mills and colleagues (1973), in a study of ibuprofen 1200 mg/day versus ketoprofen 150 mg/day, reported that, although side-effects were equal, dyspepsia was more frequent with ketoprofen. The study by Hingorani (1973) with ibuprofen 1200 mg/day versus benorylate 8000 mg/day demonstrated fewer side-effects for ibuprofen despite patient preference for benorylate, although there was no significant difference in therapeutic effect between the two drugs.

In one of the few long-term direct comparisons of ibuprofen with another NSAID, Neustadt (1997) compared ibuprofen 600 mg q.i.d. with two dosages of etodolac 150 mg b.i.d. This study was a double-blind 3-parallel-group multicentre trial (in 96 centres) in patients with active rheumatoid arthritis. While low-dose corticosteroid treatment was allowed, disease-modifying agents were not. Out of 1446 patients who were enrolled, about half completed 1 year's treatment, the dropout rates being about equal in all groups. Ibuprofen was of comparable efficacy with that of the two low dosage levels of etodolac. In long-term assessment, the higher dose of 1000 mg/day etodolac was more effective. The incidence of adverse events was the same in all three treatment groups, dyspepsia rate being slightly higher with ibuprofen than with the two dose levels of etodolac. The lack of efficacy was the main reason for discontinuation of therapy.

In general, the overall incidence and severity of side-effects due to ibuprofen is low compared to other NSAIDs (Royer *et al.*, 1984; Bird, 1985; Veltri and Rollins, 1988; Paulus, 1990; Fries *et al.*, 1991; Fries, 1995). The side-effect profile of ibuprofen has been shown to be similar to that of other NSAIDs but the incidence of gastrointestinal, renal and hepatic events is probably lower than with other NSAIDs (Rainsford and Velo, 1984; Fries, 1995; Rainsford and Quadir, 1995). There may be some variation in comparison of adverse events from ibuprofen with individul drugs. Thus, the incidence of adverse events in clinical trials with ibuprofen appears to be similar to that with tiaprofenic acid (Daymond *et al.*, 1979) and diclofenac (Stockman *et al.*, 1976; Brooks *et al.*, 1980). In contrast, Fries (1995) observed differences in the toxicity of other NSAIDs compared with ibuprofen in a review of 2747 patients with rheumatoid arthritis who had received 5642 courses of eleven NSAIDs. Toxicity was assessed by a weighted summation of symptoms, laboratory abnormalities

CHAPTER 6

and hospital admissions, based on a side-effect score of severity. Indomethacin, tolmetin and meclofenamate proved the most toxic, with intermediate toxicity for naproxen, sulindac, piroxicam, fenoprofen and ketoprofen, while the least toxic were identified to be salsalate and ibuprofen.

Epidemiological studies show that ibuprofen administered in antirheumatic doses exhibits one of the lowest profiles of toxicity in the treatment of patients with inflammatory disorders (Pavelka *et al.*, 1978; Brune, 1986; Levy, 1987; Weber, 1987; Wilholm *et al.*, 1987; Veltri and Rollins, 1988; Fries *et al.*, 1991; Carson and Strom, 1992; Rainsford and Quadir, 1995; see Table 6.1).

As noted previously, the majority of controlled double-blind clinical trials in which ibuprofen was studied in rheumatoid arthritis were of short duration (Table 6.2). It must be remembered that such trials are designed to answer the question whether the drug under study, in this case ibuprofen, at this or that dose, is superior to placebo in analgesic and anti-inflammatory effects, and how it compares to other nonsteroidal anti-inflammatory analgesics given in standard therapeutic doses. These questions therefore essentially address the pharmacological effects of ibuprofen, and to only a limited extent its toxicity. The patients who take part in such trials, because of necessary inclusion and exclusion criteria, are 'squeaky clean', so that toxicity almost certainly is less than occurs in patients with rheumatoid arthritis in the 'real world'. In order to assess the long-term therapeutic value of ibuprofen, a large number of patients need to be followed in either a double-blind or open study for a much longer period and dropout rates have to be recorded. Thus, Calin's group (1977) showed a dropout rate of 20% at 3 months of ibuprofen treatment, while Blechman and colleagues (1975) had a dropout rate of 60% at 12 months. These values are similar to the dropout rates for long-term trials of other NSAIDs (Lee *et al.*, 1976; Capell *et al.*, 1979).

Duration of use or survival data have been reported for ibuprofen 1200–2400 mg/day compared with indomethacin 75–200 mg/day, naproxen 500–100 mg/day, piroxicam 20 mg/day, sulindac 300–600 mg/day and tolmetin 800–1600 mg/day in 116 patients with rheumatoid arthritis treated with 188 courses of these treatments over a 3-year period (Luggen *et al.*, 1989). The sample size for this study was small and inevitably comprised 87.55% females with a highly variable background of disease duration, severity, and other components of clinical history. The unadjusted duration of use assessed by life table analysis showed that ibuprofen was used in a slightly greater number of subjects up to 500 days than was piroxicam but less so than sulindac and naproxen, the latter having the lowest dropout rate of all drugs. Since there were no data available with ibuprofen after 500 days of treatment, it is not possible to extend this comparison, although data were provided for the other drugs. In those patients who did not start or increase prednisolone dosage or disease-modifying drugs, the dropout rate was greater with ibuprofen than with the other drugs. The dropout from therapy can be from lack of efficacy or lack of acceptable tolerability. In this study it was not possible to establish the cause of dropout for ibuprofen. Some would suspect that the higher rate of dropout with drugs like ibuprofen reflects lack of efficacy. However, the situation can be more complex. One issue is that pain relief is progressing with time and also, coincidently, reports of gastrointestinal side-effects including ulcer perforation, bleeding and ulceration decline over several months of treatment with NSAIDs (Bolten, 1996). The issue is that the progressive decline of use of an NSAID may represent improvement having been achieved, such that the patients sees no benefit in taking the drug any longer. The decline in gastrointestinal side-effects with time would also appear at odds with the notion that dropout would increase because of this side-effect: where present, this effect is among the most serious leading to withdrawal from therapy.

Thus, in the absence of information about the cause of dropout, it is not possible to implicate any specific factors in the rates of decline from ibuprofen compared with other drugs.

Another indication of outcome in relation to the development of adverse events has come from follow-up of 13 230 members of the Group Health Cooperative of Puget Sound (Seattle, Washington State, USA) under 65 years of age who had been prescribed ibuprofen as outpatients and were reviewed within 3 months of receiving the prescription (Johnson *et al.*, 1985). The principal indication for prescription included arthritis. No serious uncommon illnesses were unequivocally attributed to the drug. In particular, no cases of acute liver or renal disease were observed. Of 15 patients hospitalized for newly diagnosed conditions that included (number of cases) agranulocytosis (1), aseptic meningitis (1), hemianopsia (1), erythema multiforme (1), peptic ulcer (1), gastritis/duodenitis (4), stomach ulcer with hemorrhage (1), hematemesis (1) and gastrointestinal bleeding (1). There were thus 8/15 cases of serious gastrointestinal adverse events that could be related to the actions of the drug. The other adverse events could be considered to be idiosyncratic for which there are no known mechanisms. The major groups that were exposed to the drug were females (79.6%) and subjects aged 30–39 years (23.8%).

6.3.4   Overall clinical outcomes

Although some clinical and *in vitro* studies (Ceuppens *et al.*, 1982; Cush *et al.*, 1990a; Menkes, 1993) have suggested a lowering of rheumatoid factor titre, and reduction in erythrocyte sedimentation rate and C-reactive protein with nonsteroidal anti-inflammatory analgesics, including ibuprofen, this has not been our clinical experience. We agree with Ward's conclusion in 1984 that doses of ibuprofen 1200 mg/day or more are as effective as aspirin and other nonsteroidal anti-inflammatory analgesics, but much less toxic (Ward, 1984).

6.4   JUVENILE RHEUMATOID ARTHRITIS

Clinical therapeutic trials of nonsteroidal anti-inflammatory analgesics have proved more difficult in children than in adults with rheumatoid arthritis. As a consequence, fewer clinical trials have been performed in juvenile rheumatoid arthritis than in the adult form of the disease. Ansell (1973) reported the first trial in 8 patients with Still's disease and observed satisfactory control with up to 32 mg/kg ibuprofen. Menon *et al.* (1973) also reported that ibuprofen was equal to aspirin in control of joint symptoms when the drug was given for 2 weeks, ibuprofen showing fewer side-effects of the two drugs. The effectiveness of Brufen™ and a liquid preparation in doses of 10–40 mg/kg body weight/day has been confirmed in both double-blind/multicentre and open studies (Sheldrake and Ansell, 1975; Brewer, 1977; Krasnova *et al.*, 1979; Brewer and Giannini, 1982; Giannini and Brewer, 1982; Giannini *et al.*, 1990; Stean *et al.*, 1990).

The Pediatric Rheumatology Collaborative Study Group in the United States has published results of studies with a number of nonsteroidal anti-inflammatory analgesics, including aspirin, fenoprofen, indomethacin, ketoprofen, meclofenamate sodium, pirprofen, oxaprozin, proquazone and tolmetin sodium in juvenile rheumatoid arthritis (Brewer and Giannini, 1982; Giannini and Brewer, 1982; Giannini *et al.*, 1990). While only minor differences in efficacy were noted, some of the drugs (e.g. aspirin, indomethacin, meclofenamate sodium and naproxen) were responsible for discontinuation from adverse events than ibuprofen or other drugs.

Ibuprofen in the liquid form has been found equipotent to aspirin, but with a better safety profile especially in the gastrointestinal tract and liver (Silver, 1988; Giannini *et al.*, 1990). It is recommended that, as with all NSAIDs, dosage should be increased stepwise, ranging from 20 to 40 mg/kg ibuprofen three to four times daily (Silver, 1988). The pharmacokinetics of ibuprofen in children is similar to that in adults, with the half-time of elimination from the plasma being approximately 2 h (Mäkelä *et al.*, 1980).

Naproxen is also available in a liquid form, but its use is limited by pseudoporphyria in fair-skinned patients (Lang and Finlayson, 1994). Although Reye's syndrome may occur as a result of metabolic disorders (Rowe *et al.*, 1988), there is little doubt that only aspirin, of the NSAIDs and analgesics used in children, is chiefly responsible for this condition. Reye's syndrome has been reported in juvenile rheumatoid arthritis and other connective-tissue diseases (Remington *et al.*, 1985; Rennebohm *et al.*, 1985; Sullivan *et al.*, 1988). For this reason it is our practice not to prescribe aspirin to children with juvenile rheumatoid arthritis or any other rheumatological disease, but to use ibuprofen as the NSAID of first choice. While it has been universal paediatric practice to use paracetamol as an antipyretic in children, it is now recognized that ibuprofen is equally as effective, or even more effective, than paracetamol in controlling fever (Kotob, 1985; Walson *et al.*, 1989; see also Chapter 7).

6.5 PRIMARY AND SECONDARY OSTEOARTHRITIS

Primary and secondary osteoarthritis result from the failure of the hyaline cartilage matrix and adjacent subchondral bone to function as a shock-absorbing or lubricating unit. The mechanisms involved in this failure and the processes that induce or modify the failure are complex, involving not only simple 'wear and tear' but active processes including cytokine-mediated and metalloprotease cartilage destruction, as well as systemic changes in growth factors that influence repair (Rainsford, 1996; March, 1997). The exact mechanism of action of NSAIDs such as ibuprofen in reducing the inflammation and pain of osteoarthritis is not entirely known, but the action probably takes place through several pathways such as inhibition of prostaglandin synthesis, inhibition of other aspects of the inflammatory process as described elsewhere (see Chapter 5), and interference with pain transmission at the free nerve endings, the dorsal horn of the spinal cord, and in the brain itself.

Osteoarthritis affects almost all of the synovial joints, although primary osteoarthritis usually appears in distinct patterns (van Sasse *et al.*, 1989; Liang and Fortin, 1991), for example the distal and proximal interphalangeal joints of the fingers, the carpometacarpal joints at the base of the thumbs, and sometimes the knees in association with the first metatarsal-phalangeal joint of the great toes. Other patterns include osteoarthritis that effects only the hip joints or only the knees.

Among the early studies of ibuprofen in osteoarthritis was one by Wagenhauser (1973), who found that 80 out of 114 patients had reduced pain when given daily doses up to 1200 mg of the drug over the course of a year. In many patients, joint tenderness and pain with exercise improved. In 1975, de Blécourt reported a double-blind crossover comparison of indomethacin versus ibuprofen in 39 patients with osteoarthritis of the hip and knee. Comparable objective improvements in joint movement were identified for the two drugs after 4 weeks. The side-effects were less with ibuprofen. Many early studies in osteoarthritis used relatively low doses. Patients studied by Boardman and colleagues (1967) did not detect therapeutic benefit or a difference between ibuprofen 600 mg/day and placebo. Sacchetti and colleagues (1978), using doses of ibuprofen of 900 mg/day, did demonstrate a response greater than placebo. Pipitone and colleagues (1973) demonstrated that ibuprofen 900 mg/day had equal effectiveness to indomethacin 75 mg/day and phenylbutazone 300 mg/day, in a double-blind trial of 21 patients with spinal osteoarthritis. The ibuprofen group had significantly fewer side-effects. A 6-month double-blind crossover study of indomethacin versus ibuprofen in 232 patients with osteoarthritis demonstrated that both compounds produced significant clinical improvement, but three times more patients withdrew owing to side-effects in the indomethacin 150 mg/day group than in the ibuprofen 1800 mg/day group. In the majority of studies in which higher doses have been used, ibuprofen is comparable to other drugs. Hingorani (1976) in a 4-week double-blind crossover study, demonstrated that ibuprofen 1600 mg/day had similar efficacy to azapropazone 1200 mg/day. Similarly, Brodie and colleagues (1980) identified that ibuprofen 1500 mg/day was similar to fenclofenac 1200 mg/day, although it was stated that fenclofenac produced superior pain relief. Bresnihan and colleagues (1978) reported no difference between diflunisal 500 mg/day and ibuprofen 1200 mg/day in a double-blind

CHAPTER 6

8-week study. No difference was identified between benoxaprofen 600 mg/day and ibuprofen 1600 mg/day in a 6-week double-blind crossover study (Highton and Grahame, 1980). Similarly, Tyson and Glynne (1980) found no difference between benoxaprofen 600 mg/day and ibuprofen 1200 mg/day in a double-blind 16-week study.

Altman (1984) provided an extensive and comprehensive review of 28 selected trials with ibuprofen that had been performed up to 1983; all but 3 of these had been double-blind, two others being single-blind and one unblinded. Where the daily dosage of ibuprofen was greater that 1200 mg, the drug gave clear benefit over placebo.

The effects of ibuprofen in osteoarthritic patients are dose-dependent (Altman, 1984; Rosenbloom et al., 1985). Approximately two-thirds of patients can be expected to respond to a daily dose of 1600–2400 mg (Rosenbloom et al., 1985). In a substantial number of double-blind controlled clinical trials, ibuprofen in doses of 1200 mg/day or more have been clearly demonstrated to be equipotent to most other nonsteroidal anti-inflammatory analgesics (Moxley et al., 1975; Andrade and Fernandez, 1978; Sacchetti et al., 1978; Cimmino et al., 1982; Klein, 1982; Caldwell et al., 1983; Umbenhauer, 1983; Altman, 1984; Cornhill and Rowley-Jones, 1984; Lambert et al., 1985; Sorkin and Brogden, 1985; Barnard-Jones et al., 1986; Di Perri et al., 1987b; Table 6.3) and paracetamol (Amadio and Cummings, 1983; Bradley et al., 1991; Griffin et al., 1995. However, these trials have been conducted on relatively few patients. A notable exception was the 3-week trial in 226 patients with osteoarthritis of the hip, knee or spine comparing naproxen 1000 mg/day to ibuprofen 1200 mg/day by the Manchester General Practitioner Group (1984). These workers found naproxen to be more effective, but noteworthy is the fact that one patient who received naproxen had a gastrointestinal bleed.

Few trials have been conducted with NSAIDs in patients with finger joint osteoarthritis (Tréves et al., 1995). In a recent critical review by Tréves et al. (1995) only 13 therapeutic trials had been performed between 1983 and 1994, seven of which were with NSAIDs; of these only two had been performed with ibuprofen. One trial was with oral ibuprofen and the other with ibuprofen administered percutaneously. Ibuprofen 600 mg/day by mouth was comparable to flurbiprofen 120 mg/day and flurbiprofen applied to the skin (Bolten, 1994). Another study by Dreiser and Tisne-Camus (1993) showed that ibuprofen 1600 mg/day b.d. was superior in pain relief to placebo in finger arthritis. However, topical nonsteroidal anti-inflammatory analgesics have a limited number of trials supporting their value (Dreiser and Tisne-Camus, 1993). In 3- to 6-week trials in 606 patients with knee osteoarthritis, glucosamine was found to be equipotent to ibuprofen, and had fewer side-effects (Rovati, 1992). Two trials of S-adenosylmethionine have shown slightly better results than with ibuprofen 1200 mg/day (Glorioso et al., 1985; Müller-Fassbender, 1987).

Sholes and co-workers (1995) compared the dropout rates in patients with osteoarthritis in a health maintenance organization (HMO) who had been prescribed four NSAIDs. They observed that rates of discontinuation with patients on NSAIDs were high after 1 year of therapy with these agents. They suggested that the rates of discontinuation were

TABLE 6.3

Summary of comparative studies of ibuprofen with other NSAIDs or placebo in osteoarthritis

Study; Joint[a]	Sample size[b]	Design[c]	Duration (days)	Outcome (drug, daily dose)[d,e]
Boardman et al. (1967)	19	DBC	14	IBU 600 mg = PLA
Wagenhauser (1973)	114	DBC	14	IBU 900 mg = IND 75 mg = PBZ. AEs IBU < IND, PBZ
Pipitone et al. (1973): Spine	21	DB	14	IBU 1200 mg = IND 75 mg
de Blécourt (1975)	39	DBC	56	IBU 1200 mg = PBZ 400 mg
Moxley et al. (1975)	144	DB	28	IBU = 1600 mg = AZA 1200 mg > PLA
Hingorani (1976): Knee	41	DBC	14	IBU 1200 mg = FBN 1800 mg. AEs IBU ≥ FBN
da Gama Moreira (1977)	29	DBP	42	IBU 900 mg > PLA
Sacchetti et al. (1977)				
Bresnihan et al. (1978): Hip, knee	30	DBP	56	For weight-bearing pain. IBU > DIF IBU 1200 mg = DIF 500 mg
Meineri et al. (1978): Knee/hip	16	DBC	14	IBU 1200 mg = PIR 600 mg. AEs IBU ≥ PIR
Brodie et al. (1980)	53	SB	84	IBU 1200–1600 mg < FEN 900–1200 mg (IBU 1500 mg = FEN 1200 mg)
Highton and Grahame (1980): Hip/knee	31	DBC	21	IBU 1600 mg = BEN 600 mg
Tyson and Glynne (1980): Hip/knee	105	DBP	28	IBU 1200 mg < BEN 600 mg
Maudsley (1980)	15	DBC	?	IBU 1600 mg > FEN 800 mg
Bonomo et al. (1981): Spine	56	DBP	14	IBU 1200 mg = PIR 600 mg. AEs IBU < PIR
Turner et al. (1982)	68	DBP	180	IBU 1200 mg = PIR 600 mg. AEs IBU ≤ PIR
Cimmino et al. (1982): Hip/knee/spine	24	DBC	21	IBU 900 mg = MEC 300 mg
Peyron and Doury (1982)	150	DBP	7	IBU 1200 mg = TIA 600 mg
Caldwell et al. (1983)	108	DBC/MCT	28–42	IBU 1600 mg < FEN 2100 mg IBU 1600 mg > ASA 3200 mg
Umbenhauer (1983)	128	DBC	28	IBU 800–1200 mg < DIF 500–750 mg. AEs IBU = DIF
Mungavin and Clarke (1983)	301	SB/P	14	IBU 1200 mg = TIA 600 mg. AEs IBU = TIA
Petera et al. (1983): Knee/hip	60	DBP	21	IBU 1200 mg = TIA 600 mg. AEs IBU = TIA
Cornhill and Rowley-Jones (1984)				
Manchester GP Group (1984)	226	SB	21	IBU 1200 mg = NAP. AEs IBU = NAP
Lambert et al. (1984)	71	DBC	14	IBU 1200 mg = TIA 600 mg. AEs IBU = TIA
Marcolongo et al. (1984)	40	NR/P	14	IBU 1200 mg ≤ TIA 600 mg. AEs IBU ≥ TIA
Glorioso et al. (1985)	150	–	30	IBU 1200 mg < SAM 1200 mg. AEs IBU > SAM
Barnard-Jones et al. (1986)	117	DBC	28	IBU 1800 mg < MEF 1500 mg. AEs IBU > MEF

TABLE 6.3 (continued)

Study: Joint[a]	Sample size[b]	Design[c]	Duration (days)	Outcome (drug, daily dose)[d,e]
Di Perri et al. (1987a)	63	DBC/MCT	30	IBU 1200 mg = IMS 2250 mg. AEs IBU = IMS
Müller-Fassbender (1987)	36	DBC	28	IBU 1200 mg < SAM 1200 mg. AEs IBU > SAM
Marcolongo et al. (1980)	30	DBC	42	IBU 1800 mg = FEN 600 mg. AEs IBU ≥ TIA
Bradley et al. (1991)	144	DB	28	IBU 1200 and 2400 mg = ACE 4000 mg. AEs IBU 1200 mg = ACE
Rovati (1992)	606	DBC	28–42	IBU = GLU > PLA. AEs IBU > GLU = PLA
Bolten (1994)	184	DBP	7	IBU 1600 mg = FLU 120
Baumgartner et al. (1996)	61	SBP/MCT	21	IBU 1600 mg = DIC 100 mg. AEs IBU < DIC
Vaz and Martins (1984): Knee	60	NR/P	14	IBU 1200 mg = TIA 600 mg. AEs IBU = TIA
Ott (1980)	70	SBP	28	IBU 1200 mg > DIC 75 mg. AEs (GI) IBU < DIC
Tausch and Fasching (1980): Knee/hip	30	CO	28	IBU 1200 mg = SUL 300 mg
Brackertz and Busson (1978): Hip/knee	35/40	SBC	14	IBU 1600 mg > SUL 200 mg > PLA. AEs IBU < SUL
Loizzi et al. (1984)	20	SBP	14	IBU 1800 mg > NAP 750 mg
Tausch and Fasching (1980): Hip/knee	30	DBC	28	IBU 1200 mg = SUL 300 mg
Tretenhan (1980): Spine	30	DBP	28	IBU 1200 mg = NAP 750 mg. AEs (GI) IBU < NAP
Giansiracusa et al. (1977)	378/437	DBC/MCT	28	IBU 1800 mg = ASA 3600 mg > PLA. AEs (GI) IBU < ASA
Levinson and Rubenstein (1983): Hip/knee	108	SBC	28	IBU 2400 mg = FEN 2400 mg > PLA
Royer et al. (1975)	232	SBP	168	IBU 900–1800 mg = IND 75–100 mg. AEs IBU < IND
Keet (1979)	35	SBP	126	IBU 1200 mg = DIF 500 mg
Rind et al. (1978): Hip/knee	25	DBC	14	IBU 800 mg = FLT 800 mg

Study	Sample size[b]	Design[c]		Outcomes[e]
Crook et al. (1981): Hip	37	DBP/DD	56	IBU 1600–2400 mg = DIC 100–150 mg
Rossi and Baroni (1975)	20	DB	14	IBU 1400–1590 mg (mean) < DIC 130–150 mg (mean)
Brooks (1980)	14	DBC	35	IBU 1200 mg < DIC 75 mg
Alarcon-Segovia (1980): Hip/knee	99	DPP	196	IBU 1200–2000 mg < BEN 400–600
Innocenti et al. (1979)	24	DBC	14	IBU 1200 mg = IDP 600 mg
Puranen and Ronty (1978): Knee	39	DB	21	IBU 1200 mg = PRQ 900 mg
Owen-Smith and Burry (1972): Hip	42	DBC	7	IBU 600 mg < IND 75. IBU = PLA
Ruoff et al. (1982)	85	DBP	35	IBU? = ASA? = PARA?
Royer et al. (1975)	167/232	DB MCT	294	IBU 900–1800 mg = IND 75–150. AEs (GI) IBU < IND
Ghosh and Rastogi (1981): Hip/knee	32	NB	84	IBU 1200 mg < SUL 400 mg
Cannella et al. (1979): Spine	121	DB/MCT	21	IBU 1300 mg (mean) = TOL 882 mg (mean)
Keet (1979): Hip/knee	34	DB	126	IBU 1200 mg = DIF 500 mg
Rgalado and Fowler (1974)	63	DB	28	IBU 1200 mg < PBZ 300 mg
Mena et al. (1976)	193	DB	42	IBU 1600 mg = FLU 80 mg
Tranmer (1978)	77	SB	14	IBU 600 mg = BNA 4500 mg
Petera et al. (1983)	60	DBP	21	IBU 1200 mg = TIA 600 mg. AEs IBU = TIA

[a] Joints specified in trial: where not mentioned, it was either mixed grouping or not clear from trial what joints were studied.

[b] Sample size: first figure represents number of patients who completed trial out of total.

[c] DB, double blind; SB, single blind; NB, not blind; DR, dose–response; PLAC, placebo; P, parallel; CO, crossover; NR, non-random; MCR, multicentre trial.

[d] AEs, adverse events; BNA, benorylate; FBN, fenbufen; FEN, fenoprofen calcium; FLT, floctafenine; IBU, ibuprofen; IDP, indoprofen; KET, ketprofen; LNX, lornoxicam; MEC, meclofenamate sodium; NAP, naproxen (acid or sodium salt); PIR, pirprofen; PPN, pirprofen; PRQ, proquazone; SAM, S-adenosylmethionine; SUL, sulindac; TIA, tiaprofenic acid.

[e] Outcomes represent majority (especially analgesic efficacy) of overall assessments comprising: anti-inflammatory efficacy; analgesic efficacy; overall estimation by physician and/or patient; functional improvement; grip strength; articular index; morning stiffness.

higher for ibuprofen and naproxen than for piroxicam. Overall, the differences in rates were relatively low and the confidence intervals appeared to overlap with each of these drugs.

6.5.1   Acceleration of cartilage destruction

Concerns have been expressed that NSAIDs, especially those that inhibit the synthesis of cartilage proteoglycans, may accelerate joint damage in osteoarthritis (Brooks *et al.*, 1982; Herman and Hess, 1984; Kalbhen, 1988; Rashad *et al.*, 1989, 1992; Dingle, 1991; Jones and Doherty, 1992; Rainsford *et al.*, 1992). The mechanisms of this accelerated joint damage may not alone arise from inhibition of proteoglycan production, but might also involve 'overuse' from the pain-relief or Charcot-type state promoted by the analgesia from the drugs (Brooks *et al.*, 1982) or the stimulation of the production of cartilage-destructive cytokines (see chapter by Rainsford, 'Pharmacology and Toxicology of Ibuprofen'). Several authors have reported that ibuprofen inhibits synthesis of cartilage proteoglycans *in vitro* (McKenzie *et al.*, 1976; Dingle, 1991). Intra-articular ibuprofen like that of several other NSAIDs has been shown to cause destruction of cartilage in rats. This effect could be a reflection of very high concentrations of free drug exposed to the cartilage as compared with the more dynamic situation following oral or parenteral administration of the drug where there is diffusion principally of protein bound drug with only small amounts of the free drug accumulating in the joint. To date no long-term studies have been performed with ibuprofen to study the effects on joint destruction and relate this to changes in pro-teoglycan concentrations or other biochemical parameters as shown in the model studies developed by Rashad and co-workers (1989, 1992). Until these definitive studies have been performed it is not possible to establish if the observed effects of ibuprofen on proteoglycan synthesis have any relevance to long-term effects of the drug in osteoarthritis.

In 1990 nonsteroidal anti-inflammatory analgesics were the most commonly pre-scribed agents in the treatment of osteoarthritis (McAlindon and Dieppe, 1990). Earlier, ibuprofen was considered as the first choice for the treatment of osteoarthritis (Busson, 1986). This was to change with the landmark paper of Bradley *et al.* (1991) the follow-ing year. These authors showed in a well-conducted double-blind controlled trial that paracetamol (acetaminophen) 4 g/day was just as effective as analgesic 1.2g/day or anti-inflammatory doses 2.4 g/day of ibuprofen in knee-joint osteoarthritis. It should be noted that corresponding comparisons of these drugs have not been performed in patients with hip, digital/hand or mixed arthropathies, so it is not possible to generalize from these studies performed in knee osteoarthritis. Furthermore, periodic or spasmodic local inflammation of the affected joint may be a major indication for an NSAID compared with use of analgesic in order to minimize the destructive effects accompanying inflammation. Since the patients in the study by Bradley *et al.* (1991) were not selected for inflammatory state, it is not possible to define the drug response to inflammatory pain separately from control of inflammatory changes or 'non-inflammatory' pain.

6.5.2   Therapeutic aspects

A number of studies have confirmed that for many patients their pain can be as adequately controlled with paracetamol 4 g/day as with nonsteroidal anti-inflammatory analgesics such as ibuprofen and naproxen (Amadio and Cummings, 1983; Mazzuca *et al.*, 1991; Williams *et al.*, 1993; March *et al.*, 1994; Griffin *et al.*, 1995). Paracetamol 4 g/day is now generally recommended as the first drug of choice for control of pain in osteoarthritis (Brandt, 1993; Cicuttini and Spector, 1995; March, 1997). However, recent concerns about the potential hepatotoxicity of paracetamol, even in doses within the therapeutic range (Benison *et al.*, 1987), have lead to re-evaluation of the apparent benefits of this drug, especially when given in the long term. This is especially important for elderly rheumatic patients, who often eat poorly and have subnormal nutrition and other complications to their disease.

Paracetamol and other analgesics, such as codeine, have been shown to enhance the effects of ibuprofen (Frame *et al.*, 1986; Vlok and van Vuren, 1987), and this may be a useful combination. When nonsteroidal anti-inflammatory analgesics are required, smaller doses have been shown to be effective: an important consideration in the elderly (Mazzuca *et al.*, 1991). In general, therefore, we agree with Jobanputra and Nuki (1994) and March (1997) that the judicious use of nonsteroidal anti-inflammatory analgesics in the management of osteoarthritis is acceptably safe. An important issue about use of NSAIDs such as ibuprofen in osteoarthritis is dosage and whether pain control is just as effective on a p.r.n. basis compared with long-term continuous dosage. In most of the trials, adequate pain control is achieved at dosages of 1200–1600 mg/day. These are much lower than required in rheumatoid arthritis, where additional anti-inflammatory effects are required. The lower dose range clearly confers safety benefit for reducing the risk of gastrointestinal and other side-effects (see Chapter 9). Our first choice therefore, of a nonsteroidal anti-inflammatory analgesic would appear to be ibuprofen, 1200–1600 mg/day (March, 1997). The choice is largely made on the basis of safety. While ibuprofen clearly has the lowest risk of upper gastrointestinal ulceration (see Chapter 9), gastroprophylaxis with misoprostol, an H_2-receptor antagonist, or H-pump blocker may be required in at-risk patients (March, 1997).

Justification for employing misoprostol for gastroprophylaxis with ibuprofen, the low ulcer risk NSAID, in elderly subjects with osteoarthritis has been provided from the study of Roth *et al.* (1993). They performed a randomized prospective multicentre endoscopic-blinded study in 171 patients with osteoarthritis over 60 years of age (148 of whom completed the trial) who received ibuprofen 2400 mg/day plus misoprostol 800 μg/day ($n = 60$) or nabumetone 100 mg/day ($n = 58$). Eight patients on ibuprofen alone developed ulcers, whereas none on ibuprofen/misoprostol developed ulcers. Nabumetone produced ulcers only in one subject. Similar results were observed in an earlier study (Roth, 1990).

6.6 FORMULATIONS

O'Connor *et al.* (1993) found that a sustained release formulation of ibuprofen was superior to conventional ibuprofen, with the former offering advantages for once-daily treatment in general practice. Sustained release ibuprofen taken for osteoarthritis in the evening resulted in improved sleep (Fernandes and Jenkins, 1994).

The use of topical formulations of NSAIDs for pain relief has been recommended during the early stages of the therapeutic tree for osteoarthritis (March, 1997). Ibuprofen, topical like other NSAIDs as gels or creams, has utility in digital or trapeziometacarpal osteoarthritis (Arendt-Nielsen *et al.*, 1994; Tréves *et al.*, 1995). The kinetics of uptake of ibuprofen into joint tissue have been detailed, but skin irritation occurs in about 1–2% of subjects being treated with percutaneous NSAIDs (Chlud, 1991).

6.7 VARIABILITY IN RESPONSE

It is well established that NSAIDs, including ibuprofen, vary considerably in therapeutic response from patient to patient as well as during the long-term treatment of rheumatic conditions with these drugs (Williams and Day, 1985, 1988; Walker *et al.*, 1997). While part of this problem is related to variations in pharmacokinetics of the drugs (Williams and Day, 1985, 1988; Walker *et al.*, 1997), it is also clear from controlled experimental studies in chronic pain states (Walker *et al.*, 1996) that part of the problem has to do with placebo effects and prior drug exposure. Even acute inflammatory responses vary from patient to patient (Walker *et al.*, 1994). Recent studies (Cush *et al.*, 1990a,b; Walker *et al.*, 1997) have highlighted the importance of the concept of 'responders' and 'nonresponders' to NSAID therapies in both rheumatoid arthritis and osteoarthritis. There is evidence of complex interplay between variations in plasma concentrations of the drugs and the status of or alterations in the levels of pro-inflammatory cytokines in response to therapy with NSAIDs. In rheumatoid arthritis pretreatment, ESR and lymphocyte counts appear to be reliable predictors of the responsiveness to NSAIDs (Walker *et al.*, 1997). Response to treatment with sustained-release ibuprofen 2400 mg/day or flurbiprofen 200 mg/day was associated with significant reduction compared with post-washout values of IgM rheumatoid factor and C-reactive protein, as well as with increases in circulating lymphocytes and decrease in circulating granulocytes (Cush *et al.*, 1990b). An additional and important finding was that the responders to these drugs showed higher initial baseline assessments of pain. This indicates that the relative difference in pain response (or the 'delta' value) may have a greater value in these patients than in nonresponders simply because these differences will inevitably be larger from a statistical viewpoint. Nonresponders show either no changes or deterioration in laboratory parameters. These studies suggest that initial pain levels and monitoring of laboratory parameters of immunoinflammatory indices may be useful in predicting the outcome of therapy with ibuprofen as well as with other NSAIDs.

6.8   RELATION OF DRUG KINETICS TO CLINICAL RESPONSE

As indicated in the previous section, the issues have been raised that (a) the variability of clinical response of ibuprofen, like that of other NSAIDs, may in part be attributed to variations in pharmacokinetics in individual patients, and (b) in the case of propionic acids that undergo metabolic inversion, there may be stereoselectivity in the accumulation of the enantiomers in synovial fluids and tissues.

Several studies have attempted to address these aspects. Day *et al.* (1988) studied the distribution into synovial fluid of (*R*)-(–)- and (*S*)-(+)-ibuprofen in patients with arthritis and chronic knee effusions following administration of 200 mg *rac*-ibuprofen tablets; most of the subjects had been receiving this drug previously. The ratio of synovial fluid concentrations of (*S*)-(+)/(*R*)-(–) ibuprofen was 2.1 ± 0.3 (mean $\pm$ S.E.M.) indicating a high concentration of the cyclooxygenase inhibitory component of the drug at the site of inflammation. Synovial fluid concentrations of the drug fluctuated much less than those in plasma. The (*R*)-(–) and (*S*)-(+) concentrations exceeded those in plasma for over 5 h.

These observations are interesting for they suggest (a) that the synovial compartment is more 'stable' than its source from the plasma; (b) plasma variations in concentration of ibuprofen may have much less significance than hitherto thought in relation to the drug concentrations at the active site in the synovium of the prostaglandin synthesis inhibitory (*S*)-(+) – form of the drug; and (c) the interpatient differences that were evident in synovial distribution of enantiomers may contribute to the interindividual variability in response to ibuprofen. Day *et al.* (1988) also showed that the enantiomers diffuse from the blood to the synovial fluid in their unbound forms and that diffusion out of the drug may be in the protein-bound form. This suggestion was made without information being provided on the protein concentration in the synovial fluid so it is difficult to ascertain the meaning of their suggestion.

In a similarly designed study, but with higher drug doses than employed by Day *et al.* (1988), Cox *et al.* (1991) studied the serum to synovial distribution of enantiomers of ibuprofen in 8 patients with knee and hip osteoarthritis who received 800 mg ibuprofen as 13 doses every 8 hours. Blood samples were withdrawn on first 8 hours after the first dose, and 10–12 h on day 5 after the last dose, being 1 day afterwards. The authors concluded from this study that synovial fluid albumin concentrations are a determining factor in controlling the study state distribution of the isomers of ibuprofen, a finding they noted that agreed with earlier studies by Whitlam *et al.* (1981) with *rac*-ibuprofen distribution into the synovium. Thus the issue of the free compared with bound concentrations of the enantiomers being important determinants controlling the rate of synovial transfer of the enantiomers is unresolved. The assessment of this factor may depend on the state of joint injury of the patients and their selection for study. The subjects selected by Day *et al.* (1988) and Cox *et al.* (1991) had effusions of the affected joint that was used for sampling of synovial fluid. Obviously these subjects represent a subgroup of those patients

CHAPTER 6

with osteoarthritis, for many may not exhibit sufficient swelling to be suitable for this type of study. Thus it is possible that the distribution of drug from plasma to synovium, may depend on (a) the degree of vascular damage in the synovial region allowing little appreciable accumulation of fluid, (b) the extent of localized bone crystal and other degraded joint components that have accumulated therein and are promoting the cycle of joint inflammation, and (c) the intrinsic kinetic properties of the drugs under study.

The above studies did not allow for the pharmacokinetics of ibuprofen to be related to clinical response in these issues. To resolve this aspect, Bradley *et al.* (1992) studied the stereospecific pharmacokinetics in 45 patients who had received *rac*-ibuprofen at either 1200 mg/day (21 subjects) or 2400 mg/day (24 subjects) for 4 weeks for the treatment of hip or knee osteoarthritis. The serum AUC of (*S*)-(+)-ibuprofen at completion of dosing correlated with improvement in disability (Standard HAQ assessment), pain at rest and physicians' global assessment. This study did not allow for study of the synovial fluid kinetics of the enantiomers, so that the issue of their relationship to clinical response is unresolved.

Trans-synovial kinetics of (*S*)-(+)-ibuprofen from doses of dexibuprofen compared with equivalent enantiomer doses of *rac*-ibuprofen do not appear to have been studied. Such studies would require corrections to be made for variations in enantiomer composition or contamination, in the case of dexibuprofen, with trace amounts of the (*R*)-(–) isomer in commercial preparations. The mean (*S*)-(+)-ibuprofen bioavailability from dexibuprofen compared with *rac*-ibuprofen is 0.66 in healthy volunteers (Gabard *et al.*, 1995). This is in general agreement with estimation of the bioconversion of (*R*)-(–)-ibuprofen to the (*S*)-(+) antipode being about 60% (see Chapter 4). Since synovial fluid concentration ratios of (*S*)-(+)- to (*R*)-(–)-ibuprofen are about 2:1 (Cox *et al.*, 1991), it would appear that the rate of bioconversion of (*R*)-(–)- to (*S*)-(+)-ibuprofen in extrasynovial compartments determines the ratio of these isomers entering and being resident on the synovial compartments.

In conclusion, the clinical pharmacokinetics of ibuprofen indicates that clinical response is related to serum or plasma concentrations of (*S*)-(+)-ibuprofen. It is evident that relatively high concentrations of both enantiomers are present in synovial fluid compared with plasma/serum concentrations and that about 60–70% of the ibuprofen present in synovial fluid is in the 'active' prostaglandin synthesis-inhibitory (*S*)-(+) form. As pointed out in Chapter 5, the (*R*)-(–) form might have appreciable pharmacological activity in regulating the actions of leukocytes and in control of pain so that the exact significance of the (*R*)-(–)-ibuprofen concentrations in synovial fluid is as yet unclear.

6.9 LOW BACK PAIN

The treatment of low back pain is virtually a therapeutic conundrum. The pathology underlying low back pain can vary from varying grades of spondylitis or physical injury to conditions where there is little or no obvious joint pathology. Therapy of this group of conditions involves use of a variety of strategies (Deyo, 1983; Spitzer *et al.*, 1987; van Tulder *et al.*, 1997), among them NSAIDs, of which use is extensive (Koes *et al.*, 1997). Unfortunately, the efficacy of treatments including the use of NSAIDs has not been rigorously evaluated (Deyo, 1983; Spitzer *et al.*, 1987; Koes *et al.*, 1997). Part of the problem of treating low back pain is that it has a variety of aetiologies, pathologies and sequelae with, in some groups of patients, a strong sociopsychological element underlying causes and responses to therapies.

There appears to be a paucity of clinical therapeutic trials of ibuprofen in the treatment of low back pain (Rosenbloom *et al.*, 1985). Recently, in an attempt to evaluate the efficacy of NSAID therapies, Koes and co-workers (1997) undertook a systematic evaluation of published randomized controlled clinical trials (RCT) of NSAID treatments in low back pain. Their literature evaluation selected 26 RCTs, which were scored for quality (maximum = 100 points) of methods in four categories comprising (a) study population, (b) interventions, (c) measurements of effect, and (d) data presentation and analysis. The method scores of the trials ranged from 27 to 83 points. The pooled odds ratios in four trials comparing NSAIDs with placebo after 1 week was 0.53 (CI = 0.32–0.89), indicating a significant effect with NSAID treatments, although this was relatively small and the authors cautioned that these did not use identical outcome measures in some trials. Two other studies showed that NSAIDs were better than paracetamol alone or with dextropropoxyphene.

Koes *et al.* (1997) identified two trials in which ibuprofen had been studied that met their criteria. A study by Hosie (1993) that had achieved the highest methods score of 83 compared ibuprofen 400 mg capsules t.i.d. (and a placebo also t.i.d.) with the topical NSAID febinac as a 3% foam t.i.d. (with placebo capsules t.i.d.) in 140 patients; the treatments lasted 14 days. There were no significant differences between these treatments and ibuprofen showed improvement (assessed as those having no or mild severity) in 84% patients after 1 week and in 76% after 2 weeks of treatment. There were no significant differences in the occurrence of side-effects in the groups.

In a less complex trial that was also evaluated by Koes *et al.* (1997), Siegmeth and Placheta (1978) compared treatment with 1200 mg/day ibuprofen with that with 75 mg/day diclofenac for 14 days in 15 subjects. Koes *et al.* (1997) gave this study a methods score of 49 and, since this was performed in 1978, the methods must be considered less rigorous than would be employed today. By 4 weeks, 6/15 patients had improved with ibuprofen and 11/15 with diclofenac. One side-effect was noted in each group. Considering the low dose of ibuprofen employed in this study, it is not surprising that the response was limited to about half the patients.

One of the approaches for therapy of low back conditions is to employ pain-relieving NSAIDs or an analgesic with muscle relaxants. Following this approach, Berry and Hutchinson (1988) conducted a trial of 105 patients with acute low back pain, employing combinations of tizanidine 4 mg t.i.d. plus ibuprofen 400 mg t.i.d. versus placebo plus ibuprofen 400 mg t.i.d. Pain was assessed by visual analogue scale recorded in patients'

CHAPTER 6

daily diaries, and by physicians' assessment at baseline, and on days 3 and 7. Earlier improvement occurred in the tizanidine/ibuprofen group with respect to pain at night and pain at rest. The doctors' assessment of helpfulness of treatment identified that tizanidine/ibuprofen was significantly better than placebo/ibuprofen at day 3 ($p = 0.05$). There were significant differences between treatments in favour of tizanidine/ibuprofen in patients with moderate and severe pain at night ($p < 0.05$), at rest ($p < 0.05$), and in those with moderate or severe sciatica ($p < 0.5$). Interestingly, there were more gastrointestinal side-effects in the placebo/ibuprofen group compared to the tizanidine/ibuprofen-treated patients ($p = 0.002$). The authors concluded that this supported previous work in animals that had shown that tizanidine mediated gastric mucosal protection against anti-inflammatory drugs. It was stated that more patients given tizanidine/ibuprofen suffered drowsiness and other central nervous system effects ($p = 0.025$). The authors emphasize that in patients with severe acute low back pain some sedation and bed rest was advantageous. The authors concluded that tizanidine/ibuprofen was more effective in the treatment of moderate or severe acute low back pain than placebo with ibuprofen.

It is our opinion that there is a need to define the role of ibuprofen in the management of low back pain by further randomized controlled trials. However, the accuracy of study of mechanical low back pain is impaired by the difficulty in examining a relatively homogeneous population with this type of disorder.

6.10   PERIARTHRITIS OF THE SHOULDER

Supraspinatus tendinitis is a common clinical problem encountered by family physicians. It is generally agreed that ibuprofen is effective in treating shoulder complaints (Friis *et al.*, 1992; Van der Windt *et al.*, 1995). Two double-blind trials have been reported, one comparing ibuprofen 1600 mg/day with diclofenac 100 mg/day (Famaey and Ginsberg, 1984), and the other 1200 mg/day ibuprofen with 150 mg/day diclofenac (Huskisson and Bryans, 1983). Both trials had adequate numbers of patients, 50 and 40 respectively, and ibuprofen was found equivalent to diclofenac in both. It would have been useful if a placebo group had been included in these studies. The methods used to diagnose the periarthritis were solely on clinical grounds.

The specific site and hence the accuracy of diagnosis of periarthritis of the shoulder can now be made much more accurately with the use of diagnostic ultrasound and/or MRI scan and/or arthrogram. It is only with the incorporation of such diagnostic techniques that a more precise study of NSAID efficacy and toxicity can be made in shoulder dysfunction.

6.11   REACTIVE ARTHRITIS (REITER'S SYNDROME)

It is our opinion that the term reactive arthritis possibly encompasses the arthritides previously referred to as the seronegative arthritides. We know of no controlled trials of ibuprofen in Reiter's syndrome or the arthritis associated with inflammatory bowel disease.

6.12   PSORIATIC ARTHRITIS

Despite an intensive search of the literature we have been unable to find a single properly designed controlled clinical trial of ibuprofen in psoriatic arthritis. A trial was reported, in which etretinate (Tigason™) combined with ibuprofen was compared to ibuprofen alone in a double-blind controlled trial in psoriatic patients (Hopkins *et al.*, 1985). Ibuprofen was compared to placebo in a randomized double-blind, crossover study in 19 psoriatic patients receiving UV-B phototherapy, which showed ibuprofen to be more effective than placebo in relieving symptoms of UV-B-induced psoriatic inflammation (Sterns and Dodgson, 1985). Again there is a need for properly designed trials of ibuprofen in patients with psoriatic arthritis.

6.13   ANKYLOSING SPONDYLITIS

There have been few trials of ibuprofen in patients with ankylosing spondylitis (Calin, 1983), although there are several with flurbiprofen that have compared favourably with phenylbutazone (Calin and Grahame, 1974; Mena and Willkens, 1977) and indomethacin (Sturrock and Hart, 1974; Good and Mena, 1977). Clearly there is a need for a properly controlled clinical trial of high-dose ibuprofen (Rosenbloom *et al.*, 1985). Calin and Elswood (1990), in a prospective nationwide cross-sectional study of nonsteroidal anti-inflammatory usage in 1331 patients with ankylosing spondylitis, identified that indomethacin was the most popular of the nonsteroidal anti-inflammatory analgesics. This was confirmed in a review of clinical trials (Gotzsche, 1989).

CHAPTER 6

6.14   GOUT

Ibupofen has been used for acute gout, although indomethacin, azapropazone and more potent NSAIDs are usually preferred. However, in elderly patients with hypertension, congestive cardiac failure or renal failure, or with a peptic ulcer, it is our policy as it is of others (Gonzalez *et al.*, 1994) to administer intra-articular or intramuscular injections of corticosteroid as indicated. Rosenbloom *et al.* (1985) were unable to find any properly conducted clinical trials of ibuprofen in acute gouty arthritis. It might be of interest to have one. Ibuprofen does not interact with probenecid (Graham, 1987), and this may be an advantage for its concurrent use with the latter, especially as indomethacin does interact with probenecid. Since urate activation of polymorphonuclear neutrophil leukocytes (PMNs) involves a major component of the pathogenesis of joint inflammation in gout, it would be instructive to establish whether ibuprofen blocks the activation of PMNs by urate. Using various inflammatory stimuli, ibuprofen has been found to inhibit aggregation and degranulation of neutrophils, although the superoxide anion generation is not always affected (Kaplan *et al.*, 1984; Abramson., 1989; Partsch *et al.*, 1990; see also Chapter 5).

6.15   FIBROMYALGIA

This intrinsically difficult state has a complex neuroendocrinological and psychological basis that makes treatment difficult (Pillemer *et al.*, 1997). White and Harth (1996) reviewed the published trials, totalling 35 in all, of the effects of a variety of agents in the treatment of fibromyalgia syndrome. Only 24 of these met the criteria for being controlled clinical trials. Two of these included randomized double-blind studies showing the efficacy of ibuprofen (Yunus *et al.*, 1989; Russell *et al.*, 1991). Combination of ibuprofen and alprazolam has also been shown to convey relief in primary fibromyalgia (Russell *et al.*, 1991).

6.16   HEMOPHILIAC ARTHRITIS

Inwood *et al.* (1983) in a 16-week double-blind study, showed clearly the superiority of ibuprofen 1600 mg/day over placebo in controlling joint pain. Perhaps more importantly, there were no side-effects. The safety and efficacy of ibuprofen in hemophiliac arthritis has been confirmed in open studies (Hasiba *et al.*, 1980; Steven *et al.*, 1985).

6.17   POSTOPERATIVE PAIN

There seems to be general agreement that ibuprofen is useful in relieving both post-operative (Slavic-Svircev *et al.*, 1984) and postpartum pain (Windle *et al.*, 1989). Several double-blind trials have been performed showing the efficacy of ibuprofen compared with placebo or other NSAIDs in relief of acute surgical pain (Table 6.4). Other studies have shown that ibuprofen is effective in relief of pain after orthopaedic surgery (Boström *et al.*, 1994), hernia repairs (Iles, 1980), tonsillectomy (Parker *et al.*, 1986), dental surgery (Gallardo and Rossi, 1980; Lokken and Skjelbred, 1980; Squires and Masson, 1981; Forbes *et al.*, 1984; Seymore and Walton, 1984; Moore *et al.*, 1985; Frame *et al.*, 1986; Giles *et al.*, 1986; Jain *et al.*, 1986; Cooper and Mardirossian, 1986; Hill *et al.*, 1987; Cooper *et al.*, 1989; Carrillo *et al.*, 1990; Table 6.4; see also Chapter 8), vasectomy (Manson, 1988), abortion (Weibe and Rawling, 1995) and episiotomy (Bloomfield *et al.*, 1974; Taina, 1981; Cater *et al.*, 1985; Norman *et al.*, 1985; Sunshine *et al.*, 1987; Schachtel *et al.*, 1989) and have demonstrated the superiority of ibuprofen over placebo. In double-blind trials, adminis-tration of ibuprofen was shown to reduce the requirement for morphine (Owen *et al.*, 1986) and augment the efficacy of methadone (Ferrer-Brechner and Ganz, 1984). In a large trial in 425 patients, Iles (1980) found 400 mg ibuprofen equivalent to a combination of 375 mg aspirin, 30 mg caffeine and 8 mg of codeine. Schachtel *et al.* (1989), in a placebo-controlled double-blind trial in 36 patients with post-episiotomy pain, found 400 mg ibuprofen superior to 1 g of paracetamol. Horneffer *et al.* (1990), in a randomized double-blind trial in 149 patients with post-pericardiotomy pain, found ibuprofen equipotent to indomethacin. However, other double-blind controlled trials found ibuprofen to be inferior to aspirin (Parker *et al.*, 1986) and indoprofen (Olstad and Skjelbred, 1986).

TABLE 6.4

Comparative effects of ibuprofen with some other NSAIDs or analgesics in control of acute pain

Study	Condition	Study design[a]	Dosage (mg)[b]	No. of patients	Duration	Efficacy result[c]
Cooper et al. (1994), also details quoted by Balfour et al. (1996)	Dental surgery	PLAC R DB	IBU 400 (×1) 400 (×2) LNX 2 (×1) 2 (×2) 8 (×1) 8 (×2)	47 51 48 52 53 48	12 h	TOTPAR IBU × 1–2 = LNX 8 × 1–2 IBU × 2 = LNX 8 × 2 > LNX 2 × 1–2
Laveneziana et al. (1996a)	Inguinal hernia surgery	PLAC R DB DD	IBU (Arg) 400 KET 30 PLC	42 41 40	6 h	Total pain relief (VAS) IBU = KET but with severe pain group IBU = KET = PLC
Pagnoni et al. (1996a)	Caesarian section	PLAC R DB DD	IBU 400 KET 30 PLC	30 30 30	6 h	Total pain relief (VAS; PID) IBU = KET > PLC
Pagnoni et al. (1996)	Suction abortion	R DB PC MCT	IBU 400 PLC	38 37	4 h	Total pain relief (VAS) IBU > PLC
Borea et al. (1986)	Dental surgery	PLAC R DB DD	IBU 400 NAP 550 PLC		12 h	IBU = NAP > PLC

[a] R, randomized; DB, double blind; PLAC, placebo controlled; DD, double dummy; MCT, multicentre trial.
[b] IBU, ibuprofen p.o.; IBU (Arg), ibuprofen arginine p.o.; LNX, lornoxicam p.o.; KET, ketorolac tromethamine i.m.; PLC, placebo; NAP, naproxen sodium p.o.; ×, number of doses.
[c] TOTPAR, total pain relief scores; VAS, visual analgoue scale; PID, pain intensity difference.

6.18 SPORTS INJURIES

Aspirin and other NSAIDs are used extensively for the relief of pain in acute injuries and also longer-term sports injuries (Weiler et al., 1987; Abramson, 1990; Buchanan and Rainsford, 1990). Ibuprofen is recommended among the standard drugs for inclusion in the physician's emergency kit for use in treating the injured athlete (Ray, 1989). This is based on the drug being well tolerated and it can be used for menstrual cramps (Ray, 1989). A key issue with sports injuries concerns the complex nature of some of these conditions

CHAPTER 6

(Weiler *et al.*, 1987; Abramson, 1990; Leadbetter *et al.*, 1990) and the assessment of therapeutic response (Weiler *et al.*, 1987). There is also the issue of the motivation of highly competitive athletes influencing the clinical response. A whole range of musculoskeletal complications can arise in these states and it is important to realize that the pathological state underlying the development of pain inevitably raises issues about the appropriate pain-relieving medications to employ in sports injuries (Weiler *et al.*, 1987; Abramson, 1990). For instance tendon injury, overuse syndromes, fibrosis, and hematoma complications can all represent complex sequelae that may be unresponsive to application of NSAIDs. Also, it is worth noting that inflammation does not play a significant role in a majority of sports injuries.

Several trials have been performed to examine the efficacy and safety of NSAIDs in a range of sports injuries seen today (Weiler *et al.*, 1987). Simple application of NSAIDs for relief of pain and swelling in soft-tissue injuries is the usual form of many trials (Abramson, 1990; Buchanan and Rainsford, 1990). There is a choice of oral or topical formulations and the latter find extensive application even though they have often not been rigorously assessed for their efficacy or safety. The latter is of particular importance, especially with respect to the development of gastrointestinal side-effects. In this respect ibuprofen would appear from its well-established safety record in the gastrointestinal tract to have particular advantages.

Ibuprofen has been found effective in double-blind placebo-controlled trials in relieving pain and swelling in both ankle (McLatchie, 1985; Sloan *et al.*, 1989) and knee injuries (Hutson *et al.*, 1986). The dose used in these trials was 2400 mg/day. In equally well-designed trials of ibuprofen in the same dosage, no superiority was observed over placebo medication (Andersson *et al.*, 1983; Jenner, 1987; Fredberg *et al.*, 1989). In a review of clinical trials of over 1000 patients, Jenner (1987) concluded that nabumetone was efficacious in the treatment of soft-tissue injury and was similarly efficacious to soluble aspirin, ibuprofen and naproxen. However, it was not possible in these studies to demonstrate a definite advantage over placebo. Clinical trials comparing ibuprofen with other non-steroidal anti-inflammatory analgesics without placebo (Hayes *et al.*, 1984) are therefore difficult to interpret. In a recent extensive review of 150 articles, 84 of which were on soft-tissue injuries, few randomized double-blind trials were identified (Ogilvie-Harris and Gilbart, 1995). The authors concluded, however, that nonsteroidal anti-inflammatory analgesics did shorten the time to recovery. The evidence is in favour of treatment with ibuprofen 2400 mg/day for soft-tissue injuries, beginning treatment as soon as possible after the injury (Sloan *et al.*, 1989). Topical application of felbinac (biphenylacetic acid) gel has recently been shown in four separate trials of soft-tissue injury and osteoarthritis to be equal to oral ibuprofen or fenbufen (Hoskie and Bird, 1994).

Williams (1983) found that 7 days' treatment with ibuprofen 1600 mg/day resulted in significant improvement in 'pain on movement' in patients with a variety of conditions described as 'soft-tissue rheumatism'. Some of these states may have originated from sports injuries.

Recently, interest has been shown in the potential of NSAIDs to *prevent* muscle soreness during exercise. Ibuprofen has been investigated for its physiological effects and effects in preventing muscle soreness (Hasson *et al.*, 1993). In this study 20 subjects were randomly assigned to receive *prophylactic* ibuprofen (400 mg t.i.d. 4 h before strenuous exercise), *therapeutic* ibuprofen (400 mg t.i.d. initially 24 h and 48 h after exercise) or control treatments. The prophylactic ibuprofen group had 40–50% less perceived muscle soreness and decline in isometric, concentric and eccentric torque at 24 h compared with the other treatments. There was no difference in muscle damage (plasma creatinine clearance) among the treatment groups, but the decline in EMG in the vastus lateralis was significantly less with ibuprofen given prophylactically.

At first sight these results would suggest that there may be therapeutic advantages in employing ibuprofen in prevention of muscle soreness. Various exercise clinics report quite extensive use of ibuprofen and other NSAIDs for preventing muscle soreness. However, there is the issue of taking a medication in competitive sport that may convey an advantage for the recipient over his or her competitors. Ibuprofen, like other NSAIDs, is acceptable for taking in competitive sports for therapy of sports injuries (Goyen, 1996) and clearly it is not in the same league as more potent drugs such as amphetamines, for which there is legal prohibition (Goyen, 1996). However, taking a drug that gives an advantage over one's competitors is not legitimate in competitive sport (Goyen, 1996). It is possible to regard the taking of an NSAID like ibuprofen to prevent muscle soreness — a serious limitation to prolonged exercise — as giving a competitive edge, and thus it could be questionable in relation to the criteria for the use of drugs in competitive sport.

A more serious aspect concerns the risk of renal injury during excess exercise while taking NSAIDs like ibuprofen. There has been a report of end-stage renal failure with ibuprofen in treatment of sports injuries (Griffiths, 1992). The drug has also been shown to induce acute renal failure during exercise (Sanders, 1995). This drug effect has its basis in the fact that exercise reduces renal blood flow and can of itself induce acute renal failure (Sanders, 1995). Renal ischemia from exercise combined with inhibition of prostaglandin production (with consequences for reduction of renal blood flow and electrolyte secretion) creates a potential combination that can lead to acute renal failure (Sanders, 1995). The case report (Sanders, 1995) was from a patient who had taken the diuretics hydrochlorothiazide and triamterene with ibuprofen. Combinations of diuretics and NSAIDs are known to affect renal function (see Chapter 10) so that the abnormal added effects of diuretics with NSAIDs and exercise represent a potentially hazardous combination. Renal effects of NSAIDs and prolonged exercise may also depend on the state of hydration of the individual, such that any appreciable water loss, as during exercise, could create stress on renal handling of electrolytes.

CHAPTER 6

6.19   OTHER PAINFUL STATES

The use of ibuprofen in the treatment of dental pain, including that from surgery, is reviewed in depth elsewhere in this book (see Chapter 8). Likewise, the non-prescription (OTC) use of ibuprofen in the treatment of minor pain conditions is reviewed in Chapter 7.

Ibuprofen 2400 mg/day and sulindac 400 mg/day were both found better than placebo in a double-blind trial in 18 patients with diabetic neuropathy (Cohen and Harris, 1987). Kaminski *et al.* (1985) found that ibuprofen reduced the pain of cholecystitis compared to placebo. It perhaps is also worth noting that nonsteroidal anti-inflammatory analgesics may prevent the formation of gallstones (Buchanan *et al.*, 1991).

Max *et al.* (1988), in a randomized double-blind crossover study of 40 patients with post-herpetic neuralgia, identified that clonidine 0.2 mg in a single dose was more effective than placebo or codeine 120 mg, or ibuprofen 800 mg. Clonidine had a higher side-effect profile. The authors added a comment that clonidine had a similar side-effect profile to codeine but had a superior analgesic effect. However, they stated that the side-effects may have contributed to clonidine analgesia by suggesting to patients that they had received a potent drug. This is a seminal paper as the authors showed that both mild and severe side-effects enhanced analgesia. This, to our knowledge, is a factor not taken into account in trials with analgesics or NSAIDs. Perhaps those who found ibuprofen less effective (e.g. in arthritis disease) may not have appreciated that it was because ibuprofen caused fewer adverse effects!

A double-blind trial failed to show efficacy of ibuprofen in herpes genitalis (Milch *et al.*, 1986).

It would appear that the best results of ibuprofen medication in 'pain states' are in the management of dental pain and dysmenorrhoea (Miller, 1981; Benvenuti *et al.*, 1984; see also Chapter 7).

6.20   CANCER

NSAIDs are useful in the control of mild to moderate pain (Gilman and Chang, 1987) and are considered to form part of the therapeutic 'ladder' employed in the control of pain in cancer patients (Ahmedzai, 1997). The NSAID of choice usually promoted is ketorolac (Ahmedzai, 1997) and no doubt this is employed because of its effectiveness when given parenterally. However, this drug is associated with an exceptionally high risk of upper GI bleeding and ulceration (Rainsford, 1996).

Ferrer-Brechner and Ganz (1984) have shown, in a randomized double-blind trial in patients with severe cancer-related pain, that the addition of ibuprofen (600 mg) to methadone significantly increases analgesia. The surprising aspect of this study was the relatively small dose of ibuprofen that was used (600 mg). Ibuprofen, like other NSAIDs, could be particularly useful in relieving pain due to bone metastases (Gilman and Chang, 1987).

Ventafridda and co-workers (1990) compared the pain relief and tolerability in 72 outpatients with unspecified cancers who received 8 NSAIDs or paracetamol in a double-blind, double-dummy, within-patient randomized study. There were a considerable number of dropouts, totalling 10 in all due to gastric and other side-effects, and 7 patients were excluded because of elevated liver enzymes. Based on the visual analogue score for pain relief, ibuprofen 1800 mg/day resulted in a 59% reduction in pain compared with naproxen 750 mg/day (71%), diclofenac 200 mg/day (67%) and indomethacin 150 mg/day (63%); these being the NSAIDs more effective in pain control than ibuprofen, based on these averaged scores. Suprofen 600 mg/day, pirprofen 1200 mg/day, aspirin 1800 mg/day, sulindac 600 mg/day and paracetamol 1500 mg/day were, in declining order, less effective than ibuprofen.

While there were no statistical analyses performed on the data for scores, the standard deviations of the values all appeared to overlap, so it is difficult to ascribe much value to these data. Likewise, the large number of dropouts/exclusions and the relatively small sizes in this 9-arm study make it very difficult to interpret the results other than to give qualitative assessments of pain relief. The absence of information on the type of cancers and the degree of pain at the presumed sites of tumours also makes for difficulties in the interpretation of this study. The adverse events were about equal among the NSAIDs, although ibuprofen and sulindac had a trend towards low GI side-effects. Clearly, more rigorously designed studies are required.

As reviewed elsewhere in this book (see Chapter 5), there is evidence that, as with other NSAIDs, therapy with ibuprofen may prevent colon and mammary cancers (Koutsos *et al.*, 1995; Harris *et al.*, 1996). Gridley *et al.* (1993) showed that there was a reduced risk of cancers of the colon, rectum and stomach in patients with rheumatoid arthritis and they suggested that this might be due to the intake of NSAIDs. Part of this effect may be due to prevention of prostaglandin-related metastatic changes as well as overcoming the prostaglandin inhibition of immune suppression (Gilman and Chang, 1987; Shiff and Rigas, 1997). NSAIDs also reduce tumour cell growth *in vitro* and in animal models *in vivo* (Gilman and Chang, 1987). Some NSAIDs have been shown to reduce tumour size in humans (Gilman and Chang, 1987; Shiff and Rigas, 1997).

6.21 POTENTIAL NON-ANALGESIC USAGE

Elmstedt *et al.* (1985) studied the effects of ibuprofen compared to placebo in 43 patients after hip arthroplasty, and showed reduction in heterotopic ossification with ibuprofen. This clearly requires further study. McCauley *et al.* (1990) have suggested that because ibuprofen reduces the systemic levels of thromboxane it might be useful in the treatment of frostbite, but it remains to be seen whether it will confer any benefit. Ibuprofen in a dose of 25 mg/kg/day had no demonstrable effect in hereditary nephrogenic diabetes insipidus (Libber *et al.*, 1986). Ibuprofen in a daily dose of 1800 mg/day has been reported

CHAPTER 6

to compromise wound repair after split-skin grafting because of its inhibition of an inflammatory response necessary for healing (Proper *et al.*, 1988).

6.22 THE ELDERLY

Because of its low toxicity profile (Royer *et al.*, 1984; Fries *et al.*, 1991), ibuprofen should probably be considered the nonsteroidal anti-inflammatory analgesic of first choice for pain relief in the elderly (Afable and Ettinger, 1993; Lamy, 1993), even with the recent tendency to use higher dosages (Busson, 1986). Although Greenblatt *et al.* (1984) reported a prolongation of ibuprofen plasma half-life ($t_{1/2}$) in elderly subjects, this does not appear to have any major clinical consequences (Albert *et al.*, 1984; Albert and Gernaat, 1984; Dollery, 1991). Like other nonsteroidal anti-inflammatory analgesics, ibuprofen needs to be used carefully in the elderly, especially the 'frail' elderly (Owens *et al.*, 1994) and those with congestive cardiac failure, hypertension and renal insufficiency (Portenoy and Farkash, 1988; Gurwitz *et al.*, 1990; Murray *et al.*, 1990; Whelton *et al.*, 1990; Weinblatt, 1991; Silagy, 1993; Girgis and Brookes, 1994; Seppälä and Sourander, 1995). In general, the dose of ibuprofen does not need to be adjusted in elderly patients (Albert *et al.*, 1984). There does not appear to be a renal risk with over-the-counter doses, but only with doses exceeding 1600 mg/day (Schlondorff, 1993). Cummings and colleagues (1988) studied 52 elderly patients, mean age 72 years, range 63–87 years, with degenerative joint disease and multiple concomitant illnesses. The patients were randomly selected to receive ibuprofen suspension 400 mg or aspirin 650 mg each q.i.d. The authors stated that there was no significant change from baseline in serum creatinine, blood urea nitrogen (BUN), weight, and blood pressure compared to values identified weekly for 6 weeks. The authors concluded that ibuprofen and aspirin administered in the above doses for 6 weeks had little effect on renal function as measured by serum creatinine and BUN in a sample of elderly patients for whom the drugs are commonly employed. Concomitant diuretic therapy did not appear to increase the risk. The authors concluded that while ibuprofen and aspirin are contraindicated in patients with severe hemodynamic insult, they should not be withheld from elderly patients who require analgesic/anti-inflammatory treatment because of concerns for renal impairment (Cummings *et al.*, 1988). In patients with pre-existing renal failure, administration of 800 mg of racemic ibuprofen resulted in acceleration of (R)-$(-)$- to (S)-$(+)$-ibuprofen conversion with reduced elimination of the (S)-$(+)$ enatiomer, and resultant elevation in plasma levels of (S)-$(+)$ enantiomer (Chen and Chen, 1994). This is a possible mechanism of ibuprofen toxicity in elderly patients with renal insufficiency, since renal clearance reduces to approximately 20% of normal by age 80 years. The (R)-$(-)$ to (S)-$(+)$ inversion is slowed and elimination is prolonged in subjects with hepatic cirrhosis (Li *et al.*, 1993).

It is worth remembering that ibuprofen, like other nonsteroidal anti-inflammatory analgesics, may cause confusion, drowsiness, behavioural disturbance, headaches and dizziness in elderly patients (Buchanan, 1990; Goodwin and Regan, 1992; Bowen and Larson, 1993).

6.23 DEXIBUPROFEN

The use of active enantiomers of racemates of drugs has been proposed by a number of authors (Howard-Lock *et al.*, 1986), especially in the use of ibuprofen in rheumatoid diseases (Klein *et al.*, 1992). The case for employing the active (S)-(+) enantiomer of ibuprofen has been based on arguments that (a) the 50% (R)-(−)-ibuprofen present in racemic ibuprofen represents a metabolic load ('ballast') on the drug-metabolizing/detoxifying and lipid metabolic pathways; (b) analogy may be made with the potential toxic reactivity of this inactive component with that of other racemic drugs (e.g. thalidomide); (c) inherent variability in response to treatment wih *rac*-ibuprofen may be reduced by employing the active enantiomers of this drug; and (d) intrinsic physicochemical differences exist between or *rac*-ibuprofen and the (S)-(+) enantiomers to that there might be differences in the pharmacokinetics of these two forms (as well as in their pharmacodynamics) (Williams and Day, 1985, 1988; Caldwell and Hutt, 1987; Kean *et al.*, 1991; Williams, 1993; Williams *et al.*, 1993; Zohman, 1994; Evans, 1996; Leising *et al.*, 1996; Mayer, 1996). The fact that evidence in support of these arguments and postulates is still wanting has not precluded extensive commercial interest in the development of the (S)-(+) enantiomer by a number of companies. Indeed one company, Gebro Broschek GmbH (Fieberbrunn, Austria) has obtained licences in several European countries for (S)-(+)-ibuprofen under the generic name dexibuprofen, (Seractil™). Several clinical trials have been reported on the use of (S)-(+)-ibuprofen, or dexibuprofen, for treating rheumatoid diseases (Stock *et al.*, 1991; Klein *et al.*, 1992; Chlud, 1995; Klein *et al.*, 1994; Rahlfs and Stat, 1996; Hawel *et al.*, 1997). The overall conclusion from these studies is that dexibuprofen provides effective pain and functional relief in a range of rheumatic diseases at daily doses ranging from 250 mg (initially) to 1800 mg with most at 600–900 mg daily (Chlud, 1995; Rahlfs and Stat, 1996; Hawel *et al.*, 1997).

One study that can be regarded as of the dose-ranging type showed that by dose adjustment the mean daily dose of (S)-(+)-ibuprofen required for the relief of symptoms over a 2-week period associated with pain and restricted movement was 1220 mg/day compared with *rac*-ibuprofen 1870 mg/day (Stock *et al.*, 1991). Longer-term studies are indicated to determine the extent of therapeutic response and dropout rates comparing these two forms of ibuprofen.

In a recent report Hawel *et al.* (1997) compared the effects of 300 mg dexibuprofen t.i.d. with 50 mg diclofenac sodium t.i.d. in a double-blind trial in 100 patients with painful osteoarthritis of the knee given the drugs for 15 days. The functional assessment was determined over the treatment period using the Lequesne Index. The mean value of improvement with dexibuprofen was 7.4, while that from diclofenac sodium was 7.4;

application of the Mann–Whitney statistical analysis showing no difference between the two treatments. Assessments of secondary criteria including pain relief, tenderness, range of movement, handicap, disease progression, global tolerance and efficacy showed a significant difference in favour of dexibuprofen because of its better tolerability. The tolerance and efficacy of dexibuprofen in post-marketing surveillance studies in 1400 patients showed the drug to be tolerated and efficacious, the daily doses being principally in the range 600–900 mg (Chlud, 1995). More recently, statistical analyses have been reported of trials in patients with a range of rheumatic/degenerative diseases where 1200 mg/day dexibuprofen (Seractil™) was compared with 2400 mg/day *rac*-ibuprofen (formulation unspecified). Again equivalence was demonstrated in these extensive statistical analyses.

Other aspects of the clinical and experimental pharmacology and toxicology of dexibuprofen are discussed elsewhere (see Chapter 5).

6.24 CONCLUSIONS

Ibuprofen has a long and well-established record of being a safe and effective therapy in a considerable range of chronic arthritic and non-arthritic states, and in treatment of acute pain, inflammatory and febrile states. Its merits are that it has a wide range of tolerability. Comparisons with other NSAIDs indicate that this drug is of intermediate potency in most painful and inflammatory states. Thus, the balance between therapeutic efficacy and tolerability is especially favourable because of the high ceiling of toxicity. In the present situation where the costs of drugs are an important consideration for long term therapy, ibuprofen also compares favourably in the cost–benefit assessment.

Ibuprofen has found application in a variety of painful and inflammatory states where the development and application of a wide range of formulations has been investigated and this will continue to be a main prospect for the application of the drug for treatment in the future. Ibuprofen is also being investigated for potential therapeutic use in a number of conditions where inflammatory responses and other, in some cases as yet undetermined, mechanisms of the drug are being exploited.

REFERENCES

AARONS, L., GRENNAN, D.M., RAJAPAKSE, C., BRINKLEY, J., SIDDIQUI, M., TAYLOR, L. and HIGHAM, C. (1983) Anti-inflammatory (ibuprofen) drug therapy in rheumatoid arthritis-rate of response and lack of dependency of plasma pharmacokinetics. *British Journal of Clinical Pharmacology* 15, 387–388.

ABERNATHY, D.R. and GREENBLATT, D.J. (1983) Ibuprofen does not impair antipyrine clearance. *Journal of Clinical Pharmacology* 23, 517–522.

ABRAMSON, S.B. (1989) Therapy and mechanisms of nonsteroidal anti-inflammatory drugs. *Current Opinion in Rheumatology* 1, 61–67.

ABRAMSON, S.B. (1990) Nonsteriodal anti-inflammatory drugs: mechanisms of action and therapeutic considerations. In: LEADBETTER, W.B., BUCKWALTER, J.A. and GORDON, S.L. (eds), *Sports-Induced Inflammation: Clinical and Basic Science Concepts*. Park Ridge (IL), American Academy of Orthopaedic Surgeons, 421–430.

ADAMS, S.S. (1987) The discovery of Brufen. *Chemistry in Britain* 1987 (Dec.), 1193–1195.

ADAMS, S.S. and BUCKLER, J.W. (1979) Ibuprofen and flurbiprofen. *Clinics in Rheumatic Diseases* 5, 359–379.

ADAMS, S.S., CLIFFE, E.E., LESSEL, B. and NICHOLSON, J.S. (1963) Some biological properties of ibufenac, a new anti-rheumatic drug. *Nature* 200, 271.

ADAMS, S.S., CLIFFE, E.E., LESSEL, B. and NICHOLSON, J.S. (1967) Some biological properties of 2-(4-isobutyrylphenyl)-propionic acid. *Journal of Pharmaceutical Sciences* 56, 1686.

ADAMS, S.S., BOUGH, R.G., CLIFFE, E.E., LESSEL, B. and MILLS, R.F.N. (1969) Absorption, distribution and toxicity of ibuprofen. *Toxicology and Applied Pharmacology* 15, 310–330.

ADAMS, S.S., BOUGH, R.G., CLIFFE, E.E., DICKINSON, W. LESSEL, B., McCULLOUGH, K.F., MILLS, R.F.N., NICHOLSON, J.S. and WILLIAMS, G.A.H. (1970) Some aspects of the pharmacology, metabolism, and toxicology of ibuprofen. *Rheumatology and Physical Medicine* 11(Symposium), 9–26.

AFABLE, R.F. and ETTINGER, W.H. (1993) Musculoskeletal disease in the aged. Diagnosis and management. *Drugs and Aging* 3, 49–59.

AHMEDZAI, S. (1997) New approaches to pain control in patients with cancer. *European Journal of Cancer* 33(Suppl. 6), S8–S14.

ALARCON-SEGOVIA, T. (1980) Long-term treatment of symptomatic osteoarthritis with benoxaprofen. Double blind comparison with aspirin and ibuprofen. *Journal of Rheumatology* 6(Suppl.), 89–99.

ALBERT, K.S. and GERNAAT, R.N. (1984) Pharmacokinetics of ibuprofen. *American Journal of Medicine* 77, 40–46.

ALBERT, K.S., GILLESPIE, W.R., WAGNER, J.G., PAU, A. and LOCKWOOD, G.F. (1984) Effects of age on the clinical pharmacokinetics of ibuprofen. *American Journal of Medicine* 77, 47–50.

ALTMAN, R.D. (1984) Review of ibuprofen for osteoarthritis. *American Journal of Medicine* 77, 10–18.

AMADIO, P.J. and CUMMINGS, D.M. (1983) Evaluation of acetaminophen in the management of osteoarthritis of the knee. *Current Medical Research* 34, 59–66.

AMERICAN MEDICAL ASSOCIATION (1995) *Drug Evaluations Annual 1995*. American Medical Association.

ANDERSON, J.A., LEE, P., WEBB, J. and BUCHANAN, W.W. (1974) Evaluation of the therapeutic potential of ketoprofen in rheumatid arthritis. *Current Medical Research and Opinion* 2, 189–197.

CHAPTER 6

ANDERSSON, S., FREDIN, H., LINDBERG, H., SANZEN, L. and WESTLIN, N. (1983) Ibuprofen, and compression bandage in the treatment of ankle sprains. *Acta Orthopaedica Scandanavica* **54**, 322–325.

ANDRADE, L. and FERNANDEZ, A. (1978) Sulindac in the treatment of osteoarthritis: a double blind 8 week study comparing sulindac with ibuprofen and 96 weeks of long term therapy. *European Journal of Rheumatology and Inflammation* **1**, 36–40.

ANSELL, B.M. (1973) Ibuprofen in the management of Still's disease. *Practitioner* **211**, 659–663.

APPELROUTH, D.J., CHODOCK, A.L., MILLER, J.L. and POWELL, W.R. (1986) A comparison of single daily doses of oxaprozin with multiple daily doses of ibuprofen for the treatment of rheumatoid arthritis. *Seminars in Arthritis and Rheumatism* **15**(Suppl. 2), 54–58.

ARENDT-NIELSEN, L., DREWES, A.M., SVENDSEN, L. and BRENNUM, J. (1994) Quantitative assessment of joint pain treatment of rheumatoid arthritis with ibuprofen cream. *Scandinavian Journal of Rheumatology* **23**, 334–337.

ARENDT-RACINE, E.C., ATKINSON, M.H., DECOTEAU, W.E., FLATT, V.L. and VARADY, J. (1978) Drug trial in rheumatoid arthritis. A new design. *Clinical Pharmacology and Therapeutics* **23**, 233–240.

AUSTRALIAN MULTICENTRE TRIAL GROUP (1980) The simultaneous assessment of four non-steroidal anti-inflammatory drugs in rheumatoid arthritis using a simple and rapid time design. *Journal of Rheumatology* **7**, 857–864.

BACHMANN, K.A., SCHWARTZ, J.I., FORNEY, R.B. JR., JUAREGUI, L. and SULLIVAN, T.J. (1986) Inability of ibuprofen to alter single dose phenytoin disposition. *British Journal of Clinical Pharmacology* **21**, 165–169.

BAKRIS, G.L., STARKE, U., HEIFETS, M., POLAK, D., SMITH, M. and LEURGAN, S. (1995) Renal effects of oral prostaglandin supplementation after ibuprofen in diabetic subjects: a double-blind, placebo-controlled, multicentre trial. *Journal of the American Society of Nephrology* **5**, 1684–1688.

BALFOUR, J.A., FITTON, A. and BARRADELL, L.B. (1996) Lornoxicam. A review of its pharma-cology and therapeutic potential in the management of painful and inflammatory conditions. *Drugs* **51**, 639–657.

BALLAS, Z.K. and DONTA, S.T. (1983) Sulindac-induced aseptic meningitis. *Archives of Internal Medicine* **142**, 165–166.

BALOGH, F., PAPAZOGLOU, S.N., MACLEOD, M. and BUCHANAN, W.W. (1979) A crossover clinical trial of piroxicam, indomethacin and ibuprofen in rheumatoid arthritis. *Current Medical Research and Opinion* **6**, 148–153.

BARNARD-JONES, K., DAVIES, R.W., LALLA, O., MANN, P.G. and WELCH, R.B. (1986) Mefenamic acid versus ibuprofen in osteoarthritis — a double-blind crossover study. *British Journal of Clinical Practice* **40**, 528–531.

BAR-SELA, S., LEVO, Y., ZEEVI, D. *et al.* (1980) A lupus-like syndrome due to ibuprofen hypersensitivity. *Journal of Rheumatology* **1**, 379–380.

BAUMGARTNER, H., SCHWARZ, H.A., BLUM, W., BRUHIN, A., GALLACHI, G., GOLDINGER, G., SAXER, M. and TROST, H. (1996) Ibuprofen and diclofenac sodium in the treatment of osteoarthritis: a comparative trial of two once-daily sustained release NSAID formulations. *Current Medical Research and Opinion* **13**, 435–444.

BENISON, H., KACZYNSKI, J. and WALLERSTEDT, S. (1987) Paracetamol medication and alcohol abuse: a dangerous combination for the liver and kidney. *Scandanavian Journal of Gastroenterology* **22**, 701–704.

BENNETT, R.M. (1986) A 12 week double-blind, multicenter study comparing diflunisal twice daily and ibuprofen four times daily in the treatment of rheumatoid arthritis. *Clinical Therapy* **9**(Suppl.), 27–36.

BENVENUTI, C., BERETTA, A., LONGONI, A. and PICKVANCE, N.J. (1984) A multi-centre general practice study evaluating the efficacy and tolerance of ibuprofen in common painful conditions. *Pharmatherapeutica* **4**, 9–12.

BERLINER, S., WEINBERGER, A., SHOENFELD, Y., SANDBANK, U., HAZAZ, B., JOSHUA, H., ROSEN, M. and PINKHAS, J. (1985) Ibuprofen may induce meningitis in (NZB × NZW) F1 mice. *Arthritis and Rheumatism* **28**, 104–107.

BERRY, H. and HUTCHINSON, D.R. (1988) Tizanidine and ibuprofen in acute low-back pain: results of a double-blind multicentre study in general practice. *Journal of International Medical Research* **16**, 83–91.

BHATTACHARYA, S.K., GOEL, R.K., BHATTACHARYA, S.K. and TANDON, R. (1991) Potentiation of gastric toxicity of ibuprofen by paracetamol in the rat. *Journal of Pharmacy and Pharmacology* **43**, 520–521.

BIRD, H.A. (1985) Impact of over the counter availability of nonsteroidal anti-inflammatory drugs. In: BROOKS, P.M., DAY, R.O., WILLIAMS, K.M. and GRAHAM, G. (eds), *Agents and Actions Supplement: Basis for Variability of Response to Antirheumatic Drugs.* Basel, Birkhauser Verlag, 55–59.

BIRD, H.A., HILL, J., LOWE, J.R. and WRIGHT, V. (1984) A double-blind comparision of tenoxicam (Tilcotil, Mobiflex) at two doses against ibuprofen in rheumatoid arthritis. *European Journal of Rheumatology and Inflammation* **7**, 28–32.

BIRKETT, D.J. (1980) The practical application of drug assays in general practice. *Australian Family Physician* **9**, 142–145.

BJARNASON, I. (1988) NSAID-induced small intestinal inflammation in man. *Records of Advances in Gastroenterology* **7**, 23–46.

BLECHMAN, W.J., SCHMID, F.R., APRIL, P.A., WILSON, C.H. and BROOKS, C.D. (1975) Ibuprofen or aspirin in rheumatoid arthritis therapy. *Journal of the American Medical Association* **233**, 336–339.

CHAPTER 6

BLOOMFIELD, S.S., BARDEN, T.P. and MITCHELL, J. (1974) Comparative efficacy of ibuprofen and aspirin in episiotomy pain. *Clinical Pharmacology and Therapeutics* **15**, 565–570.

BOARDMAN, P.L., NUKI, G. and HART, F.D. (1967) Ibuprofen in the treatment of rheumatoid arthritis and osteo-arthritis. *Annals of the Rheumatic Diseases* **26**, 560–561.

BOLTEN, W. (1994) The pharmacokinetics, pharmacodynamics and comparative efficacy of flurbiprofen, LAT. *British Journal of Clinical Practice* **48**, 190–195.

BOLTEN, W. (1996) Clinical experience with meloxicam, a selective COX-2 inhibitor. In: BAZAN, N., BOTTING, J. and VANE, J. (eds), *New Targets in Inflammation. Inhibitors of COX-2 or Adhesion Molecules*. Dordrecht, Kluwer Academic Publishers, 105–116.

BONEBERG, E.M., ZOU, M.-H. and ULLRICH, V. (1996) Inhibition of cyclooxygenase -1 and -2 by (R)-(–)- and (S)-(+)-ibuprofen. *Journal of Clinical Pharmacology* **36**(Suppl.), 16S–19S.

BONNEY, S.L., NORTHINGTON, R.S., HEDRICH, D.A. and WALKER, B.R. (1986) Renal safety of two analgesics used over the counter: ibuprofen and aspirin. *Clinical Pharmacology and Therapeutics* **40**, 373–377.

BONOMO, I., CHAHADE, W.H. and GRAMAJO, R.J. (1981) A multi-centre double-blind trial of pirprofen, ibuprofen and placebo in osteoarthritis of the spine. In: VAN DER KORST, A. (ed.), *A New Antirheumatic-Analgesic Agent: Pirprofen (Rengasil®)*. Bern, Hans Huber, 97–101.

BOREA, G., MONOPOLI, R. and COLANTONI, A. on behalf of a multicenter trial (1996) Ibuprofen arginine *vs* naproxen sodium as prophylactic oral treatment of pain due to dental surgery. A randomised double-blind, double-dummy, placebo-controlled multi centre study. *Clinical Drug Investigation* **11**(Suppl. 1), 33–40.

BOSTRÖM, A.A.S., FORBES, J.A., ADOLFSON, C., BEAVER, W.T. and BELL, W.E. (1994) Evaluation of bromfenac and ibuprofen for pain after orthopedic surgery. *Pharmacotherapy* **14**, 305–313.

BOWEN, J.D. and LARSON, E.B. (1993) Drug-induced cognitive impairment. Defining the problem and findings solutions. *Drugs and Aging* **3**, 349–357.

BOWER, R.J., UMBENHAUER, E.R. and HERCUS, V. (1979) In: WEISSMAN, G., SAMUELSSON, B. and PAOLETTI, R. (eds), *Advances in Inflammation Research*, vol. 1. New York, Raven Press, 559.

BRACKETZ, B. and BUSSON, M. (1978) Comparative study of sulindac (Clinoril) and ibuprofen (Brufen) in osteoarthritis. *British Journal of Clinical Practice* **32**, 77–80.

BRADLEY, J.G. (1991) Non-prescription drugs and hypertension. Which one affects blood pressure? *Postgraduate Medicine* **89**, 195–197.

BRADLEY, J.D., BRANDT, K.D., KATZ, B.P., KALASINSKI, L.A. and RYAN, S.I. (1991) Comparison of an anti-inflammatory dose of ibuprofen, an analgesic dose of ibuprofen, and acetaminophen in the treatment of patients with osteoarthritis of the knee. *New England Journal of Medicine* **325**, 87–91.

BRADLEY, J.D., RUDY, A.C., KATZ, B.P., RYAN, S.I., KALASINSKI, L.A., BRATER, D.C., HALL, S.D. and BRANDT, K.D. (1992) Correlation of serum concentrations of ibuprofen stereo-isomers with clinical response in the treatment of hip and knee osteoarthritis. *Journal of Rheumatology* **19**, 130–134.

BRANDT, K.D. (1993) Should nonsteroidal anti-inflammatory drugs be used to treat osteoarthritis? *Rheumatic Disease Clinics of North America* **19**, 29–44.

BRESNIHAN, B., HUGHES, G. and ESSIGMAN, W.K. (1978) Diflunisal in the treatment of osteoarthritis: a double-blind study comparing diflunisal with ibuprofen. *Current Medical Research and Opinion* **5**, 556–561.

BREWER, E.J. (1977) Therapy of the rheumatic diseases of childhood: nonsteroidal anti-inflammatory agents. *Arthritis and Rheumatism* **20**(Suppl.), 520–525.

BREWER, E.J. and GIANNINI, E.H. (1982) Standard methodology for segment I, II and III Paediatric Rheumatology Collaborative Study Group studies. I. Design. *Journal of Rheumatology* **9**, 109–113.

BRODIE, N.H., MCGHIE, R.L., O'HARA, H., O'HARA, J. and VALLE-JONES, J.C. (1980) Fenclofenac and ibuprofen in the treatment of osteoarthritis. *British Journal of Clinical Practice* **34**, 334–336.

BROOKS, C.D., SCHMID, F.R., BIUDO, J., BLAU, S., GONZALEZ-ALCOVER, R., GOWANS, J.D.C., HURD, E., PARTRIDGE, R.E.H. and TARPLEY, E.L. (1970) Ibuprofen and aspirin in the treatment of rheumatoid arthritis: a cooperative double-blind trial. *Rheumatology and Physical Medicine* **11**(Suppl.), 48–63.

BROOKS, C.D., SCHLAGEL, C.A., SEKJAR, N.C. and SOBOTA, J.T. (1973) Tolerance and pharmacology of ibuprofen. *Current Therapeutic Research* **15**, 180–190.

BROOKS, P.M., HILL, W. and GEDDES, R. (1980) Diclofenac and ibuprofen in rheumatoid arthritis and osteoarthritis. *Medical Journal of Australia* **1**, 29–30.

BROOKS, P.M., POTTER, S.R. and BUCHANAN, W.W. (1982) NSAIDs and osteoarthritis — help or hindrance? *Journal of Rheumatology* **9**, 3–5.

BROWERS, J.R.B.J. and DE SMET, P.A.G.M. (1994) Pharmacokinetic-pharmacodynamic drug interactions with nonsteroidal anti-inflammatory drugs. *Clinical Pharmacokinetics* **27**, 462–485.

BRUGUERAS, N.E., LEZOTTE, L.A. and MOXLEY, T.E. (1978) Ibuprofen: a double-blind comparison of twice-a-day therapy with four-times-a-day therapy. *Clinical Therapeutics* **2**(Suppl. 1), 13–21.

BRUNE, K. (1986) Comparative pharmacology of 'non-opoid' analgesics. [Review]. *Medical Toxicology* **1**, 1–9.

BUCHANAN, W.W. (1990) Implications of NSAID therapy in elderly patient. *Journal of Rheumatology* **17**(Suppl. 20), 29–32.

CHAPTER 6

BUCHANAN, W.W. and KASSAM, Y.B. (1986) European experience with flurbiprofen. A new anti-inflammatory/analgesic agent. *American Journal of Medicine* **80**(Suppl. 3A), 1–5.

BUCHANAN, W.W., HERNANDEZ, A., GERECZ-SIMON, E.M. and BUCHANAN, H.M. (1991) Are gallstones less prevalent in rheumatoid arthritis? *Clinical Rheumatology* **10**, 339–340.

BUCHANAN, W.W. and RAINSFORD, K.D. (1990) Nonsteriodal anti-inflammatory drugs: mechanisms of action and therapeutic considerations. In: LEADBETTER, W.B., BUCKWALTER, J.A. and GORDON, S.L. (eds), *Sports-Induced Inflammation: Clinical and Basic Science Concepts*. Park Ridge (IL), American Academy of Orthopaedic Surgeons, 431–441.

BUSSON, M. (1986) Update on ibuprofen: review article. *Journal of International Medical Research* **14**, 53–62.

BURRY, H.C. and WITHERINGTON, L. (1979) A comparison of sulindac with ibuprofen in the management of rheumatoid arthritis. *New Zealand Medical Journal* **89**, 298–300.

CALDWELL, J.R. (1986) Efficacy and safety of diclofenac sodium in rheumatoid arthritis. Experience in the United States. *American Journal of Medicine* **80**, 43–47.

CALDWELL, J. and HUTT, A.J. (1987) Biological implications of the metabolic chiral inversion of 2-arylpropionic acid nonsteroidal anti-inflammatory drugs. In: RAINSFORD, K.D. and VELO, G.P. (eds), *Side-Effects of Anti-inflammatory Drugs. Pt.1. Clinical and Epidemiological Aspects*. Lancaster, MTP Press, 217–228.

CALDWELL, J.R., CRAIN, D., HOFFMEISTER, R.T., KANTROWITZ, F., LLOYD, R.J., NUSSDORF, R.T., SCHMID, F.R. and REPICE, M.R. (1983) Four-way multicentre, crossover trial of ibuprofen, fenoprofen calcium, naproxen, and tolmetin sodium in osteoarthritis: comparative clinical profiles. *Southern Medical Journal* **76**, 706–711.

CALIN, A., BENNETT, R.M., SCHMID, F.R., GOLDMAN, A.L., MONTOYA, H.E., O'BRIEN, W.M., GUILIANO, V.J., WILLKENS, R.F. and SAKOFSKY, Y. (1976) Double-blind multicentre parallel trial of ketoprofen and ibuprofen in the treatment of rheumatoid arthritis. *Arthritis and Rheumatism* **19**, 791.

CALIN, A. (1983) Clinical use of tolmetin sodium in patients with ankylosing spondylitis: a review. *Journal of Clinical Pharmacology* **23**, 301–308.

CALIN, A. and ELSWOOD, J. (1990) A prospective nationwide cross-sectional study of NSAID usage in 1331 patients with ankylosing spondylitis. *Journal of Rheumatology* **17**, 801–803.

CALIN, A. and GRAHAME, R. (1974) Double-blind crossover trial of ibuprofen and phenylbutazone in ankylosing spondylitis. *British Medical Journal* **4**, 496–499.

CALIN, A., BENNETT, R.M., SUKHUPUNYARAKSA, S., GOLDMAN, A.L., MONTOYA, H.E., O'BRIEN, W.M., GUILIANO, V.J., SCHMID, F.R., WILLKENS, R.F. and SAKOFSKY, H.Y. (1977) Double-blind multi-centre parallel trial of ketoprofen and ibuprofen in the treatment of rheumatoid arthritis. *The Journal of Rheumatology* **4**, 153–157.

CAMU, F., VAN LERSBERGHE, C. and LAUWERS, M.H. (1992) Cardiovascular risks and benefits of perioperative nonsteroidal anti-inflammatory drug treatment. *Drugs* **44**(Suppl. 5), 42–51.

CANNELLA, J.J. (JR), BROBYN, R.D., ALBERT, M. and MORTON, G. (1979) A multiclinic comparative double blind evaluation of tolmetin sodium and ibuprofen in osteoarthritis of the spine. *Current Therapeutic Research* **25**, 447–456.

CAPELL, H.A., RENNIE, J.A.N., ROONEY, P.J., MURDOCK, R.M., HOLE, D.J., DICK, W.C. and BUCHANAN, W.W. (1979) Patient compliance: a novel method of testing nonsteroidal anti-inflammatory analgesics in rheumatoid arthritis. *Journal of Rheumatology* **6**, 584–593.

CARDOE, N. and FOWLER, P.D. (1979) Diclofenac sodium (Voltarol): a double-blind comparative study with ibuprofen in patients with rheumatoid arthritis. *Rheumatology and Rehabilitation* **2**(Suppl.), 89–99.

CARRILLO, J.S., CALATAYUD, J., MANSO, F.J., BARBERIA, E., MARTINEZ, J.M. and DONADO, M. (1990) A randomized double-blind clinical trial on the effectiveness of helium-neon laser in the prevention of pain, swelling and trismus after removal of impacted third molars. *International Dental Journal* **40**, 31–36.

CARSON, J.L. and STROM, B.L. (1992) The gastrointestinal toxicity of the nonsteroidal anti-inflammatory drugs. In: RAINSFORD, K.D. and VELO, G.P. (eds), *Side-Effects of Anti-inflammatory Drugs 3*. Lancaster, Kluwer Academic Publishers, 1–8.

CASTLES, J.J. and SKOSEY, J.L. (1980) Comparative efficacy and safety of naproxen and ibuprofen in rheumatoid arthritis. *Current Therapeutic Research* **27**, 556–564.

CATER, M., O'BRIEN, P.M. and PICKVANCE, N.J. (1985) A double-blind comparison of the new ibuprofen-codeine phosphate combination, zomepirac, and placebo in the relief of postepisiotomy pain. *Clinical Therapeutics* **7**, 442–447.

CEUPPENS, J.L., GOODWIN, J.S. and RODRIGUEZ, M.A. (1982) Nonsteroidal anti-inflammatory agents inhibit the synthesis of IgM rheumatoid factor *in vitro*. *The Lancet* **1**, 528–533.

CHALMERS, T.M. (1969) Clinical experience with ibuprofen in the treatment of rheumatoid arthritis *Annals of the Rheumatic Diseases* **28**, 513–517.

CHEN, C.Y. and CHEN, C.S. (1994) Stereoselective disposition of ibuprofen in patients with renal dysfunction. *Journal of Pharmacology and Experimental Therapeutics* **268**, 590–594.

CHLUD, K. (1991) Perkutane Therapie der schmerzhaften arthritis. *Therapeutische Umschau* **48**, 42–45.

CHLUD, K. (1995) Evaluation of tolerance and efficacy of (S)-(+)-ibuprofen (Seractil™) in daily practice: a post-marketing-surveillance study in 1400 patients. Poster Presentation *Annual Meeting of the American College of Clinical Pharmacology*, Washington DC, USA, Sept. 1995.

CHAPTER 6

CICUTTINI, F.M. and SPECTOR, T.D. (1995) Osteoarthritis in the aged. Epidemiological issues and optimal management. *Drugs and Aging* 6, 409–420.

CIMMINO, M.A., CUTOLO, M., SAMANTA, E. and ACCARDO, S. (1982) Short-term treatment of osteoarthritis: a comparison of sodium meclofenamate and ibuprofen. *Journal of International Medical Research* 10, 46–52.

COHEN, A. (1976) Intestinal blood loss after a new anti-inflammatory drug, sulindac. *Clinical Pharmacology and Therapeutics* 20, 238–240.

COHEN, K.L. and HARRIS, S. (1987) Efficacy and safety of nonsteroidal anti-inflammatory drugs in the therapy of diabetic neuropathy. *Archives of Internal Medicine* 147, 1442–1444.

COLLUM, L.M.T. and BOWEN, D.I. (1971) Ocular side-effects of ibuprofen. *British Journal of Opthalmology* 55, 472–477.

COOPER, S.A. and MARDIROSSIAN, G. (1986) Comparision of flurbiprofen and aspirin in the relief of postsurgical pain using the dental pain model. *American Journal of Medicine* 80, 36–40.

COOPER, S.A., ENGEL, J., LADOV, M., PRECHEUR, H., ROSENHECK, A. and RAUCH, A. (1982) Analgesic efficacy of an ibuprofen-codeine combination. *Pharmacotherapy* 2, 162–167.

COOPER, S.A., SCHACHTEL, B.P., GOLDMAN, E., GELB, S. and COHN, P. (1989) Ibuprofen and acetaminophen in the relief of acute pain: a randomized, double-blind, placebo-controlled study. *Journal of Clinical Pharmacology* 29, 1026–1030.

COOPER, S.A., LUCYK, D. and SMITH, B. (1994) An analgesic evaluation of lornoxicam. *95th Annual Meeting of the American Society for Clinical Pharmacology and Therapeutics*, March 31–April, 1994, New Orleans. Abstract 126.

CORNHILL, J. and ROWLEY-JONES, D. (1984) Is sustained release ibuprofen as effective as piroxicam? A comparison in patients with osteoarthritis. *European Journal of Rheumatology and Inflammation* 7, 114–121.

COX, S.R., GALL, E.P., FORBES, K.K., GRESHAM, M. and GORIS, G. (1991) Pharmacokinetics of the (R)-(–) and (S)-(+) enantiomers of ibuprofen, in the serum and synovial fluid of arthritis patients. *Journal of Clinical Pharmacology* 31, 88–94.

CROOK, P.R., FOWLER, P.D., HOTHERSALL, T.E. and CHISWELL, R.J. (1981) A study of the efficacy and tolerability of diclofenac and ibuprofen in osteoarthritis of the hip. *British Journal of Clinical Practice* 35, 309.

CUMMINGS, D.M., AMADIO, P.J., NETTLER, S. and FREEDMAN, M. (1988) Office-based evaluation of renal function in elderly patients receiving nonsteroidal anti-inflammatory drugs. *Journal of the American Board of Family Practitioners* 1, 77–80.

CUSH, J.J., JASIN, H.E., JOHNSON, R. and LIPSKY, P.E. (1990a) Relationship between clinical efficacy and laboratory correlates of inflammatory and immunologic activity in rheumatoid arthritis patients treated with nonsteroidal anti-inflammatory drugs. *Arthritis and Rheumatism* 33, 623–633.

CUSH, J.J., LIPSKY, P.E., POSTLETHWAITE, A.E., SCHROHENLOHER, R.E., SAWAY, A. and KOOPMAN, W.J. (1990b) Correlation of serologic indicators of inflammation with effectiveness of nonsteroidal anti-inflammatory drug therapy in rheumatoid arthritis. *Arthritis and Rheumatism* **33**, 19–28.

DA GAMA, G.G. and MOREIRA, C. (1976) Fenbufen in comparison to ibuprofen in patients with rheumatoid arthritis. *A Folha Medica* **73**, 625–629.

DARLINGTON, L.G. and COOMES, E.M. (1975) Comparison of benorylate and ibuprofen in the treatment of established rheumatoid arthritis. *Rheumatology and Rehabilitation* **14**, 76–80.

DAVIES, E.F. and AVERY, G.S. (1971) Ibuprofen. A review of its pharmacological properties and therapeutic efficacy in rheumatic disorders. *Drugs* **2**, 416.

DAVIES, J.G., RAWLINS, D.C. and BUSSON, M. (1988) Effect of ibuprofen on blood pressure control by propanolol and bendrofluazide. *Journal of International Medical Research* **16**, 173–181.

DAY, R.O., FURST, D.E., GRAHAM, G.G. and LEE, E. (1987) Ibuprofen, fenoprofen, ketoprofen. In: PAULUS, H.E., FURST, D.E. and DROMGOOLE, S.H. (eds), *Drugs for Rheumatic Disease*. New York, Churchill-Livingstone, 315–346.

DAY, R.O., WILLIAMS, K.M., GRAHAM, G.G., LEE, E.J., KNIHINICKI, R.D. and CHAMPION, G.D. (1988) Stereoselective disposition of ibuprofen enantiomers in synovial fluid. *Clinical Pharmacology and Therapeutics* **48**, 480–487.

DAYMOND, T.J., THOMPSON, M., AKKAR, F.A. and CHESTNEY, V. (1979) A controlled trial of tiaprofenic acid versus ibuprofen in rheumatoid arthritis. *Rheumatology and Rehabilitation* **18**, 257–260.

DEARMOND, B., FRANCISCO, C.A., LIN, J.S., HUANG, F.Y., HALLIDAY, S., BARTZEIK, R.D. and SKARE, K.L. (1995) Safety profile of over-the-counter naproxen sodium. *Current Therapeutics* **17**, 587–601.

DE BLÉCOURT, J.J. (1975a) A comparative study of ibuprofen (Brufen) and indomethacin (Indocid) in uncomplicated gonarthrosis and coxarthrosis. *Current Medical Research and Opinion* **3**, 477–480.

DE BLÉCOURT, J.J. (1975b) A comparative study of inbuprofen (Brufen) and indomethacin in uncomplicated arthrosis. *Nederlands Tijdschrift voor Geneeskunde* **119**(Suppl. 51), 2032–2034.

DEODHAR, S.D., DICK, W.C., HODGKINSON, R. and BUCHANAN, W.W. (1973) Measurement of clinical response to anti-inflammatory drugs in rheumatoid arthritis. *Quarterly Journal of Medicine* **42**, 387–401.

DEYO, R.A. (1983) Conservative therapy for low back pain: distinguishing useful from useless therapy. *Journal of the American Medical Association* **250**, 1057–1062.

CHAPTER 6

DICK, W.C., NUKI, G., WHALEY, K., DEODHAR, S. and BUCHANAN, W.W. (1970) Some aspects in the quantitation of inflammation in joints of patients suffering from rheumatoid arthritis. *Rheumatology and Physical Medicine* 11(Suppl.), 40–47.

DICK-SMITH, J.B. (1969) Ibuprofen, aspirin and placebo in treatment of rheumatoid arthritis. A double-blind clinical trial. *Medical Journal of Australia* 853–859.

DINGLE, J.T. (1991) Cartilage maintenace in osteoarthritis: interaction of cytokines, NSAIDs and prostaglandins in articular cartilage damage and repair. *Journal of Rheumatology* 18(Suppl. 28), 30–37.

DIONNE, R.A., CAMPBELL, R.A., COOPER, S.A., HALL, D.L. and BUCKINGHAM, B. (1983) Suppression of postoperative pain by preoperative administration of ibuprofen in comparison to placebo, acetaminophen, and acetaminophen plus codeine. *Journal of Clinical Pharmacology* 23, 37–43.

DI PERRI, T., AUTERI, A., FUMAGALLI, M., GANDINI, R., GIORDANO, A., GIORDANO, M., SCARICARBAROZZI, I., VAIANI, G. and VATTI, M. (1987a) Multicentre double-blind randomized clinical trial of imidazole salicylate versus ibuprofen in patients with rheumatoid arthritis. *International Journal of Clinical Pharmacology Therapeutics and Toxicology* 25, 443–447.

DI PERRI, T., AUTERI, A., CARUSO, I., CORVETTA, A., DANIELI, G., SARZI PUTTINI, P.C. and SCARICABAROZZI, I. (1987b) Multicenter double-blind randomized clinical trial of imidazole salicylate versus ibuprofen in patients with osteoarthritis. *International Journal of Clinical Pharmacology Therapeutics and Toxicology* 25, 479–482.

DOLLERY, C. (1991) *Therapeutic Drugs*. Edinburgh, Churchill Livingstone, 11–16.

DORNAN, J. and REYNOLDS, W.J. (1974) Comparison of ibuprofen and acetylsalicylic acid in the treatment of rheumatoid arthritis. *Canadian Medical Association Journal* **110**, 1370–1372.

DREISER, R.L. and TISNE-CAMUS, M. (1993) DHEP plasters as a topical treatment of knee OA — a double-blind placebo-controlled study. *Drugs under Experimental and Clinical Research* 19, 117–123.

EASTMOND, C.J., HOPKINS, R. and WRIGHT, V. (1982) A comparative controlled study of tiaprofenic acid ('Surgam') and naproxen in the treatment of rheumatoid arthritis. *Current Medical Research and Opinion* 7(Suppl. 9), 605–609.

EHRLICH, G.E., MILLER, S.B. and ZEIDERS, R.S. (1980) Choline magnesium trisalicylate versus ibuprofen in rheumatoid arthritis. *Rheumatology and Rehabiliation* 19, 30–41.

ELMSTEDT, E., LINDHOLM, T.S., NILSSON, O.S. and TORNKVIST, H. (1985) Effect of ibuprofen on heterotopic ossification after hip replacement. *Acta Orthopaedica Scandinavica* 56, 25–27.

EVANS, A.M. (1996) Pharmacodynamics and pharmacokinetics of the profens: enantioselectivity, clinical implications and special reference to (S)-(+)-ibuprofen. *Journal of Clinical Pharmacology* 36(Suppl.), 7S–15S.

EVANS, R.G., VAL-MEJIAS, J.E., KULEVICH, J., FISCHER, V.W. and MUELLER, H.S. (1985) Evaluation of a rat model for assessing interventions to salvage ischaemic myocardium: effects of ibuprofen and verapamil. *Cardiovascular Research* **19**, 132–8.

EWERT, B.H. (1989) Ibuprofen-associated meningitis in a woman with only serological evidence of a rheumatologic disorder. *American Journal of Medical Sciences* **297**, 326–327.

FAMAEY, J.P. and GINSBERG, F. (1984) Treatment of periarthritis of the shoulder: a comparision of ibuprofen and diclofenac. *Journal of International Medical Research* **12**, 238–243.

FAMAEY, J.P. and HUSKISSON, E.C. (eds) (1988) Symposium on therapeutic aspects of tiaprofenic acid. *Drugs* **35**(Suppl. 1), 1–111.

FASCHING, U. (1983) Diflunisal versus ibuprofen in rheumatoid arthritis. *Wiener Klinische Wochenschrift* **95**, 859–872.

FERNANDEZ, L. and JENKINS, R. (1994) Investigation into the duration of action of sustained release ibuprofen in osteoarthritis and rheumatoid arthritis. *Current Medical Research and Opinion* **13**, 242–250.

FERRER-BRECHNER, T. and GANZ, P. (1984) Combination therapy with ibuprofen and methadone for chronic cancer pain. *American Journal of Medicine* **77**, 78–83.

FORBES, J.A., BARKASZI, B.A., RAGLAND, R.N. and HANKLE, J.J. (1984) Analgesic effect of fendosal, ibuprofen, and aspirin in postoperative oral surgery pain. *Pharmacotherapy* **4**, 385–391.

FRACASSO, M.E., FRANCO, L., GASPERINI, R. and VELO, G.P. (1992) Effects of NSAIDs on liver microsomal mono-oxygenase system and products of oxidative metabolism of arachidonic acid. In: RAINSFORD, K.D. and VELO, G.P. (eds), *Side-effects of Anti-inflammatory Drugs*. Lancaster, Kluwer Academic Publishers, 204–211.

FRAME, J.W., FISHER, S.E., PICKVANCE, N.J. and SKENE, A.M. (1986) A double-blind placebo-controlled comparision of three ibuprofen/codeine combinations and aspirin. *British Journal of Oral and Maxillofacial Surgery* **24**, 122–129.

FREDBERG, U., HANSEN, P.A. and SKINHOJ, A. (1989) Ibuprofen in the treatment of acute ankle joint injuries. A double-blind study. *American Journal of Sports Medicine* **17**, 564–566.

FRIEDEL, H.A., LANGTRY, H.D. and BUCKLEY, M.M. (1993) Nabumetone. A reappraisal of its pharmacology and therapeutic use in rheumatic diseases. *Drugs* **45**, 131–156.

FRIES, J.F. (1995) ARAMIS and toxicity measurement. *Journal of Rheumatology* **22**, 995–997.

FRIES, J.F., WILLIAMS, C.A. and BLOCH, D.A. (1991) The relative toxicity of nonsteroidal anti-inflammatory drugs. *Arthritis and Rheumatism* **34**, 1353–1360.

FRIIS, J., JARNER, D., TOFT, B., CHRISTENSEN, K., CHRISOPHERSEN, J., IBFELDT, H.H., KORSGAARD, J., SKINHOF, A. and ANDERSEN, F. (1992) Comparison of two ibuprofen formulations in the treatement of shoulder tendonitis. *Clinical Rheumatology* **11**, 105–108.

CHAPTER 6

GABARD, B., NIRENBERGER, G., SCHIEL, H., MASKEV, H., KIKUTA, C. and MAYER, J.M. (1995) Comparision of the bioavailability of dexibuprofen administered above or as part of racemic ibuprofen. *European Journal of Clinical Pharmacology* **48**, 505–511.

GABB, G.M. (1996) Fatal outcome of interaction between warfarin and a nonsteroidal anti-inflammatory drug. *Medical Journal of Australia* **164**, 700–701.

GABRIEL, S.E., JAAKKIMAINEN, L. and BOMBARDIER, C. (1991) Risk of serious gastrointestinal complications related to use of nonsteroidal anti-inflammatory drugs. A meta-analysis. *Annals of Internal Medicine* **115**, 787–796.

GALL, E.P., CAPERTON, E.M., McCOMB, J.E., MESSNER, R., MULTZ, C.V., O'HANLAN, M. and WILKENS, R.F. (1982) Clinical comparison of ibuprofen, fenoprofen calcium, naproxen and tolmetin sodium in rheumatoid arthritis. *Journal of Rheumatology* **9**, 402–407.

GALLARDO, F. and ROSSI, E. (1980) Double-blind evaluation of naproxen and ibuprofen in periodontal surgery. *Pharmacology and Therapeutic Dentistry* **5**, 69–72.

GARCIA RODRIGUEZ, L.A. and JICK, H. (1994) Risk of upper gastrointestinal bleeding and perforation associated with individual nonsteroidal anti-inflammatory drugs. *The Lancet* **343**, 1075–1078.

GARCIA RUBIO, R. (1976) Diclofenac sodium and ibuprofen in rheumatoid arthritis: a double-blind comparative study. *Prensa Medicine Mexico* **41**, 270–272.

GHOSH, A.K. and RASTOGI, A.K. (1981) A randomized comparison between sulindac and ibuprofen in osteoarthritis of the aged. *Current Medical Research and Opinion* **7**, 482–487.

GIANNINI, E.H. and BREWER, E.J. (1982) Standard methodology for segment I, II and III. Paediatric Rheumatology Collaborative Study Group studies. II. Analysis and presentation of data. *Journal of Rheumatology* **9**, 114–122.

GIANNINI, E.H., BREWER, E.J., MILLER, M.L. *et al.* for the Paediatric Rheumatology Collaborative Study Group (1990) Ibuprofen suspension in the treatment of juvenile rheumatoid arthritis. *Journal of Paediatrics* **117**, 645–652.

GIANSIRACUSA, J.E., DONALDSON, M.S., KOONCE, M.L., LEFTON, T.E., RUOFF, G.E. and BROOKS, C.D. (1977) Ibuprofen in osteoarthritis. *Southern Medical Journal* **70**, 49–52.

GIANSIRACUSA, D.F., BLUMBERG, S. and KANTROWITZ, F.G. (1980) Aseptic meningitis associated with ibuprofen. *Archives of Internal Medicine* **140**, 1533.

GILES, A.D., HILL, C.M., SHEPHERD, J.P., STEWART, D.J. and PICKVANCE, N.J. (1986) A single dose assessment of an ibuprofen/codeine combination in postoperative dental pain. *International Journal of Oral and Maxillofacial Surgery* **15**, 727–732.

GILMAN, S.C. and CHANG, J. (1987) Nonsteroidal anti-inflammatory drugs in cancer therapy. In: LEWIS, A.J. and FURST, D.E. (eds), *Nonsteroidal Anti-inflammatory Drugs. Mechanisms and Clinical Use.* New York, Marcel Dekker, 157–179.

GIRGIS, L. and BROOKS, P. (1994) Nonsteroidal anti-inflammatory drugs. Differential use in older patients. *Drugs and Aging* 6, 101–112.

GLASS, R.C. and SWANNELL, A.J. (1978) Concentration of ibuprofen in serum and synovial fluid from patients with arthritis. *British Journal of Clinical Pharmacology* 6, 453P–454P.

GLORIOSO, S., TODESCO, S., MAZZI, A., MARCOLONGO, R., GIORDANO, M. and COLOMBO, B. (1985) Double-blind multicentre study of the activity of S-adenosylmethionine in hip and knee osteoarthritis. *International Journal of Clinical Pharmacology Research* 5, 39–49.

GODFREY, R.G. and DE LA CRUZ, S. (1975) Effect of ibuprofen dosage on patient response in rheumatoid arthritis. *Arthritis and Rheumatism* 18, 135–137.

GODFREY, K.E. and SWAIN, M.C. (1985) Fenclofenac. In: RAINSFORD, K.D. (ed.), *Anti-Inflammatory and Anti-Rheumatic Drugs. Volume II: Newer Anti-Inflammatory Drugs.* Boca Raton (FL), CRC Press, 105–136.

GONZALEZ, E.B., MILLER, S.B. and AGUDELO, C.A. (1994) Optimal management of gout in older patient. *Drugs and Aging* 4, 128–134.

GOOD, A. and MENA, H. (1977) Treatment of ankylosing spondylitis with flurbiprofen and indomethacin. *Current Medical Research and Opinion* 5, 117–121.

GOODWIN, J.S. and REGAN, M. (1982) Cognitive dysfunction associated with naproxen and ibuprofen in the elderly. *Arthritis and Rheumatism* 25, 1013–1015.

GOTZSCHE, P.C. (1989) Patients' preference in indomethacin trials: an overview. *The Lancet* 1, 88–91.

GOYEN, M. (1996) *The Australian Guide to Medications, Including Prescription and Non-Prescription Drugs*, 3rd edn. Sydney, The Watermark Press.

GRAHAM, G.G. (1987) Pharmacokinetics and metabolism of nonsteroidal anti-inflammatory drugs. *Medical Journal of Australia* 147, 597–602.

GREENBLATT, D.J., ABERNATHY, D.R., MATLIS, R., HARMATZ, J.S. and SHADER, R.I. (1984) Absorption and disposition of ibuprofen in the elderly. *Arthritis and Rheumatism* 27, 1066–1069.

GRENNAN, D.M., FERRY, D.G., ASHWORTH, M.E., KENNY, R.E. and McKINNON, M. (1979) The aspirin–ibuprofen interaction in rheumatoid arthritis. *British Journal of Clinical Pharmacology* 8, 497–503.

GRENNAN, D.M., AARONS, L., SIDDIQUI, M., RICHARDS, M., THOMPSON, R. and HIGHAM, C. (1983) Dose response study with ibuprofen in rheumatoid arthritis: clinical and pharmacokinetic findings. *British Journal of Clinical Pharmacology* 15, 311–316.

GRIDLEY, G., McLAUGHLIN, J.K., EKBOM, A., KLARESKOG, L., ADAMI, H.-O., HACKER, D.G., HOOVER, R. and FRAUMENI, J.F. JR (1993) Incidence of cancer among patients with rheumatoid arthritis. *Journal of the National Cancer Institute* 85, 307–311.

CHAPTER 6

GRIFFIN, M.R., RAY, W.A. and SCHAFFNER, W. (1988) Nonsteroidal anti-inflammatory drug use and death from peptic ulcer in elderly persons. *Annals of Internal Medicine* **109** 359–363.

GRIFFIN, M.R., PIPER, J.M., DAUGHERTY, J.R., SNOWDEN, M. and RAY, W. (1991) Nonsteroidal anti-inflammatory drug use and increased risk for peptic ulcer disease in elderly persons. *Annals of Internal Medicine* **114**, 257–264.

GRIFFIN, M.R., BRANDT, K.D., LIANG, M.H., PINCUS, T. and RAY, W.A. (1995) Practical management of osteoarthritis. Integration of pharmacological and nonpharmacologic measures. *Archives of Family Medicine* **4**, 1049–1055.

GRIFFITHS, M.L. (1992) End-stage renal failure caused by regular use of anti-inflammatory analgesic medication in minor sports injuries. A case report. *South African Medical Journal* **81**, 377–378.

GUM, O.B. (1980) Long-term efficacy and safety of benoxaprofen: comparison with aspirin and ibuprofen in patients with active rheumatoid arthritis. *Journal of Rheumatology* **7**(Suppl. 6), 76–88.

GURWITZ, J.H., AVORN, J., ROSS-DEGAN, D. and LIPSITZ, L.A. (1990) Nonsteroidal anti-inflammatory drug-associated azotemia in the very old. *Journal of the American Medical Association* **264**, 471–475.

HADIDI, T., ASAR, D.K. and ESMAT, A. (1972) A double-blind crossover study of ibuprofen, metiazinic acid, aspirin and a placebo in rheumatoid arthritis. *Journal of International Medical Research* **1**, 18–21.

HALL, E.D. (1985) Beneficial effects of acute intravenous ibuprofen on neurologica recovery of head-injured mice: comparision of cyclooxygenase inhibition with inhibition of thromboxane A_2 synthetase or 5-lipoxygenase. *Central Nervous System Trauma* **2**, 75–83.

HANSEN, P.D. (1979) *Drug Interactions*. Philadelphia: Lea and Febiger.

HARRIS, R.E., NAMBOODIRI, K.K. and FARRAR, W.B. (1996) Nonsteroidal anti-inflammatory drugs and breast cancer. *Epidemiology* **7**, 203–205.

HASIBA, U., SCRANTON, P.E., LEWIS, J.H. and SPERO, J.A. (1980) Efficacy and safety of ibuprofen for hemophiliac arthropathy. *Archives of Internal Medicine* **140**, 1583–1585.

HASSON, S.M., DANIELS, J.C., DIVINE, J.G., NIEBUHR, B.R., RICHMOND, S., STEIN, P.G. and WILLIAMS, J.H. (1993) Effect of ibuprofen use on muscle soreness, damage, and performance: a preliminary investigation. *Medical Science in Sports and Exercise* **25**, 9–17.

HAWELL, R., KLEIN, G., MITTERHUBER, J. and BRUGGER, A. (1997) Doppelblinde Studie zum Vergleich der Wirksamkeit und Vertraeglichkeit von 900 mg Dexibuprofen und 150 mg Diclofenac-Natrium bei Patienten mit schmerzhafter Gonarthrose **109**, 53–59.

HAYES, T.B., FYVIE, A., JANKE, P.G., VANDENBURG, M.J. and CURRY, W.J. (1984) Sulindac versus ibuprofen in sprains and strains. *British Journal of Sports Medicine* 18, 30–33.

HEATON, J.M. and BOURKE (1976) Papillary necrosis associated with calyceal arthritis. *Nephron* 16, 57–66.

HERMAN, J.H. and HESS, E.V. (1984) Nonsteroidal anti-inflammatory drugs and modulation of cartilagenous changes in osteoarthritis and rheumatoid arthritis. *American Journal of Medicine* 77, 16–25.

HIGHTON, J. and GRAHAME, R. (1980) Benoxaprofen in the treatment of osteoarthritis — A comparison with ibuprofen. *Journal of Rheumatology* 7(Suppl.), 125–131.

HILL, C.M., CAROLL, M.J., GILES, A.D. and PICKVANCE, N. (1987) Ibuprofen given pre- and post-operatively for the relief of pain. *International Journal of Oral and Maxillofacial Surgery* 16, 420–424.

HILL, J., BIRD, H.A., FENN, C.C., LEE, C.E., WOODWARD, M. and WRIGHT, V. (1990) A double-blind crossover study to compare lysine acetyl salicylate (Apergic) with ibuprofen in the treatment of rheumatoid arthritis. *Journal of Clinical Pharmacology* 15, 205–211.

HINGORANI, K. (1970) Double-blind crossover comparing ibuprofen with flufenamic acid in rheumatoid arthritis. *Rheumatology and Physical Medicine* 11(Suppl.), 76–82.

HINGORANI, K. (1973) Double-blind study of benorylate and ibuprofen in rheumatoid arthritis. *Rheumatology and Rehabilitation* 11(Suppl.), 39–47.

HINGORANI, K. (1976) A comparative study of azapropazone and ibuprofen in the treatment of osteoarthritis of the knee. *Current Medical Research and Opinion* 4, 57–64.

HOPKINS, R., BIRD, H.A., JONES, H., HILL, J., SURRALL, K.E., ASTBURY, C., MILLER, A. and WRIGHT, V. (1985) A double-blind controlled trial of etretinate (Tigason) and ibuprofen in psoriatic arthritis. *Annals of the Rheumatic Diseases* 44, 189–193.

HORNEFFER, P.J., MILLER, R.H., PEARSON, T.A., RYKIEL, M.F., REITZ, B.A. and GARDNER, T.J. (1990) The effective treatment of postpericardiotomy syndrome after cardiac operations. A randomized placebo-controlled trial. *Journal of Thoracic and Cardiovascular Surgery* 100, 292–296.

HOSIE, G.A.C. (1993) The topical NSAID, felbinac, versus oral ibuprofen: a comparison of efficacy in the treatment of acute lower back injury. *British Journal of Clinical Research* 4, 5–17.

HOSKIE, G. and BIRD, H. (1994) The topical NSAID felbinac versus oral NSAIDS: a critical review. *European Journal of Rheumatology and Inflammation* 14, 21–28.

HOUSTON, M.C., WEIR, M., GRAY, J., GINSBERG, D., SZETO, C., KAIHLENEN, P.M., SUGIMOTO, D., RUNDE, M. and LEFKOWITZ, M. (1995) The effects of nonsteroidal anti-inflammatory drugs on blood pressures of patients with hypertension controlled by verapamil. *Archives of Internal Medicine* 155, 1049–1054.

CHAPTER 6

HOWARD-LOCK, H.E., LOCK, C.J.L. and KEAN, W.F. (1986) Does the left hand know what the right hand is doing? Or clinical pharmacology: The use of optically pure (*R* or *S*) forms of chiral drugs rather than racemic mixtures. *Journal of Rheumatology* **13**, 1000–1003.

HUBSCHER, J.A. and WALKER, B.R. (1983) Oxaprozin once daily and ibuprofen four times daily in the treatment of rheumatoid arthritis: a multicentre study. *Clinical Pharmacology and Therapeutics* **33**, 267.

HUSKISSON, E.C. and BRYANS, R. (1983) Diclofenac sodium in the treatment of painful stiff shoulder. *Current Medical Research and Opinion* **8**, 350–353.

HUSKISSON, E.C. and SCOTT, J. (1979) Analgesic and anti-inflammatory properties of indoprofen. *Rheumatology and Rehabilitation* **18**, 49–52.

HUSKISSON, E.C., SHENFIELD, G.M., TAYLOR, R.T. and HART, F.D. (1970) A new look at ibuprofen. *Rheumatology and Physical Medicine* **11**(Suppl.), 88–92.

HUSKISSON, E.C., WOOLF, D.L., BALME, H.W., SCOTT, J. and FRANKLYN, S. (1976) Four new anti-inflammatory drugs, responses and variations. *British Medical Journal* **1**, 1048–1049.

HUTSON, M.A. (1986) A double-blind study comparing ibuprofen 1800 mg or 2400 mg daily and placebo in sports injuries. *Journal of International Medical Research* **14**, 142–147.

ILES, J.D. (1980) Relief of postoperative pain by ibuprofen: a report of two studies. *Canadian Journal of Surgery* **23**, 288–290.

INCHIOSA, M.A.J. and SMITH, C.M. (1990) Effects of ibuprofen on doxorubicin toxicity. *Research Communications in Chemical Pathology and Pharmacology* **67**, 63–78.

INNOCENTI, P.F., BRUNI, G., MANDELLI, V. and FERRATI, G.C. (1979) Indoprufen versus ibuprofen in osteoarthritis: a short-term, double-blind, crossover trial. *Current Medical Research and Opinion* **5**, 791–798.

INWOOD, M.J., KILLACKEY, B. and STARTUP, S.J. (1983) The use and safety of ibuprofen in the hemophiliac. *Blood* **61**, 709–711.

JAIN, A.K., RYAN, J.R., MCMAHON, F.G. and SMITH, G. (1986) Analgesic efficacy of low-dose ibuprofen in dental extraction pain. *Pharmacotherapy* **6**, 318–322.

JAIN, S. (1994) Ibuprofen-induced thrombocytopenia. *British Journal of Clinical Practice* **48**, 51.

JASANI, M.K., DOWNIE, W.W., SAMUELS, B.M. and BUCHANAN, W.W. (1968) Ibuprofen in rheumatoid arthritis. *Annals of the Rheumatic Diseases* **27**, 457–462.

JASZEWSKI, R., GRAHAM, D.Y. and STROMATT, S.C. (1992) Treatment of nonsteroidal anti-inflammatory drug-induced gastric ulcers with misoprostol. *Digestive Diseases and Sciences* **37**, 1820–1824.

JENNER, P.N. (1987) Nabumetone in the treatment of skin and soft tissue injury. *American Journal of Medicine* **83**, 101–106.

JOBANPUTRA, P. and NUKI, G. (1994) Nonsteroidal anti-inflammatory drugs in the treatment of osteoarthritis. *Current Opinion in Rheumatology* **6**, 433–439.

JOHNSON, A.G., NGUYEN, T.V. and DAY, R.O. (1994a) Do nonsteroidal anti-inflammatory drugs affect blood pressure? *Annals of Internal Medicine* **121**, 289–300.

JOHNSON, A.G., SEIDEMANN, P. and DAY, R.O. (1994b) NSAID-related adverse drug interactions with clinical relevance. *International Journal of Clinical Pharmacology and Therapeutics* **32**, 509–532.

JOHNSON, J.H., JICK, H., HUNTER, J.R. and DICKSON, J.F. (1985) A followup study of ibuprofen users. *Journal of Rheumatology* **12**, 549–552.

JONES, A.C. and DOHERTY, M. (1992) The treatment of osteoarthritis. *British Journal of Clinical Pharmacology* **33**, 357–363.

JORGENSEN, H.S., CHRISTENSEN, H.R. and KAMPMANN, J.P. (1991) Interaction between digoxin and indomethacin or ibuprofen. *British Journal of Clinical Pharmacology* **31**, 108–110.

JOSEF, H., CHAHADE, W.H. and CHAUDRI, H.A. (1981) A comparative trial of pirprofen and ibuprofen in rheumatoid arthritis. In: VAN DER KORST, A. (ed.) *A New Antirheumatic-Analgesic Agent: Pirprofen (Regasil™)*. Bern, Hans Huber, 114–118.

KALBHEN, D.A. (1988) The influence of NSAIDs on morphology of articular cartilage. *Scandinavian Journal of Rheumatology* **77**(Suppl.), 13–22.

KAMINSKI, D.L., DESHPANDE, Y., THOMAS, L., QUALY, J. and BLANK, W. (1985) Effect of oral ibuprofen on formation of prostaglandins E and F by human gallbladder muscle and mucosa. *Digestive Diseases and Sciences* **30**, 933–940.

KANTOR, G.T. (1979) Ibuprofen. *Annals of Internal Medicine* **91**, 877–882.

KANTOR, G.T. (1986) Ketoprofen: a review of its pharmacological and clinical properties. *Pharmacotherapy* **6**, 93–103.

KAPLAN, H.B., EDELSON, H.S., KORCHAK, H.M., GIVEN, W.P., ABRAMSON, S. and WEISSMAN, G. (1984) Effects of nonsteroidal anti-inflammatory agents on human neutrophil functions *in vitro* and *in vivo*. *Biochemical Pharmacology* **33**, 371–378.

KARSH, J., KIMBERLY, R.P., STAHL, N.I., PLOTZ, P.H. and DECKER, J.L. (1980) Comparative effects of aspirin and ibuprofen in the management of systemic lupus erythematosus. *Arthritis and Rheumatism* **23**, 1401–1404.

KATONA, B.G., WIGLEY, F.M., WALTERS, J.K. and CASPI, M. (1988) Aseptic meningitis from over-the-counter ibuprofen. *The Lancet* **1**, 59.

KATONA, S. and BURGOS-VARGOS, R. (1981) A new derivative of propionic acid, tiaprofenic acid and its efficacy in the treatment of rheumatoid arthritis: comparative studies with ibuprofen. *Current Therapeutic Research* **29**, 1–11.

CHAPTER 6

KEAN, W.F., LOCK, C.J.L. and HOWARD-LOCK, H.E. (1991) Chirality in antirheumatic drugs. *The Lancet* **338**, 1565–1568.

KEET, J.G.M. (1979) A comparative clinical trial of diflunisal and ibuprofen in the control of pain in osteoarthritis. *The Journal of International Medical Research* **7**, 272–276.

KHOURY, M.I. (1989) Ulcerative proctitis in juvenile SLE after ibuprofen treatment. *Journal of Rheumatology* **16**, 217–218.

KLEIN, B. (1982) Carprofen in osteoarthrosis. *European Journal of Rheumatology and Inflammation* **5**, 507–513.

KLEIN, G., NEFF, H. and KULLICH, W. (1992) (S)-(+) versus racemic ibuprofen. *The Lancet* **i**, 681.

KLEIN, G., HAWEL, R., WALLNER, H. and KULLICH, W. (1994) NSAR-Therapy: Schliesst Wirksamkeit Vertraeglichkeit aus? Klinische Erfahrungen mit dem neuen Anti-rheumatikum Dexibuprofen. *Der Praktische Arzt* **48**, 3–7.

KOES, B.W., SHOLTEN, R.J.P.M., MENS, J.M.A. and BOUTER, L.M. (1997) Efficacy of nonsteroidal anti-inflammatory drugs for low back pain: a systematic review of randomised clinical trials. *Annals of the Rheumatic Diseases* **56**, 214–223.

KOOPMANS, P.P., THIEN, T. and GRIBNAU, F.W.J. (1987) The influence of ibuprofen, diclofenac and sulindac on the blood pressure lowering effect of hydrochlorothiazide. *European Journal of Clinical Pharmacology* **31**, 553–557.

KOTOB, A. (1985) A comparative study of two dosage levels of ibuprofen syrup in children with pyrexia. *Journal of International Medical Research* **13**, 122–126.

KOUTSOS, M., SHIFF, S.J. and RIGAS, B. (1995) Can nonsteroidal anti-inflammatory drugs be recommended to prevent colon cancer in high risk elderly patients? *Drugs and Aging* **6**, 421–425.

KRASNOVA, K.N., CHENCHIKOVA, E.P. and SHKARENKOVA, L.V. (1979) Treatment of rheumatoid arthritis in children with Brufen. *Vorp Okhr Materin Det* **24**, 22–24.

KREMER, I., RITZ, R. and BRUMMER, F. (1983) Aseptic meningitis as an adverse effect of co-trimoxazole. *New England Journal of Medicine* **308**, 1481.

LAMBERT, J.R., CARDOE, N., SIMPSON, N.R., OLDHAM, P., NICOL, P.E. and MARTIN, L. (1984) A controlled comparison of tiaprofenic acid and ibuprofen in osteoarthritis. (Abstract). *International Conference on Inflammation, Antirheumatics, Analgesics and Immuno-modulators*, Venice 16–18 April 1984.

LAMBERT, J.R., CARDOE, N., SIMPSON, N.R., OLDHAM, P., NICHOL, P.E. and MARTIN, L. (1985) A controlled comparison of tiaprofenic acid and ibuprofen in osteoarthritis. *International Journal of Clinical Pharmacology Research* **5**, 161–164.

LAMY, P.P. (1993) Institutionalisation and drug use in older adults in the US. *Drugs and Aging* **3**, 232–237.

LANEUVILLE, O., BREUER, D.K., DEWITT, D.L., HLA, T., FUNK, C.D. and SMITH, W.L. (1994) Differential inhibition of human prostaglandin endoperoxide H syntheses-1 and -2 by nonsteroidal anti-inflammatory drugs. *Journal of Pharmacology and Experimental Therapeutics* **271**, 927–934.

LANG, B.A. and FINLAYSON, L.A. (1994) Naproxen-induced pseudoporphyria in patients with juvenile rheumatoid arthritis. *Journal of Pediatrics* **124**, 639–642.

LANGMAN, M.J.S., WEIL, J., WAINWRIGHT, P., LAWSON, D.H., RAWLINS, M.D., LOGAN, R.F.A., MURPHY, M., VESSEY, M.P. and COLIN-JONES, D.G. (1994) Risk of bleeding peptic ulcer associated with individual nonsteroidal anti-inflammatory drugs. *The Lancet* **343**, 1075–1078.

LANZA, F.L., ROYER, G.L., NELSON, R.S., RACK, M.F., SECKMAN, C.E. and SCHWARTZ, J.H. (1986) Effect of acetaminophen on human gastric mucosal injury caused by ibuprofen. *Gut* **27**, 440–443.

LASKA, E.M., SUNSHINE, A., MARRERO, I., OLSON, N., SIEGEL, C. and McCORMICK, N. (1986) The correlation between blood levels of ibuprofen and clinical analgesic response. *Clinical Pharmacology and Therapeutics* **40**, 1–7.

LAVENEZIANA, D., RIVA, A., BONAZZI, M., CIPOLLA, M. and MIGLIAVACCA, S. (1996) Comparative efficacy of oral ibuprofen arginine and intramuscular ketolorac in patients with postoperative pain. *Clinical Drug Investigation* **11**(Suppl. 1), 8–14.

LEADBETTER, W.B., BUCKWALTER, J.A. and GORDON, S.L. (eds) (1990) *Sports-Induced Inflammation: Clinical and Basic Science Concepts*. Park Ridge (IL), American Academy of Orthpaedic Surgeons.

LEE, P., ANDERSON, J.A., MILLER, J., WEBB, J. and BUCHANAN, W.W. (1976) Evaluation of analgesic action and efficacy of antirheumatic drugs: Study of 10 drugs in 684 patients with rheumatoid arthritis. *Journal of Rheumatology* **3**, 283–294.

LEE, R.P., KING, E.G. and RUSSEL, A.S. (1983) Ibuprofen: a severe systemic reaction. *Canadian Medical Association Journal* **129**, 854–855.

LEISING, G., RESEL, R., STELTZER, F., TASH, S., LANGINER, A. and HANTICH, G. (1996) Physical aspects of dexibuprofen and racemic ibuprofen. *Journal of Clinical Pharmacology* **36**, 3S–6S.

LESLIE, R.D.G. (1977) Mefenamic acid compared with ibuprofen in the treatment of rheumatoid arthritis. *Journal of International Medical Research* **5**, 161–163.

LEVINSON, D.J. and RUBINSTEIN, H.M. (1983) Double blind comparison of fenoprofen calcium and ibuprofen in osteoarthritis of large joints. *Current Therapeutic Research* **34**, 280–284.

LEVY, M. (1987) Pyrazolone-induced agranulocytosis: an epidemiological evaluation. In: RAINSFORD, K.D. and VELO, G.P. (eds), *Side-effects of Anti-inflammatory Drugs 1: Clinical and Epidemiological Aspects*. Lancaster, MTP Press, 99–104.

CHAPTER 6

LI, G., TREIBER, G., MAIER, K., WALKER, S. and KLOTZ, U. (1993) Disposition of ibuprofen in patients with liver cirrhosis. Stereochemical considerations. *Clinical Pharmacokinetics* **25**, 154–63.

LIANG, N.M. and FORTIN, P. (1991) Management of osteoarthritis of the hip and knee. *New England Journal of Medicine* **325**, 125–127.

LIBBER, S., HARRISON, H. and SPECTOR, D. (1986) Treatment of nephrogenic diabetes insipidus with prostaglandin synthesis inhibitors. *Journal of Pediatrics* **108**, 305–311.

LOIZZI, S., FASTELLO, V. and BERETTA, A. (1984) A new dosage regimen of ibuprofen in the treatment of osteoarthrosis. *1st World Conference on Inflammation, Analgesics, Immunomodulators*, Venice 15–18 April 1984.

LOKKEN, P. and SKJELBRED, P. (1980) Analgesic and anti-inflammatory effects of para-cetamol evaluated by bilateral oral surgery. *British Journal of Clinical Pharmacology* **10**(Suppl. 2), 253S–260S.

LUGGEN, M.E., GARTSIDE, P.S. and HESS, E.V. (1989) Nonsteroidal anti-inflammatory drugs in rheumatoid arthritis: duration of use as a measure of relative value. *Journal of Rheumatology* **16**, 1565–1569.

MÄKELÄ, A.-L., LEMPIÄINEN, M. and YRJÄNÄ, T. (1980) Ibuprofen in the treatment of juvenile rheumatoid arthritis: metabolism and concentrations in synovial fluid. *British Journal of Clinical Practice* (Suppl. 6), 23–27.

MAKISARA, P. and NUOTIO, P. (1978) Piroxicam and rheumatoid arthritis. Comparative study of piroxicam and ibuprofen. *Royal Society of Medicine International Congress Symposium Series I* **1**, 65–70.

Manchester General Practitioner Group (1984) A study of naproxen and ibuprofen in patients with osteoarthritis seen in general practice. *Current Medical Research and Opinion* **9**, 41–46.

MANSON, A.L. (1988) Trial of ibuprofen to prevent post-vasectomy complications. *Journal of Urology* **139**, 965–966.

MARCH, L.M. (1997) Osteoarthritis. *Medical Journal of Australia* **166**, 98–103.

MARCH, L., IRWIG, L., SCHWARZ, J., SIMPSON, J., CHOCK, C. and BROOKS, P. (1994) N of 1 trial comparing a nonsteroidal drug with paracetamol in osteoarthritis. *British Medical Journal* **309**, 1041–1045.

MARCOLONGO, R., FIORAVANTI, A., GIORDANO, N., FRATI, E. and MARUANI, A.M. (1984) Tiaprofenic acid in the treatment of osteoarthritis of the knee. In: BERRY, H. and FRANCHIMONTI, P. (eds), *Tiaprofenic Acid Symposium: 10th European Congress of Rheumatology*. Geneva, Exerpta Medica, 82–87.

MATTHEWSON, K., PUGH, S. and NORTHFIELD, T.C. (1988) Which peptic ulcer patients bleed? *Gut* **29**, 70–74.

MAWDSLEY, P. (1980) A survey of clinical trials with fenbufen. *Arzneimittel-Forschung* **30**, 740.

MAX, M.B., SCHAFER, S.C., CULNANE, M., DUBNER, R. and GRACELY, R.H. (1988) Association of pain relief with drug side-effects in postherpetic neuralgia: a single-dose study of clonidine, codeine, ibuprofen, and placebo. *Clinical Pharmacology and Therapeutics* **43**, 363–371.

MAYER, J.M. (1996) Ibuprofen enantiomers and lipid metabolism. *Journal of Clinical Pharmacology* **36**(Suppl.), 27–32.

MAYER, J.M., BARTOLUCCI, C., MAITRE, J.M. and TESTA, B. (1988) Metabolic chiral inversion of anti-inflammatory 2-arylpropionates: lack of reaction in liver homogenates, and study of methine proton acidity. *Xenobiotica* **18**, 533–543.

MAZZUCA, S.A., BRANDT, K.D., ANDERSON, S.E., MUSICK, B.S. and KATZ, B.P. (1991) The therapeutic approaches of community based primary care practitioners to osteoarthritis of the hip in the elderly patient. *Journal of Rheumatology* **18**, 1593–1600.

MCARTHUR, A.W., FERRY, D.J. and PALMER, D.G. (1979) A comparative study of indomethacin and ibuprofen. *Medical Journal of Australia* **1**, 25–27.

MCALINDON, T. and DIEPPE, P. (1990) The medical management of osteoarthritis of the knee: an inflammatory issue? *British Journal of Rheumatology* **29**, 471–473.

MCCAULEY, R.L., HEGGERS, J.P. and ROBON, M.C. (1990) Frostbite. Methods to minimize tissue loss. *Postgraduate Medicine* **88**, 67–68.

MCKENZIE, L.S., HORSBURGH, B.A., GHOSH, P. and TAYLOR, T.K.F. (1976) Effect of anti-inflammatory drugs on sulfated glycosaminoglycan synthesis in aged human articular cartilage. *Annals of the Rheumatic Diseases* **35**, 487–497.

MCLATCHIE, G.R., ALLISTER, C., MACEWEN, C., HAMILTON, G., McGREGOR, H., COLQUHUON, I. and PICKVANCE, N.J. (1985) Variable scheduled of ibuprofen for ankle sprains. *British Journal of Sports Medicine* **19**, 203–206.

MCLAUGHLIN, G.E. (1985) A double-blind comparative study of piroxicam and ibuprofen in the treatment of rheumatoid arthritis. *Seminars in Arthritis and Rheumatism* **14**, 11–13.

MCMILLEN, J.I. (1977) Tolmetin sodium vs ibuprofen in rheumatoid arthritic patients previously untreated with either drug: a double-blind crossover study. *Current Therapeutic Research* **22**, 266–275.

MCMILLEN, J.I. (1982) Rheumatoid arthritis: A double-blind study comparing tolmetin sodium with ibuprofen in patients untreated with either drug previously. *Current Therapeutic Research* **31**, 813–818.

MEINERI, C., LESTANI, J. and GENTILETTI, A. (1978) Ensayo de un nuevo analgesico-anti-inflamatorio: C 21'524-Su en osteoarthritis de cadera y de rodilla. *Orientacion Medica* **27**, 365–367.

MEINICKE, J. and DANNESKIOLD-SAMSØE, B. (1980) Diclofenac sodium (Voltaren) and ibuprofen in rheumatoid arthritis. *Scandinavian Journal of Rheumatology* (Suppl. 35), 2–8.

MENA, H.R. and WILLKENS, R.F. (1977) Treatment of ankylosing spondylitis with fluribiprofen or phenylbutazone. *European Journal of Clinical Pharmacology* 11, 263–266.

MENA, H.R., EHRLICH, G.E., GIANSIRACUSA, J., WARD, J. and GRAY, J. (1976) Response of osteoarthritis to ibuprofen or flurbiprofen. *Journal of International Medical Research* 4, 152–157.

MENA, H.R., WARD, J.R., ZUCKNER, J., WOLSKI, K.P., BRINEY, W.G. and GIANSIRACUSA, J. (1977) Treatment of rheumatoid arthritis with flurbiprofen or ibuprofen. *Journal of Clinical Pharmacology* 17, 56–62.

MENKES, C.J. (1993) Effects of disease-modifying antirheumatic drugs, steroids and non-steroidal anti-inflammatory drugs on acute-phase proteins in rheumatoid arthritis. *British Journal of Rheumatology* 32(Suppl. 3), 14–18.

MENON, N.D., WHELTON, J.J., ANSELL, B.M. and GOLDBERG, A.A.J. (1973) A comparative study of ibuprofen and aspirin in Still's Disease (juvenile rheumatoid polyarthritis). *XIIIth International Congress of Rheumatology, Kyoto*, Abstract Volume 1, 17–18.

MEYER, T., HERMANN, C., WIEGAND, V., MALHAIS, B., KIEFEL, V. and MUELLER-ECKHARDT, C. (1993) Immune thrombocytopenia associated with hemorrhagic diathesis due to ibuprofen administration. *Clinical Investigation* 71, 413–415.

MENZEL-SOGLOWEK, S., GEISSLINGER, G. and BRUNE, K. (1993) Metabolic chiral inversion of 2-arylpropionates in different tumor cell lines. In: BROOKS, P.M., DAY, R.O., GRAHAM, G.G. and WILLIAMS, L.M. (eds), *Variability in Response to Anti-Rheumatic Drugs (Agents and Actions Supplement)*. Basel, Birkhauser Verlag, 23–29.

MILCH, P.O., MONHEIT, A.G., ROCHELSON, B.L., METZ, G. and BAKER, D.A. (1986) Failure of ibuprofen in treatment of herpes genitalis. *American Journal of Obstetrics and Gynecology* 155, 399–400.

MILLER, R.R. (1981) Evaluation of the analgesic efficacy of ibuprofen. *Pharmacotherapy* 1, 21–27.

MILLS, S.B., BLOCK, M. and BRUCKNER, F.E. (1973) A double-blind crossover study of ketoprofen and ibuprofen in management of rheumatoid arthritis. *British Medical Journal* 4, 82–84.

MINOCHA, A., BARTH, J.T., HEROLD, D.A., GIDEON, D.A. and SPIKER, D.A. (1986) Modulations of ethanol-induced central nervous system depression by ibuprofen. *Clinical Pharmacology and Therapeutics* 39, 123–127.

MONTRONE, F., FUMAGALLI, M., PELLEGRINI, P., RATTI, G., SALA, G., LIVERTA, C., POLLINI, C.V. and PONTIROLI, A.E. (1979) A double-blind crossover evaluation of ketoprofen (Orudis) and ibuprofen in the management of rheumatoid arthritis. *Rheumatology and Rehabilitation* 18, 114–118.

MOORE, P.A., ACS, G. and HARGREAVES, J.A. (1985) Postextraction pain relief in children; a clinical trial of liquid analgesics. *International Journal of Clinical Pharmacology Therapeutics and Toxicology* **23**, 573–577.

MORGAN, G.J., POLAND, M. and DELAPP, R.E. (1993) Efficacy and safety of nabumetone versus diclofenac, naproxen, ibuprofen, and piroxicam. *American Journal of Medicine* **95**(Suppl. 2A), 19S–27S.

MOXLEY, T.E., ROYER, G.L., HEARRON, M.S., DONOVAN, J.F. and LEVI, L. (1975) Ibuprofen versus buffered phenylbutazone in the treatment of osteoarthritis: double-blind trial. *Journal of the American Geriatric Society* **23**, 343–349.

MÜLLER-FASSBENDER, H. (1987) Double-blind clinical trial of S-adenosylmethionine versus ibuprofen in the treatment of osteoarthritis. *American Journal of Medicine* **83**, 81–83.

MUNGAVIN, J.M. and CLARKE, T.K. (1983) A multi-centre study of tiaprofenic acid (Surgam) and five comparative drugs in rheumatoid arthritis and osteoarthritis in general practice. *Current Medical Research and Opinion* **8**, 461–471.

MURPHY, P.J., BADIA, P., MYERS, B.L., BOECKER, M.R. and WRIGHT, K.P. (1994) Nonsteroidal anti-inflammatory drugs affect normal sleep patterns in humans. *Physiology and Behavior* **55**, 1063–1066.

MURRAY, M.D., BRATER, D.C., TIERNEY, W.M., HUI, S.L. and McDONALD, C.J. (1990) Ibuprofen-associated renal impairment in a large general internal medicine practice. *American Journal of Medical Sciences* **299**, 222–229.

MURRAY, M.D., LAZARIDIS, E.N., BRIZENDINE, E., HAAG, K., BECKER, P. and BRATER, D.C. (1997) The effect of nonsteroidal anti-inflammatory drugs on electrolyte homeostasis and blood pressure in young and elderly persons with and without renal insufficiency. *American Journal of the Medical Sciences* **314**, 80–88.

NAHATA, M.C., DURRELL, D.E., POWELL, D.A. and GUPTA, N. (1991) Pharmacokinetics of ibuprofen in febrile children. *European Journal of Clinical Pharmacology* **40**, 427–428.

NARANJO, C.A. and BREMNER, K.E. (1993a) Behavioural correlates of alcohol intoxications, *Addiction* **88**, 31–41.

NARANJO, C.A. and BREMNER, K.E. (1993b) Clinical pharmacology of serotonin-altering medications for decreasing alcohol consumption. *Alcohol and Alcoholism* **2**(Suppl.), 221–229.

NEUSTADT, D.H. (1997) Double blind evaluation of the longterm effects of etodolac versus ibuprofen in patients with rheumatoid arthritis. *Journal of Rheumatology* **24**(Suppl. 47), 17–22.

NEUVONEN, P.J. (1991) The effect of magnesium hydroxide on the oral absorption of ibuprofen, ketoprofen and diclofenac. *British Journal of Clinical Pharmacology* **31**, 263–266.

CHAPTER 6

NICHOLSON, J.S. (1982) Ibuprofen. In: BINDRA, J.S. and LEDNICER, D. (eds), *Chronicles of Drug Discovery*, Vol. 1. New York, Wiley, 149–171.

NORMAN, S.L., JEAVONS, B.I., O'BRIEN, P.M. *et al.* (1985) A double-blind comparision of a new ibuprofen–codeine phosphate combination, codeine phosphate, and placebo in the relief of postepisiotomy pain. *Clinical Therapeutics* **7**, 549–554.

NOVAK, S.N. (1975) Side-effect of ibuprofen therapy. *Arthritis and Rheumatism* **18**, 628.

O'CONNOR, T.P., ANDERSON, A.M., LENNOX, B. and MULDOON, C. (1993) A novel sustained release formulation of ibuprofen provides effective once-daily therapy in the treatment of rheumatoid arthritis and osteo-arthritis. *British Journal of Clinical Practice* **47**, 10–13.

OGILVIE-HARRIS, D.J. and GILBART, M. (1995) Treatment modalities for soft tissue injuries of the ankle: a critical review. *Clinical Journal of Sports Medicine* **5**, 175–186.

OLDSTAD, O.A. and SKJELBRED, P. (1986) The effects of indoprofen vs paracetamol on swelling, pain and other events after surgery. *International Journal of Clinical Pharmacology, Therapeutics and Toxicology* **24**, 34–38.

O'NEILL, G.P., MANCINI, J.A., KARGMAN, S. *et al.* (1993) Over expression of human prostaglandin G/H synthase-1 and -2 by recombinant vaccinia virus: inhibition by non-steroidal anti-inflammatory drugs and biosynthesis of 15-hydroxy-eicosatetraenoic acid. *Molecular Pharmacology* **45**, 245–254.

ØSTENSEN, M. (1994) Optimisation of antirheumatic drug treatment in pregnancy. *Clinical Pharmacokinetics* **27**, 486–503.

OTT, H. (1979) Ibuprofen versus diclofenac in osteoarthrosis — a clinical comparison. Brufen under Review, IXth European Congress of Rheumatology, Wiesbaden 1979. *British Journal of Clinical Practice* **6**(Suppl.), 32–39.

OWEN, H., GLAVIN, R.J. and SHAW, N.A. (1986) Ibuprofen in the management of post-operative pain. *British Journal of Anaesthesiology* **58**, 1371–1375.

OWENS, N.J., FRETWELL, M.D., WILLEY, C. and MURPHY, S.S. (1994) Distinguishing between the fit and frail elderly, and optimising pharmacotherapy. *Drugs and Aging* **4**, 47–55.

OWEN-SMITH, B.D. and BURRY, H.C. (1992) Ibuprofen in the management of osteoarthrosis of the hip. *Rheumatology and Physical Medicine* **11**, 281–286.

PAGNONI, B., VIGNALI, M., COLELLA, S., MONOPOLI, R. and TIENGO, M. (1996a) Comparative efficacy of oral ibuprofen arginine with intramuscular ketolorac in patients with post-caesarian section pain. *Clinical Drug Investigation* **11**(Suppl. 1), 15–21.

PAGNONI, B., RAVENELLI, A., DEGRADI, L., ROSSI, R. and TIENGO, M. (1996b) Clinical efficacy of ibuprofen arginine in the management of postoperative pain associated with suction termination of pregnancy. A double-blind placebo-controlled study. *Clinical Drug Investigation* **11**(Suppl. 1), 27–32.

PALMER, D.G., FERRY, D.G., GIBBINS, B.L., HALL, S.M., GRENNAN, D.M., LUM, J. and MYERS, D.B. (1981) Ibuprofen and difunisal in rheumatoid arthritis: a double-blind comparative trial. *New Zealand Medical Journal* **94**, 45–47.

PARKER, D.A., GIBBIN, K.P. and NOYELLE, R.M. (1986) Syrup formulations for post-tonsillectomy analgesia: a double-blind study comparing ibuprofen, aspirin and placebo. *Journal of Laryngology and Otology* **100**, 1055–1060.

PARTSCH, G., SCHWARZER, C. and BERI, R. (1990) The effects of ibuprofen and diclofenac on the chemotaxis and adenosine triphosphate level of polymorphonuclear cells *in vitro*. *Journal of Rheumatology* **17**, 583–588.

PASSMORE, A.P., COPELAND, S. and JOHNSTON, G.D. (1990) The effects of ibuprofen and indomethacin on renal function in the presence of fursemide in healthy volunteers on a restricted sodium diet. *British Journal of Clinical Pharmacology* **29**, 311–319.

PAULUS, H.E. (1990) FDA arthritis advisory committee meeting: guidelines for approving nonsteroidal anti-inflammatory drugs for over-the-counter use. *Arthritis and Rheumatism* **33**, 1056–1058.

PAVELKA, K., SUSTA, A., VOJTISEK, D., BREMOVA, A., KANKOVA, D., HANDLOVA, D. and MALECEK, J. (1973) Double-blind comparison of ibuprofen and phenylbutazone in a short-term treatment of rheumatoid arthritis. *Arzneimittel-Forschung* **23**, 842–846.

PAVELKA, K., VOJTISEK, O., SUSTA, A., KANKOVA, D., BREMOVA, A. and KRALOVA, M. (1978) Experience with high doses of ibuprofen in the long-term management of rheumatoid arthritis. *Journal of International Medical Research* **6**, 355–364.

PENNER, J.A. and ALBRECHT, P.H. (1975) Lack of interaction between ibuprofen and warfarin. *Current Therapeutic Research* **18**, 862–871.

PETERA, P., TAUSCH, G. and EBERL, R. (1983) Doppelblindstudie mit Tiaprofensäure (Surgam^R) gegen Ibuprofen (Brufen^R) bei Patienten mit Arthrose der Knie- und Hüftgelenke. *Wiener Medizinsche Wochenschrift* **133**, 409–412.

PEYRON, J. and DOURY, P. (1982) Comparative study of pirprofen and ketoprofen in the treatment of OA of the hip and of the knee (French). *Nouvelle Presse Medicale* **11**, 2497–2499.

PIERUCCI, A. and PATRONO, C. (1992) NSAIDs in renal impairment and dialysis. In: FAMEY, J.P. and POWLESS, H.E. (eds), *Therapeutic Application of NSAID. Subpopulation and New Formulations*. New York, Marcel Dekker, 211–246.

PILLEMER, S.R., BRADLEY, L.A., CROFFORD, L.J., MOLDOFSKY, H. and CHROUSOS, G.P. (1997) The neuroscience and endocrinology of fibromyalgia. *Arthritis and Rheumatism* **40**, 1928–1939.

PIPITONE, V., CARROZZO, M. and LOIZZI, P. (1973) A clinical study of Brufen in comparison with phenylbutazone and indomethacin. *Abstracts of XIII International Congress of Rheumatology, Kyoto*, p. 134.

CHAPTER 6

POILEY, J., SPINDLER, J.S., CLARKE, J.P. and BRAINE, C.L. (1986) Nonsteroidal anti-inflammatory drug therapy in rheumatoid arthritis: a comparison of oxaprozin and ibuprofen. *Seminars in Arthritis and Rheumatism* **15**(Suppl. 2), 59–65.

PORTENOY, R.K. and FARKASH, A.F. (1988) Practical management of non-malignant pain in the elderly. *Geriatrics* **43**, 29–47.

PROPER, S.A., FENSKE, N.A., BURNETT, S.M. and LURIA, L.W. (1988) Compromised wound repair caused by perioperative use of ibuprofen. *Journal of the American Academy of Dermatology* **18**(Suppl. 2), 1173–1178.

PURANEN, J. and RONTY, J. (1978) A new anti-inflammatory drug, proquazone and ibuprofen in the treatment of degenerative joint disease of the knee (gonarthrosis). *Scandinavian Journal of Rheumatology* **21**(Suppl.), 21–24.

QUINN, J.P., WEINSTEIN, R.A. and CAPLAN, L.R. (1984) Eosinophilic meningitis and ibuprofen therapy. *Neurology* **34**, 108–109.

RADACK, K.L., DECK, C.C. and BLOOMFIELD, S.S. (1987) Ibuprofen interferes with the efficacy of antihypertensive drugs. A randomized, double-blind, placebo controlled trial of ibuprofen compared with acetaminophen. *Annals of Internal Medicine* **107**, 628–635.

RAHLFS, V.W. and STAT, C. (1996) Reevaluation of some double-blind, randomized studies of dexibuprofen (Seractil): a state-of-the-art overview. Studies in patients with lumbar vertebral column syndrome, rheumatoid arthritis, distortion of the ankle joint, gonarthrosis, ankylosing spondylitis, and activated coxarthrosis. *Journal of Clinical Pharmacology* **36**, 33S–40S.

RAINSFORD, K.D. (1994) Diclofenac (Voltaren:Voltarol)-associated hepatotoxicity, *Inflammopharmacology* **2**, 333–336.

RAINSFORD, K.D. (1995) Gastric ulcerogenicity in mice of enantiomers of nonsteroidal anti-inflammatory drugs having differing potency as prostaglandin synthesis inhibitors, *Pharmaceutical Sciences* **1**, 169–171.

RAINSFORD, K.D. (1996) Mode of action, uses, and side-effects of anti-inflammatory drugs. In: RAINSFORD, K.D. (ed.), *Advances in Anti-Rheumatic Therapy*. Boca Raton FL, CRC Press, 59–111.

RAINSFORD, K.D. (1977) The comparative gastric ulcerogenic activities of nonsteroidal anti-inflammatory drugs. *Agents and Actions* **7**, 575–577.

RAINSFORD, K.D. and QUADIR, M. (1995) Gastrointestinal damage and bleeding from nonsteroidal anti-inflammatory drugs. I. Clinical and epidemiological aspects. *Inflammopharmocology* **3**, 169–190.

RAINSFORD, K.D. and VELO, G.P. (eds) (1984) *Side-Effects of Anti-inflammatory/Analgesic Drugs*. New York, Raven Press.

RAINSFORD, K.D. and VELO, G.P. (eds) (1992) *Side-Effects of Anti-Inflammatory Drugs 3*. Dordrecht, Kluwer Academic Publishers.

RAINSFORD, K.D., RASHAD, S.Y., REVELL, P.A., LOW, F.M., HEMINGWAY, A.P. and WALKER, F.S. (1992) Effects of NSAIDs on cartilage proteoglycan and synovial prostaglandin metabolism in relation to progression of joint deterioration in osteoarthritis. In: BÁLINT, G., GÖMÖR, B. and HÓDINKA, L. (eds), *Rheumatology, State of the Art*. Amsterdam, Elsevier, 177–183.

RANDALL, C.L., BECKER, H.C. and ANTON, R.F. (1991) Effect of ibuprofen on alcohol-induced teratogenesis in mice. *Alcoholism, Clinical and Experimental Research* **15**, 673–677.

RASHAD, S., REVELL, P., HEMINGWAY, A., LOW, F., RAINSFORD, K. and WALKER, F. (1989) Effect of nonsteroidal anti-inflammatory drugs on the course of osteoarthritis. *Lancet* **2**, 519–522.

RASHAD, S., RAINSFORD, K., REVELL, P., LOW, F., HEMINGWAY, A. and WALKER, F. (1992) Effects of NSAIDs on the course of osteoarthritis. In: BÁLINT, G., GÖMÖR, B. and HÓDINKA, L. (eds), *Rheumatology, State of the Art*. Amsterdam, Elsevier, 184–188.

RAY, R.L. (ed.) (1989) *Clinics in Sports Medicine*. Philadelphia, W.B. Saunders, 140.

RAZA, K. and HARDING, J.J. (1991) Non-enzymic modification of lens proteins by glucose and fructose: effects of ibuprofen. *Experimental Eye Research* **52**, 205–212.

REGALDO, R.G. and FOWLER, P.D. (1974) Butacote and Brufen in the treatment of rheumatic diseases. *Journal of International Medical Research* **2**, 115–124.

REMINGTON, R.L., SHABINO, C.L., McGEE, H., PRESTON, G., SARNIAK, A.P. and HALL, W.N. (1985) Reye's syndrome and juvenile rheumatoid arthritis in Michigan. *American Journal of Diseases of Children* **139**, 870–872.

RENNEBOHM, R.M., HEUBI, J.E., DOUGHERTY, C.C. and DANIELS, S.R. (1985) Reye's syndrome in children receiving salicylate therapy for connective tissue disease. *Journal of Pediatrics* **107**, 877–880.

REYNOLDS, J.E.F. (ed.) (1996) *Martindale. The Extra Pharmacopoeia*, 31st edn. London, Royal Pharmaceutical Society.

REYNOLDS, P.M.G. and WHORWELL, P.J. (1974) A single-blind crossover comparison of fenoprofen, ibuprofen and naproxen in rheumatoid arthritis. *Current Medical Research and Opinion* **2**, 461–464.

RIDDER, W.H. III and TOMLINSON, A. (1992) Effect of ibuprofen on contrast sensitivity. *Optometry and Vision Science* **69**, 652–655.

RIND, V.M., LEATHAM, P.A., WRIGHT, V., AKBAR, F.A. and DOWNIE, W.W. (1978) A comparative study of flocafenine (Idarac) and ibuprofen in the treatment of osteoarthritis. *Journal of International Medical Research* **6**, 11–13.

RODRIGUEZ, L.A.G., WILLIAMS, R., DERBY, L.E., DEAN, A.D. and JICK, H. (1994) Acute liver injury associated with nonsteroidal anti-inflammatory drugs and the role of risk factors. *Archives of Internal Medicine* **154**, 311–316.

CHAPTER 6

ROSENBLOOM, D., BROOKS, P., BELLAMY, N. and BUCHANAN, W.W. (1985) *Clinical Trials in the Rheumatic Diseases. A Selected Critical Review.* New York, Praeger.

ROSSI, F.A. and BARONI, L. (1975) A double-blind comparison between diclofenac sodium and ibuprofen in osteoarthritis. *Journal of International Medical Research* 3, 267–274.

ROTH, S.H. (1990) Misoprostol in the prevention of NSAID-induced gastric ulcer: a multi-center double-blind, placebo-controlled trial. *Journal of Rheumatology* 20(Suppl.), 20–24.

ROTH, S.H., TINDALL, E.A., JAIN, A.K., MCMAHON, F.G., APRIL, P.A., BOCKOW, B.I., COHEN, S.B. and FLEISCHMANN, R.M. (1993) A controlled study comparing the effects of nabumetone, ibuprofen, and ibuprofen plus misoprostol on the upper gastrointestinal mucosa. *Archives of Internal Medicine* 153, 2565–2571.

ROVATI, L.C. (1992) Clinical research in osteoarthritis: design and results of short-term and long-term trials with disease-modifying drugs. *International Journal of Tissue Reactions* 14, 243–251.

ROWE, P.C., VALLE, D. and BRUISLOW, S.W. (1988) Inborn errors of metabolism in children referred with Reye's syndrome. A changing pattern. *Journal of the American Medical Association* 260, 3168–3171.

ROYER, G.L., SECKMAN, C.E. and WELSHMAN, M.S. (1984) Safety profile: fifteen years of clinical experience with ibuprofen. *American Journal of Medicine* 77, 25–34.

ROYER, G.L., MOXLEY, T.E., HEARRON, M.S., MIYARA, A. and DONOVAN, J.F. (1975) A six-month double-blind trial of ibuprofen and indomethacin in osteoarthritis. *Current Therapeutic Research* 17, 234–248.

RUDY, A.C., KNIGHT, P.M., BRATER, D.C. and HALL, S.D. (1991) Stereoselective metabolism of R-, S- and racemic ibuprofen. *Journal of Pharmacology and Experimental Therapeutics* 259, 1133–1139.

RUOFF, G., WILLIAMS, S., COOPER, W. (JR) and PROCACCINI, R.L. (1982) Aspirin-acetaminophen vs ibuprofen in a controlled multicenter double-blind study in patients experiencing pain associated with osteoarthritis. *Current Therapeutic Research* 31, 821–831.

RUOTSI, A. and SKRIFVARS, B. (1978) A long-term double-blind comparative study on proquazone (Biarison) and ibuprofen in rheumatoid arthritis. *Scandinavian Journal of Rheumatology* (Suppl. 21), 28–32.

RUPPERT, G.B. and BARTH, W.F. (1981) Tolmetin-induced aseptic meningitis. *Journal of the American Medical Association* 245, 67–68.

RUSSELL, I.J., FLETCHER, E.M., MICHALEK, J.E., MCBROOM, P.C. and HESTER, G.G. (1991) Treatment of primary fibrosis/fibromyalgia syndrome with ibuprofen and alprazolam. A double blind, placebo-controlled study. *Arthritis and Rheumatism* 34, 552–560.

SACCHETTI, G., DIMURRO, R., MANDELLI, V. and GALLICO, S. (1978) Clinical testing of indoprofen in osteoarthritis: a controlled trial using a balanced incomplete block design. *Current Therapeutic Research* **24**, 274–283.

SANDERS, L.R. (1995) Exercise-induced renal failure associated with ibuprofen, hydrochlorothiazide, and triamterene. *Journal of the American Society of Nephrology* **5**, 2020–2023.

SANFORD-DRISCOLL, M. and KNODEL, L.C. (1986) Induction of hemolytic anemia by NSAID. *Drug Intelligence and Clinical Pharmacy* **20**, 925–934.

SASAKI, S. (1970) Clinical trials of ibuprofen in Japan. *Rheumatology and Physical Medicine* **11**(Suppl.), 32–39.

SAXENA, R.P. and SAXENA, U. (1978) A comparative trial of ketoprofen and ibuprofen in patients with rheumatic disease. *Current Medical Research and Opinion* **5**, 484–488.

SCALIE, J.J. and RIVELIS, L. (1981) Double-blind crossover study of indoprofen versus ibuprofen and placebo in rheumatoid arthritis patients. *European Journal of Rheumatology and Inflammation* **4**, 93–96.

SCHACHTEL, B.P., THODEN, W.R. and BAYBUTT, R.I. (1989) Ibuprofen and acetaminophen in the relief of postpartum episiotomy pain. *Journal of Clinical Pharmacology* **29**, 550–553.

SCHLONDORFF, D. (1993) Renal complications of nonsteroidal anti-inflammatory drugs. *Kidney International* **44**, 643–653.

SEMBLE, E.L., WU, W.C. and CASTELL, D.O. (1989) Nonsteroidal anti-inflammatory drugs and esophageal injury. *Seminars in Arthritis Rheumatism* **19**, 99–109.

SEPPÄLÄ, M. and SOURANDER, L. (1995) A practical guide to prescribing in nursing homes avoiding the pit falls. *Drugs and Aging* **6**, 426–435.

SEYMOUR, R.A. and WALTON, J.G. (1984) Pain control after third molar surgery. *International Journal of Oral Surgery* **13**, 457–485.

SHAH, S.J., BHANDARKAR, S.D. and SATOSKAR, R.S. (1984) Drug interaction between chlorpropamid and nonsteroidal anti-inflammatory drugs ibuprofen and phenylbutazone. *International Journal of Clinical Pharmacology Therapy and Toxicology* **22**, 470–472.

SHELDRAKE, F.E. and ANSELL, B.M. (1975) The use of 'Brufen' (ibuprofen) in the treatment of juvenile chronic polyarthritis. *Current Medical Research and Opinion* **3**, 604–606.

SHIFF, S.J. and RIGAS, B. (1997) Nonsteroidal anti-inflammatory drugs and colorectal cancer: evolving concepts of their chemopreventive actions. *Gastroenterology* **113**, 1992–1998.

SHIRLEY, M.A., GUAN, X., KAISER, D.G., HALSTEAD, G.W. and BAILLIE, T.A. (1994) Taurine conjugation of ibuprofen in humans and in rat liver *in vitro*. Relationship to metabolic chiral inversion. *Journal of Pharmacology and Expimental Therapeutics* **269**, 1166–1174.

■
CHAPTER 6
■

SHOENFELD, Y., LIVNI, E., SHAKLAIM, M. and PINCHAS, J. (1980) Sensitization to ibuprofen in systemic lupus erythematosus. *Journal of the American Medical Association* **244**, 547–548.

SIEGMETH, W. and PLACHETA, W. (1978) A comparison of short-term effects of ibuprofen and diclofenac in spondylitis. *Journal of International Medical Research* **6**, 369–377.

SILAGY, C. (1993) Aspirin and the elderly current status. *Drugs and Aging* **3**, 301–307.

SILVER, R.M. (1988) Nonsteroidal anti-inflammatory drugs in the management of juvenile arthritis. *Journal of Clinical Pharmacology* **28**, 566–570.

SLAVIC-SVIRCEV, V., HEIDRICH, G., KAIKO, R.F. and RUSY, B.F. (1984) Ibuprofen in the treatment of postoperative pain. *American Journal of Medicine* **77**(1A), 84–86.

SLOAN, J.P., HAIN, R. and POWNALL, R. (1989) Benefits of early anti-inflammatory medication following acute ankle injury. *Injury* **20**, 81–83.

SMITH, W.L., MEADE, E.A. and DEWITT, D.L. (1994) Interactions of PGH synthase isozymes-1 and -2 with NSAIDs. *Annals of the New York Academy of Sciences* **744**, 50–57.

SONEBLICK, M. and ABRAHAM, A.F. (1978) Ibuprofen hypersensitivity in systemic lupus erythematosus. *British Medical Journal* **1**, 619–20.

SORKIN, E.M. and BROGDEN, R.N. (1985) Tiaprofenic acid. A review of its pharmacological efficacy in rheumatic diseases and pain states. *Drugs* **29**, 208–235.

SPITZER, W.O., LEBLANC, F.E. and DUPUIS, M. (eds) (1987) Scientific approach to the assessment and management of activity related spinal disorders. *Spine* **7**(Suppl.), 1–59.

SQUIRES, D.J. and MASSON, E.L. (1981) A double-blind comparison of ibuprofen, ASA–codeine–caffeine compound and placebo in the treatment of dental surgery pain. *Journal of International Medical Research* **9**, 257–260.

STEANS, A., MANNERS, P.J. and ROBINSON, I.G. (1990) A multicentre long-term evaluation of the safety and efficacy of ibuprofen syrup in children with juvenile chronic arthritis. *British Journal of Clinical Practice* **44**, 172–175.

STERNS, R.S. and DODSON, T.B. (1985) Ibuprofen in the treatment of UV-B-induced inflammation. *Archives of Dermatology* **12**, 508–512.

STEVEN, M.M., SMALL, M., PINKERTON, L., MADDOK, R., STURROCK, R.D. and FORBES, C.D. (1985) Nonsteroidal anti-inflammatory drugs in hemophilic arthritis. A clinical and laboratory study. *Hemostasis* **15**, 204–209.

STEWART, W.F., KAWAS, C., CORRADA, M. and METTER, E.J. (1997) Risk of Alzheimer's disease and duration of NSAID use. *Neurology* **48**, 626–632.

STOCK, K.P., GEISSLINGER, G., LOEW, D., BECK, W.S., BACH, G.L. and BRUNE, K. (1991) (S)-Ibuprofen versus ibuprofen-racemate. A randomized double-blind study in patients with rheumatoid arthritis. *Rheumatology International* **11**, 199–202.

STOCKMAN, A., VARIGOS, J.A. and MUIRDEN, K.D. (1976) Comparison of effectiveness of mefenamic acid and ibuprofen in treatment of rheumatoid arthritis. *Medical Journal of Australia* **2**, 819–821.

STRATTON, M.A. (1985) Drug induced systemic lupus. *Clinical Pharmacy* **4**, 457–463.

STURROCK, R.D. and HART, F.D. (1974) Double-blind crossover comparision of indomethacin, flubiprofen, and placebo in ankylosing spondylitis. *Annals of the Rheumatic Diseases* **33**, 129–131.

STURROCK, R.D., GRENNAN, D., LEE, P., CANESI, B.A. and BUCHANAN, W.W. (1975) Eine Bewertung der Phenylalkanoinsäure-Derivate in der Behandlung rheumatischer Erkrankungen sowie einige Erläuterungen zur Lehre der klinischen Versuchsmethodene. *Zeitschrift für Rheumatologie* **34**, 55–57.

SUDLOW, G., BIRKETT, D.J. and WADE, D.N. (1975) Spectroscopic techniques in the study of protein binding. A fluorescence technique for the evaluation of the albumin binding and displacement of warafin and warafin-alcohol. *Clinical and Experimental Pharmacology and Physiology* **2**, 129–140.

SUDLOW, G., BIRKETT, D.J. and WADE, D.N. (1976) Further characterization of specific drug binding sites on human serum albumin. *Molecular Pharmacology* **12**, 1052–1061.

SULLIVAN, K.M., REMINGTON, P.L., HURWITZ, E.S. and HALPIN, T.J. (1988) Reye's syndrome among patients with juvenile rheumatoid arthritis. *Journal of the American Medical Association* **260**, 3434–3435.

SUNSHINE, A., ROURE, C., OLSON, N., LASKA, E.M., ZORRILLA, C. and RIVERS, J. (1987) Analgesic efficacy of two ibuprofen–codeine combinations for the treatment of postepisiotomy and postoperative pain. *Clinical Pharmacology and Therapeutics* **42**, 374–380.

SUWA, T., URANO, H., KOHNO, Y., SUZUKI, A. and AMANO, T. (1987) Comparative studies on the gastrointestinal lesions caused by several nonsteroidal anti-inflammatory agents in rats. *Agents and Actions* **21**, 167–172.

Symposium on Ibuprofen (1970) *Rheumatology and Physical Medicine* **11**(Suppl.), 1–107.

Symposium on Ibuprofen ('Brufen') (1975) *Current Medical Research and Opinion* **3**, 473–606.

TABORN, J., ANDERSON, S., GOLDBERG, M., KANTROWITZ, F., MENANDER-HUBER, K. and GROSS, J. (1985) Relief of morning stiffness: a comparative study of naproxen and ibuprofen. *Current Medical Research and Opinion* **9**, 350–365.

TAINA, E. (1981) Ibuprofen versus placebo in the relief of post-episiotomy pain. *Current Medical Research and Opinion* **7**, 423–428.

TANNER, A.R. and RAGHUNATH, R. (1988) Colonic inflammation and NSAID administration. *Digestion* **41**, 116–120.

CHAPTER 6

TAUSCH, T.E. and FASCHING, U. (1980) A further clinical comparison of ibuprofen and sulindac in osteoarthrosis. Brufen under Review, IXth European Congress of Rheumatology, Wiesbaden 1979. *British Journal of Clinical Practice* (Suppl. 6), 53–61.

THOMPSON, M., STEPHENSON, P. and PERCY, S. (1964) Ibufenac in the treatment of arthritis. *Annals of the Rheumatic Diseases* 23, 397.

THOMPSON, M., FOX, H. and NEWELL, D.H. (1968) Ibuprofen in the treatment of arthritis. *Medical Proceedings (South Africa)* 14, 579–582.

TODD, P.A. and BERESFORD, R. (1986) Pirprofen. A review of its pharmacodynamic and pharmacokinetic properties, and therapeutic efficacy. *Drugs* 32, 509–537.

TODD, P.A. and CLISSOLD, S.P. (1990) Naproxen. A reappraisal of its pharmacology, and therapeutic use in rheumatic diseases and pain states. *Drugs* 40, 91–137.

TODD, P.A. and CLISSOLD, S.P. (1991) Tenoxicam. An update of its pharmacology and therapeutic efficacy in rheumatic diseases. *Drugs* 41, 625–646.

TODD, P.A. and HEEL, R.C. (1985) Suprofen: a review of its pharmacodynamic and pharmacokinetic properties. *Drugs* 30, 514–538.

TRACY, T.S., WIRTHEIM, D.P. and HALL, S.D. (1993) Metabolic inversion of (R)-ibuprofen. Formation of ibuprofenyl-coenzyme A. *Drug Metabolism and Disposition* 21, 114–120.

TRANMER, C. (1978) Benorylate versus ibuprofen in the treatment of osteoarthritis. *Rheumatology and Rehabilitation* 17, 91–94.

TRETENHAN, W. (1980) A comparison between ibuprofen and naproxen in osteoarthrosis of the spine. Brufen under Review, IXth European Congress of Rheumatology, Wiesbaden 1979. *British Journal of Clinical Practice* (Suppl. 6), 45–52.

TRÉVES, R., MAHEU, E. and DREISER, R.L. (1995) Therapeutic trials in digital osteoarthritis. A critical review. *Revue du Rhumatologie English Edition* 62(Suppl.), 33S–41S.

TURNER, R.A., APRIL, P.A. and ROBBINS, D.L. (1982) Double-blind multi-centre study comparing piroxicam and ibuprofen in the treatment of rheumatoid arthritis. *American Journal of Medicine* 72(Suppl.), 34–38.

TYSON, V.C.H. and GLYNNE, A. (1980) A comparative study of benoxaprofen and ibuprofen in osteoarthritis general practice. *Journal of Rheumatology* 7(Suppl.), 132–138.

UMBENHAUER, E.R. (1983) Diflunisal in the treatment of the pain of osteoarthritis. Summary of clinical studies. *Pharmacotherapy* 3, 55S–60S.

VAN DER WINDT, D.A.W.M., VAN DER HEIJDEN, G.J.M.G., SCHOLTEN, R.J.P.M., KOES, B.W. and BOUTER, L.M. (1995) The efficacy of nonsteroidal anti-inflammatory drugs (NSAIDs) for shoulder complaints. A systematic review. *Journal of Clinical Epidemiology* 48, 691–704.

VANE, J.R. and BOTTING, R.M. (1995) New insights into the mode of action of anti-inflammatory drugs. *Inflammation Research* 44, 1–10.

VAN SAASE, J.L.C.M., VAN ROMUNDE, L.K.J., CATS, A., VANDENBROUCHE, J.P. and VALKENBURG, H.A. (1989) Epidemiology of oasteoarthritis: Zoetermeer survey: comparisons of radiological osteoarthritis in a Dutch population with that in 10 other populations. *Annals of the Rheumatic Diseases* **48**, 271–280.

VAN TULDER, M.W., KOES, B.W., BOUTER, L.M. and METSEMAKERS, J. (1997) Management of chronic, nonspecific low-back pain in general practice: a descriptive study. *Spine* **22**, 76–82.

VAZ, A.L. and MARTINS, D. (1984) A comparative controlled study of tiaprofenic acid and ibuprofen in the treatment of osteoarthritis of the knee. In: BERRY, H. and FRANCHIMONTI, P. (eds), *Tiaprofenic Acid Symposium, 10th European Congress of Rheumatology, Moscow.* Geneva, Exerpta Medica, 77–81.

VELO, G.P., MINUZ, P., AROSIO, E., CAPAZZO, M.G., COVI, G. and LECHI, A. (1987) Interactions between nonsteroidal anti-inflammatory drugs and angiotensin-converting enzyme inhibitors in man. In: RAINSFORD, K.D. and VELO, G.P. (eds), *Side-Effects of Anti-inflammatory Drugs 1: Clinical and Epidemiological Aspects.* Lancaster, MTP Press, 195–201.

VELTRI, J.C. and ROLLINS, D.E. (1988) A comparison of the frequency and severity of poisoning cases for ingestion of acetaminophen, aspirin, and ibuprofen. *American Journal of Emergency Medicine* **6**, 104–107.

VENTAFRIDDA, V., DE CONNO, F., PANERAI, A.E., MARESCA, V., MONZA, G.C. and RIPAMONTI, C. (1990) Nonsteroidal anti-inflammatory drugs as the first step in cancer pain therapy: double-blind, within patient study comparing nine drugs. *Journal of International Medical Research* **18**, 21–29.

VLOK, G.J. and VAN VUREN, J.P. (1987) Comparison of a standard ibuprofen treatment regimen with a new ibuprofen/paracetamol/codeine combination in chronic osteoarthritis. *South African Medical Journal* **4**(1; Pt 1), 1–6.

WAGENHAUSER, F.J. (1973) Long-term study with Brufen. *Abstracts of XIII International Congress of Rheumatology*, Kyoto, 106.

WALKER, J.S., NGUYEN, T.V. and DAY, R.O. (1994) Clinical response to nonsteroidal anti-inflammatory drugs in urate-crystal induced inflammation: a simulataneous study of intersubject and intrasubject variability. *British Journal of Clinical Pharmacology* **38**, 341–347.

WALKER, J.S., LOCKTON, A.I., NGUYEN, T.V. and DAY, R.O. (1996) Analgesic effect of ibuprofen after single and multiple doses in chronic spinal pain patients. *Analgesia* **2**, 93–101.

WALKER, J.S., SHEATHER-REID, R.B., CARMODY, J.J., VIAL, J.H. and DAY, R.O. (1997) Nonsteroidal anti-inflammatory drugs in rheumatoid arthritis and osteoarthritis. Support for the concept of 'responders' and 'nonresponders'. *Arthritis and Rheumatism* **40**, 1944–1954.

CHAPTER 6

WARD, J.R. (1984) Update on ibuprofen for rheumatoid arthritis. *American Journal of Medicine* 77, 3–9.

WALSON, P.D., GALLETTA, G., BRADEN, N.J. and ALEXANDER (1989) Ibuprofen, acetaminophen, and placebo treatment of febrile children. *Clinical Pharmacology and Therapeutics* 46, 9–17.

WEBER, J.C.P. (1987) Epidemiology in the United Kingdom of adverse drug reactions from non-steroidal anti-inflammatory drugs. In: RAINSFORD, K.D. and VELO, G.P. (eds), *Side-effects of Anti-Inflammatory Drugs 1: Clinical and Epidemiological Aspects*. Lancaster, MTP Press, 27–35.

WEIBE, E.R. and RAWLING, M. (1995) Pain control in abortion. *International Journal of Gynecology and Obstetrics* 50, 41–46.

WEILER, J.M., ALBRIGHT, J.P. and BUCKWALTER, J.A. (1987) Nonsteriodal anti-inflammatory drugs in sports medicine. In: LEWIS, A.J. and FURST, D.E. (eds), *Nonsteroidal Anti-Inflammatory Drugs. Mechanisms and Clinical Use*. New York, Marcel Dekker, 71–88.

WEINBLATT, M.E. (1991) Nonsteroidal anti-inflammatory drug toxicity: increased risk in the elderly. *Scandinavian Journal of Rheumatology* 91(Suppl.), 9–17.

WHELTON, A., STOUT, R.L., SPILMAN, P.S. and KLASSEN, D.K. (1990) Renal effects of ibuprofen, piroxicam, and sulindac in patients with asymptomatic renal failure. *Annals of Internal Medicine* 112, 568–576.

WHITLAM, J.B., BROWN, K.F., CROOKS, M.S. and ROOM, G.F.W. (1981) Trans-synovial distribution of ibuprofen in arthritis patients. *Clinical Pharmacology and Therapeutics* 29, 487–492.

WHITE, K.P. and HARTH, M. (1996) An analytical review of 24 controlled clinical trials for fibromyalgia syndrome (FMS). *Pain* 64, 211–219.

WHITEHOUSE, M.W. and RAINSFORD, K.D. (1987) Why are non-steroidal drugs so gastrotoxic, even when given orally as solubilized salt formulations or parenterally? In: RAINSFORD, K.D. and VELO, G.P. (eds), *Side-effects of Anti-Inflammatory Drugs, 2. Studies in Major Organ Systems*. Lancaster, Kluwer Academic Publishers, 55–65.

WILHOLM, B.E., MYRHED, M. and EKMAN, E. (1987) Trends and patterns in adverse drug reactions to non-steroidal anti-inflammatory drugs reported in Sweden. In: RAINSFORD, K.D. and VELO, G.P. (eds), *Side-effects of Anti-Inflammatory Drugs 1: Clinical and Epidemiological Aspects*. Lancaster, MTP Press, 55–72.

WILLETT, L.R., CARSON, J.L. and STROM, B.L. (1994) Epidemiology of gastrointestinal damage associated with nonsteroidal anti-inflammatory drugs. *Drug Safety* 10, 170–181.

WILLIAMS, J. and STURROCK, R.D. (1976) An opthalmic study of ibuprofen in rheumatoid conditions. *Current Medical Research and Opinion* 4, 128–131.

WILLIAMS, K.M. (1993) Chiral NSAIDs: so what? In: BROOKS, P.M., DAY, R.O., GRAHAM, G.G. and WILLIAMS, K.M. (eds), *Variability in Response to Anti-rheumatic Drugs*. Basel, Birkhäuser, 15–22.

WILLIAMS, K.M. and DAY, R.O. (1985) Stereoselective disposition — basis for variability in response to NSAIDs. In: BROOKS, P.M. and DAY, R.O. (eds), *Basis for Variability in Response*. Basel, Birkhäuser, 119–127.

WILLIAMS, K.M. and DAY, R.O. (1988) The contribution of enantiomers to variability in response to anti-inflammatory drugs. In: BROOKS, P.M., DAY, R.O., WILLIAMS, K. and GRAHAM, G. (eds), *Basis for Variability of Response to Anti-Rheumatic Drugs*. Proceedings of a Satellite Meeting of the Xth International Congress of Pharmacology, Basel, Birkhäuser, 76–84.

WILLIAMS, K., DAY, R., KNIHINICKI, R. and DUFFIELD, A. (1986) The stereoselective uptake of ibuprofen enantiomers into adipose tissue. *Biochemical Pharmacology* **35**, 3405–3409.

WILLIAMS, H.J., WARD, J.R., EGGER, M.J. *et al.* (1993) Comparison of naproxen and aceta-minophen in a two year study of treatment of osteoarthritis of the knee. *Arthritis and Rheumatism* **36**, 1196–1206.

WILLIAMS, W.R. (1983) Comparison between fenoprofen and ibuprofen in the treatment of soft-tissue rheumatism. *Journal of International Medical Research* **11**, 349–353.

WINDLE, M.L., BOOKER, L.A. and RAYBURN, W.F. (1989) Postpartum pain after vaginal delivery. A review of comparative analgesic trials. *Journal of Reproductive Medicine* **34**, 891–895.

WISEMAN, E.H. and NOGUCHI, Y. (1987) Limitations of laboratory models in predicting gastrointestinal toleration of oxicams and other anti-inflammatory drugs. In: RAINSFORD, K.D. and VELO, G.P. (eds), *Side-effects of Anti-inflammatory Drugs 2: Studies in Major Organ Systems*. Lancaster, Kluwer Academic Publishers, 41–54.

YUNUS, M.B., MASI, A.T. and ALDAG, J.C. (1989) Short term effects of ibuprofen in primary fibromyalgia syndrome: a double blind, placebo controlled trial. *Journal of Rheumatology* **16**, 527–532.

ZOHMANN, A. (1994) Stereochemie in der Praxis-Mythos oder Optimierung? *Der Praktische Arzt* **48**, 3–6.

ZWAIFLER, N. (1989) A review of the antiarthritic efficacy and safety of etodolac. *Clinical Rheumatology* **8**(Suppl. 1), 43–53.

ZUCKNER, J. (1986) International experience with diclofenac in rheumatoid arthritis. *American Journal of Medicine* **80**(Suppl. 4B), 39–42.

CHAPTER 6

Safety and Efficacy of Non-prescription (OTC) Ibuprofen

K D RAINSFORD

Division of Biomedical Sciences and Biomedical Research Centre,
Sheffield Hallam University, Pond Street, Sheffield S1 1WB, UK

Contents

7.1 INTRODUCTION

Ibuprofen is used on a non-prescription, or over-the-counter (OTC), basis for management of mild to moderate pain, soft-tissue inflammation including dysmenorrhoea, migraine, postoperative pain, dental pain, musculoskeletal conditions, and the relief of fever (Dollery, 1991; Reynolds, 1996). It is probably the safest anti-inflammatory/analgesic drug available today. This drug stands out for its safety in comparison with aspirin or paracetamol as well as the newer nonsteroidal anti-inflammatory drugs (NSAIDs), e.g. naproxen and ketoprofen. Furthermore, the toxicity at high dosages of ibuprofen is very low in comparison with these drugs and paracetamol (Veltri and Rollins, 1988; see Chapter 12). The evidence for the favourable safety record of ibuprofen comes from (a) clinical trial data in which the adverse effects of this drug have been compared with paracetamol, aspirin and other NSAIDs; (b) spontaneous reports to manufacturers and drug regulatory authorities of adverse events; (c) epidemiological studies performed in populations exposed to OTC dosages of the drug; and (d) toxicological data from incidents where the drug has been ingested accidentally or as an agent for (para)suicide. The last has been reviewed at length by Volans, Chapter 12. Here the safety of the ibuprofen is considered from evidence in studies categorized in the studies (a) to (c) above. Extensive studies on the effects of ibuprofen in comparison with other reference drugs are also reviewed. Thus, it is possible to give an assessment of the efficacy of the drug in relation to its safety.

There have been some studies and reviews on the safety and efficacy of ibuprofen and some other OTC NSAIDs and non-narcotic analgesics, to which the reader is referred (Rainsford, 1984, 1996; Bird, 1985; Brune, 1986; Busson, 1986; Fowler, 1987; Forster *et al.*, 1992; Furey *et al.*, 1992; Baker, 1996; Moore *et al.*, 1996; Prescott, 1996; Rainsford *et al.*, 1997; Rainsford and Powanda, 1998). The 'Special Report on Clinical Safety of OTC Analgesics' (sponsored by McNiel Consumer Products Company — a company producing paracetamol/acetaminophen) gives an overview of the safety and efficay of paracetamol, aspirin and ibuprofen (Baker, 1996). The proceedings have been published of a symposium on OTC NSAIDs and analgesics held in 1997 together with a debate among international experts regarding some of the major issues concerning the safety and efficacy of these drugs (Rainsford and Powanda, 1998).

Ibuprofen was the first of the new generation of NSAIDs and the first analgesic after paracetamol (acetaminophen) to be given OTC status (Adams and Marchant, 1984; see also Chapter 1). This approval was initially granted in the United Kingdom in 1983 by the UK Department of Health following review by the Committee on the Safety of Medicines. It was followed closely by approval in 1984 in the United States by the Food and Drug Administration (FDA). The direct sale to the public of ibuprofen was a milestone decision by both these authorities as it established a basis that allowed drugs to progress ('switch') from prescription-only to OTC status. The prime consideration for granting of OTC status in the United States was safety in prescription doses, since efficacy was granted (Paulus,

1990). This has continued to be the basis for approval of NSAIDs (ketoprofen, naproxen) and other drugs for OTC by the FDA and many other drug-regulatory authorities.

Recently, this basis was, in effect, challenged by an application by the Bayer Company (USA) for the (S)-$(+)$ isomer of ibuprofen, or dexibuprofen, to be made available OTC without substantial data from prescription dosage of this drug. This company made the case that since half of the conventional *rac*-ibuprofen is composed of (R)-$(-)$-ibuprofen, this is an inactive drug. However, the combined FDA Advisory Committee and the consumer group were of the view that dexibuprofen was in effect a new drug and therefore would be required to have substantial safety data before approval could be granted for OTC use. Thus, the FDA in effect reinforced the earlier decision that safety based on experience with prescription dosage was the primary basis for approval.

7.2   ANALYSIS OF CLINICAL TRIALS

A considerable number of clinical trials have been performed in which ibuprofen has been examined for its efficacy in different pain states and the adverse reactions recorded. In various studies ibuprofen has been compared with placebo, other NSAIDs, paracetamol or other analgesics. These studies have served as a useful database for assessing the adverse reactions from ibuprofen with those from other analgesics taken at OTC doses. Recently, a comparison was reported of the adverse reactions from ibuprofen with those from paracetamol, each taken at their recommended OTC doses in clinical trials (Table 7.1) (Rainsford *et al.*, 1997). There was particular interest in this study in comparing the adverse reactions from ibuprofen with those from paracetamol as the latter drug is regarded as a 'bench standard' for its low ulcerogenic acivity (Loebl *et al.*, 1977; Johnson and Driscoll, 1981; Lanza *et al.*, 1986; Prescott, 1996). There is considerable evidence that ibuprofen is among the NSAIDs with lowest risk of upper GI bleeding and ulcerogenicity (Ivey and Settree, 1976; Ivey *et al.*, 1978; Warrington *et al.*, 1982; Konturek *et al.*, 1984; Royer *et al.*, 1984; Weber, 1984, 1987; Wilholm *et al.*, 1987; Aabakken *et al.*, 1989; Carson and Strom, 1992; Johnson *et al.*, 1994; Rainsford and Quadir, 1995). Even low-dose aspirin used for the prevention of thrombo-embolic conditions has an appreciable risk for development of GI bleeding and ulceration (Steering Committe of the Physicians' Health Study Group, 1989; Dutch TIA Trial Study Group, 1991; SALT Collaborative Group, 1991; Camu *et al.*, 1992; Kimmey, 1996).

There has also been concern that taking NSAIDs and non-narcotic analgesics may increase the risk of renal disorders, e.g. fluid retention, acute renal failure, nephrotic syndrome or renal papillary necrosis (Bonney *et al.*, 1986; Prescott, 1996; Whelton, 1996; see also Chapter 10). This is esepcially so in subjects who may be considered to be at risk, e.g. the elderly or patients with subnormal hepatorenal function (Whelton, 1996). Thus, it is important to know what the risks are for the population taking OTC analgesics and NSAIDs under controlled clinical trial conditions.

TABLE 7.1

Recommended non-prescription (OTC) dosages of ibuprofen and paracetamol

	Unit single dose	Maximum daily dose	Period[a]
Ibuprofen			
Adults	400 mg	1200 mg	< 10 days
Children[b]			
1–12 years divided doses	20 mg/kg each		
1–2 years	50 mg	200 mg	
3–7 years	100 mg	400 mg	
8–12 years	200 mg	800 mg	
Paracetamol			
Adults	1 g	4 g	< 10 days
Children:			
< 3 months	5–10 mg/kg		
3–12 months	60 mg	120 mg	
1–4 years	120 mg	480 mg	
1–5 years	250 mg	1 g	
6–12 years	500 mg	2 g	

The data here are those that were used as the basis for the study by Rainsford *et al.* (1997) comparing the safety of ibuprofen with that of paracetamol from published reports of criteria-selected clinical trials from 1981. The inclusion criteria set for the study were: (a) the studies should have been prospective, controlled (or in some few cases uncontrolled) with respect to placebo, blinded (or in a few cases unblinded) studies in which one of the two drug treatments was the primary interest; (b) single or multiple daily continuous dosing was employed with the drugs given orally (or in a few cases rectally) taken at the recommended OTC doses (as above); and (c) the adverse events should have been monitored. Exclusion criteria were: (a) use of one of the drugs as a rescue analgesic; (b) perioperative use where there was a risk that prior or concurrent medications could have interfered with the actions of the drugs being analyzed; (c) paracetamol used as a marker of gastric emptying; (d) where the adverse events were not specifically monitored or not satisfactorily so; and (e) where there was use of combinations of medications with the two study drugs.

[a] The total period recommended for continuous dosage in most countries. For later data analysis this was for conservative reasons taken to be 7 days (Tables 7.3–7.5).

[b] In some countries ibuprofen can be given to children younger than 1 year.

Among the more serious adverse reactions associated with intake of high, toxic doses of paracetamol is the development of severe, sometimes irreversible, hepatitis that can culminate in liver failure and rarely in death (Freeland *et al.*, 1988; Campbell and Oates, 1992; Friis and Andreasen, 1992; Prescott, 1992, 1996; Boelsterli *et al.*, 1995). This problem is of particular concern with children who may consume the drug accidentally (Hawkins and Goldring, 1995; Webster *et al.*, 1996). Thus, the major question to be considered with paracetamol taken under OTC dosage conditions is whether there is, albeit rarely, development of hepatic reactions (e.g. elevated liver enzymes, hepaptitis).

It, therefore, appeared important to determine the incidence of these and other side-effects associated with use of ibuprofen or paracetamol (Agus *et al.*, 1990; Johnson *et al.*, 1994; Prescott, 1992, 1996; Østensen, 1994) in controlled clinical trials where the drugs were taken at their recommended OTC dosages. Thus, for the analysis of the published data, Rainsford *et al.* (1997) selected trials in published studies from conventional on-line records (Medline, Excerta Medica, BIDS) as well as from a manual search of those clinical

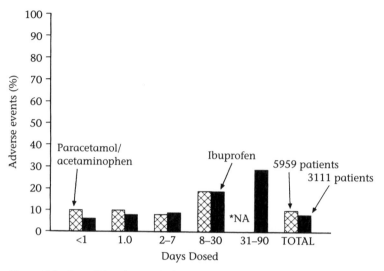

Figure 7.1: Overall incidence of adverse events recorded in published literature reports of 96 trials in which ibuprofen and/or paracetamol were analyzed. There were no data available for paracetamol/acetaminophen for treatment periods ranging from 31 to 90 days (*NA). From Rainsford (1998), reproduced with permission of Kluwer Academic Publishers.

trials published after 1981. Studies were selected from these reports that fulfilled specific inclusion and exclusion criteria that would enable analysis of the side-effects attributable to ibuprofen or paracetamol without confounding variables such as intake of other drugs. Reports were included where the studies had been performed for periods longer than the recommended OTC dosage period of 7–10 days because this enabled time-dependent effects to be determined. It was also recognized that often patients take analgesics available OTC for much longer periods than recommended. Of 730 potentially useful publications, 111 fulfilled the essential criteria and 96 were from trials that were randomized and double-blinded. The other studies were included because they were considered useful and they did not unduly affect the statistical analysis.

Figure 7.1 shows the overall incidence of adverse events that were obtained in the selected studies. It was found that, overall, there were no statistically significant differences in the adverse events recorded in those studies where either ibuprofen or paracetamol was employed for up to 30 days' treatment. Unfortunately, data were not available from subjects given paracetamol for 30–90 days, so a direct comparison could not be made of the adverse events from ibuprofen with paracetamol for this period of treatment. Where direct comparisons were made of the adverse events from the two drugs for up to 28 days of treatment, it was found that there were no differences in the number of subjects with adverse events or the total number of adverse reactions (Table 7.2; Rainsford *et al.*, 1997).

A detailed analysis of the adverse events in different organ systems (Table 7.3; Rainsford *et al.*, 1997) showed that (a) there were no statistically significant differences (as

TABLE 7.2

Adverse events in trials where ibuprofen and paracetamol were compared

Days dosed	Drug	Percentage with adverse events	Number with adverse events[a]	No. of patients	Total exposure[b]	Number of adverse events[c]	Reference
<1	Ibuprofen	2	21	878	0	3	Furey et al. (1992)
<1	Paracetamol	3	27	849	0	31	Furey et al. (1992)
<1	Ibuprofen	0	0	39	0	0	Schachtel and Thoden (1993)
<1	Paracetamol	0	0	38	0	0	Schachtel and Thoden (1993)
<1	Ibuprofen	9	27	306	0	27	Mehlisch et al. (1990)
<1	Paracetamol	10	32	306	0	33	Mehlisch et al. (1990)
<1	Ibuprofen	0	0	36	0	0	Schachtel et al. (1989)
<1	Paracetamol	0	0	37	0	0	Schachtel et al. (1989)
<1	Ibuprofen	8	5	61	0	6	Cooper et al. (1989)
<1	Paracetamol	19	11	59	0	13	Cooper et al. (1989)
<1	Ibuprofen	0	0	20	0	0	Kauffman et al. (1992)
<1	Paracetamol	0	0	8	0	0	Kauffman et al. (1992)
<1	Ibuprofen	0	0	39	0	0	Schachtel et al. (1988)
<1	Paracetamol	0	0	40	0	0	Schachtel et al. (1988)
<1	Ibuprofen	0	0	14	0	0	Moore et al. (1985)
<1	Paracetamol	0	0	11	0	0	Moore et al. (1985)
1	Ibuprofen	18	6	34	34	6	Van Esch et al. (1995)
1	Paracetamol	22	8	36	36	8	Van Esch et al. (1995)
7	Ibuprofen	0	0	8	56	0	Furey et al. (1993)
7	Paracetamol	0	0	8	56	0	Furey et al. (1993)
21	Ibuprofen	33	4	12	252	4	Radack et al. (1987)
21	Paracetamol	20	3	15	315	3	Radack et al. (1987)
28	Ibuprofen	26	16	62	1736	16	Bradley (1991)
28	Paracetamol	31	19	61	1708	19	Bradley (1991)

[a] Adverse events grouped as total number of patients having these events.
[b] Number of patient days.
[c] Adverse events grouped as the total of recorded adverse events.
From Rainsford et al. (1997), reproduced with permission of the Editor of the *Journal of Pharmacy and Pharmacology*.

■ CHAPTER 7 ■

TABLE 7.3

Adverse events by Costart term

Days dosed	Indication	Total adverse events	Costart term[a]	Reference
A. With ibuprofen				
<1	Pain	23	Rash (1; 4%), paraesthesia circumoral (1; 4%), neck rigid (1; 4%), headache (5; 22%), dizziness (1; 4%), somnolence (6; 26%), gastrointestinal dis. (8; 35%)	Furey et al. (1992)
<1	Dental extractions	12	Vasodilatation (1; 8%), asthenia (1; 8%), somnolence (8; 67%), abnormal thoughts (1; 8%), tinnitus (1; 8%)	Cooper et al. (1982)
<1	Dental extractions	8	Headache (2; 25%), somnolence (1; 13%), nausea (1; 13%), asthenia (1; 13%), agitation (1; 13%), dizziness (1; 13%), nervousness (1; 13%)	Forbes et al. (1991b)
<1	Dental extractions	35	Bleeding (2; 6%), dizziness (2; 6%), dyspepsia (1; 3%), oedema general (2; 6%), fever (3; 9%), headache (6; 17%), nausea (6; 17%), somnolence (10; 29%), vomiting (3; 9%)	Jain et al. (1986a)
<1	Volunteers	4	Mucous membrane dis. (4; 100%)	Bergmann et al. (1992)
<1	Oral surgery	27	Dizziness (3; 11%), somnolence (6; 22%), headache (2; 7%), gastrointestinal dis. (16; 59%)	Mehlisch et al. (1990)
<1	Volunteers	4	Asthenia (2; 50%), headache (2; 50%)	Karttunen et al. (1990)
<1	Dental extractions	1	Asthenia (1; 100%)	Ahlstrom et al. (1993)
<1	Dental extractions	6	Headache (2; 33%), somnolence (4; 67%)	Cooper et al. (1989)
<1	Dental extractions	27	Nervousness (3; 11%), dizziness (1; 4%), vomiting (3; 11%), tinnitus (1; 4%), somnolence (6; 22%), ear pain (1; 4%), nausea (1; 4%), insomnia (1; 4%), fainting (1; 4%), asthenia (1; 4%), agitation (1; 4%), headache (7; 26%)	Forbes et al. (1991a)
<1	Dental extractions	8	Dizziness (2; 25%), somnolence (1; 13%), abdominal pain (1; 13%), headache (1; 13%), asthenia (1; 13%), amblyopia (1; 13%), nervousness (1; 13%)	Forbes et al. (1992)

<1	Dental extractions	Anxiety (1; 9%), nausea (1; 9%), somnolence (5; 45%), vasodilation (1; 9%), vomiting (1; 9%), dizziness (1; 9%), headaches (1; 9%)	Hersh et al. (1993)
1	Fever	Rash (1; 100%)	Marriott et al. (1991)
1	Febrile seizures	Hypothermia (2; 33%), insomnia (1; 17%), rash (1; 17%), convulsions (2; 33%)	Van Esch et al. (1995)
1	Coxarthrosis	Nausea (3; 38%)	Quiding et al. (1992)
1	Dental extractions	Asthenia (1; 14%), sweat (1; 14%), nausea (3; 43%), headache (1; 14%), hypotension postural (1; 14%)	Petersen et al. (1993)
2	Foot surgery	Headache (1; 14%), nausea (1; 14%), pruritus (1; 14%), tinnitus (2; 29%), urticaria (1; 14%), constipation (1; 14%)	Wittenberg et al. (1984)
3	Dental extractions	Nausea (1; 25%), somnolence (1; 25%), dizziness (1; 25%), headache (1; 25%)	McQuay et al. (1989)
6	Dental extractions	Bleeding (2; 15%), headache (3; 23%), nausea (3; 23%), somnolence (3; 23%), sweating (1; 8%); vomiting (1; 8%)	McQuay et al. (1993)
7	Sports injuries	Gastroenteritis (1; 100%)	Walker et al. (1984)
7	Volunteers	Dyspepsia (1; 25%), nausea (1; 25%), abdominal pain (2; 50%)	Puscas et al. (1989)
14	Rheumatoid arthritis	Nausea, vomiting (1; 100%)	Hill et al. (1990)
14	Osteoarthritis	Rash (1; 6%), abnormal dreams (1; 6%)	Lambert et al. (1985)
21	Hypertension	Somnolence (1; 25%), flatulence (1; 25%), pruritus (1; 25%), rash (1; 25%)	Radack et al. (1987)
28	Osteoarthritis	Nervous system (7; 44%), oedema general (2; 13%), gastrointestinal dis. (5; 31%)	Bradley (1991)
28	Osteoarthritis	Dyspepsia (1; 33%), somnolence (2; 67%)	Vlok and van Vuren (1987)
30	Osteoarthritis	Gastrointestinal dis. (7; 88%), rash (1; 13%)	Di Perri et al. (1987)
40	Menstrual bleeding	Nausea (2; 18%), headache (2; 18%), dyspepsia (1; 9%), diarrhoea (1; 9%), dizziness (1; 9%)	Mäkäläinen and Ylikorkala (1986a)
56	Rheumatoid arthritis	Abdominal pain (3; 100%)	Alam and Kabir (1983)

TABLE 7.3 (*continued*)

Days dosed	Indication	Total adverse events	Costart term[a]	Reference
60	Osteoarthritis	9	Sweat (1; 11%), rash (1; 11%), abdominal pain (3; 33%), nausea (1; 11%), dyspepsia (3; 33%)	Kaik et al. (1991)
84	Osteoarthritis	5	Urea clearance decrease (1; 20%), creatinine increase (1; 20%), hypertension (1; 20%), phosphatase alk. (1; 20%), rash (1; 20%)	Admani and Verma (1983)
90	Non-articular rheumatism	12	Dyspepsia (7; 58%), flatulence (1; 8%), nausea (2; 17%), abdominal pain (1; 8%), constipation (1; 8%)	Valle-Jones et al. (1984)
B. With paracetamol				
<1	Strabismus surgery	2	Nausea, vomiting (2; 100%)	Morrison and Repka (1994)
<1	Dental extractions	3	Headache (1; 33%), nausea (1; 33%), somnolence (1; 33%)	Forbes et al. (1989)
<1	Acute pain	31	Diarrhoea (1; 3%), somnolence (13; 42%), eye pain (1; 3%), nervousness (1; 3%), headache (1; 3%), dizziness (4; 13%), ataxia (1; 3%), anxiety (1; 3%), gastrointestinal dis. (8; 26%)	Furey et al. (1992)
<1	Episiotomy	6	Dizziness (3; 50%), somnolence (3; 50%)	Rubin and Winter (1984)
<1	Dental extractions	2	Pain (1; 50%), headache (1; 50%)	Forbes et al. (1984a)
<1	General surgery	15	Sweat (3; 20%), somnolence (5; 33%), vomiting (1; 7%), abdominal pain (2; 13%), nausea (3; 20%), pharyngitis (1; 7%)	Gertzbein et al. (1986)
<1	Headache	13	Gastroenteritis (7; 54%)	Peters et al. (1983)
<1	Dental extractions	9	Nausea, vomiting (2; 22%), somnolence (4; 44%), headache (1; 11%)	Dionne et al. (1994)
<1	Muscle contraction headache	5	Nausea (1; 20%), somnolence (1; 20%), insomnia (1; 20%), dry mouth (1; 20%), diarrhoea (1; 20%)	Miller et al. (1987)
<1	Oral surgery	33	Dizziness (6; 18%), gastrointestinal dis. (13; 39%), headache (4; 12%), somnolence (10; 30%)	Mehlisch et al. (1990)
<1	Dental extractions	13	Nausea (2; 15%), nervousness (1; 8%), dizziness (2; 15%), somnolence (8; 62%)	Cooper et al. (1989)

<1	Episiotomy or dental surgery	27	Dizziness (6; 22%), gastrointestinal dis. (2; 7%), somnolence (19; 70%)	McMahon et al. (1987)
<1	Oral surgery	31	Nausea (7; 23%), vomiting (6; 19%), vertigo (1; 3%), appetite change (1; 3%), somnolence (5; 16%), hypotension postwal (1; 3%), headache (1; 3%), hallucinations (1; 3%), gastroenteritis (1; 3%), abnormal dreams (1; 3%), dizziness (5; 16%), tinnitus (1; 3%)	Bentley and Head (1987)
<1	General surgery	10	Somnolence (7; 70%), nervousness (1; 10%), headache (1; 10%), depression (1; 10%)	Forbes et al. (1984b)
<1	Orthopaedic surgery	43	Headache (8; 19%), nausea (8; 19%), sweat (2; 5%), thirst (3; 7%), vomiting (4; 9%), amblyopia (1; 2%)	McQuay et al. (1986)
<1	Surgery	9	Headache (2; 22%), somnolence (7; 78%)	Jain et al. (1986b)
<1	Dental extractions	1	Headache (1; 100%)	Sunshine et al. (1986)
<1	Headache	226	Dizziness (33; 15%), dyspepsia (112; 50%), nervousness (23; 10%)	Migliardi et al. (1994)
1	Dental extractions	16	Urination (1; 6%), chills (3; 19%), fever (1; 6%), headache (5; 31%), nausea (1; 6%); somnolence (3; 19%), vomiting (1; 6%), bleeding (1; 6%)	Nystrom et al. (1988)
1	Dental extractions	7	Somnolence (1; 14%), abdominal pain (1; 14%), nausea (2; 29%), headache (1; 14%), agitation (1; 14%), dizziness (1; 14%)	Quiding et al. (1982b)
1	Dental extractions	6	Somnolence (2; 33%), headache (1; 17%), abdominal pain (1; 17%), back pain (1; 17%), ear pain (2; 33%)	Quiding et al. (1982a)
1	Migraine	3	Nausea (1; 33%), vomiting (1; 33%), dyspepsia (1; 33%)	Pearce et al. (1983)
1	Febrile seizure	8	Hypothermia (1; 13%), rash (2; 25%), convulsions (3; 38%), gastrointestinal dis. (2; 25%)	Van Esch et al. (1995)
1	Dental extractions	3	Asthenia (1; 33%), headache (2; 67%)	Quiding et al. (1981)
1	Oral surgery	5	Somnolence (2; 40%), nausea (1; 20%), dry mouth (1; 20%), headache (1; 20%)	Gallardo and Rossi (1990)
1	Migraine	1	Somnolence (1; 100%)	MacGregor et al. (1993)

TABLE 7.3 (*continued*)

Days dosed	Indication	Total adverse events	Costart term[a]	Reference
2	Tonsillitis, pharyngitis	3	Nausea (3; 100%)	Bertin et al. (1991)
2	Fever	2	Vomiting (2; 100%)	Weippl et al. (1985a)
3	Dental extractions	11	Headache (5; 45%), nausea (1; 9%), somnolence (4; 36%), vomiting (1; 9%)	Skoglund and Skjelbred (1984)
4	Rheumatoid arthritis	1	Site reaction (1; 100%)	Di Munno and Sarchi (1982)
5	Upper respiratory tract infection	14	Abdominal pain (1; 7%), somnolence (5; 36%), dry mouth (2; 14%), dizziness (1; 7%), gastrointestinal dis. (5; 36%)	Middleton (1981)
5	Acute migraine	7	Somnolence (1; 14%), dizziness (1; 14%), constipation (1; 14%), diarrhoea (1; 14%), chest pain (1; 14%), sleep dis. (1; 14%), asthenia (1; 14%)	Million et al. (1984)
7	Lung disease	12	Somnolence (4; 33%), vomiting (1; 8%), pneumonia (1; 8%), pain (1; 8%), nausea (2; 17%), dyspnoea (2; 17%), diarrhoea (1; 8%)	Munck et al. (1990)
7	Cancer (Note: some adverse events might be related to disease state)	26	Dizziness (1; 4%), nausea (1; 4%), vertigo (2; 8%), tremor (2; 8%), sweating (3; 12%), somnolence (3; 12%), pruritus (2; 8%), gastrointestinal dis. (1; 4%), agitation (2; 8%), dry mouth (3; 12%), constipation (1; 4%), dyspepsia (3; 12%), headache (2; 8%)	Ventafridda et al. (1990)
13	Stable chronic liver disease	1	Rash (1; 100%)	Benson (1983)
21	Hypertension	3	Headache (1; 33%), nervousness (1; 33%), abnormal thoughts (1; 33%)	Radack et al. (1987)
28	Osteoarthritis	19	Renal (1; 5%), rash (1; 5%), oedema general (1; 5%), nervous system (4; 21%), hematological (1; 5%), genitourinary (1; 5%), gastrointestinal dis. (10; 53%)	Bradley (1991)
30	Osteoarthritis	16	Diarrhoea (1; 6%), headache (1; 6%), nausea, vomiting (5; 31%), abdominal pain (6; 38%), pruritis (1; 6%), rash (1; 6%), anorexia (1; 6%)	Glorioso et al. (1985)

[a] Values in brackets are number of adverse events and percentage of the total number of adverse events.
From Rainsford, K.D. (1997), reproduced with permission of the Editor of *Journal of Pharmacy and Pharmacology*.

determined by analysis of variance, or by calculation of the odds ratios) in the adverse events recorded in the major organ systems (Costart dictionary coded) from treatment with the two drugs (Table 7.4); (b) the adverse events were all minor (Table 7.3) and would be reversible upon cessation of the drug; (c) the adverse reactions in the gastrointestinal system from ibuprofen were not statistically significantly different from those from paracetamol, and no clinically significant gastrointestinal bleeding or malaena was observed with ibuprofen (Table 7.5); (d) there were no deaths or hospitalizations such as would be required for treatment of severe reactions; and (e) there were no differences in the adverse events with age (even with children or the elderly) or sex of the individuals (Rainsford *et al.*, 1997).

Calculations of the odds ratios (OR) where ibuprofen was directly compared with paracetamol (the drugs being taken for ≤ 7 days in ≥ 40 subjects) yielded data for the gastrointestinal (GI) system as a whole with an OR = 1.00 (Rainsford and Brown, 1997, unpublished studies). With the individual GI adverse events, the odds ratio for abdominal discomfort was 0.45, for nausea 1.03, for heartburn 0.77 and for abdominal pain 3.1. This last suggests that ibuprofen may have been responsible for more abdominal discomfort than was paracetamol, but the data were not significantly different. This was borne out when all of the data for the two drug groups were compared, which yielded an OR value of 1.35.

The only other data of clinical significance were those in the central nervous system which, when the two drugs were compared directly, yielded an OR value of 0.59. There were no reports of serious kidney adverse events in these studies.

Thus, it can be concluded from these data from clinical trials under controlled conditions that both ibuprofen and paracetamol are relatively safe when taken in their recommended doses even for periods exceeding the times (7–10 days) recommended for self-administration.

7.3   OTHER TRIALS

In an evaluation of 15 double-blind trials in 878 patients of OTC doses of ibuprofen 200 or 400 mg used to treat painful conditions (headache, sore throat, dental or episiostomy pain) the overall rate of adverse reactions was 2.4% (Furey *et al.*, 1992). This was comparable with that of paracetamol 650 or 1000 mg (3.2% in 849 patients) and placebo (2.1% in 852 patients) (Furey *et al.*, 1992). The side-effects from all three treatments were most frequent in the gastrointestinal tract and central nervous system. The majority of gastrointestinal symptoms were stomach upset, indigestion and nausea, and thus can be considered to be mild. The adverse reactions in the central nervous system were principally drowsiness or tiredness and headache. More adverse reactions were observed in subjects who received the drug for dental compared with non-dental pain, suggesting that the stress from dental pain may exacerbate the likelihood of adverse reactions.

■ CHAPTER 7 ■

TABLE 7.4

Detailed comparison of study type, treatments and adverse events recorded in studies where there were ≥ 40 subjects and where treatments were for ≤ 7 days. Adverse drug reaction events expressed as percentage of total number of subjects

Dose regimen [Study duration] Study type (* = Clinical trial)	(Formulation) [Comparator(s)]: (A) Aspirin, (B) Bromfenac, (C) Codeine, (D) Diclofenac, (F) Fenprofen, (I) Ibuprofen, (K) Ketoprofen, (M) Meclofenamate, (N) Naproxen, (P) Paracetamol, (S) Sulindac	Comments (M) More, (L) Less effective than comparator, (E) Equiactive, (N) No effect	No of Subjects	GI Blood loss (BL), Heartburn (H), Diarrhoea/constipation (DC), Discomfort (SD), General (G) (%)	GI Nausea (N), Vomiting (V) (%)	GI Total (%)	CNS Total (%)	Other Total (%)	Total	Total ADR events	Total ADR subjects	Study
Ibuprofen												
400 mg t.i.d. [5 d] GI blood loss	[A; clonixinate lysine]	GI blood loss from ^{51}Cr-RBCs	6	Observed DC; SD; H	0.00	0.00	0.00	0.00	?	7	6	Bidlingmaier et al. (1995)
200 mg [2 h] Sore throat*	(Motrin); 2 doses	Ibuprofen effective; lower time for re-medication	9	0.00	0.00	0.00	0.00	0.00	0.00	0	0	Schachtel et al. (1994)
400 mg*	(As above)	(As above)	10	0.00	0.00	0.00	0.00	0.00	0.00	0	0	(As above)
400 mg [ns] Pressure headache at high altitude*	–	1/12 Vomited with drug; 1/12 with placebo	20	0.00	5.00 V	5.00	10.00	0.00	15	3	2	Broome et al. (1994)
25 mg t.i.d.[4 h] Antipyretic efficacy in uncomplicated falciparum malaria*	[P 4 × 1000 mg/day]	Pre-treated with mefloquine (750 and 500 mg); M	21	0.00	0.00	0.00	0.00	0.00	0	0	0	Wilairatana and Looaresuwan (1994)
400 mg [1.5 h] Pain from CO_2 gas applied inside nostril*	(Aktren)	–	18	0	0	0	0	0	0	0	0	Kobal et al. (1994)
800 mg*	(As above)	–	18	0	0	0	0	0	0	0	0	(As above)

Drug / dose; indication		Code										Reference
400 mg [3 h] 3rd molar extraction*	[D Na 50 mg]	5 ADR events observed; data insufficient; L (onset)	80 @	?	?	?	?	?	?	?	6	Bakshi et al. (1994)
200 mg [8 h] 3rd molar extraction*	[M 50 and 100 mg]	—	51 @	0.00	0.00	0.00	7.84	0.00	7.84	4	4	Hersh et al. (1993)
400 mg (As above)*	(As above)	—	49 @	0.00	2.04 V; 2.04 N	4.08	8.16	2.04	14.28	7	6	(As above)
5 × 200 mg/day, 6 × 200 mg/day × 6 d (As above)*	(As above)	E (highest dose and high dose meclofenamate	59 @	0.00	1.69 V; 10.17 N	11.86	30.50	3.38	45.74	27	19	(As above)
5 × 400 mg/day, 6 × 400 mg/day × 6 d (As above)*	(As above)	Bleeding at surgical site	57 @	1.75 DC; 1.75 SD	1.75 V; 14.04 N	19.29	28.06	10.51	57.86	33	18	(As above)
3 × 200 mg [12 h] Dental surgery impaction*	[C 30 mg]	M	45 @	?	11.11 N	11.11	?	?	11.11	30	?	Cooper et al. (1993)
600 mg (Controlled release)* (As above)	(I-CRT) (As above)	Controlled-release superior analgesic	38	?	2.22 N	2.22	?	?	2.22	16	?	(As above)
2 × 400 mg [10 h] 3rd molar extraction*	[I + C 60 mg]	L	69 @	0.00	4.35 N	4.35	4.35	0.00	8.7	7	6	Petersen et al. (1993)
≤ 4 × 400 mg/day [10 h], ≤ 6 d (As required) 3rd molar extraction*	(Boots) [dihydro-C 30, 60 mg]	M	41 @	0.00	2.44 V; 7.32 N	9.76	14.64	7.32	31.72	13	8	McQuay et al. (1993)
200 mg [4 h] Dental extraction*	(Aluminium) [P 240 or 360 mg; P 240 mg + C 24 mg]	E	14	0.00	0.00	0.00	0.00	0.00	0	0	0	Moore et al. (1985)
400 mg [6 h] Sore throat*	[P 1000 mg]	M	39	0.00	0.00	0.00	0.00	0.00	0	0	0	Schactel et al. (1988)
1200 mg/day t.i.d. × 4 d [4 d] Joint sprains*	(Brufen) [S 400 mg b.d.]	E	83 @	0.00	0.00	0.00	0.00	0.00	0	0	0	Bouchier-Hayes et al. (1984)
10 mg/kg t.i.d. × 2 d. Tonsillitis/pharyngitis*	(Microgranules or Sparklets) [P 10 mg/kg t.i.d. × 2 d]	M	77 @	Observed SD	Observed	0.00	0.00	?	?	?	5	Bertin et al. (1991)

TABLE 7.4 (continued)

Dose regimen [Study duration] Study type (* = Clinical trial)	(Formulation) [Comparator(s)]: (A) Aspirin, (B) Bromfenac, (C) Codeine, (D) Diclofenac, (F) Fenprofen, (I) Ibuprofen, (K) Ketoprofen, (M) Meclofenamate, (N) Naproxen, (P) Paracetamol, (S) Sulindac	Comments [(M) More, (L) Less effective than comparator, (E) Equiactive, (N) No effect]	No of Subjects	GI — Blood loss (BL), Heartburn (H), Diarrohea/constipation (DC), Discomfort (SD), General (G) (%)	Nausea (N), Vomiting (V) (%)	Total (%)	CNS Total (%)	Other Total (%)	Total	Total ADR events	Total ADR subjects	Study
400 mg [8 h] 3rd molar extraction*	[A 650 mg, B 10–100 mg]	M (to all but higher doses of bromfenac)	45 @	2.22 SD	0.00	2.22	13.32	2.22	17.76	8	4	Forbes et al. (1992)
2.5/5/10 mg/kg q.i.d. × 1–2 d Antipyretic in febrile children*	[P 4 × 15 mg/kg/day × 1–2 d]	E	48 @	6.25 SD; 14.58 G	6.25 V; 6.25 N	33.33	0.00	16.67	50	16	?	Walson et al. (1992)
7.5/10 mg/kg [8 h] Fever reduction in febrile children*	[P 10 mg/kg]	M	20	0.00	0.00	0.00	0.00	0.00	0	0	0	Kauffman et al. (1992)
400 mg [6 h]; post orthopedic surgery*	[P 300 mg + C 30 mg]	M; overall occurrence of ADR's = 15%	40 @	0.00	?	?	?	?	?	?	?	Heidrich et al. (1985)
50 mg [8 h] 3rd molar extraction*	[I 100 mg + caffeine 100 mg; I 200 mg + caffeine 100 mg]	L	63 @	0.00	1.59 V; 1.59 N	3.18	17.46	3.18	23.82	15	10	Forbes et al. (1991a)
100 mg* (As above)	(As above)		62 @	0.00	0.00	0.00	9.68	0.00	9.68	6	5	(As above)
200 mg* (As above)	(As above)		60 @	0.00	3.33 V	3.33	6.67	0.00	10	6	6	(As above)
400 mg [2 h] 3rd molar extraction*	[2 × P 500 mg + C 8 mg + caffeine 30 mg (Solpadeine); 2 × A 300 mg + 30 mg caffeine (Anadin); dihydro-C tartrate 30 mg]	E (combinations) M (dihydro-C)	26	0.00	0.00	0.00	0.00	0.00	0	0	0	Habib et al. (1990)
400 mg [6 h] Dental impaction surgery*	[P 1000 mg]	M	63 @	0.00	0.00	0.00	11.11	0.00	11.11	6	5	Cooper et al. (1989)

Reference									n	Comment	Formulation	Regimen
Ahlstrom et al. (1993)	3	?	3.13	0.00	3.13	?	?	?	32	E	[D dispersible 50 mg]	400 mg [6 h] 3rd molar extraction*
Schactel and Thoden (1988)	0	0	0	0.00	0.00	0.00	0.00	0.00	35	Early onset of action	–	400 mg [2 h] Muscle contraction headaches*
Schactel et al. (1989)	0	0	0	0.00	0.00	0.00	0.00	0.00	36	M	[P 1000 mg]	400 mg [4 h] Pain after episiotomy*
McQuay et al. (1989)	3	4	17.4	0.00	13.05	4.35	4.35 N	0.00	23	L	[C base 20 mg + I 400 mg]	400 mg/day t.i.d. × 6 d As required [6 d] 3rd molar extraction*
Seymour et al. (1991)	0	0	0	0.00	0.00	0.00	0.00	0.00	93 @	–	[Soft gelatin/tabs (Nurofen)/ soluble]	400 mg [6 h] 3rd molar extraction*
Karttunen et al. (1990)	2	2	20	0.00	20.00	0.00	0.00	0.00	10	L (Iburo absorbtion)	(Iburo/Burana)	400 mg [1 d] Pharmacokinetic study
Mehlisch et al. (1990)	31	27	8.72	0.00	3.56	5.16	0.00	5.16 G	310 @	M	[P 1000 mg]	400 mg [6 h] Oral surgery*
Ventafridda et al. (1990)	?	21	161.52	69.23	53.83	38.46	7.69 N	7.69 BL; 23.08 H	13	M (paracetamol); Naproxen, diclofenac, indomethacin highly effective and well tolerated	[A 600 mg t.i.d.; P 500 mg t.i.d.; D s.r. b.d. + placebo; indomethacin 50 mg t.i.d.; pirprofen 400 mg t.i.d.; S 300 mg b.d. + placebo; N 250 mg t.i.d.; suprofen 200 mg]	600 mg t.i.d. × 7 d [7 d] Cancer*
Quiding et al. (1992)	?	5	11.54	0.00	0.00	11.54	11.54 N	Observed SD	26	L	[I 200 mg + C 30 mg]	6 × 200 mg/day [24 h] Coxarthrosis*
Bergmann et al. (1992)	?	?	?	?	?	?	?	?	12	Mucosal lesions lower with I and K than A	[K 25 mg; A 500 mg]	200 mg [2 h] Endoscopic evaluation of gastroduodenal mucosa
Sunshine et al. (1987)	0	0	0	0.00	0.00	0.00	0.00	0.00	38	L (high dose combination), E (low); M (C-sulfate)	[I 400 mg + C 60 mg; I 200 mg + C 30 mg; C-sulfate]	400 mg [4 h] Episiotomy, caesarean section, or gynaecological surgery*
Van Esch et al. (1995)	0	6	8.82	5.88	2.94	0.00	0.00	0.00	34	M	(Syrup) [P (syrup) 10 mg/kg/day]	5 mg/kg q.i.d. × 1–3 d Antipyretic in febrile children*

TABLE 7.4 (continued)

Dose regimen [Study duration] Study type (* = Clinical trial)	(Formulation) [Comparator(s)]: (A) Aspirin, (B) Bromfenac, (C) Codeine, (D) Diclofenac, (F) Fenprofen, (I) Ibuprofen, (K) Ketoprofen, (M) Meclofenamate, (N) Naproxen, (P) Paracetamol, (S) Sulindac	No of Subjects	Comments (M) More, (L) Less effective than comparator, (E) Equiactive, (N) No effect	GI — Blood loss (BL), Heartburn (H), Diarrohea/constipation (DC), Discomfort (SD), General (G) (%)	Nausea (N), Vomiting (V) (%)	Total (%)	CNS Total (%)	Other Total (%)	Total	Total ADR events	Total ADR subjects	Study
0.625 mg/kg [3 h] Antipyretic*	(Suspension)	26	Dose-related antipyretic effect	0.00	3.85 N	3.85	0.00	0.00	3.85	2	2	Marriott et al. (1991)
1.25 mg/kg (As above)	(As above)	24	(As above)	0.00	0.00	0.00	8.34	0.00	8.34	3	3	(As above)
2.5 mg/kg (As above)	(As above)	26	(As above)	0.00	3.85 N	3.85	15.39	3.85	23.09	7	6	(As above)
5.0 mg/kg (As above)	(As above)	24	(As above)	4.17 DC	12.50 N	16.67	4.17	0.00	20.84	7	6	(As above)
10 mg/kg [6 h] Sore throat*	[P 15 mg/kg]	39	E	0	2.56 V	0	0	0	0	1	1	Schactel and Thoden (1993)
400 mg/day t.i.d. [48 h] Sleep patterns	[A 650 mg t.i.d.; P 650 mg t.i.d]	9	Disrupted sleep patterns	?	?	?	?	?	?	?	?	Murphy et al. (1994)
400 mg t.i.d. [7 d] Primary dysmenorrhoea*	(Motrin) [Indomethacin (Indocin) 25 mg]	31	M	0.00	0.00	0.00	0.00	0.00	0	0	0	Gookin et al. (1983)
100 mg [6 h] Impacted tooth extraction*	[A 650 mg]	39	E	2.56 H	5.13 V; 7.69 N	15.38	17.96	5.12	38.46	15	13	Jain et al. (1986a)
200 mg (As above)	(As above)	47 @	(As above)	0.00	6.38 N	6.38	4.26	6.39	17.03	8	6	(As above)
400 mg (As above)	(As above)	49 @	(As above)	0.00	2.04 V	2.04	18.36	4.08	24.48	12	10	(As above)
400 mg [8 h] 3rd molar extraction*	[B 5/10/25 mg; A 650 mg]	43 @	M (all but bromfenac 25 mg)	0.00	2.33 N	2.33	16.30	0.00	18.63	8	7	Forbes et al. (1991b)
600 mg t.i.d. × 7 d [7 d]; endoscopic study	[A 500 mg; Indomethacin 25 mg; phenylbutazone 200 mg]	5	All produced dyspeptic symptoms	?	?	?	?	?	?	?	?	Puscus et al. (1989)

Dose/indication	Comparator	Comments	n									Reference
400 mg/day t.i.d. × 7 d [7 d] Renal function in rheumatoid arthritis	[Suprofen 200 mg t.i.d. × 7 d]	Renal function unimpaired; decreases in prostaglandin levels	11	?	?	?	?	?	?	?	?	Malandrino et al. (1987)
400 mg/day t.i.d. × 7 d [7 d] Renovascular effects	[A 650 mg t.i.d. × 7 d; P 650 mg t.i.d. × 7 d]	N	8	0.00	0.00	0.00	0.00	0.00	0.00	0	0	Furey et al. (1993)
400 mg [4 h] Dental impaction surgery*	[C 60 mg; A 650 mg; I 400 mg; A 650 mg + C 60 mg; I 400 mg + C 60 mg]	M (aspirin)	38	0.00	0.00	0.00	26.31	5.26	31.57	12	11	Cooper et al. (1982)
400 mg t.i.d. × 7 d [7 d] Sports injury*	[S 200 mg b.d. × 7 d]	L	14	7.14 G	0.00	7.14	0.00	0.00	7.14	1	1	Walker et al. (1984)
1–12 × 400 mg Within 4 d as required [4 d] Postoperative foot pain*	[1–12 × P 300 mg + C 30 mg within 4 d as required]	E	36	2.78 DC	2.78 N	5.56	2.78	11.12	19.46	7	4	Wittenberg et al. (1984)
200 mg [6 h] SE profile	[P 650/1000 mg]	–	171@	2.34 SD; 2.34 H	2.34 N	7.02	2.33	1.16	10.51	9	8	Furey et al. (1992)
400 mg (As above)	(As above)		707@	0.57 SD; 0.57 H	0.57 N	1.70	1.98	0.14	3.82	17	13	(As above)
600 mg [5 h] Strabismus surgery*	[P 650 mg; ketorolac 60 mg i.v.]	L	20	0.00	10.00 N	10.00	0.00	0.00	10	1	1	Morrison and Repka (1994)
400 mg/6 h [72 h] Postinstrumentation of root canals*	(Motrin) [A 650 mg; P (Tylenol) 650 mg; K (Orudis) 50 mg; P 325 mg + C 60 mg (Phenaphen #4); penicillin (Veetids) 500 mg; erythromycin base 500 mg; penicillin 500 mg + I 400 mg; methylprednisolone (MedRol) 2 mg + penicillin 500 mg]	1.8% of subjects had ADRs though data insufficient to categorize; N (with mild pain)	57	?	?	?	?	?	?	?	?	Torabinejad et al. (1994)
400 mg [4 h] Suction termination pregnancy*	(l-arginine)	N	38	0.00	2.632 V	2.63	0.00	0.00	2.63	1	1	Pagnoni et al. (1996a)

TABLE 7.4 (*continued*)

Dose regimen [Study duration] Study type (* = Clinical trial)	(Formulation) [Comparator(s)]: (A) Aspirin, (B) Bromfenac, (C) Codeine, (D) Diclofenac, (F) Fenprofen, (I) Ibuprofen, (K) Ketoprofen, (M) Meclofenamate, (N) Naproxen, (P) Paracetamol, (S) Sulindac	Comments (M) More, (L) Less effective than comparator, (E) Equiactive, (N) No effect	No of Subjects	GI — Blood loss (BL), Heartburn (H), Diarrhoea/constipation (DC), Discomfort (SD), General (G) (%)	Nausea (N), Vomiting (V) (%)	Total (%)	CNS Total (%)	Other Total (%)	Total	Total ADR events	Total ADR subjects	Study
Dose? [4 h] tension-type headache*	(l-arginine, sachet) [beta-cyclodextrin piroxicam dose?]	E; those with nausea usually suffered it with headache anyway	26	0.00	3.85 N	3.85	0.00	0.00	3.85	1	1	Laveneziana et al. (1996a)
400 mg [6 h] Caesarean section*	(l-arginine) [ketorolac 30 mg i.m.]		30	0.00	0.00	0.00	0.00	0.00	0	0	0	Pagnoni et al. (1996b)
400 mg [6 h] Postoperative pain*	(l-arginine) [ketorolac 30 mg i.m.]		42 @	0.00	0.00	0.00	0.00	0.00	0	0	0	Laveneziana et al. (1996b)
400 mg q.i.d. × 7 d [7 d] Rheumatism*	[F-calcium 4 × 600 mg/day × 7 d]	N (except where limitation of movement concerned)	50 @	2.00 SD	1.00 V; 4.00 N	13.00	0.00	0.00	13	7	4	Williams (1983)
400 mg [5 h] Dental surgery*	(l-arginine, sachet) [N-sodium 550 mg]	E; Involved some bone surgery	46 @	0.00	0.00	0.00	2.17	0.00	2.17	1	1	Borea et al. (1996)
400 mg t.i.d. [7 d] Rheumatoid arthritis*	[Indomethacin s.r. 50 mg b.d.]	Reduction in duration of morning stiffness; aspirin used as rescue analgesic	22	4.55 SD	4.55 V; 4.55 N	13.64	13.64	0.00	27.28	6	5	Gordin et al. (1985)
TOTALS:			3571							395	253	

	Comparator	Type	n									Reference
MEAN%:				0.14 BL; 0.15 DC; 0.34 SD; 0.47 G; 0.49 H	1.60 (0.72 V; 2.46 N)	4.66	6.54	2.63	13.45			
SD:				1.03 BL; 0.69 DC; 1.12 SD; 2.23 G; 3.05 H	3.02 (1.50 V; 3.80 N)	7.61	10.10	9.33	23.28			
MEDIAN:				0.00 BL, DC, SD, G, H	0.00 V, N	2.04	2.08	0.00	8.52			
MAX:				7.69 BL; 4.17 DC; 6.25 SD; 14.58 G; 23.08 H	14.04 (6.25 V; 14.04 N)	38.46	53.83	69.23	161.5			
MIN:				0.00 BL, DC, SD, G, H	0.00 V, N	0.00	0.00	0.00	0.00			
Paracetamol												
1000 mg [4 h] Tension headache*	[P 500 mg + A 500 mg + caffeine 130 mg; P 1000 mg + caffeine 130 mg]	L	2091 @	5.36 SD	0.00	5.36	2.68	10.81	18.85	3	226	Migliardi et al. (1994)
650 mg [8 h] Antipyretic in endotoxin-induced fever*	[ketorolac 15/30/60 mg i.m.]	E: 378 ADR events observed but unable to relate cause with type	30	?	?	?	?	?	?	?	?	Vargas et al. (1994)
100 mg q.i.d. [4 h] Antipyretic in uncomplicated falciparum malaria*	[125 mg t.i.d.]	L; Pre-treated with mefloquine (750 and 500 mg)	21	0.00	0.00	0.00	0.00	0.00	0	0	0	Wilairatana and Looaresuwan (1994)
1000 mg/4 h/Attack (≤ 4 ×) as required [24 h] migraine*	[Domperidone 30 mg + P 1000 mg/4 h/attack (max. 4 ×) as required; domperidone 20 mg + P 1000 mg/4 h/attack (max. 4 ×) as required]	L	46 @	0.00	0.00	0.00	2.17	0.00	2.17	1	1	MacGregor et al. (1993)
10 mg/kg/day/6 h ≤ 360 mg/day max. [5 d] Influenza A infection*	[Rimantadine 6.6 mg/kg/day/12 h up to 200 mg/day max.]	E	34	0.00	2.94 N	2.94	0.00	2.94	5.88	2	2	Thompson et al. (1987)

TABLE 7.4 (continued)

Dose regimen [Study duration] Study type (* = Clinical trial)	(Formulation) [Comparator(s)]: (A) Aspirin, (B) Bromfenac, (C) Codeine, (D) Diclofenac, (F) Fenprofen, (I) Ibuprofen, (K) Ketoprofen, (M) Meclofenamate, (N) Naproxen, (P) Paracetamol, (S) Sulindac	Comments effective than comparator, (M) More, (L) Less effective than comparator, (E) Equiactive, (N) No effect	No of Subjects	GI Blood loss (BL), Heartburn (H), Diarrhoea/constipation (DC), Discomfort (SD), General (G) (%)	Nausea (N), Vomiting (V) (%)	Total (%)	CNS Total (%)	Other Total (%)	Total	Total ADR events	Total ADR subjects	Study
500 mg [4 d] Wisdom tooth extraction*	[Suprofen 200 mg (Suprocil)]	(As above)	29	0.00	0.00	0.00	3.45	3.45	6.9	2	2	Reijntjes et al. (1987)
1000 mg t.i.d. Followed by 4 × 500 mg/day × 2 d [7 d] oral surgery*	[Methylprednisolone (Medrol) 24/20/16/12/8/4 mg in decreasing doses up to 1 d post surgery]	> 3 ADR events observed, but data insufficient to relate drug with event; M	24	?	?	?	?	?	?	?	3	Olstad and Skjelbred (1986)
650 mg [6 h] 3rd molar extraction*	[Flurbiprofen (Ansaid) 50/100 mg; zomepirac sodium 100 mg; P 650 mg + C-phosphate 60 mg]	E combination L (others)	30	0.00	0.00	0.00	3.33	0.00	3.33	1	1	Sunshine et al. (1986)
650 mg [6 h] Postoperative pain*	[Nalbuphine 30 mg; P 650 mg + nalbuphine 30 mg]	L	30	0.00	0.00	3.33	26.66	3.33	33.32	9	9	Jain et al. (1986b)
50/200/400 mg (t.i.d. max.) Depending on age and weight [6 h] Antipyretic activity*	[Suprofen (Suprol) syrup 50/100/200 mg (t.i.d. max.) depending on age and weight]	L	59 @	0.00	5.08 V	5.08	0.00	0.00	5.08	3	3	Weippe et al. (1985a)
125/250/250 + 125/ 500/500 + 125/500 + 250 mg (t.i.d. max.) Depending on weight [6 h] Antipyretic activity*	[Suprofen (Suprol) suppository 50/100/100 + 50/200/200 + 50 mg (t.i.d. max.) depending on weight]	2 ADR events observed, but data insufficient; L	60 @	?	?	?	?	?	?	?	?	Weippe et al. (1985b)

Dose and indication	Drug											Reference
500 mg [6 h] Pain from orthopaedic operation*	[ketorolac 5/10/20 mg]		30	0.00	3.33 V; 6.67 N	10.00	10.00	40.00	60	18	15	McQuay et al. (1986)
1000 mg (As above)	(As above)	L (high doses of ketoprofen)	30	0.00	10.00 V; 20.00 N	30.00	16.67	36.66	83.33	25	17	(As above)
240/360 mg [4 h]; dental extraction in children*	[I (Aluminium); P 240 mg + C 24 mg]	E	11	0.00	0.00	0.00	0.00	0.00	0	0	0	Moore et al. (1985)
Up to 1000 mg q.i.d. × 5 d [5 d] migraine*	[Flupirtine maleate up to 100 mg/day × 5 d as required]	L	20	10.00 DC	0.00	10.00	20.00	5.00	35	7	5	Million et al. (1984)
1000 mg [6 h] Sore throat*	[I 400 mg]	L	40 @	0.00	0.00	0.00	0.00	0.00	0	0	0	Schactel et al. (1988)
1000 mg q.i.d., then 500 mg q.i.d. × 2 d [4 d] Oral surgery*	(Panadol) [2 × P 1000 mg + P-N-acetyl-DL-methionate (SUR2647) 2146 mg/day followed by 2 × P 500 mg + SUR2647 1073 mg/day × 2 d]	L	26	0.00	3.85 V; 3.85 N	7.70	34.61	0.00	42.31	11	8	Skoglund and Skjelbred (1984)
650 mg [4 h] Postoperative pain*	[Nalbuphine hydrochloride 30 mg; nalbuphine HCl 30 mg + P 650 mg]	Analgesic efficacy of combination additive	33	0.00	0.00	0.00	30.30	0.00	30.3	10	9	Forbes et al. (1984b)
1000 mg [5 h] Oral surgery*	[C 60 mg; P 1000 mg + C 60 mg]	L	42 @	2.38 SD	14.29 V; 16.67 N	33.34	38.08	2.38	73.8	31	21	Bentley and Head (1987)
650 mg [6 h] Episiotomy, surgical or dental proceedures*	[Flupirtine 100/200/300 mg; C 60 mg; pentazocine 50 mg/oxycodone 10 mg + P 650 mg]		?	Observed G	?	?	?	?	?	?	18	McMahon et al. (1987)
10 mg/kg/ t.i.d. × 2 d [2 d] Tonsillitis/ pharyngitis*	[I 10 mg/kg t.i.d. × 2 d (Microgranules or Sparklets)]	L	78 @	0.00	3.85 N	3.85	0.00	0.00	3.85	3	3	Bertin et al. (1991)
1000 mg [4 h] Muscle contraction headache*	[A 1000 mg + caffeine 64 mg]	L	100 @	0.00	0.00	0.00	0.00	0.00	0	0	0	Schactel et al. (1991)
15 mg/kg q.i.d. × 1–2 d Antipyretic*	[4 × 2.5/5/10 mg/kg/day × 1-2 d]	E	16	18.75 SD	0.00	18.75	18.75	18.75	56.25	9	?	Walson et al. (1992)
10 mg/kg [8 h] Antipyretic*	[I 7.5/10 mg/kg]	L	8	0.00	0.00	0.00	0.00	0.00	0.00	0	0	Kauffman et al. (1992)

TABLE 7.4 (continued)

Dose regimen [Study duration] Study type (* = Clinical trial)	(Formulation) [Comparator(s)]: (A) Aspirin, (B) Bromfenac, (C) Codeine, (D) Diclofenac, (F) Fenprofen, (I) Ibuprofen, (K) Ketoprofen, (M) Meclofenamate, (N) Naproxen, (P) Paracetamol, (S) Sulindac	Comments effective than comparator, (M) More, (L) Less effective than comparator, (E) Equiactive, (N) No effect	No of Subjects	GI Blood loss (BL), Heartburn (H), Diarrhoea/constipation (DC), Discomfort (SD), General (G) (%)	Nausea (N), Vomiting (V) (%)	Total (%)	CNS Total (%)	Other Total (%)	Total	Total ADR events	Total ADR subjects	Study
2 × 1000 mg [10 h] 3rd molar extraction*	[Diflunisal 500 mg]	One dose paracetamol pre- and one 4 h post-operative, diflusinal pre-operative; N	35	0.00	0.00	0.00	0.00	0.00	0	0	0	Rodrigo et al. (1989)
1000 mg [6 h] Dental impaction surgery*	[I 400 mg]	L	63 @	0.00	3.17 N	3.17	15.87	0.00	19.04	13	11	Cooper et al. (1989)
650 mg [6 h] Episiotomy*	[P 650 mg + Phenyltoloxamine citrate 60 mg]	L	75 @	0.00	0.00	0.00	0.00	0.00	0	0	0	Sunshine et al. (1989)
1000 mg [4 h] Episiotomy*	[I 400 mg]	L	37	0.00	0.00	0.00	0.00	0.00	0	0	0	Schactel et al. (1989)
1000 mg [6 h] Oral surgery*	[I 400 mg]	L	307 @	4.23 G	0.00	4.23	6.51	0.00	10.74	33	32	Mehlisch et al. (1990)
500 mg/day t.i.d. × 7 d Cancer*	[I 600 mg t.i.d.; A 600 mg t.i.d.; D s.r. b.d. + placebo; indomethacin 50 mg t.i.d.; pirprofen 400 mg t.i.d.; sulindac 300 mg b.d. + placebo; N 250 mg t.i.d.; suprofen 200 mg t.i.d. all × 7 d]	L	13	7.69 DC; 30.77 H	7.69 N	46.15	69.22	76.91	192.3	26	?	Ventafridda et al. (1990)
1000 mg [7 d] Chronic obstructive lung disease*	[C 60 mg + P 1000 mg]	More GI SE in combination	18	5.56 DC	5.56 V; 11.11 N	22.23	22.22	22.23	66.68	12	10	Munck et al. (1990)

Dose [interval] indication	Comparator											Reference
500 mg q.i.d. × 1 d [24 h] Periodontal surgery*	[4 × 100 mg/1 d Flubiprofen]	L	15	0.00	6.67 N	6.67	20.00	6.67	33.34	5	?	Gallardo and Rossi (1990)
10 mg/kg × 5 d [5 d] Infection by influenza A*	[6.6 mg/kg × 5 d Rimantadine]	L	32	0	0	0	0	0	0	0	0	Bresse Hall et al. (1987)
650 mg [12 h] Muscle contraction headache*	(Tylenol) [N-sodium (Anaprox) 550 mg]	L	50@	2.00 DC	2.00 N	4.00	4.00	2.00	10	5	4	Miller et al. (1987)
250 mg q.i.d. × 5 d [5 d] Common cold/upper respiratory tract infection*	[3 × P 500 mg + phenylpropanolamine 25 mg and 1 × P 500 mg + diphenydramine hydrochloride 25 mg/day ('Benylin Day and Night') × 5 d]	L	90@	1.11 DC; 6.67 SD; 5.56 H	5.56 N	18.90	6.67	2.22	27.79	14	11	Middleton (1981)
1000 mg [6 h] Orthopaedic operations*	[Tiaramide hydrochloride 100 mg/200 mg]	M	21	0.00	4.76 N	4.76	0.00	0.00	4.76	1	1	Winnem et al. (1981)
500 mg/2 h × 10 h as required lower wisdom tooth removal*	[5 × C-phosphate 30 mg + A 300 mg + P 200 mg + caffeine 50 mg + magnesium oxide 25 mg (Staralgin)/2 h × 10 h as required; 5 × dextro-propoxyphene napsylate 100 mg + A 350 mg + phenazone 150 mg (Doleron novum)/2 h × 10 h as required]	L (Doleron novum); E (codeine)	27	0.00	3.70 N	3.70	11.11	0.00	14.81	4	3	Quiding et al. (1981)
650 mg [6 h] 3rd molar extraction*	[Flurbiprofen 50/100 mg; P 650 mg + C 60 mg]	L (Flurbiprofen); E (combination)	27	0.00	7.41 N	7.41	18.51	7.41	33.33	9	7	Dionne et al. (1994)
10 mg/kg q.i.d. × 1–3 d Antipyretic*	[I 4 × 5 mg/kg/day × 1–3 d]	L	36	5.56 G	0.00	5.56	0.00	2.78	8.34	8	0	Van Esch et al. (1995)
15 mg/kg [6 h] Sore throat*	[I 10 mg/kg]	E	38	0	0	0	0	0	0	0	0	Schactel and Thoden (1993)

TABLE 7.4 (continued)

Dose regimen [Study duration] Study type (* = Clinical trial)	(Formulation) [Comparator(s)]: (A) Aspirin, (B) Bromfenac, (C) Codeine, (D) Diclofenac, (F) Fenprofen, (I) Ibuprofen, (K) Ketoprofen, (M) Meclofenamate, (N) Naproxen, (P) Paracetamol, (S) Sulindac	Comments More (M), Less (L), Equiactive (E), No effect (N) effective than comparator	No of Subjects	GI Blood loss (BL), Heartburn (H), Diarrohea/constipation (DC), Discomfort (SD), General (G) (%)	GI Nausea (N), Vomiting (V) (%)	GI Total (%)	CNS Total (%)	Other Total (%)	Total	Total ADR events	Total ADR subjects	Study
650 mg/day t.i.d. [48 h] Effect on sleep patterns	[I 400 mg/day t.i.d.] Effect on sleep patterns	Effect on sleep patterns	9	?	?	?	?	?	?	?	?	Murphy et al. (1994)
1000 mg [6 h] Headache*	[A 650 mg]		87 @	8.05 G	0.00	8.05	0.00	6.90	14.95	13	?	Peters et al. (1983)
500 mg/2 h × 10 h As required lower wisdom tooth extraction*	[500 mg Phenazone/2 h × 10 h; 500 mg phenazone + 100 mg dextropropoxyphene napsylate/2 h × 10 h]	E	33	3.03 SD	0.00	3.03	15.15	9.09	27.27	9	5	Quiding et al. (1982a)
500 mg/2 h × 10 h As required lower wisdom tooth extraction*	[P 500 mg + C 20 mg/2 h × 10 h; P 500 mg + C 30 mg/2 h × 10 h; P 500 mg + C 40 mg/2 h × 10 h]		66 @	1.52 G	3.03 N	4.55	6.08	0.00	10.63	7	6	Quiding et al. (1982b)
1000 mg [5 h] Postoperative pain*	[C-phosphate 60 mg; P 1000 mg + C-phosphate 60 mg]		46 @	2.17 SD; 2.17 H	2.17 V; 6.52 N	13.03	10.87	6.52	30.42	0	0	Gertzbein et al. (1986)
500 mg q.i.d. × 4 d [4 d] Post-endodontic periodontitis secondary to infiltrative/abscessed pulpitis*	[100 mg Fentiazac q.i.d. × 4 d]	L (in patient, though not in investigators' assessment of induced pain)	14	0.00	0.00	0.00	0.00	0.00	0	0	0	Leguen (1985)
1000 mg q.i.d. × 2 d Immune response to influenza vaccine*	None	N	39	0.00	0.00	0.00	0.00	10.25	10.25	4	4	Gross et al. (1994)

Dose / indication	Drug / treatment	Comment	n								Reference
650 mg [6 h] Post-episiotomal pain*	[Aceclofenac 100 mg]	L	30	0.00	0.00	0.00	0.00	0.00	0	0	Movilia (1989)
650 mg/day t.i.d. × 7 d; renovascular effects	[I 400 mg/day t.i.d. × 7 d]	N	8	0.00	0.00	0.00	0.00	0.00	0	0	Furey et al. (1993)
650 mg [6 h] Oral surgery*	[Phenyltoloxamine 60 mg; P 650 mg + phenyltoloxamine 60 mg]	M	43 @	0.00	0.00	2.33	0.00	2.33	2	1	Forbes et al. (1984a)
1000 mg [4 h] Post-partum pain*	[A 800 mg + caffeine 65 mg; P 648 mg + A 648 mg]	(As above)	123 @	0.00	0.00	4.88	0.00	4.88	6	6	Rubin and Winter (1984)
650 mg [6 h] SE profile	[I 200/400 mg]		237 @	0.42 DC; 2.11 SD; 2.11 H	2.11 N	6.75	0.42	13.5	20	15	Furey et al. (1992)
1000 mg (As above)	(As above)		612 @	1.27 SD; 1.27 H	1.27 N	3.81	0.00	11.83	17	12	(As above)
2000 mg/day × 4 d [4 d] Grip strength in rheumatoid arthritis	[Tolmetin 1200 mg/day × 4 d]	L	12	0.00	0.00	0.00	0.00	0	0	0	Di Munno and Sarchi (1982)
600 mg [12 h] 3rd molar extraction*	[Flurbiprofen 100 mg; P 600 mg + C 60 mg]	L	26	0.00	3.85 N	3.85	7.70	0.00	11.55	3	3	Forbes et al. (1989)
650 mg [5 h] Post-strabismus surgery*	[I 600 mg; Ketorolac 60 mg i.v.]	L (Ketorolac)	20	0.00	10.00 N	10.00	0.00	0.00	10	1	1	Morrison and Repka (1994)
2 × 500 mg/10 h as required lower wisdom tooth extraction*	[500 mg Diflunisal]	L	45 @	0.00	2.22 N	2.22	2.22	6.66	11.1	6	5	Nystrom et al. (1988)
2 × 1000 mg/10 h as required* (As above)	(As above)	(As above)	46 @	0.00	2.17 V	2.17	13.04	6.52	21.73	10	7	(As above)
650 mg/6 h [72 h] Postinstrumentation of root canals*	[(Tylenol) [A 650 mg; I (Motrin) 400 mg; K (Orudis) 50 mg; P 325 mg + C 60 mg (Phenaphen #4); penicillin (Veetids) 500 mg; erythromycin base 500 mg; penicillin 500 mg + I 400 mg; methylprednisolone (MedRol) 2 mg + penicillin 500 mg]	1.8% Of subjects had ADRs though data insufficient to catagorize; E (with mild pain)	50 @	?	?	?	?	?	?	?	Torabinejad et al. (1994)
1000 mg q.i.d. × 5 d Laser-induced pain*	(Plain)	Effective analgesic	15	0.00	0.00	0.00	0.00	0.00	0	0	Nielsen et al. (1991)

TABLE 7.4 (*continued*)

Dose regimen [Study duration] Study type (* = Clinical trial)	(Formulation) [Comparator(s)]: (A) Aspirin, (B) Bromfenac, (C) Codeine, (D) Diclofenac, (F) Fenprofen, (I) Ibuprofen, (K) Ketoprofen, (M) Meclofenamate, (N) Naproxen, (P) Paracetamol, (S) Sulindac	Comments (M) More, (L) Less effective than comparator, (E) Equiactive, (N) No effect	No of Subjects	GI			CNS Total (%)	Other Total (%)	Total	Total ADR events	Total ADR subjects	Study
				Blood loss (BL), Heartburn (H), Diarrohea/constipation (DC), Discomfort (SD), General (G) (%)	Nausea (N), Vomiting (V) (%)	Total (%)						
2000 mg b.d. × 5 d (As above)	(s.r.)	(As above)	15	0.00	6.67 N	6.67	6.67	0.00	13.34	2	1	(As above)
		TOTALS:	5348							365	488	
		MEAN%:		0.00 BL; 0.49 DC; 0.76 SD; 0.35 G; 0.76 H	1.71 (0.84 V; 2.58 N)	5.84	8.44	5.27	19.55			
		SD:		0.00 BL; 1.84 DC; 2.78 SD; 1.42 G; 4.21 H	3.61 (2.57 V; 4.26 N)	9.15	12.79	12.79	31.16			
		MEDIAN:		0.00 BL, DC, SD, G, H	0.00 V, N	3.33	3.33	0.00	10.25			
		MAX:		0.00 BL; 10.00 DC; 18.75 SD; 8.05 G; 30.77 H	20.00 (14.29V; 20.00 N)	46.15	69.22	76.91	192.3			
		MIN:		0.00 BL, DC, SD, G, H	0.00 V, N	0.00	0.00	0.00	0.00			

= N ≥ 40;
? = No adverse drug reactions (ADRs) mentioned.
Reproduced from Rainsford *et al.* (1997), with permission of the Editor of the *Journal of Pharmacy and Pharmacology*.

TABLE 7.5

Statistical comparisons (analysis of variance; Fisher's F-test) of adverse events from the data shown in Table 7.4 where the treatment with either ibuprofen or paracetamol was for ≤ 7 days and number of subjects per group, n ≥ 40 (this data is indicated by @ in Table 7.4). In these analyses the overall data is shown in Part A while that from direct comparisons of ibuprofen with paracetamol is shown in Part B.

Part A. All data:

Adverse events	F	P	
Gastrointestinal			
Constipation	0.563	0.457	N/S
Vomiting	0.048	0.827	N/S
Discomfort	0.336	0.565	N/S
Nausea	0.460	0.501	N/S
Heartburn	0.161	0.690	N/S
General	0.044	0.835	N/S
Gastrointestinal total	0.0003	0.987	N/S
CNS total	0.704	0.406	N/S
Other total	0.055	0.816	N/S
Total	0.351	0.557	N/S

N/S, Not significant; analysis of variance single factor, level of significance set at p < 0.05.

Part B. Data from studies where ibuprofen was directly compared with paracetamol:

Adverse events	F	P	
Gastrointestinal			
Constipation	1.000	0.341	N/S
Vomiting	1.225	0.297	N/S
Discomfort	1.227	0.297	N/S
Nausea	0.006	0.941	N/S
Heartburn	0.001	0.975	N/S
General	1.060	0.328	N/S
Gastrointestinal total	0.639	0.443	N/S
CNS total	1.013	0.338	N/S
Other total	1.138	0.311	N/S
Total	0.733	0.414	N/S

N/S, Not significant; analysis of variance single factor, level of significance set at p < 0.05.

Overall, the rates of adverse effects of ibuprofen 200–400 mg have been found to be comparable with those of naproxen 440 mg and paracetamol 500–1000 mg (De Armond *et al.*, 1995).

In a 2-year study in 421 patients, Wilcox and co-workers (1994) observed that ibuprofen can be associated, albeit rarely, with gastrointestinal reactions. These may be exacerbated in elderly patients with osteoarthritis (Liang and Fortin, 1991).

Kaufman and co-workers (1997) found in a case-controlled study of hospitalized patients in the United States, Sweden and Hungary that alcohol was a major risk factor for major upper gastrointestinal bleeding with intake of OTC doses of aspirin, ibuprofen and naproxen. The mutivariate relative risks for aspirin, ibuprofen and naproxen did not vary according to the level of alcohol consumed. For aspirin taken regularly at doses ≤ 325 mg in the week before the index date, the relative risk was 3.2, while with 325 mg of the drug it was 2.3, and at up to 1000 mg it was 4.4. Among drinkers (≥ 21 drinks/week) the risk with aspirin at ≥ 325 mg regularly was 4.9. For regular intake of ibuprofen the risk with alcohol was 2.7, and with regular naproxen it was 6.1. These and other data provided by the authors highlight the pronounced risk of serious gastrointestinal reactions from large quantities of alcohol consumed with regular doses of NSAIDs such as ibuprofen.

Ibuprofen at high OTC doses has been found to elevate blood pressure slightly (Bradley, 1991); this is a feature with other NSAIDs. This may, in part, arise from renal complications since these are also seen with NSAIDs (Schlondorff, 1993). Moreover, Whelton and colleagues (1990) observed that ibuprofen 800 mg t.i.d. in patients with asymptomatic, chronic renal failure resulted in reversible acute renal failure that recurred upon re-challenge. While the risk of renal complications with ibuprofen at OTC doses is small (Mann *et al.*, 1993; see also Chapter 10), it appears to be greater in patients on diuretics (Bonney *et al.*, 1986). Thus, as with all NSAIDs, combinations of these drugs with diuretics should be avoided. Reversible renal failure from ibuprofen has been associated with a bout of binge drinking (Elsasser *et al.*, 1988; Wen *et al.*, 1992).

Mitchell and Lesko (1995) stated that there is a need to provide valid and statistical risk estimates of adverse effects of ibuprofen, both over-the-counter and prescribed, in children.

Of the more serious adverse recations reported, there is one of a child who developed a metabolic acidosis after an acute massive overdosage of ibuprofen 800 mg tablets (Linden and Townsend, 1987). In general most clinical reports indicate a low incidence and severity of adverse reactions in children (Bertin *et al.*, 1991; McIntyre and Hull, 1996).

In an assessment of the tolerability in the GI tract of a liquigel formulation of ibuprofen with that of an equivalent dose of 200 mg of the ibuprofen tablet formulation (Doyle *et al.*, 1997), in a multicentre, double-blind, randomized, age-stratified, parallel study, it was found that faecal occult blood and adverse reactions in 1246 subjects who took ibuprofen tablets and the liquigel formulation at the dose of 1200 mg/day did not differ from those with placebo or among the treatment groups. Also, the dropouts due to adverse reactions did not differ among these treatments. The symptomatic adverse reactions were all minor and comparable with those reported in the study by Rainsford *et al.* (1997; Table 7.4).

Thus, these clinical trials show that under OTC dosage conditions ibuprofen has a low incidence of adverse reactions, and this is evident with formulations that would be expected to enhance absorption from the GI tract.

7.4 PHARMACOEPIDEMIOLOGICAL DATA

Moore, Noblet and Breemeersch (1996) reviewed the pharmacovigilance data available worldwide for adverse events recorded from ibuprofen. The spontaneous reports suggests that the rate in the United Kingdom is 1 per 5.31 million 200 mg tablets sold. In the United States the rate appears lower and is 1 per 25 million 200 mg tablets.

Clinical and post-marketing studies reviewed by Moore *et al.* (1996) showed that the frequency of adverse events from ibuprofen was similar to that from paracetamol and placebo.

Using what is probably the largest available manufacturer's database on spontaneous reports, Ewell *et al.* (1997) studied the adverse reaction from ibuprofen (Advil™; Whitehall-Robins, Madison, NJ, USA) over the 13-year period since the start of OTC marketing of this drug in the United States. The data were analyzed using secular trend analysis of all reports. The adverse reactions were graded into (a) 15-day reports (rated as serious, unexpected reports, total 142); (b) documented serious reports (total 213); and (c) non-serious reports (total 1375). The pattern of adverse events from these data is shown in Figure 7.2 in comparison with the cumulative tablet distribution which, up to 1997, totalled about 6 billion 200 mg tablets. It should be noted that this latter statistic should not be confused with tablet intake; it only represents the overall distribution of the tablets from the manufacturer, but is a useful indication of the availability of the drug to the population at large in the United States.

A total of 16 death reports had been received over the 13-year period of the analysis, of which, upon medical review, 7 may have been causally related to ingestion of ibuprofen. One of these was assigned to a category in which the amount of drug taken was greater than 800 mg or a higher dose category.

When the data were analyzed according to body system (using the Cosart Dictionary organ systems), 77% of serious reports were in Costart categories of Body as a Whole, Digestive, Urinogenital, and Skin and Integumentary. Of the non-serious reports, 80% were in the Costart categories of Body as a Whole, Digestive, Skin and Integumentary and Nervous. High-dose intake (> 600 mg daily dose) accounted for 35% of reports and about half of these resulted in hospitalization.

These data attest to the high safety profile of ibuprofen in the population at large. The relatively low death rate and incidence of serious adverse reactions is testament to the safety of ibuprofen.

CHAPTER 7

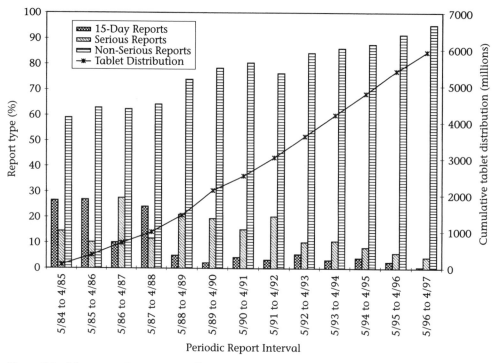

Figure 7.2: Adverse event reports according to reporting year and cumulative ibuprofen distribution.

7.5 EFFICACY

The summary of published studies shown in Table 7.4 shows the range and type of conditions treated with ibuprofen in comparison with paracetamol and other analgesics. In the main, these trials showed that ibuprofen had therapeutic benefit in relief of mild to moderate pain, inflammation or fever comparable with, or sometimes better than, that observed with other analgesics/antipyretics. In the following some of the trials are discussed in which the effects of ibuprofen were studied in various acute conditions.

7.5.1 Upper respiratory tract infections and ENT conditions

Ibuprofen is effective at recommended OTC doses for the relief of symptoms of mild to moderate upper respiratory tract infections such as colds and influenza (Reynolds, 1996). Ibuprofen controls the febrile responses and may also reduce the inflammatory reactions in the throat and airways. The analgesic and antipyretic activity of OTC ibuprofen in children is claimed to be comparable with that of paracetamol (Henretig, 1996), although this is not borne out by analysis of dose for weight comparisons. Moreover, recent studies suggest that ibuprofen is actually superior to paracetamol in relief of pain associated with throat infections (Schachtel and Thoden, 1993; Boureau, 1998).

Sperber *et al.* (1989), in a trial in 58 patients, observed that ibuprofen 200 mg significantly reduced the nasal symptoms compared with placebo in subjects with colds.

Shachtel and Thoden (1993) found that ibuprofen 10 mg/kg was superior in relief of sore throat in children over a 6 h period compared with paracetamol 15 mg/kg, although the initial response with paracetamol at 1 h was better than that with ibuprofen. Both treatments were appreciably better than placebo. A recent carefully controlled study by Boureau (1998) also concluded that ibuprofen was superior to paracetamol in relief of symptoms of sore throat associated with tonsillitis.

In a study of fever in children, Walson and colleagues (1989) found that ibuprofen 10 mg/kg was more effective than placebo and was favoured over paracetamol 10 mg/kg. At initial temperatures greater than 39.2°C (102.5°F), a dose-response was evident with ibuprofen 5–10 mg/kg in both the percentage of fever reduction and the rate of temperature decline from the initial 2 h period. The antipyretic efficacy of ibuprofen 10 mg/kg for temperatures in excess of 39.2°C was greater than at 5 mg/kg of the drug, which in turn was superior to paracetamol 10 mg/kg, all treatments being significantly better than placebo. All treatments were well tolerated and no significant clinical or laboratory abnormalities were recorded. It has been concluded from this and a later study (Walson *et al.*, 1992) that ibuprofen is a safe and effective antipyretic in children.

Ibuprofen was found to be less effective in the treatment of symptoms of otitis media than trimethoprim-sulfamethoxazole or prednisolone in a randomized controlled clinical trial conducted in 76 children (Giebink *et al.*, 1990). In some respects this is not surprising since antimicrobial treatment is the norm for this condition. Combinations of antimicrobial agents and an analgesic–anti-inflammatory such as ibuprofen would be expected to have particular benefit in otitis media.

7.5.2 Dysmenorrhoea

Ibuprofen, like some other NSAIDs, is an established therapy for relief of pain in primary dysmenorrhoea (Reynolds, 1996). Its advantage is that it has low incidence and severity of side-effects and does not produce excessive bleeding as in the case of aspirin.

Ibuprofen but not placebo has been shown to decrease menstrual prostaglandin release (Chan *et al.*, 1981; Mäkäläinen and Ylikorkala, 1986a). In doses ranging from 400 to 800 mg ibuprofen has been shown in several double-blind randomized trials to be superior to placebo in reducing menstrual pain (Morrison *et al.*, 1980; Furniss, 1982; Arnold *et al.*, 1983; Goökin *et al.*, 1983; Mehlisch *et al.*, 1988; Dawood and Ramos, 1990). In doses of 400 mg, ibuprofen has been shown to be superior in pain relief to propoxyphene hydrochloride 64 mg (Morrison *et al.*, 1980) and paracetamol 500 mg and naproxen 250 mg (Milsom and Andersch, 1984), and equal to piroxicam 20 mg and 40 mg (Pasquale *et al.*, 1988) and fenoprofen 200 mg (Arnold *et al.*, 1983). However, in a review of 51 trials, fenamates appeared to be more effective than ibuprofen, indomethacin and naproxen

CHAPTER 7

(Owen, 1984). Further studies are clearly required, especially to determine the relative value of larger doses of ibuprofen compared to other nonsteroidal anti-inflammatory analgesics, in particular in relation to development of adverse effects. Ibuprofen in a dose of 1200 mg/day has also proved effective in treating primary menorrhagia and reducing blood loss following insertion of copper-releasing intrauterine devices (Mäkäläinen and Ylikorkala, 1986b).

7.5.3 Migraine

Ibuprofen, like other NSAIDs, has been found to be useful in the treatment of migraine (Diamond, 1994). In brief, several NSAIDs have been shown to be superior to placebo and to standard reference drugs in the majority of double-blind trials (Diamond, 1994). However, the effects were marginal or without clinical relevance in some studies (Pfaffenrath and Scherzer, 1995). Ibuprofen 400–800 mg has been shown to be effective in some studies of migraine.

Havanka-Kaniainen (1989) compared ibuprofen, in an initial dose of 800 mg supplemented if necessary by 400 mg, with placebo in a double-blind trial in 40 patients. Ibuprofen 200 mg was found to be superior to paracetamol 450 mg for the relief of migraine. Doses of 400–800 mg have generally been shown to be effective in helping to relieve an acute attack of migraine (Pearce *et al.*, 1983; Pfaffenrath and Scherzer, 1995; Stewart and Lipton, 1998). In children, ibuprofen 10 mg/kg was found by Hämäläinen *et al.* (1997) to be superior to paracetamol 15 mg/kg in relief of migraine. Moreover, ibuprofen was twice as likely as paracetamol to abort a migraine attack at 2 h (Hämäläinen *et al.*, 1997).

Stewart and Lipton (1998) showed that combining ibuprofen with caffeine conferred only marginal benefit over ibuprofen alone for the relief of migraine.

7.6 CONCLUSIONS

The overall assessment from the published reports suggests that ibuprofen is a safe and effective drug for the treatment of mild to moderate pain, inflammatory states and fever in a wide section of the population when taken under recommended OTC dosage conditions.

ACKNOWLEDGEMENTS

My thanks to Dr Anthony Ewell for information on the adverse reactions from ibuprofen in the United States (Figure 7.2). The data in Tables 7.2–7.4 are reproduced with permission of the Editor of the *Journal of Pharmacy and Pharmacology*.

REFERENCES

AABAKKEN, L., DYBDAHL, J.H., LARSEN, S., MOWINCKEL, P., OSNES, M. and QUIDING, H. (1989) A double-blind comparison of gastrointestinal effects of ibuprofen sustained release assessed by means of endoscopy and 51-Cr-labelled erythrocytes. *Scandinavian Journal of Rheumatology* **18**, 307–313.

ADAMS, S.S. and MARCHANT, B. (1984) . . . and the ibuprofen story. *Pharmaceutical Journal* 1984 (24 Nov.); 646.

ADMANI, A.K. and VERMA, S. (1983) A study of sulindac versus ibuprofen in elderley patients with osteoarthritis. *Current Medical Research and Opinion* **8**, 315–320.

AGUS, B., NELSON, J., KRAMER, N., MAHAL, S.S. and ROSENSTEIN, E.D. (1990) Acute central nervous system symptoms caused by ibuprofen in connective tissue disease. *Journal of Rheumatology* **17**, 1094–1096.

AHLSTROM, U., BAKSHI, R., NILSSON, P. and WAHLANDER, L. (1993) The analgesic efficacy of diclofenac, dispersible and ibuprofen in postoperative pain after dental extraction. *European Journal of Clinical Pharmacology* **44**, 587–588.

ALAM, M.N. and KABIR, M.Z. (1983) Comparative study of piroxicam and ibuprofen in rheumatoid arthritis. *Bangladesh Medical Research Council Bulletin* **9**, 54–59.

ARNOLD, J.D., IBER, F.L., BURT, R.A. and GRUBER, C.M. JR. (1983) Comparison of fenoprofen calcium, ibuprofen and placebo in primary dysmenorrhea. *Journal of Medicine* **14**, 337–350.

BAKER, J.R. (ed.) (1996) Clinical safety of OTC analgesics. *Postgraduate Medicine. Special Report* 4–84.

BAKSHI, R., FRENKEL, G., DIETLEIN, G., MEURER-WITT, B., SCHNEIDER, B. and SINTERHAUF, U. (1994) A placebo-controlled comparative evaluation of diclofenac dispersible versus ibuprofen in postoperative pain after third molar surgery. *Journal of Clinical Pharmacology* **34**, 225–230.

BENSON, G.D. (1983) Acetaminophen in chronic liver disease. *Clinical Pharmacology and Therapeutics* **33**, 95–101.

BENTLEY, K.C. and HEAD, T.W. (1987) The additive analgesic efficacy of acetominophen, 1000 mg, and codeine, 60 mg, in dental pain. *Clinical Pharmacology and Therapeutics* **42**, 634–640.

BERGMANN, J.F., CHASSANY, O., GENEVE, J., ABITEBOUL, M., CAULIN, C. and SEGRESTAA, J.M. (1992) Endoscopic evaluation of the effect of ketoprofen, ibuprofen and aspirin on the gastroduodenal mucosa. *European Journal of Clinical Pharmacology* **42**, 685–688.

BERTIN, L., PONS, G., D'ATHIS, P., LASFARGUES, G., MAUDELONDE, C., DUHAMEL, J.F. and OLIVE, G. (1991) Randomized, double-blind, multicenter, controlled trial of ibuprofen versus acetominophen (paracetamol) and placebo for treatment of symptoms of tonsillitis and pharyngitis in children. *Journal of Pediatrics* **119**, 811–814.

BHATTACHARYA, S.K., GOEL, R.K., BHATTACHARYA, S.K. and TANDON, R. (1991) Potentiaton of gastric toxicity of ibuprofen by paracetamol in the rat. *Journal of Pharmacy and Pharmacology* **43**, 520–521.

BIDLINGMAIER, A., HAMMERMAIER, A., NAGYIVANYI, P., PABST, G. and WAITZINGER, J. (1995) Gastrointestinal blood loss induced by three different nonsteroidal anti-inflammatory drugs. *Arzneimittel-Forschung/Drug Research* **45**, 491–493.

BIRD, H.A. (1985) Impact of over the counter availability of nonsteroidal anti-inflammatory drugs. In: BROOKS, P.M., DAY, R.O., WILLIAMS, K.M. and GRAHAM, G. (eds), Agents and Actions Supplements: *Basis for Variability of Response to Anti-Rheumatic Drugs.* Birkhauser Verlag, Basel, 55–59.

BOELSTERLI, U.A., ZIMMERMAN, H.J. and KRETZ-ROMMEL (1995) Idiosyncratic liver toxicity of nonsteroidal anti-inflammatory drugs: molecular mechanisms and pathology. *Critical Reviews in Toxicology* **25**, 207–235.

BONNEY, S.L., NORTHINGTON, R.S., HEDRICH, D.A. and WALKER, B.R. (1986) Renal safety of two analgesics used over the counter: ibuprofen and aspirin. *Clinical Pharmacology and Therapeutics* **40**, 373–377.

BOREA, G., MONOPOLI, R. and COLANTONI, A. (1996) Ibuprofen arginine vs naproxen sodium as prophylactic oral treatment of pain due to dental surgery. *Clinical Drug Investigation* **11**, 33–40.

BOUREAU, F. (1998) Multicentre study of the efficacy of ibuprofen compared with paracetamol in throat pain associated with tonsilitis. In: RAINSFORD, K.D. and POWANDA, M.C. (eds), *Safety and Efficacy of OTC Non-prescription NSAIDs and Analgesics.* Dordrecht, Kluwer Academic Publishers, 119–121.

BOUCHIER-HAYES, T., FYVIE, A., JANKE, P.G., VANDENBURG, M.J. and CURRIE, W.J.C. (1984) Sulindac versus ibuprofen in sprains and strains. *British Journal of Sports Medicine* **18**, 30–33.

BRADLEY, J.G. (1991) Non-prescription drugs and hypertension. Which one affects blood pressure? *Postgraduate Medicine* **89**, 195–197.

BRADLEY, J.D., BRANDT, K.D., KATZ, B.P., KALINSKI, L.A. and RYAN, S.I. (1991) Comparison of an anti-inflammatory dose of ibuprofen and acetaminophen in treatment of patients with osteoarthritis of the knee. *New England Journal of Medicine* **325**, 87–91.

BRESSE-HALL, C., DOLIN, R., GALA, C.L. *et al.* (1987) Children with influenza A infection: treatment with rimantadine. *Pediatrics* **80**, 275–282.

BROOME, J.R., STONEHAM, M.D., BEELEY, J.M., MILLEDGE, J.S. and HUGHES, A.S. (1994) High altitude headache: treatment with ibuprofen. *Aviation, Space and Environmental Medicine* **65**, 19–20.

BRUNE, K. (1986) Comparative pharmacology of 'non-opioid' analgesics. [Review]. *Medical Toxicology* **1**, 1–9.

BRUNE, K. and MCCORMACK, K. (1994) The over-the-counter use of nonsteroidal anti-inflammatory drugs and other antipyretic agents. In: LEWIS, A.J. and FURST, D.E. (eds), *Nonsteroidal Anti-Inflammatory Drugs. Mechanisms and Clinical Uses.* New York, Marcel Dekker, 97–126.

BUSSON, M. (1986) Update on ibuprofen: review article. *Journal of International Medical Research* **14**, 53–61.

CAMPBELL, D. and OATES, R.K. (1992) Childhood poisoning — a changing profile with scope for prevention. *Medical Journal of Australia* **156**, 238–240.

CAMU, F., VAN LERSBERGHE, C. and LAUWERS, M.H. (1992) Cardiovascular risks and benefits of perioperative nonsteroidal anti-inflammatory drug treatment. [Review]. *Drugs* **44**, 42–51.

CARSON, J.L. and STROM, B.L. (1992) The gastrointestinal toxicity of the nonsteroidal anti-inflammatory drugs. In: RAINSFORD, K.D. and VELO, G.P. (eds), *Side-Effects of Anti-inflammatory Drugs 3: Inflammation and Drug Therapy.* Kluwer Academic Publishers, Lancaster, 1–8.

CHAN, W.Y., DAWOOD, M.Y. and FUCHS, F. (1981) Prostaglandins in primary dysmenorrhea. Comparison of prophylactic and non-prophylactic treatment with ibuprofen and use of oral contraceptives. *American Journal of Medicine* **70**, 535–541.

COOPER, S.A., SCHACHTEL, B.P., GOLDMAN, E., GELB, S. and COHN, P. (1989) Ibuprofen and acetaminophen in the relief of acute pain: a randomized, double-blind, placebo-controlled study. *Journal of Clinical Pharmacology* **29**, 1026–1030.

COOPER, S.A., ENGEL, J., LADOV, M., PRECHEUR, H., ROSENHECK, A. and RAUCH, D. (1982) Analgesic efficacy of an ibuprofen-codeine combination. *Pharmacotherapy* **2**, 162–167.

COOPER, S.A., QUINN, P.D., MACAFEE, K., HERSH, E.V., SULLIVAN, D. and LAMP, C. (1993) Ibuprofen controlled release formulation. A clinical trial in dental impaction pain. *Oral Surgery, Oral Medicine and Oral Pathology* **75**, 677–683.

DAVIS, R., YARKER, Y.E. and GOA, K.L. (1995) Diclofenac/misoprostol. A review of its pharmacology and therapeutic efficacy in painful inflammatory conditions. [Review]. *Drugs and Aging* **7**, 372–393.

DAWOOD, M.Y. (1984) Ibuprofen and dysmenorrhea. *American Journal of Medicine* **77**, 87–94.

CHAPTER 7

DAWOOD, M.Y. and RAMOS, J. (1990) Transcutaneous electrical nerve stimulation (TENS) for the treatment of primary dysmenorrhea: a randomized crossover comparison with placebo TENS and ibuprofen. *Obstetrics and Gynecology* **75**, 656–60.

DEARMOND, B., FRANCISCO, C.A., LIN, J.S. *et al.* (1995) Safety profile of over-the-counter naproxen sodium. *Clinical Therapeutics* **17**, 587–601.

DIAMOND, S. (1994) Nonsteroidal anti-inflammatory drugs in migraine. In: LEWIS, A.J. and FURST, D.E. (eds), *Nonsteroidal Anti-Inflammatory Drugs. Mechanisms and Clinical Uses.* 2nd edn. New York, Marcel Dekker, 27–42.

DI MUNNO, O. and SARCHI, C. (1982) Effectiveness of tolmetin in rheumatoid arthritis: evaluation by means of a new method. Methods Find. *Experimental Clinical Pharmacology* **4**, 203–206.

DIONNE, R.A., SNYDER, J. and HARGREAVES, K.M. (1994) Analgesic efficacy of flubiprofen in comparison with acetaminophen plus codeine, and placebo after impacted third molar removal. *Journal of Oral and Maxillofacial Surgery* **52**, 919–924.

DOLLERY, C. (1991) *Therapeutic Drugs.* Edinburgh, Churchill Livingstone, 11–16.

DOYLE, G.A., BAIRD, L.A. and COOPER, S.A. (1997) Evaluation of the gastrointestinal safety profile of a 200 mg ibuprofen liquigel formulation. *Journal of Clinical Pharmacology* **37**, 871 (Abstract No. 56).

DUTCH TIA TRIAL STUDY GROUP (1991) A comparison of two doses of aspirin (30 mg vs 283 mg a day) in patients after a transient ischemic attack or minor ischemic stroke. *New England Journal of Medicine* **325**, 1261–1266.

ELSASSER, G.N., LOPEZ, L., EVANS, E. *et al.* (1988) Reversible acute renal failure associated with ibuprofen ingestion and binge drinking. *Journal of Family Practice* **27**, 221–222.

EWELL, A., TOTH, F., WOLFE, B., PERELSON, A. and PAUL, K. (1997) Thirteen year secular trend analysis of manufacturer-received Advil® spontaneous adverse experience reports. *Pharmacoepidemiology and Drug Safety* **7**(Suppl. 2), S101.

FORBES, J.A., BARKASZI, B.A., RAGLAND, R.N. and HANKLE, J.J. (1984a) Analgesic effect of acetominophen, phenyltoloxamine and their combination in postoperative oral surgery pain. *Pharmacotherapy* **4**, 221–226.

FORBES, J.A., KOLODNY, A.L., CHACHICH, B.M. and BEAVER, W.T. (1984b) Nalbuphine, acetaminophen, and their combination in postoperative pain. *Clinical Pharmacology and Therapeutics* **35**, 843–851.

FORBES, J.A., BUTTERWORTH, G.A., BURCHFIELD, W.H., YORIO, R.N., SELINGER, L.R., ROSENMERTZ, S.K. and BEAVER, W.T. (1989) Evaluation of flubiprofen, acetominophen and acetaminophen–codeine combination, and placebo in postoperative oral surgery pain. *Pharmacotherapy* **9**, 322–330.

FORBES, J.A., BEAVER, W.T., JONES, K.F., KEHM, C.J., KING SMITH, W., GONGLOFF, C.M., ZELEZNOCK, J.R. and SMITH, J.W. (1991a) Effect of caffeine on ibuprofen analgesia in postoperative oral surgery pain. *Clinical Pharmacology and Therapeutics* **49**, 674–684.

FORBES, J.A., EDQUIST, I.A., SMITH, F.G., SCHWARTZ, M.K. and BEAVER, W.T. (1991b) Evaluation of bromfenac, aspirin, and ibuprofen in postoperative oral surgery pain. *Pharmacotherapy* **11**, 64–70.

FORBES, J.A., BEAVER, W.T., JONES, K.F., EDQUIST, R.N., GONGLOFF, C.M., KING SMITH, W., SMITH, F.G. and SCHWARTZ, M.K. (1992) Analgesic efficacy of bromfenac, ibuprofen, and aspirin in postoperative oral surgery pain. *Clinical Pharmacology and Therapeutics* **52**, 343–352.

FORSTER, C., MAGERL, W., BECK, A., GEISSLINGER, G., GALL, T., BRUNE, K. and HANDWERKER, H.O. (1992) Differential effects of dipyrone, ibuprofen, and paracetamol on experimentally induced pain in man. *Agents and Actions* **35**, 112–121.

FOWLER, P.D. (1987) Aspirin, paracetamol and non-steroidal anti-inflammatory drugs. A comparative review of side-effects. *Medical Toxicology* **2**, 338–366.

FREELAND, G.R., NORTHINGTON, R.S., HEDRICH, D.A. and WALKER, B.R. (1988) Hepatic safety of two analgesics used over the counter: ibuprofen and aspirin. *Clinical Pharmacology and Therapeutics* **43**, 473–479.

FRIES, J.F., WILLIAMS, C.A. and BLOCH, D.A. (1991) The relative toxicity of nonsteroidal anti-inflammatory drugs. *Arthritis and Rheumatism* **34**, 1353–1360.

FRIIS, H. and ANDREASEN, P.B. (1992) Drug-induced hepatic injury: an analysis of 1100 cases reported to The Danish Committee on adverse drug reactions between 1978 and 1987. *Journal of Internal Medicine* **232**, 133–138.

FUREY, S.A., WAKSMAN, J.A. and DASH, B.H. (1992) Non-prescription ibuprofen: side-effect profile. *Pharmacotherapy* **12**, 403–407.

FUREY, S.A., VARGAS, R. and McMAHON, F.G. (1993) Renovascular effects of non-prescription ibuprofen in elderly hypertensive patients with mild renal impairment. *Pharmacotherapy* **13**, 143–148.

FURNISS, L.D. (1982) Nonsteroidal anti-inflammatory agents in the treatment of primary dysmenorrhea. *Clinical Pharmacy* **1**, 327–333.

GALLARDO, F. and ROSSI, E. (1990) Analgesic efficacy of flurbiprofen as compared to acetaminophen and placebo after periodontal surgery. *Journal of Periodontology* **61**, 224–227.

GERTZBEIN, S.D., TILE, M.D., McMURTY, R.Y., KELLAM, J.F., HUNTER, G.A., KEITH, R.G., HARSANYI, Z. and LUFFMAN, J. (1986) Analysis of the analgesic efficacy of acetaminophen 1000 mg, codeine phosphate 60 mg, and the combination of acetaminophen 1000 mg and codeine phosphate 60 mg, in the relief of postoperative pain. *Pharmacotherapy* **6**, 104–107.

CHAPTER 7

GIEBINK, G.S., BATALDEN, P.B., LE, C.T. *et al.* (1990) A controlled trial comparing three treatments for chronic otitis media with effusion. *Pediatric Infectious Diseases Journal* **9**, 33–40.

GLORIOSO, S., TODESCO, S., MAZZI, A., MARCOLONGO, R., GIORDANO, M., COLOMBO, B., CHERIE-LIGNIERE, G., MATTARA, L., LEARDINI, G., PASSERI, M. and CICINOTTA, D. (1985) Double-blind multicentre study of the activity of S-adenosylmethionine in hip and knee osteoarthritis. *International Journal of Clinical Pharmacy Research* **5**, 39–49.

GOÖKIN, K.S., FORMAN, E.S., VECCHIO, T.J., WISER, W.L. and MORRISON, J.C. (1983) Comparative efficacy of ibuprofen, indomethacin, and placebo in the treatment of primary dysmenorrhea. *Southern Medical Journal* **76**, 1361–1362.

GORDIN, A., SAARELAINEN, P., RISTOLA, M. and NUUTILA, J. (1985) Comparison of a slow-release indomethacin tablet and ibuprofen in rheumatoid arthritis. *Current Therapeutic Research* **37**, 406–411.

GOULSTON, K. and SKYRING, A. (1964) Effect of paracetamol (*N*-acetyl-*p*-aminophenol) on gastrointestinal bleeding. *Gut* **5**, 463–466.

GRAHAM, N.M.H., BURRELL, C.J., DOUGLAS, R.M., DEBELLE, P. and DAVIES, L. (1990) Adverse effects of aspirin, acetaminophen, and ibuprofen on immune function, viral shedding, and clinical status in rhinovirus-infected volunteers. *Journal of Infectious Diseases* **162**, 1277–1282.

GROSS, P.A., LEVANDOWSKI, R.A., RUSSO, C., WEKSLER, M., BONELLI, J., DRAN, S., MUNK, G., DEICHMILLER, S., HILSEN, R. and PANUSH, R.F. (1994) Vaccine immune response and side-effects with the use of acetaminophen with influenza vaccine. *Clinical and Diagnostic Laboratory Immunology* **1**, 134–138.

HABIB, S., MATTHEWS, R.W., SCULLY, C., LEVERS, B.G.H. and SHEPHERD, J.P. (1990) A study of the comparative efficacy of four common analgesics in the control of postsurgical dental pain. *Oral Surgery, Oral Medicine and Oral Pathology* **70**, 559–563.

HÄMÄLÄINEN, M.J., HOPPU, K., VALKEILA, E. and SANTAVUORI, P. (1997) Ibuprofen or acetaminophen for the acute treatment of migraine in children: a double-blind, randomized, placebo-controlled, crossover study. *Neurology* **48**, 103–107.

HASSON, S.M., DANIELS, J.C., DIVINE, J.G., NIEBUHR, B.R., RICHMOND, S., STEIN, P.G. and WILLIAMS, J.H. (1993) Effect of ibuprofen use on muscle soreness, damage, and performance: a preliminary investigation. *Medical Science in Sports and Exercise* **25**, 9–17.

HAVANKA-KANNIAINEN, H. (1989) Treatment of acute migraine attack: ibuprofen and placebo compared. *Headache* **29**, 507–509.

HAWKINS, N. and GOLDRING, J.; The ALSPAC Survey Team (1995) A survey of the administration of drugs to young infants. *British Journal of Clinical Pharmacology* **40**, 79–82.

HEIDRICH, G., SLAVIC-SVIRCEV, V. and KAIKO, R.F. (1985) Efficacy and quality of ibuprofen and acetaminophen plus codeine analgesia. *Pain* **22**, 385–397.

HENRETIG, F.M. (1996) Appropriate use of OTC analgesics in paediatric patients. *Postgraduate Medicine. A Special Report. Clinical Safety of Analgesics*, 1996 (Dec.), 68–74.

HERSH, E.V., COOPER, S., BETTS, N., WEDELL, D., MACAFEE, K., QUINN, P., LAMP, C., GASTON, G., BERGMAN, S. and HENRY, E. (1993) Single dose and multidose analgesic study of ibuprofen and meclofenamate sodium after third molar surgery. *Oral Surgery, Oral Medicine and Oral Pathology* **76**, 680–687.

HILL, J., BIRD, H.A., FENN, G.C., LEE, C.E., WOODWARD, M. and WRIGHT, V. (1990) A double-blind crossover study to compare lysine acetylsalicylate (aspergesic) with ibuprofen in the treatment of rheumatoid arthritis. *Journal of Clinical Pharmacology and Therapeutics* **15**, 205–211.

HOLLINGWORTH, P. (1993) The use of non-steroidal anti-inflammatory drugs in paediatric rheumatic diseases. [Review]. *British Journal of Rheumatology* **32**, 73–77.

IVEY, K.J. and SETTREE, P. (1976) Effect of paracetamol (acetaminophen) on gastric ionic fluxes and potential difference in man. *Journal of the British Society of Gastroenterology* **17**, 916–919.

IVEY, K.J., SILVOSO, G.R. and KRAUSE, W.J. (1978) Effect of paracetamol on gastric mucosa. *British Medical Journal* **1**, 1586–1588.

JAIN, A.K., RYAN, J.R., MCMAHON, F.G., KUEBEL, J.O., WALTERS, P.J. and NOVECK, C. (1986a) Analgesic efficacy of low-dose ibuprofen in dental extraction pain. *Pharmacotherapy* **6**, 318–322.

JAIN, A.K., RYAN, J.R., MCMAHON, F.G. and SMITH, G. (1986b) Comparison of oral nalbuphine, acetaminophen, and their combination in postoperative pain. *Clinical Pharmacology and Therapeutics* **39**, 295–299.

JOHNSON, A.G., SEIDEMANN, P. and DAY, R.O. (1994) NSAID-related adverse drug interactions with clinical relevance. *International Journal of Clinical Pharmacology and Therapeutics* **32**, 509–532.

JOHNSON, P.C. and DRISCOLL, T. (1981) Comparison of plain and buffered aspirin with acetaminophen in regard to gastrointestinal bleeding. *Current Therapeutic Research* **30**, 79–84.

JORGENSEN, H.S., CHRISTENSEN, H.R. and KAMPMANN, J.P. (1991) Interaction between digoxin and indomethacin or ibuprofen. *British Journal of Clinical Pharmacology* **31**, 108–110.

KAIK, B., BAUER, K. and BROLL, H. (1991) Double-blind randomized clinical trial on imidazole salicylate vs ibuprofen in osteoarthritis. *International Journal of Clinical Pharmacology, Therapeutics and Toxicology* **32**, 509–532.

CHAPTER 7

KARTTUNEN, P., SAANO, V., PARONEN, P., PEURA, P. and VIDGREN, M. (1990) Pharmacokinetics of ibuprofen in man: a single-dose comparison of two over-the-counter, 200 mg preparations. *International Journal of Clinical Pharmacology, Therapeutics and Toxicology* **28**, 251–255.

KAUFFMAN, R.E., SAWYER, L.A. and SCHEINBAUM, M.L. (1992) Antipyretic efficacy of ibuprofen vs acetaminophen. *American Journal of Diseases of Children* **146**, 622–625.

KAUFMAN, D.W., KELLY, J.P., SHEEHAN, J., WIHOLM, B.-E., LASZLO, A., ALFREDSSON, L., KOFF, R. and SHAPIRO, S. (1997) The risk of major upper gastro-intestinal bleeding among users of non-steroidal anti-inflammatory drugs at various levels of alcohol consumption. *Pharmacoepidemiology and Drug Safety* **6**(Suppl. 2), S104 (Abstract 215).

KIMMEY, M.B. (1996) Aspirin and nonaspirin NSAIDs in OTC doses. *Postgraduate Medicine, A Special Report. Clinical Safety of OTC Analgesics*, 1996 (Dec.), 7–14.

KOBAL, G., HUMMEL, C., GRUBER, M., GEISSLINGER, G. and HUMMEL, T. (1994) Dose-related effects of ibuprofen on pain-related potentials. *British Journal of Clinical Pharmacology* **37**, 445–452.

KONTUREK, S.J., OBTULOWICZ, W., KWIECIEN, N. and OLEKSY, J. (1984) Generation of prostaglandins in gastric mucosa of patients with peptic ulcer disease: effect of non-steroidal anti-inflammatory compounds. *Scandinavian Journal of Gastroenterology* **19**, 75–77.

LAMBERT, J.R., CARDOE, N., SIMPSON, N.R., OLDHAM, P., NICHOL, P.E. and MARTIN, L. (1985) A controlled comparison of tiaprofenic acid and ibuprofen in osteoarthritis. *International Journal of Clinical Pharmacology Research* **5**, 161–164.

LANZA, F.L., ROYER, G.L., NELSON, R.S., RACK, M.F., SECKMAN, C.E. and SCHWARTZ, J.H. (1986) Effect of acetaminophen on human gastric mucosal injury caused by ibuprofen. *Gut* **27**, 440–443.

LAVENEZIANA, D., SPERANZA, R., RAULLI, P. and PAREDI, G. (1996a) Comparative efficacy of ibuprofen arginine and beta-cyclodextrin piroxicam as treatment for tension-type headache. *Clinical Drug Investigations* **11**, 22–26.

LAVENEZIANA, D., RIVA, A., BONAZZI, M., CIPOLLA, M. and MIGLIAVACCA, S. (1996b) Comparative efficacy of oral ibuprofen arginine and intramuscular ketorolac in patients with postoperative pain. *Clinical Drug Investigations* **11**, 8–14.

LEGUEN, M.A. (1985) Single-blind clinical trial comparing use of fentiazac and paracetamol in postendodontic periodontitis. *Clinical Therapeutics* **7**, 145–150.

LEVY, M. (1987) Pyrazolone-induced agranulocytosis: an epidemiological evaluation. In: RAINSFORD, K.D. and VELO, G.P. (eds), *Side-effects of Anti-inflammatory Drugs 1: Clinical and Epidemiological Aspects*. Lancaster, MTP Press, 99–104.

LIANG, N.M. and FORTIN, P. (1991) Management of osteoarthritis of the hip and knee. *New England Journal of Medicine* **325**, 125–127.

LINDEN, C.H. and TOWNSEND, P.L. (1987) Metabolic acidosis after acute ibuprofen overdose. *Journal of Pediatrics* **111**, 922–925.

LOEBL, D.H., CRAIG, R.M., CULIC, D.D., RIDOLFO, A.S., FALK, J. and SCHMID, F.R. (1977) Gastrointestinal blood loss. Effect of aspirin, fenoprofen, and acetaminophen in rheumatoid arthritis as determined by sequential gastroscopy and radioactive fecal markers. *Journal of the American Medical Association* **237**, 976–981.

MACGREGOR, E.A., WILKINSON, M. and BANCROFT, K. (1993) Domperidone plus paracetamol in the treatment of migraine. *Cephalagia* **13**, 124–127.

MÄKÄLÄINEN, L. and YLIKORKALA, O. (1986a) Primary and myoma-associated menorrhagia: role of prostaglandins and effects of ibuprofen. *British Journal of Obstetrics and Gynaecology* **93**, 974–978.

MÄKÄLÄINEN, L. and YLIKORKALA, O. (1986b) Ibuprofen prevents IUCD-induced increases in menstrual blood loss. *British Journal of Obstetrics and Gynaecology* **93**, 285–288.

MALANDRINO, S., ANGLINI, M., BALDINI, L., BARENGHI, L., BORSA, M., CARRABBA, M., CERIOTTI, F. and TONON, G.C. (1987) Effects of suprofen on renal function in patients with rheumatoid arthritis. *Internation Journal of Clinical Pharmacology Research* **7**, 259–263.

MANN, J.F.E., GOERIG, M., BRUNE, K. and LUFT, F.C. (1993) Ibuprofen as an over the counter drug: is there a risk for renal injury? *Clinical Nephrology* **39**, 1–6.

MARCH, L., IRWIG, L., SCHWARZ, J., SIMPSON, J., CHOCK, C. and BROOKS, P. (1994) n Of 1 trials comparing a nonsteroidal anti-inflammatory drug with paracetamol in osteoarthritis. *British Medical Journal* **309**, 1041–1045.

MARRIOTT, S.C., STEPHENSON, T.J., HULL, D., POWNALL, R., SMITH, C.M. and BUTLER, A. (1991) A dose ranging study of ibuprofen suspension as an antipyretic. *Archives of Disease in Childhood* **66**, 1037–1042.

MARTINEZ-MIR, I., GARCIA-LOPEZ, M., PALOP, V., FERRER, J.M., ESTAN, L., RUBIO, E. and MORALES-OLIVAS, F.J. (1996) A prospective study of adverse drug reactions as a cause of admission to a paediatric hospital. *British Journal of Pharmacology* **42**, 319–324.

MAYER, J.M., BARTOLUCCI, C., MAITRE, J.M. and TESTA, B. (1988) Metabolic chiral inversion of anti-inflammatory 2-arylpropionates: lack of reaction in liver homogenates, and study of methine proton acidity. *Xenobiotica* **18**, 533–543.

MCINTYRE, J. and HULL, D. (1996) Comparing efficacy and tolerability of ibuprofen and paracetamol in fever. *Archives of Diseases in Childhood* **74**, 164–167.

MCMAHON, F.G., ARNDT, W.F., NEWTON, J.J., MONTGOMERY, P.A. and PERHACH, J.L. (1987) Clinical experience with flupirtine in the US. *Postgraduate Medical Journal* **63**, 81–85.

MCQUAY, H.J., POPPLETON, P., CARROLL, D., SUMMERFIELD, R.J., BULLINGHAM, R.E.S. and MOORE, R.A. (1986) Ketorolac and acetominophen for orthopedic postoperative pain. *Clinical Pharmacology and Therapeutics* **39**, 89–93.

CHAPTER 7

McQUAY, H.J., CARROL, D., WATTS, P.G., JUNIPER, R.P. and MOORE, R.A. (1989) Codeine 20 mg increases pain relief from ibuprofen 400 mg after third molar surgery. A repeat-dosing comparison of ibuprofen and an ibuprofen–codeine combination. *Pain* 37, 7–13.

McQUAY, H.J., CARROLL, D., GUEST, P.G., ROBSON, S., WIFFEN, P.J. and JUNIPER, R.P. (1993) A multiple dose comparison of ibuprofen and dihydrocodeine after third molar surgery. *British Journal of Oral and Maxillofacial Surgery* 31, 95–100.

MEHLISCH, D.R., SOLLECITO, W.A., HELFRICK, J.F., LEIBOLD, D.G., MARKOWITZ, R., SCHOW, C.E. JR., SHULTZ, R. and WAITE, D.E. (1990) Multicenter clinical trial of ibuprofen and acetaminophen in the treatment of postoperative dental pain. *Journal of the American Dental Association* 121, 257–263.

MIDDLETON, R.S.W. (1981) Double blind trial in general practice comparing the efficacy of 'Benylin Day and Night' and paracetamol in the treatment of the common cold. *British Journal of Clinical Practice* 35, 297–300.

MIGLIARDI, J.R., ARMELLINO, J.J., FREIDMAN, M., GILLINGS, D.B. and BEAVER, W.T. (1994) Caffeine as an analgesic adjuvant in tension headache. *Clinical Pharmacology and Therapeutics* 56, 576–586.

MILLER, D.S., TALBOT, C.A., SIMPSON, W. and KOREY, A. (1987) A comparison of naproxen sodium, acetaminophen and placebo in the treatment of muscle contraction headache. *Headache* 27, 392–396.

MILLION, R., FINLAY, B.R. and WHITTINGTON, J.R. (1984) Clinical trial of flupirtine maleate in patients with migraine. *Current Medical Research and Opinion* 9, 204–212.

MILSOM, I. and ANDERSCH, B. (1984) Effect of ibuprofen, naproxen sodium and paracetamol on intrauterine pressure, and menstrual pain in dysmenorrhoea. *British Journal of Obstetrics and Gynecology* 91, 1129–1135.

MITCHELL, A.A. and LESKO, S.M. (1995) When a randomized controlled trial is needed to assess drug safety. The case of paediatric ibuprofen. *Drug Safety* 13, 15–24.

MOORE, N., NOBLET, C. and BREEMEERSCH, C. (1996) Mise au point sur la sécurité de l'ibuprofen à dose antalgique-antipyrètique. *Thérapie* 51, 458–463.

MOORE, P.A., ACS, G. and HARGREAVES, J.A. (1985) Postextraction pain relief in children: a clinical trial of liquid analgesics. *International Journal of Clinical Pharmacology, Therapeutics and Toxicology* 23, 573–577.

MOORE, U.J., MARSH, V.R., ASHTON, C.H., SEYMOR, R.A. (1995) Effects of peripherally and centrally acting analgesics on somato-sensory evoked potentials. *British Journal of Clinical Pharmacology* 40, 111–117.

MORRISON, J.C., LING, F.W., FORMAN, E.K., BATES, G.W., BLAKE, P.G., VECCHIO, T.J., LINDEN, C.V. and O'CONNELL, M.J. (1980) Analgesic efficacy of ibuprofen for treatment of primary dysmenorrhea. *Southern Medical Journal* 73, 999–1002.

Morrison, N.A. and Repka, M.X. (1994) Ketorolac versus acetaminophen of ibuprofen in controlling postoperative pain in patients with strabismus. *Opthalmology* **101**, 915–918.

Movilia, P.G. (1989) Evaluation of the analgesic activity and tolerability of aceclofenac in the treatment of post-episiotomy pain. *Drugs under Experimental and Clinical Research* **15**, 47–51.

Munck, L.K., Christensen, C.B., Pedersen, L., Larsen, U., Branebjerg, P.E. and Kampmann, J.P. (1990) Codeine in analgesic doses does not depress respiration in patients with severe chronic obstructive lung disease. *Pharmacology and Toxicology* **66**, 335–340.

Murphy, P.J., Badia, P., Myers, B.L., Boecker, M.R. and Wright, K.P. Jr (1994) Non-steroidal anti-inflammatory drugs affect normal sleep patterns in humans. *Physiology and Behavior* **55**, 1063–1066

Nielsen, J.C., Bjerring, P. and Arendt-Nielsen, L. (1991) A comparison of the hypoalgesic effect of paracetamol in slow-release and plain tablets on laser-induced pain. *British Journal of Clinical Pharmacology* **31**, 267–270.

Nystrom, E., Gustafsson, I. and Quiding, H. (1988) The pain intensity at analgesic intake, and the efficacy of diflunisal in single doses and effervescent acetaminophen in single and repeated doses. *Pharmacotherapy* **8**, 201–209.

Ochs, H.R., Greenblatt, D.J. and Verburg-Ochs, B. (1985) Ibuprofen kinetics in patients with renal insufficiency who are receiving maintenance hemodialysis. *Arthritis and Rheumatism* **28**, 1430–1434.

Olstad, O.A. and Skjelbred, P. (1986) Comparison of the analgesic effect of a corticosteroid and paracetamol in patients with pain after oral surgery. *British Journal of Clinical Pharmacology* **22**, 437–442.

Østensen, M. (1994) Optimisation of antirheumatic drug treatment in pregnancy. *Clinical Pharmacokinetics* **27**, 486–503.

Owen, P.R. (1984) Prostaglandin synthetase inhibitors in the treatment of primary dysmenorrhea. Outcome trials reviewed. *American Journal of Obstetrics and Gynecology* **148**, 96–103.

Pagnoni, B., Ravanelli, A., Degradi, L., Rossi, R. and Tiengo, M. (1996a) Clinical efficacy of ibuprofen arginine in the management of postoperative pain associated with suction termination of pregnancy. *Clinical Drug Investigation* **11**, 27–32.

Pagnoni, B., Vignali, M., Colella, S., Monopoly, R. and Tiengo, M. (1996b) Comparative efficacy of oral ibuprofen arginine and intramuscular ketorolac in patients with post-caesarian section pain. *Clinical Drug Investigation* **11**, 15–21.

Pasquale, S.A., Rathauser, R. and Dolese, H.M. (1988) A double-blind, placebo-controlled study comparing three single-dose regimes of piroxicam and ibuprofen in patients with primary dysmenorrhea. *American Journal of Medicine* **84**(5A), 30–34.

CHAPTER 7

PAULUS, H.E. (1990) FDA arthritis advisory committee meeting: guidelines for approving nonsteroidal anti-inflammatory drugs for over-the-counter use. *Arthritis and Rheumatism* **33**, 1056–1058.

PEARCE, I., FRANK, G.J. and PEARCE, J.M. (1983) Ibuprofen compared with paracetamol in migraine. *Practitioner* **227**, 465–467.

PENNA, A. and BUCHANAN, N. (1991) Paracetamol poisoning in children and hepatotoxicity. *British Journal of Clinical Pharmacology* **32**, 143–149.

PETERS, B.H., FRAIM, C.J. and MASEL, B.E. (1983) Comparison of 650 mg aspirin and 1000 mg acetaminophen with each other, and with placebo in moderately severe headache. *American Journal of Medicine* **74**, 36–42.

PETERSEN, J.K., HANSSON, F. and STRID, S. (1993) The effect of an ibuprofen–codeine combination for the treatment of patients with pain after removal of lower third molars. *Journal of Oral and Maxillofacial Surgery* **51**, 637–640.

PFAFFENRATH, V. and SCHERZER, S. (1995) Analgesics and NSAIDs in the treatment of the acute migraine attack. *Cephalalgia* **15**(Suppl. 15), 14–20.

PRESCOTT, L.F. (1992) The hepatotoxicity of non-steroidal anti-inflammatory drugs. In: RAINSFORD, K.D. and VELO, G.P. (eds), *Side-Effects of Anti-inflammatory Drugs 3: Inflammation and Drug Therapy*. Lancaster, Kluwer Academic Publishers, 176–187.

PRESCOTT, L.F. (1996) *Paracetamol (Acetaminophen). A Critical Bibliographic Review*. London, Taylor and Francis.

PUSCUS, I., HAJDU, A., BUZAS, G. and BERNATH, Z. (1989) Prevention of non-steroidal anti-inflammatory agents induced acute gastric mucosal lesions by carbonic anhydrase inhibitors. An endoscopic study. *Acta Physiologica Hungarica* **73**, 279–283.

QUIDING, H., OKSALA, E., HAPPONEN, R.P., LEHTIMAKI, K. and OJALA, T. (1981) The visual analog scale in multiple-dose evaluations of analgesics. *Journal of Clinical Pharmacology* **21**, 424–429.

QUIDING, H., OIKARINEN, V., HUITFELDT, B., KOSKIMO, M., LEIKOMAA, H. and NYMAN, C. (1982a) An analgesic study with repeated doses of phenazone, phenazone plus dextropropoxyphene, and paracetamol, using a visual analogue scale. *International Journal of Oral Surgery* **11**, 304–309.

QUIDING, H., PERSSON, G., AHLSTROM, U., BANGENS, S., HELLEM, S., JOHANSSON, G., JONSSON, E. and NORDH, P.G. (1982b) Paracetamol plus supplementary doses of codeine. An analgesic study of repeated doses. *European Journal of Clinical Pharmacology* **23**, 315–319.

QUIDING, H., GRIMSTAD, J., RUSTEN, K., STUBHAUG, A., BREMNES, J. and BREIVIK, H. (1992) Ibuprofen plus codeine, ibuprofen, and placebo in a single- and multidose cross-over comparison for coxarthrosis pain. *Pain* **50**, 303–307.

QUINN, J.P., WEINSTEIN, R.A. and CAPLAN, L.R. (1984) Eosinophilic meningitis and ibuprofen therapy. *Neurology* **34**, 108–109.

RADACK, K.L., DECK, C.C. and BLOOMFIELD, S.S. (1987) Ibuprofen interferes with the efficacy of antihypertensive drugs. *Annals of Internal Medicine* **107**, 628–635.

RAINSFORD, K.D. (1984) *Aspirin and the Salicylates*. London, Butterworths.

RAINSFORD, K.D. (1996) Mode of action, uses, and side-effects of anti-inflammatory drugs. In: RAINSFORD, K.D. (ed.), *Advances in Anti-Rheumatic Therapy*. Boca Raton, CRC Press, 59–111.

RAINSFORD, K.D. and POWANDA, M.C. (eds) (1998) *Safety and Efficacy of OTC Non-prescription NSAIDs and Analgesics*. Dordrecht, Kluwer Academic Publishers.

RAINSFORD, K.D. and QUADIR, M. (1995) Gastrointestinal damage and bleeding from non-steroidal anti-inflammatory drugs. I. Clinical and epidemiological aspects. *Inflammopharmacology* **3**, 169–190.

RAINSFORD, K.D., ROBERTS, S.C. and BROWN, S. (1997) Ibuprofen and paracetamol: relative safety in non-prescription doses. *Journal of Pharmacy and Pharmacology* **49**, 345–376.

REIJNTJES, R.J., BOERING, G., WESSELING, H. and VAN RIJN, L.J. (1987) Suprofen versus paracetamol after oral surgery. *International Journal of Oral and Maxillofacial Surgery* **16**, 45–49.

REYNOLDS, J.E.F. (ed.) (1996) *Martindale. The Extra Pharmacopoeia*, 31st edn. London, Royal Pharmaceutical Society.

RODRIGO, C., CHAU, M. and ROSENQUIST, J. (1989) A comparison of paracetamol and diflunisal for pain control following 3rd molar surgery. *International Journal of Oral and Maxillofacial Surgery* **18**, 130–132.

ROYER, G.L., SECKMAN, C.E. and WELSHMAN, M.S. (1984) Saftey profile: fifteen years of clinical experience with ibuprofen. *American Journal of Medicine* **77**, 25–34.

ROYER, G.L., SECKMAN, C.E., SCHWARTZ, J.H. and BENNETT, K.P. (1985) Effects of ibuprofen on normal subjects: clinical and routine and special laboratory assessments. *Current Therapeutic Research* **37**, 412–426.

RUBIN, A. and WINTER, L. JR (1984) A double-blind randomized study of an aspirin/caffeine combination versus acetaminophen/aspirin combination versus acetaminophen verses placebo in patients with moderate to severe post-partum pain. *Journal of International Medical Research* **12**, 338–345.

SALT COLLABORATIVE GROUP (1991) Swedish aspirin low-dose trial (SALT) of 75 mg aspirin as secondary prophylaxis after cerebrovascular ischemic events. *Lancet* **338**, 1345–1349.

SCHACHTEL, B.P. and THODEN, W.R. (1988) Onset of action of ibuprofen in the treatment of muscle-contraction headache. *Headache* **28**, 471–474.

CHAPTER 7

SCHACHTEL, B.P. and THODEN, W.R. (1993) A placebo-controlled model for assaying systemic analgesics in children. *Clinical Pharmacology and Therapeutics* **53**, 593–601.

SCHACHTEL, B.P., FILLINGIM, J.M., THODEN, W.R., LANE, A.C. and BAYBUTT, R.I. (1988) Sore throat pain in the evaluation of mild analgesics. *Clinical Pharmacology and Therapeutics* **44**, 704–711.

SCHACHTEL, B.P., THODEN, W.R. and BAYBUTT, R.I. (1989) Ibuprofen and acetaminophen in the relief of postpartum episiotomy pain. *Journal of Clinical Pharmacology* **29**, 550–553.

SCHACHTEL, B.P., THODEN, W.R., KONERMAN, J.P., BROWN, A. and CHAING, D.S. (1991) Headache pain model for assessing and comparing the efficacy of over-the-counter analgesic agents. *Clinical Pharmacology and Therapeutics* **50**, 322–329.

SCHACHTEL, B.P., CLEVES, G.S., KONERMAN, J.P., BROWN, A.T. and MARKHAM, R.N. (1994) A placebo-controlled model to assay the onset of action of nonprescription-strength analgesic drugs. *Clinical Pharmacology and Therapeutics* **55**, 464–470.

SCHLONDORFF, D. (1993) Renal complications of nonsteroidal anti-inflammatory drugs. *Kidney International* **44**, 643–653.

SEYMOUR, R.A., HAWKESFORD, J.E., WELDON, M. and BREWSTER, D. (1991) An evaluation of different ibuprofen preparations in the control of postoperative pain after third molar surgery. *British Journal of Clinical Pharmacology* **31**, 83–87.

SEYMOUR, R.A., KELLY, P.J. and HAWKESFORD, J.E. (1996) The efficacy of ketoprofen and paracetamol (acetaminophen) in postoperative pain after third molar surgery. *British Journal of Clinical Pharmacology* **41**, 581–585.

SKOGLUND, L.A. and SKJELBRED, P. (1984) Comparison of a traditional paracetamol medication and a new paracetamol/paracetamol–methionine ester combination. *European Journal of Clinical Pharmacology* **26**, 573–577.

SPERBER, S.J., SORRENTINO, J.V., RIKER, D.K., *et al.* (1989) Evaluation of an alpha agonist alone and in combination with a nonsteroidal anti-inflammatory agent in the treatment of experimental rhinovirus colds. *Bulletin of the New York Academy of Medicine* **65**, 145–160.

Steering Committee of the Physicians' Health Study Research Group (1989) Final report on the aspirin component of the ongoing physicians' health study. *New England Journal of Medicine* **321**, 129–135.

STEINECK, G., WILHOLM, B.E. and DE VERDIER, G.M. (1995) Acetaminophen, some other drugs, some diseases and the risk of transitional cell carcinoma. *Acta Oncologica* **34**, 741–748.

STEINFATH, M., LAVICKY, J., SCHMITZ, W., SCHOLZ, H., DÖRING, V. and KALMÁR, P. (1993) Changes in cardiac beta-adrenoceptors in human heart diseases; relationship to the degree of heart failure and further evidence for etiology-related regulation of beta 1 and beta 2 subtypes. *Journal of Cardiothorac Vascular Anesthetic* **6**, 668–673.

STEWART, W.F. and LIPTON, R.B. (1998) Ibuprofen plus caffeine in the treatment of migraine. In: RAINSFORD, K.D. and POWANDA, M.C. (eds), *Safety and Efficacy of Non-Prescription (OTC) Analgesics and NSAIDs*. Dordrecht, Kluwer Academic Publishers, 123–124.

SUNSHINE, A., MARRERO, I., OLSON, N., McCORMICK, N. and LASKA, E. (1986) Comparative study of flurbiprofen, zomepirac sodium, acetaminophen plus codeine, and aceto-minophen for the relief of postsurgical dental pain. *American Journal of Medicine* **80**, 50–54.

SUNSHINE, A., ROURE, C., OLSON, N., LASKA, E.M., ZORRILLA, C. and RIVERA, J. (1987) Analgesic efficacy of two ibuprofen-codeine combinations for the treatment of postepisiotomy and postoperative pain. *Clinical Pharmacology and Therapeutics* **42**, 374–380.

SUNSHINE, A., ZIGHELBOIM, I., DE CASTRO, A., SORRENTINO, J.V., SMITH, D.S., BARTIZEK, R.D. and OLSON, N.Z. (1989) Augmentation of acetaminophen analgesia by the antihistamine phenyltoloxamine. *Journal of Clinical Pharmacology* **29**, 660–664.

THOMPSON, J., FLEET, W., LAWRENCE, E., PIERCE, E., MORRIS, L. and WRIGHT, P. (1987) A comparison of acetaminophen and rimantadine in the treatment of influenza A infection in children. *Journal of Medical Virology* **21**, 249–255.

TORABINEJAD, M., CYMERMAM, J.J., FRANKSON, M., LEMON, R.R., MAGGIO, J.D. and SCHILDER, H. (1994) Effectiveness of various medications on postoperative pain following complete instrumentation. *Journal of Endodontics* **20**, 345–354.

URQUHART, E. (1994) Analgesic agents and strategies in the dental pain model. [Review]. *Journal of Dentistry* **22**, 336–341.

VALLE-JONES, J.C., SMITH, J. and ROWLEY-JONES, D. (1984) A comparison in general practice of once and twice daily sustained release ibuprofen and standard ibuprofen in the treatment of non-articular rhematism. *British Journal of Clinical Practice* 353–358.

VAN ESCH, A., VAN STEENSEL-MOLL, H.A., STEYERBERG, E.W., OFFRINGA, M., HABBEMA, J.D.F. and DERKSEN-LUBSEN, G. (1995) Antipyretic efficacy of ibuprofen and acetaminophen in children with febrile seizures. *Archives of Pediatric and Adolescent Medicine* **149**, 632–637.

VANE, J.R. and BOTTING, R.M. (1995) New insights into the mode of action of anti-inflammatory drugs. *Inflammation Research* **44**, 1–10.

VARGAS, R., MANEATIS, T., BYNUM, L., PETERSON, C. and McMAHON, F.G. (1994) Evaluation of the antipyretic effect of ketorolac, acetaminophen, and placebo in endotoxin-induced fever. *Journal of Clinical Pharmacology* **34**, 848–853.

VELO, G.P., MINUZ, P., AROSIO, E., CAPAZZO, M.G., COVI, G. and LECHI, A. (1987) Interactions between non-steroidal anti-inflammatory drugs and angiotensin-converting enzyme inhibitors in man. In: RAINSFORD, K.D. and VELO, G.P. (eds), *Side-Effects of*

■

CHAPTER 7

■

Anti-inflammatory Drugs, Pt 1. Clinical and Epidemiological Aspects. Lancaster, MTP Press, 195–201.

VELTRI, J.C. and ROLLINS, D.E. (1988) A comparison of the frequency and severity of poisoning cases for ingestion of acetaminophen, aspirin and ibuprofen. *American Journal of Emergency Medicine* 6, 104–107.

VENTAFRIDDA, V., DE CONNO, F., PANERAI, A.E., MARESCA, V., MONZA, G.C. and RIPAMONTI, C. (1990) Non-steroidal anti-inflammatory drugs as the first step in cancer pain therapy: double-blind, within-patient study comparing nine drugs. *Journal of International Medical Research* 18, 21–29.

VLOK, G.J. and VAN VUREN, J.P. (1987) Comparison of a standard ibuprofen treatment regimen with a new ibuprofen/codeine combination in chronic osteoarthritis. *South African Medical Journal* Suppl P1, 1–6.

WALKER, J.S., NGUYEN, T.V. and DAY, R.O. (1994) Clinical response to non-steroidal anti-inflammatory drugs in urate-crystal induced inflammation: a simultaneous study of intersubject and intrasubject variability. *British Journal of Clinical Pharmacology* 38, 341–347.

WALKER, J.W., VANDENBURG, M.J. and CURRIE, W.J.C. (1984) Differential efficacy of two non-steroidal anti-inflammatory drugs in the treatment of sports injuries. *Current Medical Research and Opinion* 9, 119–123.

WALSON, P.D., GALLETTA, G., BRADEN, N.J. and ALEXANDER, L. (1989) Ibuprofen, aceta-minophen, and placebo treatment of febrile children. *Clinical Pharmacology and Therapeutics* 46, 9–17.

WALSON, P.D., GALLETTA, G., CHOMILO, F., BRADEN, N.J., SAWYER, L.A. and SCHEINBAUM, M.L. (1992) Comparison of multidose ibuprofen and acetominophen therapy in febrile children. *American Journal of Diseases of Children* 146, 626–632.

WARD, M.C., KIRWAN, J.R., NORRIS, P. and MURRAY, N. (1986) Paracetamol and diclofenac in the painful shoulder syndrome. *British Journal of Rheumatology* 25, 412–420.

WARRINGTON, S.J., HALSEY, A. and O'DONNEL, L. (1982) A comparison of gastrointestinal bleeding in healthy volunteers treated with tiaprofenic acid, aspirin or ibuprofen. *Rheumatology* 7, 107–110.

WEBER, J.C.P. (1984) Epidemiology of adverse reactions to non-steroidal anti-inflammatory drugs. In: RAINSFORD, K.D. and VELO, G.P. (eds), *Side-Effects of Anti-inflammatory/ Analgesic Drugs, Advances in Inflammation Research*. New York, Raven Press, 1–7.

WEBER, J.C.P. (1987) Epidemiology in the United Kingdom of adverse drug reactions from non-steroidal anti-inflammatory drugs. In: RAINSFORD, K.D. and VELO, G.P. (eds), *Side-effects of Anti-inflammatory Drugs 1: Clinical and Epidemiological Aspects*. Lancaster, MTP Press, 27–35.

WEBSTER, P.A., ROBERTS, D.W., BENSON, R.W. and KEARNS, G.L. (1996) Acetaminophen toxicity in children: diagnostic confirmation using a specific antigenic biomarker. *Journal of Clinical Pharmacology* **36**, 397–402.

WEIPPL, G., MICHOS, M., SUNDAL, E.J. and STOCKER, H. (1985a) Clinical experience and results of treatment with suprofen in paediatrics. 2nd communication: use of suprofen suppositories as an antipyretic in children with fever due to acute infections/a single-blind controlled study of suprofen versus paracetamol. *Arzneimittel-Forschung/Drug Research* **35**, 1724–1727.

WEIPPL, G., MICHOS, M., SUNDAL, E.J. and STOCKER, H. (1985b) Clinical experience and results of treatment with suprofen in paediatrics. 3rd communication: antipyretic effect and tolerability of repeat doses of suprofen and paracetamol syrup in hospitalized children/a single-blind study. *Arzneimittel-Forschung/Drug Research* **35**, 1728–1731.

WEN, S.F., PARTHASARATHY, R., ILIOPOULOS, O. and OBERLEY, T.D. (1992) Acute renal failure following binge drinking and nonsteroidal anti-inflammatory drugs. *American Journal of Kidney Diseases* **20**, 281–285.

WHELTON, A. (1996) Renal effects of OTC analgesics. *Postgraduate Medicine, A Special Report. Clinical Safety of OTC Analgesics* 1996 (Dec.), 34–41.

WHELTON, A., STOUT, R.L., SPILMAN, P.S. and KLAUSSEN, D.K. (1990) Renal effects of ibuprofen, piroxicam, and sulindac in patients with asymptomatic renal failure. A prospective, randomized, crossover comparison. *Annals of Internal Medicine* **112**, 568–576.

WILAIRATANA, P. and LOOARESUWAN, S. (1994) Antipyretic efficacy of indomethacin and acetominophen in uncomplicated falciparum malaria. *Annals of Tropical Medicine and Parasitology* **88**, 359–363.

WILCOX, C.M., SHALEK, K.A. and COTSONIS, G. (1994) Striking prevalence of over-the-counter nonsteroidal anti-inflammatory drug use in patients with upper gastrointestinal hemorrhage. *Archives of Internal Medicine* **154**, 42–46.

WILHOLM, B.E., MYRHED, M. and EKMAN, E. (1987) Trends and patterns in adverse drug reactions to non-steroidal anti-inflammatory drugs reported in Sweden. In: RAINSFORD, K.D. and VELO, G.P. (eds), *Side-effects of Anti-inflammatory Drugs 1: Clinical and Epidemiological Aspects*. Lancaster, MTP Press, 55–72.

WILLIAMS, W.R. (1983) Comparison between fenoprofen and ibuprofen in the treatment of soft-tissue rheumatism. *Journal of International Medical Research* **11**, 349–353.

WINNEM, B., SAMSTAD, B. and BREIVIK, H. (1981) Paracetamol, tiaramide and placebo for pain relief after orthopedic surgery. *Acta Anaesthesiologica Scandinavica* **25**, 209–214.

WITTENBERG, M., KINNEY, K.W. and BLACK, J.R. (1984) Comparison of ibuprofen and acetaminophen-codeine in postoperative foot pain. *Journal of the American Pediatry Association* **74**, 233–237.

CHAPTER 7

Use of Ibuprofen in Dentistry

RAYMOND A DIONNE[1] AND STEPHEN A COOPER[2]

[1]Pain and Neurosensory Mechanisms Branch, NIDR, National Institutes of Health, Bethesda, Maryland, USA; [2]Whitehall-Robins Health Care, Madison, New Jersey, USA

Contents

8.1   INTRODUCTION

The management of acute pain in dentistry has several unique features. Pain not only signals tissue injury, but it also acts as an impediment to most dental procedures, delays the resumption of normal activities following dental surgical procedures, and lessens the likelihood of patients seeking dental procedures in the future. While pain during therapy is usually adequately controlled by local anaesthesia, postoperative pain control is often inadequate either because of insufficient relief of pain or because of unacceptable side-effects. Side-effects such as drowsiness, nausea, and vomiting from opioids occur with greater frequency in ambulatory dental patients than in non-ambulatory hospitalized patients. In addition, inadequate pain control during the immediate postoperative period may contribute to the development of hyperalgesia (Gordon *et al.*, 1997a), leading to greater pain at later times during recovery. Pain associated with dentistry is also recognized to contribute to apprehension about future dental care such that patients frequently report themselves as very nervous or terrified at the prospects of dental care (Gordon and Dionne, 1997b). These considerations indicate that optimal analgesic therapy for ambulatory dental patients should be efficacious, with a minimum incidence of side-effects and, ideally, should lessen the prospects for pain associated with future dental therapy.

Knowledge of the clinical pharmacology of ibuprofen is based in large part on studies performed in the oral surgery model (Cooper and Beaver, 1976). The drug has demonstrated analgesic activity over a dose range from 200 to 800 mg with a duration of activity from 4 to 6 hours (Cooper, 1977). When given prior to pain onset, it suppresses the onset of pain and lessens the severity (Dionne and Cooper, 1978; Dionne *et al.*, 1983). Ibuprofen suppresses swelling over the 2- to 3-day postoperative course when oedema formation associated with the inflammatory process is most prominent. Interactions with the release of β-endorphin have been demonstrated both intraoperatively during surgical stress and during postoperative pain, suggesting that NSAIDs can modify the neurohumoral responses to pain (Dionne and McCullagh, 1997; Troullos *et al.*, 1997). Conversely, ibuprofen appears ineffective when administered chronically for orofacial pain, possibly suggesting that inflammation is not a prominent component of long-standing pain associated with temporomandibular disorders. The wealth of data from clinical trials using ibuprofen is supportive of these generalizations and makes ibuprofen one of the best-studied drugs for acute pain in ambulatory patients.

CHAPTER 8

8.2   ANALGESIA

Ibuprofen is the prototype of the NSAID class of analgesics, being first introduced into clinical practice in the United States in 1974. It is particularly useful for conditions in which aspirin or acetaminophen does not result in adequate pain relief or where the use of opioid-containing combinations would likely result in central nervous system or gastrointestinal side-effects. It is widely used for acute and chronic orofacial pain by prescription in doses of 600–800 mg, and as a non-prescription analgesic in 200–400 mg doses.

Ibuprofen in a dose of 400 mg has been found superior to 650 mg of aspirin, 600–1000 mg acetaminophen, and combinations of aspirin and acetaminophen plus 60 mg of codeine (Cooper *et al.*, 1977; Forbes *et al.*, 1984; Jain *et al.*, 1986), as well as dextropropoxyphene 65 mg (Winter *et al.*, 1978). A single dose of ibuprofen 400 mg or administration of multiple doses up to 5 days postoperatively was superior to 30 mg of dihydrocodeine in the oral surgery model (Frame *et al.*, 1989; McQuay *et al.*, 1993). Administration of doses greater than 400 mg is not likely to result in greater peak relief, but increased drug blood levels may prolong the duration of effects (Laska *et al.*, 1986).

Ibuprofen appears comparable to other NSAIDs when evaluated in the oral surgery model. Ibuprofen 400 mg produced analgesia similar to that of 100 mg of meclofenamate sodium but with a lower incidence of stomach pain and diarrhoea (Hersh *et al.*, 1993). Ibuprofen 200 mg results in similar onset and peak analgesia, but a shorter duration than 220 mg of naproxen sodium when evaluated up to 12 h following a single dose (Kiersch *et al.*, 1993). The shorter duration demonstrated would have little clinical significance, as the normal dosing interval for low-dose ibuprofen is every 4 to 6 h. The 400 mg dose of ibuprofen was also similar to a suspension formulation of diclofenac in a study with large sample sizes ($n = 80$–83) sufficient to detect differences (Bakshi *et al.*, 1994). No advantage could be demonstrated between tablets and soluble formulations of 200 mg, 400 mg and 600 mg ibuprofen evaluated up to 6 h postoperatively (Seymour *et al.*, 1996). No dose-related difference could be demonstrated in this study between the 400 mg and 600 mg doses of either formulation, leading the authors to conclude that there is little advantage in increasing the dose to 600 mg.

Ibuprofen has also been evaluated for dental pain other than from oral surgery. Periodontal surgery involves elevation of a surgical flap (often extending over a quarter of the mouth or more), osseous reshaping and implantation of materials to replace bone lost to the disease process, and can last 2–3 h. Ibuprofen in doses of 200 and 400 mg was demonstrated to be superior to placebo in a single-dose, 6-h observation following periodontal surgery, with a low incidence of adverse effects (Vogel and Gross, 1984). Comparison of ibuprofen 600 mg given either immediately prior to periodontal surgery or following the procedure demonstrated a suppression of pain intensity in comparison to placebo over the first 8 h postoperatively (Vogel *et al.*, 1992). Dosing after surgery appeared to result in greater pain suppression over the last 4 h of the observation period, consistent with the expected 6-h duration of ibuprofen 600 mg and the duration of the intervening surgery (2–3 h).

Patients undergoing orthodontic tooth movement can experience varying degrees of discomfort, especially over the first few days following placement or adjustment of orthodontic devices. Administration of a single dose of ibuprofen 400 mg in comparison to aspirin 650 mg and placebo demonstrated that both active drugs suppressed pain in comparison to placebo for up to 7 days following placement of orthodontic devices (Ngan *et al.*, 1994). Ibuprofen was superior to aspirin at most time points over the first 2 days, suggesting that it is suppressing the inflammatory response normally seen following orthodontic adjustments.

Ibuprofen was compared to a wide variety of treatments following an endodontic procedure (root canal obturation), but none of the nine active treatments could be differentiated from placebo (Torabinejad *et al.*, 1994a). This may reflect a lack of assay sensitivity for this model, as only 4% of the patient sample ($n = 411$) developed moderate or severe pain, the remainder reporting no pain or mild pain. Endodontic pain has previously been demonstrated as being sensitive to the effects of NSAIDs (Flath *et al.*, 1987), but only when subjects who were symptomatic prior to the procedure were included in the analyses; most subjects who are pain-free prior to an endodontic procedure report little pain postoperatively (Torabinejad *et al.*, 1994b).

8.2.1 Preventive analgesia

Most studies in which ibuprofen is administered after pain onset demonstrate an onset in activity within 30 min and peak analgesic activity at 2 to 3 h post drug administration. An early attempt to optimize ibuprofen analgesia in the immediate postoperative period following local anaesthesia offset involved administration of the drug prior to oral surgery. This allows sufficient time for drug absorption during the surgical procedure and the 1–2 h postoperative duration of standard local anaesthetics. Preoperative administration of 400 mg ibuprofen was demonstrated to increase the time to the first postoperative dose of analgesic by approximately 2 h in comparison to placebo pretreatment (Dionne and Cooper, 1978). A subsequent study demonstrated that preoperative administration of 800 mg ibuprofen significantly lowered pain intensity over the first 3 h postoperatively (Figure 8.1) as the residual effects of the local anaesthetic dissipated (Dionne *et al.*, 1983). Administration of a second dose of ibuprofen 4 h after the initial dose extended this preventive analgesic effect to result in less pain than with placebo, acetaminophen (given both pre- and postoperatively), or acetaminophen plus 60 mg codeine (administered postoperatively). The ability to suppress the onset and lower the intensity of postoperative pain up to 8 h is replicable (Hill *et al.*, 1987; Troullos *et al.*, 1990; Berthold and Dionne, 1993) and extends to the use of other NSAIDs such as flurbiprofen (Dionne, 1986).

Comparison of administration of ibuprofen prior to periodontal surgery versus administration immediately following surgery demonstrated that both groups experienced a significant delay in pain onset in comparison to placebo (Vogel *et al.*, 1992). A similar study in the oral surgery model using naproxen also could not differentiate between pre- or postoperative administration (Sisk and Grover, 1990), suggesting that preoperative administration is not critical for suppressing pain onset. Recognition of the induction of cyclooxygenase (COX)-2 in the postoperative period (Siebert *et al.*, 1994) suggests that

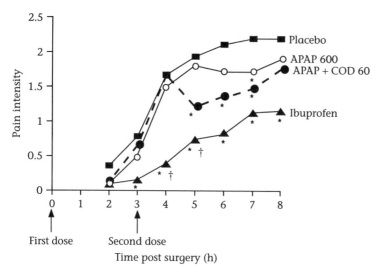

Figure 8.1: Suppression of postoperative pain following administration of ibuprofen, both prior to and following oral surgery, in comparison to placebo, acetaminophen 600 mg administered on the same schedule, and postoperative administration only of acetaminophen (APAP) 600 mg plus codeine (COD) 60 mg. *$p < 0.05$ vs placebo; †$p < 0.05$ vs acetaminophen 60 mg.

blockade of the formation of prostanoids released during surgery by constitutive COX-1 is less important than suppression of COX-2 and prostanoid release during the postoperative period. This is supported by preliminary observations that levels of prostaglandin E_2 in the first immediate postoperative sample (presumably reflective of surgical trauma) collected from the extraction site by microdialysis are detectable, decrease over the first 60 min post-operatively, and then start to increase over the next 60–120 min coincident with the onset of postoperative pain (Dionne *et al.*, 1996). Consistent with this observation is the demon-stration that both preoperative and postoperative administration of 800 mg ibuprofen are equally effective at suppressing pain and prostaglandin E_2 levels at the extraction site (Roszowski *et al.*, 1997). These observations support the administration of ibuprofen, and other NSAIDs, prior to the induction of COX-2 and subsequent release of prostanoids as a preventive analgesic strategy for suppressing pain in the immediate postoperative period as well as to inhibit peripheral and central hyperalgesia leading to pain at later times.

8.2.2 Analgesic activity of ibuprofen isomers

The biological actions of NSAIDs often reside partly or exclusively in one of the enan-tiomers (Ariens, 1983). When 2-arylpropionic acids, such as ibuprofen, are tested for cyclooxygenase inhibition *in vitro*, the activity resides almost exclusively in the (S)-(+) isomer (Caldwell *et al.*, 1988). Ibuprofen is synthesized and administered clinically as a racemic mixture of the (S)-(+) and (R)-(–) isomers; a unidirectional conversion of the inactive (R)-(–) isomer to the pharmacologically active (S)-(+) isomer results in metabolic

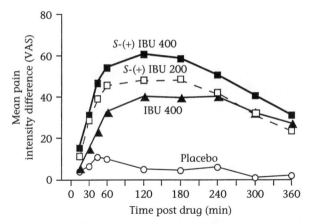

Figure 8.2: Pain intensity difference following postoperative administration of the (*S*)-(+) isomer of ibuprofen ((*S*)-(+) IBU) in doses of 200 mg and 400 mg in comparison to racemic ibuprofen (IBU) 400 mg and placebo. VAS, visual analogue scale.

activation of the racemic drug (Lee *et al.*, 1985). When given in equal amounts of the (*S*)-(+) isomer, i.e. 400 mg racemic ibuprofen versus 200 mg of the (*S*)-(+) isomer, both drugs should be essentially the same. The racemic mixture may even have a slightly longer duration of action due to conversion of the (*R*)-(–) isomer to the (*S*)-(+) isomer over time. Conversely, conversion of racemic ibuprofen to the active (*S*)-(+) isomer may contribute to variability in analgesia across individuals and may explain the poor relationship observed between plasma concentrations of ibuprofen and clinical response for acute pain (Laska *et al.*, 1986) and rheumatoid arthritis (Grennan *et al.*, 1983).

The analgesic efficacy of 200 and 400 mg of the (*S*)-(+) isomer of ibuprofen was compared to that of 400 mg of racemic ibuprofen and placebo for postoperative pain in the oral surgery model (Dionne and McCullagh, 1997). Analgesia was detectable by 15 min for both doses of (*S*)-(+)-ibuprofen in comparison to placebo and was significantly better than either placebo or racemic ibuprofen over the first 60 min (Figure 8.2), with the 400 mg dose of the (*S*)-(+) isomer producing greater analgesia than racemic ibuprofen up to 180 min post drug. Total pain relief over the 6-h observation period was greater for the 400 mg dose of (*S*)-(+) isomer in comparison to both placebo and the 400 mg racemic dose. Onset of analgesic activity, as measured by patients subjective report, was significantly faster for both doses of the (*S*)-(+) isomer in comparison to the racemic formulation. Despite these encouraging findings, replication is needed to determine whether the advantage for the (*S*)-(+) isomer was due to the greater intrinsic activity of the isomer or a difference between the racemic formulation and the (*S*)-(+) ibuprofen formulation.

Recognition of the differential effects of the two enantiomers of ibuprofen suggest that any delay in onset associated with administration of racemic ibuprofen is due to giving less of the (*S*)-(+) enantiomer and the resulting delay in hepatic conversion of the inactive form to result in therapeutic levels of the active isomer (Geisslinger *et al.*, 1990). Similarly,

CHAPTER 8

■ 413

the peak analgesic effect of racemic ibuprofen may be limited by the concentration of the (S)-(+) isomer achieved by the balance between the amount administered in the racemic mixture, incomplete conversion of the (R)-(−) isomer to the (S)-(+) isomer (Lee *et al.*, 1985; Geisslinger *et al.*, 1990), and faster renal elimination of the (R)-(−) isomer than for the (S)-(+) isomer (Ahn *et al.*, 1991). Interindividual differences in the therapeutic response to racemic ibuprofen may be related to variability in the pharmacokinetic activation of the active isomer of ibuprofen.

8.2.3 Ibuprofen-containing combinations

Ibuprofen plus codeine

While ibuprofen and related NSAIDs have proved very effective for dental pain, the inability to enhance analgesia with increasing dose has led to attempts at additive analgesia by combining ibuprofen with orally effective opioids, a reinvention of the classic analgesic combination. Results, however, have been generally disappointing. Cooper *et al.* (1982) evaluated the combination of a single dose of 400 mg ibuprofen plus 60 mg codeine in comparison to each drug alone, placebo, and the combination of aspirin 650 mg plus codeine 60 mg. While the ibuprofen plus codeine combination resulted in slightly higher mean hourly analgesic scores and produced substantially greater analgesia than codeine 60 mg, the combination did not produce significantly greater analgesia than ibuprofen 400 mg alone. Comparison of ibuprofen 400 mg plus codeine 60 mg with ibuprofen 400 mg in another study demonstrated significant differences on several, but not all, derived measures of analgesic activity (Petersen *et al.*, 1993). Side-effects were more frequent following the opioid-containing combination but consisted of minor adverse events such as drowsiness and 'faintness'. McQuay *et al.* (1989) demonstrated a 30% increase in analgesic effect with the addition of 20 mg codeine to 400 mg ibuprofen in a crossover study with two doses of the drugs being evaluated (Figure 8.3). With this lower dose of codeine, no tendency for greater incidence of adverse effects was detected and more than 70% of subjects expressed a preference for the combination.

These and other similar studies provide a basis for adding codeine to a 400 mg dose of ibuprofen as needed to produce additive analgesia, but with a dose-related increase in side-effects. It is not clear what is the minimum dose of codeine needed for additive analgesic activity and the dose that produces unacceptable side-effect liability. An additive analgesic effect for a 15 mg dose of codeine in combination with ibuprofen 200 mg could not be demonstrated with a sample size ($n = 36$–37 per group) usually sufficient to separate treatments in the oral surgery model (Giles *et al.*, 1986). The combination of 20 mg codeine and a 300 mg sustained-release formulation of ibuprofen also did not produce additive analgesia in comparison to the ibuprofen formulation alone (Walton and Rood, 1990). The duration of the observation period following drug administration (11 h) exceeds the expected duration of oral codeine (2–3 h), so that it is unlikely that any

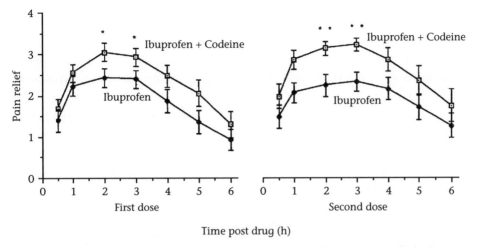

Figure 8.3: Pain relief as measured by five point category scale (10 = none, 1 = a little, 2 = some, 3 = a lot, 4 = complete) following administration of ibuprofen 400 mg or ibuprofen 400 mg plus 20 mg codeine in the oral surgery model. *Significant difference P<0.05 vs. ibuprofen 400 mg. ** significant difference P<0.02. (McQuay *et al.* 1989a)

transient advantage to the codeine would be reflected in summary measures of analgesic activity. A comparison of three dose formulations of ibuprofen plus codeine suggested an optimal balance between additive analgesia and side-effects with a 30 mg dose of codeine in combination with 400 mg ibuprofen (Frame *et al.*, 1986). The relationship between additive analgesic activity and increasing codeine dose was confounded by the increasing dose of ibuprofen, i.e. 15 mg codeine plus 200 mg ibuprofen, 30 mg codeine plus 400 mg ibuprofen, or 60 mg codeine plus 800 mg ibuprofen, so that the contribution of codeine cannot be reliably assessed with this design. The combination of ibuprofen 400 mg plus codeine 60 mg was also compared to a similar combination containing 30 mg of codeine without clearly separating the two combinations from each other in terms of analgesic activity or side-effect liability (Giles and Pickvance, 1985).

While equivocal, these data suggest that a minimum dose of 20–30 mg of codeine is needed in combination with 400 mg ibuprofen to produce detectable additive analgesia with minimal side-effects. Administration of a traditional dose of 60 mg codeine will usually produce additive analgesia, but for relatively short duration (1–2 h) in comparison to the usual duration of ibuprofen (4–6 h) while producing a significant increase in the incidence of side-effects. In the absence of a fixed dose combination, it may be more practical to initiate analgesic treatment with 400–600 mg ibuprofen on a fixed schedule and dispense 30 mg tablets of codeine to be taken as needed for pain not adequately controlled by the NSAID. This strategy will result in exposure to the side-effect liability of the opioid only for those patients in need of additional pain relief, thus resulting in a more favourable therapeutic ratio than that obtained by exposing all patients to opioids side-effects even if the additional analgesia is not clinically needed.

CHAPTER 8

Ibuprofen plus oxycodone

Analgesic combinations containing oxycodone (Percocet, Percodan, Tylox) have gener-ally been perceived as more effective than codeine-containing combinations. This appears logical on the basis of the 10–12-fold greater oral potency attributed to oxycodone in comparison to codeine (Beaver et al., 1978) but is questionable if the recommended dose of oxycodone in these combinations, 5 mg every 6 h, is administered. This should result in the same analgesia as 50–60 mg of codeine, the dose usually administered in combina-tion with aspirin or acetaminophen, while administration of two tablets of a fixed dose combination should result in even greater additive analgesia. The additive analgesia associated with 10 mg oxycodone has been demonstrated to result in adverse effects in approximately 64% of subjects receiving an oxycodone–acetaminophen combination following oral surgery (Cooper et al., 1980).

A dose–response evaluation of 2.5, 5 and 10 mg of oxycodone in combination with 400 mg ibuprofen failed to demonstrate any additive effects for the two lower oxycodone doses (Dionne, 1993). The 10 mg oxycodone dose produced greater analgesia but only over the initial 2 h of the study when ibuprofen reached its peak effect (Figure 8.4a). The addition of oxycodone was accompanied by a dose-related increase in side-effects (Figure 8.4b), with only 5 of 30 subjects at the 10 mg dose level not reporting a complaint. Conversely, Cooper et al. (1993) found a significant effect for 5 mg oxycodone plus 400 mg ibuprofen in comparison to ibuprofen alone for pain relief at later times (4–6 h post drug) and for area under the pain intensity difference (PID) time–action curve. The oxycodone combination also had a higher incidence of side-effects.

The small body of data for oxycodone plus ibuprofen in the oral surgery model limits generalization regarding the potential utility of such a combination in dentistry. Administration of 5 mg oxycodone may produce additive analgesia, probably no greater than that seen for 60 mg codeine, while resulting in the usual opioid side-effects in ambulatory patients: drowsiness, nausea and vomiting. Increasing the oxycodone dose to 10 mg will likely result in additive analgesia, but with a marked increase in side-effects. The lack of an ibuprofen plus oxycodone combination, and the regulatory restrictions placed on oxycodone when prescribed as a single entity, make the clinical utility of this combination for use in dentistry questionable.

Ibuprofen plus hydrocodone

Hydrocodone is a derivative of codeine with good oral efficacy and a duration of effect of 3–4 h. Two clinical studies have demonstrated that 10 mg of hydrocodone is at least as effective as 60 mg of codeine (Beaver and McMillan, 1980). At equieffective doses, the incidence and severity of adverse effects of hydrocodone and codeine are similar (Hopkinson, 1978a,b). A proposed dose combination of hydrocodone and ibuprofen may

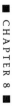

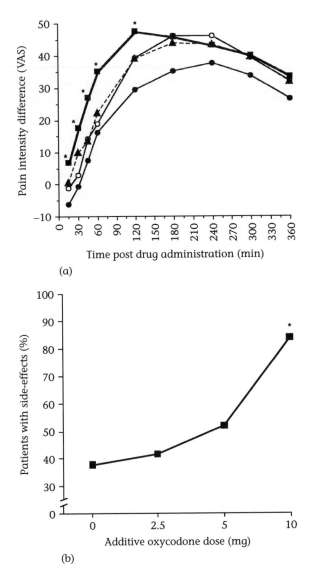

Figure 8.4: (a) Pain intensity difference following administration of 400 mg ibuprofen in combination with 0, 2.5, 5 or 10 mg of oxycodone following oral surgery. ○ , No oxycodone; ● , 2.5 mg oxycodone; ▲ , 5 mg oxycodone; ■ , 10 mg oxycodone. *$p < 0.05$ vs no oxycodone. (b) increased incidence of side-effects with increasing oxycodone dose in the same study. *$p < 0.05$ vs no oxycodone.

provide additive analgesia, but no studies have been published evaluating the formulation for dental pain. If the combination enjoys the same regulatory status in the United States as the acetaminophen plus hydrocodone combination currently available, a convenience will be the ability to prescribe this combination by telephone.

■ CHAPTER 8 ■

8.2.4   Ibuprofen formulations

Formulations of ibuprofen have been developed to enhance onset, potentiate analgesia, and extend the duration of action. The lysine salt of ibuprofen demonstrated faster onset, greater peak analgesia, and a longer duration of action than 500 mg of aspirin for moderate to severe dental pain (Nelson *et al.*, 1994). Ibuprofen lysine had a significantly faster onset of action and greater peak analgesia than 1000 mg of acetaminophen in a similar dental pain study (Mehlisch *et al.*, 1995). The lack of a direct comparison in these studies with the usual racemic ibuprofen formulation does not permit any conclusion regarding the possible clinical advantage of the lysine salt. Cooper *et al.* (1994) evaluated the relationship between analgesic efficacy and drug levels of the (S)-(+) isomer of ibuprofen lysine (400 mg), 400 mg of racemic ibuprofen lysine, and 400 mg of racemic ibuprofen in the oral surgery model. At 30 min post drug, both (S)-(+)-ibuprofen lysine and racemic ibuprofen lysine resulted in significantly greater pain relief than racemic ibuprofen. The lysine salts both resulted in greater peak analgesia and total analgesic scores over the first 3 h in comparison to racemic ibuprofen. This latter study suggests that the lysine salt of ibuprofen may enhance the onset normally seen following administration of racemic ibuprofen yet produce greater peak analgesia and comparable duration of action. Formulation differences between the two preparations may explain the apparent analgesic advantage, and caution is needed in the absence of further data.

Ibuprofen has been evaulated in the dental pain model in combination with caffeine to potentiate the effects of low ibuprofen doses (100–200 mg). A combination of 200 mg ibuprofen plus 100 mg caffeine enhanced the analgesic effect of 200 mg ibuprofen to result in analgesia comparable to that of 400 mg of ibuprofen (McQuay *et al.*, 1996) but without any increased frequency of side-effects. A relative potency comparison of ibuprofen alone to ibuprofen in combination with 100 mg caffeine demonstrated a 2- to 3-fold potentiation of analgesic efficacy over this dose range (Forbes *et al.*, 1991). While demonstration of caffeine's potentiation of ibuprofen analgesic activity may be useful for extrapolation to the use of ibuprofen as a non-prescription analgesic for mild pain, the advantage of this combination for dental pain is not clear. Administration of the usual therapeutic dose of 400 mg of ibuprofen should result in similar analgesia and less side-effect liability.

A controlled release formulation of ibuprofen that releases 200 mg of drug immediately followed by release of the remaining drug over 12 h has been evaluated in the oral surgery model. Cooper *et al.* (1993) demonstrated that controlled release ibuprofen had a comparable onset to ibuprofen, had a higher peak effect, and was significantly more effective 4 h after administration than was 200 mg of ibuprofen. Similar overall effects were reported in a similar study, with the ibuprofen controlled release formulation providing greater analgesia at 3, 4 and 5 h post drug than three doses of 200 mg ibuprofen every 4 h (Desjardins *et al.*, 1991). These data indicate that the controlled release formulation of ibuprofen is effective for long-acting analgesia without the therapeutic variability associated with the offset of one dose and onset of the next dose. The effective dose of ibuprofen in this formulation, 200 mg over 4 h, is below the normal therapeutic range of ibuprofen for dental pain — 400–600 mg every 4 h. While the demonstration of sustained efficacy may extrapolate to other therapeutic uses of ibuprofen, comparisons with repeated doses of 400–600 mg are needed to determine whether a controlled release formulation provides analgesia comparable to by-the-clock administration of the usual ibuprofen dose for moderate to severe pain.

8.3 EFFECTS ON OEDEMA

The acute postoperative sequelae of dental procedures include other signs of inflammation due to tissue injury, most prominently oedema. While synthetic analogues of endogenous corticosteroids are used extensively to control the sequelae of both acute and chronic inflammation, their use postoperatively is tempered by their ability to suppress the immune system, thereby increasing the risk of infection. NSAIDs have a more selective mechanism of action than glucocorticoids and a more favourable side-effect profile, suggesting that drugs of this class may inhibit inflammation without the risks of corticosteroid administration. Ibuprofen produced a trend for reduced swelling in comparison to placebo when given for 3 days at a dose of 400 mg three times daily (Lokken *et al.*, 1975). Administration of 600 mg ibuprofen four times a day for 2 days also showed a trend towards suppressed oedema formation at 48 h following oral surgery (Troullos *et al.*, 1990). A retrospective analysis of the data from two studies done in series (Figure 8.5) evaluating the effects of two NSAIDs (ibuprofen and flurbiprofen) permitted the conclusion that NSAIDs significantly suppress oedema formation following oral surgery in comparison to placebo (Troullos *et al.*, 1990). A more recent study concluded that the

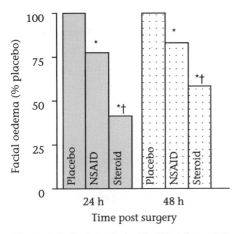

Figure 8.5: Suppression of facial oedema following oral surgery by an NSAID (ibuprofen or flurbiprofen) in comparison to placebo and a steroid (methylprednisolone) administered as a positive control. $*p < 0.05$ vs placebo; $^{\dagger}p < 0.05$ vs NSAID.

combination of ibuprofen 400 mg three times per day and 32 mg of methylprednisolone reduced swelling by greater than 50% in comparison to placebo (Schultze-Mosgau *et al.*, 1995). The lack of separate groups receiving either ibuprofen alone or methylprednisolone does not permit any conclusion about the contribution of ibuprofen to the total effect on swelling reported.

While somewhat inconclusive, the observations from the two studies in which ibuprofen was administered alone demonstrated a reduction in swelling in comparison to placebo, with minimal side-effects and no evidence of interference with healing or perioperative bleeding.

8.4   INTERACTIONS WITH PLASMA β-ENDORPHIN

Pain activates the pituitary–adrenal axis with subsequent pituitary secretion of β-endorphin, leading to elevated circulating β-endorphin levels. Clinical studies in the oral surgery model demonstrate that β-endorphin is released in response to surgical stress in conscious patients (Hargreaves *et al.*, 1986; Troullos *et al.*, 1997) and during postoperative pain (Hargreaves *et al.*, 1986; Hargreaves *et al.*, 1987a,b). Plasma β-endorphin levels are also elevated during surgery performed under general anaesthesia but remain stable if regional or spinal anaesthesia is administered prior to surgery (Figure 8.6a), demonstrating that peripheral nociceptive input activates supraspinal sites leading to pituitary β-endorphin secretion even in unconscious patients not perceiving pain (Janicki *et al.*, 1993; Gordon *et al.*, 1997a,b). These observations suggest that increased β-endorphin is an index of nociceptive input into the central nervous system.

Ibuprofen affects the release of β-endorphin during both surgical stress and postoperative pain. Administration of ibuprofen 600 mg before oral surgery results in increased release of β-endorphin intraoperatively in comparison to the elevated levels seen during surgery in a placebo group (Figure 8.6b). Parallel *in vivo* and *in vitro* studies indicate that ibuprofen potentiation of endorphin release is mediated at the level of the pituitary corticotroph cell, possibly by interfering with ultrashort feedback inhibition modulated by prostaglandins (Troullos *et al.*, 1997). The time course of this enhanced release seems to coincide with the duration of surgery such that β-endorphin levels decrease in samples collected after surgery and return to baseline within 60 min after the completion of surgery. The use of local anaesthetic should largely block the perception of pain during surgery and any residual unpleasant sensations would be similar in the placebo group. Thus, the interaction demonstrated between ibuprofen and elevated β-endorphin levels during surgery can likely be attributed to potentiation of stress-induced release.

Administration of the (*S*)-(+) isomer of ibuprofen following pain onset in the oral surgery model results in a decrease in plasma β-endorphin levels (Dionne and McCullagh, 1997) coincident with a reduction in pain (Figure 8.6c). Levels were also reduced to a lesser extent in a parallel group receiving racemic ibuprofen, consistent with the lower levels of

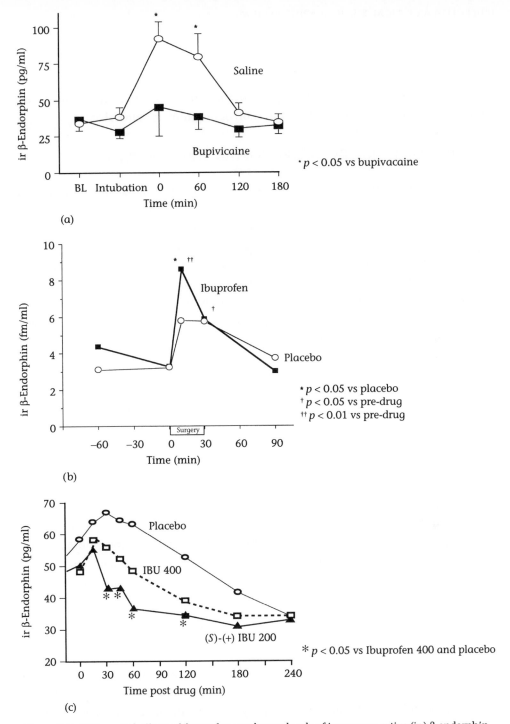

Figure 8.6: Differential effects of ibuprofen on plasma levels of immunoreactive (ir.) β-endorphin levels in humans undergoing oral surgery. (a) Plasma β-endorphin release is elevated during oral surgery performed under general anaesthesia. (b) Increased intraoperative release during surgical stress in conscious patients following ibuprofen pretreatment. (c) Suppression of β-endorphin release coincident with suppression of pain following oral surgery (lower panel).

the (S)-(+) isomer in the racemic ibuprofen group in comparison to the group receiving the pure (S)-(+) isomer. These observations suggest that ibuprofen administration in patients reporting acute pain suppresses pituitary β-endorphin release coincident with analgesia, presumably by decreasing nociceptive activation of the pituitary–adrenal axis.

8.5   USE FOR CHRONIC TEMPOROMANDIBULAR PAIN

Pharmacological intervention in the management of chronic orofacial pain is usually considered adjunctive to definitive treatment on the assumption that more definitive treatments will eventually correct the underlying pathophysiological process. It is now recognized that many putative dental and surgical therapies for temporomandibular disorders have not withstood scientific scrutiny; this has led to the use of drugs as the primary intervention for some forms of chronic orofacial pain. Palliative management of intractable pain may also be considered as an indication for pharmacological management when pain is poorly controlled following failed treatments, such as surgical interventions, or when no other treatment is available.

While the use of analgesics for acute orofacial pain is well documented through hundreds of controlled clinical trials, the use of a broad spectrum of drugs for chronic pain is based on very few studies. Even in the absence of a therapeutic benefit, however, toxicity associated with chronic administration of the drug can still occur. Recognition of the chronic adverse renal and gastrointestinal effects of NSAIDs indicates a need to examine critically their use for chronic pain conditions such as temporomandibular disorders (TMD).

A meta-analysis of the literature on TMD published from 1980 to 1992 identified more than 4000 references (Antczak-Buckoms, 1995), but only 1% ($n = 55$) were randomized controlled trials. Five of the controlled trials were drug studies, providing an extremely small body of evidence upon which to base generalizations regarding efficacy and toxicity. In addition, many of the studies evaluating pharmacological treatments are methodologically flawed, with heterogeneous patient samples, lack of an adequate control group, and a failure to use standardized methods for measurement of pain and dysfunction.

A comprehensive review of the primary literature reveals little scientific support for the idea that the daily use of NSAIDs offers benefit for chronic orofacial pain (Truelove, 1994). Standard texts (Dworkin *et al.*, 1990) and summaries of expert opinion (McNeill, 1993) often provide recommendations or extrapolate from chronic inflammatory conditions such as arthritis. Yet the results of two placebo-controlled studies suggest that NSAIDs are ineffective for chronic orofacial pain. The analgesic effects of ibuprofen 2400 mg per day for 4 weeks could not be separated from placebo in a group of patients with chronic orofacial pain characterized as myogenic in origin (Singer and Dionne, 1997). A similar comparison of piroxicam 20 mg daily for 12 days with placebo for TMD pain also failed to demonstrate any therapeutic advantage for the NSAID (Gordon *et al.*, 1990).

Both clinical and animal studies suggest that tolerance to NSAIDs can develop with repeated administration. The mean reduction in chronic lower back pain intensity following an intitial dose of 1200 mg ibuprofen was 23% (Walker *et al.*, 1996). After 2 weeks of 2400 mg per day of ibuprofen or placebo, the mean reduction in pain intensity for the last dose was 4-fold lower in the drug group. The initial low level of response (23%) suggests that low back pain is not particulary sensitive to ibuprofen and may explain, in part, the poor response seen for chronic musculoskeletal pain in the orofacial area. The development of tolerance over 2 weeks would suggest a similar process for TMD pain, which could make the analgesic response negligible by the end of 4 weeks. Tolerance to diflunisal with repeated adminstration has been demonstrated in animals without a reduction in the amount of drug in the blood over time following administration of the first dose in comparison to a dose given following 3 days of diflunisal (Walker and Levy, 1990). This suggests a functional change in the pharmacological response rather than enhanced pharmacokinetic disposition such that the same amount of drug elicits less analgesia.

The lack of clinical studies to support the efficacy of ibuprofen for TMD contrasts with the growing body of evidence on the potentially serious toxic effects of NSAIDs when given chronically at high doses. A short trial of an NSAID may be considered in patients with an apparent inflammatory component to their pain complaint. A lack of therapeutic effect after a 7–10-day trial, or the development of any gastrointestinal symptoms, should prompt discontinuation of the NSAID.

8.6 RECOMMENDATIONS FOR THE USE OF IBUPROFEN IN DENTISTRY

Ibuprofen is one of the most widely used drugs for dental pain along with aspirin, acetaminophen and codeine. It is more efficacious than these standard drugs in most studies, presumably owing to the inflammatory aetiology of most dental pain and ibuprofen's prominent anti-inflammatory effects. A single dose of 400–600 mg of ibuprofen is usually more effective than combinations of aspirin or acetaminophen plus an opioid (usually codeine or oxycodone), with fewer side effects — making it preferable for ambulatory patients who generally experience a higher incidence of side-effects following an opioid. Ibuprofen also exerts a modest suppression of swelling following surgical procedures, providing additional therapeutic benefit but without the potential liabilities of administering a steroid. These considerations and the vast experience gained through 25 years of clinical use make ibuprofen the drug of choice for dental pain in patients who do not have a contraindications to its use.

Limitations to ibuprofen for dental pain include delayed onset when compared to an injectable opioid, the inability to consistently relieve very severe pain, and its apparent lack of effectiveness when given repeatedly for chronic orofacial pain. The best strategy for minimizing pain onset is administration of the drug prior to the induction of COX-2

CHAPTER 8

postoperatively or co-administration of ibuprofen with an opioid. In patients who do not receive satisfactory relief from ibuprofen alone, combining it with an opioid may provide additive analgesia but will also be accompanied by more frequent side-effects. The optimal balance for individual patients can best be achieved by supplying them with ibuprofen 400–600 mg to be taken by-the-clock and a separate prescription for codeine 30 mg to be taken if needed and titrated between one and two tablets to achieve pain relief with minimal side-effects. Oxycodone can be given in combination with ibuprofen in a similar manner, while a fixed dose combination of ibuprofen 200 mg and hydrocodone 7.5 mg is now available in the US market.

The use of repeated, high doses of ibuprofen for chronic orofacial pain should be re-evaluated in light of its apparent lack of efficacy, the potential for serious gastrointestinal and renal toxicity with repeated dosing, and its potential for tolerance with repeated dosing. The lack of suitable alternatives predicts the continued use of ibuprofen and other NSAIDs for this patient population; their use should be limited to a short trial and discontinued if signs of gastrointestinal or renal toxicity are noted.

REFERENCES

AHN, H.Y., JAMALI, F., COX, S.R., KITTAYONOND, D. and SMITH, D.E. (1991) Stereoselective disposition of ibuprofen enantiomers in the isolated perfused rat kidney. *Pharmacology Research* **12**, 1520–1524.

ANTCZAK-BUCKOMS, A. (1995) Reaction paper to chapters 12 and 13. In: SESSLE, B.J., BRYANT, P. and DIONNE, R.A. (eds), *Temporomandibular Disorders and Related Pain Conditions*. Seattle, IASP Press, 237–245.

ARIENS, E.J. (1983) Stereoselectivity of bioactive agents: general aspects. In: ARIENS, E.J., SOUDIJN, W. and TIMMERMAN, P.B.M.W.M. (eds), *Stereochemistry and Biological Activity of Drugs*. Oxford, Blackwell, 11–32.

BAKSHI, R., FRENKEL, G., DIETLEIN, G., MEURER-WITT, B., SCHNEIDER, B. and SINTERHAUF, U. (1994) A placebo-controlled comparative evaluation of diclofenac dispersible versus ibuprofen in postoperative pain after third molar surgery. *Journal of Clinical Pharmacology* **34**, 225–230.

BEAVER, W.T. and McMILLAN, D. (1980) Methodical considerations in the evaluation of analgesic combinations: acetaminophen (paracetamol) and hydrocodone in post-partum pain. *British Journal of Clinical Pharmacology* **10**, 215S–223S.

BEAVER, W.T., WALLENSTEIN, S.L., ROGERS, A. *et al.* (1978) Analgesic studies of codeine and oxycodone in patients with cancer. I: Comparison of oral with intramuscular codeine and of oral with intramuscular oxycodone. *Journal of Pharmacology and Experimental Therapeutics* **207**, 92–100.

BERTHOLD, C.W. and DIONNE, R.A. (1993) Clinical evaluation of H1 receptor and H2 receptor antagonists for acute postoperative pain. *Journal of Clinical Pharmacology* **33**, 944–948.

CALDWELL, J., HUTT, A.J. and FOURNEL-GIGLEUX, S. (1988) The metabolic chiral inversion and dispositional enantioselectivity of the 2-arylpropionic acids and their biological consequences. *Biochemical Pharmacology* **37**, 105–114.

COOPER, S.A. (1984) Five studies on ibuprofen for postsurgical dental pain. *The American Journal of Medicine* **77A**, 70–77.

COOPER, S.A. and BEAVER, W.T. (1976) A model to evaluate mild analgesics in oral surgery outpatients. *Clinical Pharmacology and Therapeutics* **20**, 241–250.

COOPER, S.A., NEEDLE, S.E. and KRUGER, G.O. (1977) Comparative analgesic potency of aspirin and ibuprofen. *Journal of Oral Surgery* **35**, 898–903.

COOPER, S.A., ENGLE, J., LADOV, M., PRECHEUR, H., ROSENHECK, A. and RAUCH, D. (1982) Analgesic efficacy of an ibuprofen–codeine combination. *Pharmacotherapy* **2**, 162–167.

COOPER, S.A., QUINN, P.D., MacAFEE, K., HERSH, E.V., SULLIVAN, D. and LAMP, C. (1993) Ibuprofen controlled-release formulation. *Oral Surgery, Oral Medicine and Oral Pathology* **75**, 677–683.

COOPER, S.A., REYNOLDS, D.C., GALLEGOS, L.T., REYNOLDS, B., LAROUCHE, S., DEMETRIADES, J. and STRUBLE, W.E. (1994) A PK/PD study of ibuprofen formulations. *Clinical Pharmacology and Therapeutics* **55**, 126 (Abstract).

DESJARDINS, P.J., MILLES, M., FREY, V., GUBITOSA, L., MARDIROSSIAN, G. and SCHNEIDER, R. (1991) Controlled release ibuprofen vs multiple dose ibuprofen in dental impaction pain. *Clinical Pharmacology and Therapeutics* **49**, 182 (Abstract).

DIONNE, R.A. (1986) Suppression of dental pain by the preoperative administration of flurbiprofen. *The American Journal of Medicine* **80**(Suppl. 3A), 41–49.

DIONNE, R.A. (1993) Additive effects of oxycodone and ibuprofen for postoperative pain. *Journal of Dental Research* **72**, 186 (Abstract).

DIONNE, R.A. and COOPER, S.A. (1978) Evaluation of preoperative ibuprofen on postoperative pain after impaction surgery. *Oral Surgery, Oral Medicine and Oral Pathology* **45**, 851–856.

DIONNE, R.A. and McCULLAGH, L. (1997) The (S)-(+) isomer of ibuprofen supresses plasma β-endorphin coincident with analgesia in humans. *Clinical Pharmacology and Therapeutics* **63**, 694–701, 1998.

DIONNE, R.A., CAMPBELL, R.L., COOPER, S.A., HALL, D.L. and BUCKINGHAM, B. (1983) Suppression of postoperative pain by pre-operative administration of ibuprofen in comparison to placebo, acetaminophen and acetaminophen plus codeine. *Journal of Clinical Pharmacology* **23**, 37–43.

CHAPTER 8

DIONNE, R.A., GORDON, S.M. and DUBNER, R. (1996) Relationship of prostaglandin E_2 to acute pain and analgesia. *Journal of Dental Research* **75**, 137 (Abstract).

DWORKIN, S.F., TRUELOVE, E.L., BONICA, J.J. and SOLA, A. (1990) Facial and head pain caused by myofacial and temporomandibular disorders. In: BONICA, J.J. (ed.), *The Management of Pain*. Philadelphia, Lea and Febiger, 727–745.

FLATH, R.K., HICKS, M.L., DIONNE, R.A. and PELLEU, G.B. (1987) Pain suppression after pulpectomy with preoperative flurbiprofen. *Journal of Endodontics* **13**, 339–347.

FLOWER, R.J., MONCADA, S. and VANE, J.R. (1985) Analgesic-antipyretics and anti-inflammatory agents: drugs employed in the treatment of gout. In: GILMAN, A.G., GOODMAN, L.S. and GILMAN, A. (eds), *The Pharmacological Basis of Therapeutics*. New York, Macmillan, 674.

FORBES, J.A., BARKASZI, B.A., RAGLAND, R.N. and HANKLE, J.J. (1984) Analgesic effect of fendosal, ibuprofen and aspirin in postoperative oral surgery pain. *Pharmacotherapy* **4**, 385–391.

FORBES, J.A., BEAVER, W.T., JONES, K.F., KEHM, C.J., SMITH, W.K., GONGLOFF, C.M., ZELENOCK, J.R. and SMITH, J.W. (1991) Effect of caffeine in ibuprofen analgesia in postoperative oral surgery pain. *Clinical Pharmacology and Therapeutics* **49**, 674–84.

FRAME, J.W., FISHER, S.E., PICKVANCE, N.J. and SKENE, A.M. (1986) A double-blind placebo-controlled comparison of three ibuprofen/codeine combinations and aspirin. *British Journal of Oral and Maxillofacial Surgery* **24**, 122–129.

FRAME, J.W., EVANS, C.R.H., FLAUM, G.R., LANGFORD, R. and ROUT, P.G.J. (1989) A comparison of ibuprofen and dihydrocodeine in relieving pain following wisdom teeth removal. *British Dental Journal* **166**, 121–124.

GEISSLINGER, G., SCHUSTRER, O., STOCK, K.P., LOEW, D., BACH, G.L. and BRUNE, K. (1990) Pharmacokinetics of (S)-(+)-ibuprofen and (R)-(–)-ibuprofen in volunteers and first clinical experience of (S)-(+)-ibuprofen in rheumatoid arthritis. *European Journal of Clinical Pharmacology* **38**, 493–497.

GILES, A.D. and PICKVANCE, N.J. (1985) Combination analgesia following oral surgery: a double-blind comparison of ibuprofen, codeine phosphate, and two combination ratios. *Clinical Trials Journal* **22**, 300–313.

GILES, A.D., HILL, C.M., SHEPHERD, J.P., STEWART, D.J. and PICKVANCE, N.J. (1986) A single dose assessment of an ibuprofen/codeine combination in postoperative dental pain. *International Journal of Oral and Maxillofacial Surgery* **15**, 727–732.

GORDON, S.M., MONTGOMERY, M.T. and JONES, D. (1990) Comparative efficacy of piroxicam versus placebo for temporomandibular pain. *Journal of Dental Research* **69**, 218 (Abstract).

GORDON, S.M., DIONNE, R.A., BRAHIM, J., JABIR, F. and DUBNER, R. (1997a) Blockade of peripheral neuronal barrage reduces postoperative pain. *Pain* **70**, 209–215.

GORDON, S.M. and DIONNE, R.A. (1997b) Prevention of pain. *Compendium* **18**, 239–251.

GORDON, S.M., DIONNE, R.A., BRAHIM, J.S., SANG, C.N. and DUBNER, R. (1997c) Differential effects of local anaesthesia on central hyperalgesia. *Journal of Dental Research* **76** (Special Issue), 153.

GRENNAN, D.M., AARONS, L., SIDDIQUI, M., RICHARDS, M., THOMPSON, R. and HIGHAM, C. (1983) Dose–response study with ibuprofen in rheumatoid arthritis: clinical and pharmacokinetic findings. *British Journal of Clinical Pharmacology* **15**, 311–316.

HARGREAVES, K.M., DIONNE, R.A., MUELLER, G.P., GOLDSTEIN, D.S. and DUBNER, R. (1986) Naloxone, fentanyl, and diazepam modify plasma beta-endorphin levels during surgery. *Clinical Pharmacology and Therapeutics* **40**, 165–171.

HARGREAVES, K.M., MUELLER, G.P., DUBNER, R., GOLDSTEIN, D. and DIONNE, R.A. (1987a) Corticotropin-releasing factor (CRF) produces analgesia in humans and rats. *Brain Research* **422**, 154–157.

HARGREAVES, K.M., SCHMIDT, E., MUELLER, G.P. and DIONNE, R.A. (1987b) Dexamethasone alters plasma levels of β-endorphin and postoperative pain. *Clinical Pharmacology and Therapeutics* **42**, 601–607.

HERSH, E.V., COOPER, S.A., BEETS, N., WEDELL, D., MACAFEE, K., QUINN, P., LAMP, C., GASTON, G., BERGMAN, S. and HENRY, E. (1993) Single dose and multidose analgesic study of ibuprofen and meclofenamate sodium after third molar surgery. *Oral Surgery, Oral Medicine and Oral Pathology* **76**, 680–687.

HILL, C.M., CARROLL, M.J., GILES, A.D. and PICKVANCE, N. (1987) Ibuprofen given pre- and post-operatively for the relief of pain. *International Journal of Oral and Maxillofacial Surgery* **16**, 420–424.

HOPKINSON, J.H. (1978a) Hydrocodone — a unique challenge for an established drug: comparison of repeated oral doses of hydrocodone (10 mg) and codeine (60 mg) in the treatment of post partum pain. *Current Therapeutic Research* **24**, 503–516.

HOPKINSON, J.H. (1978b) Vicodin, a new analgesic: clinical evaluation of the efficacy and safety of repeated doses. *Current Therapeutic Research* **24**, 633–645.

JAIN, A.K., RYAN, J.R., McMAHON, G., KUEBEL, J.O., WALTERS, P.J. and NOVECK, C. (1986) Analgesic efficacy of low-dose ibuprofen in dental extraction. *Pharmacotherapy* **6**, 318–322.

JANIKI, P.K., ERSKINE, R. and VAN DER WATT, M.L. (1993) Plasma concentrations of immunoreactive beta-endorphin and substance P in patients undergoing surgery under general vs spinal anaesthesia. *Hormone and Metabolic Research* **25**, 131–133.

KIERSCH, T.A., HALLADAY, S.C. and KOSCHIK, M. (1993) A double-blind, randomized study of naproxen sodium, ibuprofen, and placebo in postoperative dental pain. *Clinical Therapeutics* **15**, 845–854.

CHAPTER 8

LASKA, E.M., SUNSHINE, A., MARRERO, I., OLSON, N., SIEGEL, C. and MCCORMICK, N. (1986) The correlation between blood levels of ibuprofen and clinical analgesic response. *Clinical Pharmacology and Therapeutics* **40**, 1–7.

LEE, E.J.D., WILLIAMS, K., DAY, R., GRAHAM, G. and CHAMPION, D. (1985) Stereoselective disposition of ibuprofen enantiomers in man. *British Journal of Clinical Pharmacology* **19**, 669–674.

LOKKEN, P., OLSEN, I., BRUASET, I. and NORMAN-PEDERSEN, K. (1975) Bilateral surgical removal of impacted third molar teeth as a model for drug evaluation: a test with ibuprofen. *European Journal of Clinical Pharmacology* **8**, 209–216.

MCNEILL, C. (1993) *Temporomandibular Disorders*. Chicago, Quintessence, 87.

MCQUAY, H.J., CARROLL, D., WATTS, P.G., JUNIPER, R.P. and MOORE, R.A. (1989) Codeine 20 mg increases pain relief from ibuprofen 400 mg after third molar surgery. A repeat dosing comparison of ibuprofen and an ibuprofen–codeine combination. *Pain* **37**, 7–13.

MCQUAY, H.J., CARROLL, D., GUEST, P.G., ROBSON, S., WIFFEN, P.J. and JUNIPER, R.P. (1993) A multiple dose comparison of ibuprofen and dihydrocodeine after third molar surgery. *British Journal of Oral and Maxillofacial Surgery* **31**, 95–100.

MCQUAY, H.J., ANGELL, K., CARROLL, D., MOORE, R.A. and JUNIPER, R.P. (1996) Ibuprofen compared with ibuprofen plus caffeine after third molar surgery. *Pain* **66**, 247–251.

MEHLISCH, D.R., JASPER, R.D., BROWN, P., KORN, S.H., MCCARROLL, K. and MURAKAMI, A.A. (1995) Comparative study of ibuprofen lysine and acetaminophen in patients with postoperative dental pain. *Clinical Therapeutics* **17**, 852–860.

NELSON, S.L., BRAHIM, J.S., KORN, S.H., GREENE, S.S. and SUCHOWER, L.J. (1994) Comparison of single-dose ibuprofen lysine, acetylsalicylic acid, and placebo for moderate-to-severe postoperative dental pain. *Clinical Therapeutics* **16**, 458–465.

NGAN, P., WILSON, S., SHANFELD, J. and AMINI, A. (1994) The effect of ibuprofen on the level of discomfort in patients undergoing orthodontic treatment. *American Journal of Orthodontics and Dentofacial Orthopedics* **106**, 88–95.

PETERSEN, J.K., HANSSON, F. and STRID, S. (1993) The effect of an ibuprofen–codeine combination for the treatment of patients with pain after removal of lower third molars. *Journal of Oral and Maxillofacial Surgery* **51**, 637–640.

ROSZKOWSKI, M.T., SWIFT, J.Q. and HARGREAVES, K.M. (1997) Effect of NSAID administration on tissue levels of immunoreactive prostaglandin E2, leukotriene B4, and (s)-fluribiprofen following extraction of impacted third molars. *Pain* **73**, 339–345.

SCHULTZE-MOSGAU, S., SCHMELZEISEN, R., FROLICH, J.C. and SCHMELE, H. (1995) Use of ibuprofen and methylprednisolone for the prevention of pain and swelling after removal of impacted third molars. *Journal of Oral and Maxillofacial Surgery* **53**, 2–7.

SEIBERT, K., ZHANG, Y., LEAHY, K., HAUSER, S., MASFERRER, J., PERKINS, W., LEE, L. and ISAKSON, P. (1994) Pharmacological and biochemical demonstration of the role of cyclooxygenase 2 in inflammation and pain. *Proceedings of the National Academy of Sciences of the USA* **91**, 12013–12017.

SEYMOUR, R.A., WARD-BOOTH, P. and KELLY, P.J. (1996) Evaluation of different doses of soluble ibuprofen and ibuprofen tablets in postoperative dental pain. *British Journal of Oral and Maxillofacial Surgery* **34**, 110–114.

SINGER, E. and DIONNE, R.A. (1997) A controlled evaluation of ibuprofen and diazepam for chronic orofacial muscle pain. *Journal of Orofacial Pain* **11**, 139–146.

SISK, A.L. and GROVER, B.J. (1990) A comparison of preoperative and postoperative naproxen sodium for suppression of postoperative pain. *Journal of Oral and Maxillofacial Surgery* **48**, 674–678.

TORABINEJAD, M., CYMERMAN, J.J., FRANKSON, M., LEMON, R.R., MAGGIO, J.D. and SCHILDER, H. (1994a) Effectiveness of various medications on postoperative pain following complete instrumentation. *Journal of Endodontics* **20**, 345–354.

TORABINEJAD, M., DORN, S.O., ELEAZER, P.D., FRANKSON, M., JOUHARI, B., MULLIN, R.K. and SOLUTI, A. (1994b) Effectiveness of various medications on postoperative pain following root canal obturation. *Journal of Endodontics* **20**, 427–431.

TROULLOS, E.S., HARGREAVES, K.M., BUTLER, D.P. and DIONNE, R.A. (1990) Comparison of non-steroidal anti-inflammatory drugs, ibuprofen and flurbiprofen, to methylprednisolone and placebo for acute pain, swelling, and trismus. *Journal of Oral and Maxillofacial Surgery* **48**, 945–952.

TROULLOS, E., HARGREAVES, K.M. and DIONNE, R.A. (1997) Ibuprofen elevates β-endorphin levels in humans during surgical stress. *Clinical Pharmacology and Therapeutics* **62**, 74–81.

TRUELOVE, E.L. (1994) The chemotherapeutic management of chronic and persistent orofacial pain. *Dental Clinics of North America* **38**, 669–88.

VOGEL, R.I. and GROSS, J.I. (1984) The effects of nonsteroidal anti-inflammatory analgesics on pain after periodontal surgery. *Journal of the American Dental Association* **109**, 731–734.

VOGEL, R.I., DESJARDINS, P.J. and MAJOR, K.V.O. (1992) Comparison of presurgical and immediate postsurgical ibuprofen on postoperative periodontal pain. *Journal of Periodontology* **63**, 914–918.

WALKER, J.S. and LEVY, G. (1990) Effect of multiple dosing on the analgesic action of diflunisal in rats. *Life Sciences* **46**, 737–742.

WALKER, J.S., LOCKTON, A.I., NGUYEN, T.V. and DAY, R.O. (1996) Analgesic effect of ibuprofen after single and multiple doses in chronic spinal pain patients. *Analgesia* **2**, 93–101.

CHAPTER 8

WALTON, G.M. and ROOD, J.P. (1990) A comparison of ibuprofen and ibuprofen–codeine combination in the relief of post-operative oral surgery pain. *British Dental Journal* **169**, 245–247.

WIDEMAN, G.L., KEFFER, M.W., KARPOW, S.A. *et al.* (1992) Analgesic efficacy of ibuprofen with hydrocodone vs ibuprofen alone in postoperative pain. *Clinical Pharmacology and Therapeutics* **51**, 146 (Abstract).

WINTER, L., BASS, E., RECANT, B. and CAHALY, J.F. (1978) Analgesic activity of ibuprofen (Motrin) in postoperative oral surgical pain. *Oral Surgery, Oral Medicine and Oral Pathology* **45**, 159–166.

9

Gastrointestinal Adverse Drug Reactions Attributed to Ibuprofen

DAVID HENRY[1], ANNA DREW[2] AND SCOTT BEUZEVILLE[3]

[1]Discipline of Clinical Pharmacology, Faculty of Medicine and Health Sciences, [2]Department of Clinical Toxicology, and [3]Department of General Medicine, Newcastle Mater Hospital, Newcastle, New South Wales, Australia

Contents

This chapter is reproduced here in a modified form from that which appeared in the proceedings of an International Symposium on 'Safety and Efficacy of Nonprescription (OTC) NSAIDs and Analgesics', edited by K D Rainsford and M C Powanda, with permission of Kluwer Academic Publishers, Dordrecht and Lancaster.

9.1 BACKGROUND

Concern about the capacity of nonsteroidal anti-inflammatory drugs (NSAIDs) to cause damage to the upper gastrointestinal tract goes back to the 1930s and 1940s when the first associations between ingestion of aspirin and gastrointestinal bleeding were reported (Douthwaite and Lintott, 1938; Muir and Cossan, 1955). These were relatively small case series, but the association was believed to be quite strong, and it was appreciated, even then, that widespread use of aspirin in the community might be responsible for large numbers of cases of gastrointestinal bleeding (Douthwaite and Lintott, 1938). The development of newer NSAIDs such as phenylbutazone and indomethacin followed. More recently introduced drugs, such as naproxen and ibuprofen, were thought to have lessened the risk of damage to the stomach and duodenum (Langman, 1970). The belief in the lower risk of these newer drugs was quite strong; so much so that the entity of NSAID-induced gastrointestinal bleeding became controversial (Langman *et al.*, 1974; Henry and Langman, 1981). Surprisingly, in view of the widespread use of these drugs, there were very few properly controlled pharmacoepidemiological studies performed until the mid 1980s (Somerville *et al.*, 1986; Carson *et al.*, 1987). Since then the effects of NSAIDs on the upper gastrointestinal tract have been the subject of quite intense investigation (Somerville *et al.*, 1986; Carson *et al.*, 1987; Gabriel *et al.*, 1991; Griffin *et al.*, 1991; Laporte *et al.*, 1991; Bollini *et al.*, 1992; Garcia-Rodriguez *et al.*, 1992; Nobili *et al.*, 1992; Abenhaim and Moride, 1993; Henry *et al.*, 1993; Kaufman *et al.*, 1993; Savage *et al.*, 1993; Garcia-Rodriguez and Jick, 1994; Langman *et al.*, 1994; Perez-Gutthann *et al.*, 1994; Henry *et al.*, 1996). In fact, other than oral contraceptives and hormone replacement therapy, it is doubtful whether any single group of drugs has been so extensively investigated using epidemiological methods.

The modern epidemiological studies performed between 1985 and 1994 have defined, beyond doubt, the level of risk of gastrointestinal bleeding and ulcer perforation. The factors that are associated with a variation in the level of this risk and, most relevantly for this chapter, the extent to which the risk apparently varies between different members of the class of NSAIDs have also been investigated.

The main purpose of this chapter is to review the comparative toxicity of ibuprofen and other NSAIDs on the upper gastrointestinal tract. It has been claimed that this particular drug is safer than other NSAIDs (Langman *et al.*, 1994). If true, this claim is important as it can translate into a substantial public health benefit through lowered gastrointestinal toxicity. However, the issues that have to be faced in making this judgement are complex and need to be reviewed in a systematic manner. In this chapter we have tried to do this. An initial literature search was based on a review of papers retrieved in previously published meta-analyzes (Gabriel *et al.*, 1991; Bollini *et al.*, 1992; Henry *et al.*, 1996). This was supplemented by an updated literature search of Medline from 1981 through 1996. We included studies of the mechanisms of gastrointestinal toxicity with this class of drugs,

CHAPTER 9

endoscopic surveys that give pointers to the relative toxicity of different members of this class, reviews of voluntary adverse reaction reports, and major pharmacoepidemiological studies that investigated the relationship between ingestion of NSAIDs and development of upper gastrointestinal bleeding and ulcer perforation. The strengths and weaknesses of the different methological approaches will be discussed, as will the evidence supporting the contention that there are differences between the individual members of class. Finally, we will try to pull together these different strands of evidence to determine whether there is a correlation with respect to ranking by risk for individual drugs between the data that are obtained by these different methods.

9.2 METHODS

9.2.1 Literature search

In preparing this chapter we performed an extensive search of Medline. Details of the searching algorithms are available from the authors. The search was broad and uncovered many studies of little relevance to the topic of this chapter. In total, 1687 articles were retrieved. These were sorted by reading titles and abstracts, and 195 papers form the basis of the data and conclusions in this chapter. Meta-analytical techniques were used at different stages, such as pooling of the relative risks from epidemiological studies and ranking the same studies for risk with individual drugs. More detail is provided in the relevant sections below. Despite these efforts, this review is incomplete. The work involved in tracking down every study of gastrointestinal toxicity from NSAIDs that has been performed would be monumental and is outside the scope of this chapter. However, studies have been selected here on the basis of their methodological rigour rather than their results, so the conclusions should be reasonably free of bias.

9.3 RESULTS

9.3.1 Mechanisms of gastrointestinal toxicity

These will be considered only briefly here. NSAIDs may have local and systemic effects on the gastrointestinal mucosa. The former probably accounts for the widespread acute mucosal damage seen soon after ingestion. NSAIDs, as a class, inhibit the activity of two forms of cyclooxygenase, COX-1 and COX-2 (Vane and Botting, 1997). COX-1 is present in the upper gastrointestinal mucosa, but tissue at this site does not express COX-2. COX-1 produces prostaglandins (PGs) that have important roles in maintaining the integrity of the upper gastrointestinal mucosa. This enzyme is also present in the kidney, where PGs maintain renal blood flow during times of hemodynamic stress (Clive and

Stoff, 1984). Inhibition of COX-1 leads to deleterious effects in the upper gastrointestinal mucosa. A number of mechanisms have been proposed but, surprisingly, the precise mode of action is still unclear. However, the action of PGs in maintaining vascular integrity and enabling cellular restitution after superficial injury seem to be central to the ability of the mucosa to repair itself (Gyömber *et al.*, 1996). Diminution of this activity may be what leads to frank ulceration.

COX-2 is an inducible form of cyclooxygenase that is synthesized in response to various inflammatory stimuli (Vane and Botting, 1997). PGs produced by this enzyme augment pain and participate in the inflammatory response. Various experimental systems have been used to classify the different NSAIDs according to their COX-1 and COX-2 inhibitory actions. At least in theory, drugs that are selective for COX-2 may result in therapeutic benefit with a reduced degree of gastrointestinal toxicity. One difficulty in assessing this claim is the lack of agreement on the best way of measuring these activities. The second difficulty is knowing which manifestation of clinical toxicity with which to correlate these measures. However, there does seem to be some relationship between COX-1 activity and the degree of clinically significant injury that is produced by treatment. This is discussed later in the section on epidemiological studies.

There has been intense interest in the interaction between NSAID-induced damage and the presence of the organism *Helicobacter pylori* (HP) (Meta *et al.*, 1992; Janssen *et al.*, 1994; Taha *et al.*, 1994, 1995; Laine *et al.*, 1995a; Santucci *et al.*, 1995; el-Assi, 1996; Graham, 1996; Lipscombe *et al.*, 1996; Svanes *et al.*, 1996). Most peptic ulcers are now thought to be due to infection with HP or direct damage by NSAIDs. As they are very common risk factors, patients are frequently exposed to both. A question then arises as to the interaction between these independent risk factors. In epidemiology an 'interaction' is said to exist if the risk of the outcome with joint exposure to risk factors *is greater than* the sum, (or the product) of the individual probabilities associated with the separate risk factors (depending on whether the relationship is believed to be additive or multiplicative). In other words, it is assumed that there will always be some increase in risk due to joint exposure to two independent risk factors. If there were not, it would imply that one factor was protecting against the full effects of the other, which in the case of HP and NSAIDs seems unlikely. Unfortunately the epidemiological studies that have been performed are of insufficient size and quality to explore possible interactions between these two risk factors. A summary of the best papers that have been published is summarized in Table 9.1. As can be seen, although some of the studies are prospective and even randomized, the numbers of subjects included have been small, and normal volunteers have been recruited. The conclusions of the studies appear contradictory. Meta-analysis is not useful in this situation as a means of resolving apparent conflict because of the small number of good-quality studies. To resolve this dilemma it would be necessary to perform quite large prospective studies with subjects categorized at the outset as being HP positive or negative, and then assigned to NSAIDs or an untreated control group. Subjects would have to be ulcer

CHAPTER 9

TABLE 9.1

Endoscopic studies of *Helicobacter pylori* (HP) and NSAIDs

Author	Study subjects	Intervention	Study method	Outcomes	Conclusions
al-Assi *et al.* (1996)	10 subjects with DU, and 145 with GU	None	Cross-sectional endoscopic study	HP status, location of ulcer	Gastric ulcers in HP$^+$ NSAID$^-$ subjects were more likely to be on the lesser curve than in HP$^-$ NSAID$^+$ subjects. Latter were more likely to be on a greater curve. NSAIDS used by 74% of subjects with UGIB and were an important cause of bleeding complications
Lipscomb *et al.* (1996)	24 healthy volunteers. 12 HP$^+$ and 12 HP$^-$	Nap 500 mg b.d. for 28 days	Prospects of endoscopic study	Gastric-mucosal damage at 1, 7 and 28 days	Adaptation to NSAID-induced damage seen equally in HP$^+$ and HP$^-$ individuals
Santucci *et al.* (1995)	51 health volunteers	Comparison of pirox, melox and placebo	Prospective random masked endoscopic study	Ulcers and erosions at 28 days	Severity of mucosal damage greater in HP$^+$ than HP$^-$ individuals
Lane *et al.* (1995a)	52 health volunteers	Nap or etodol or placebo	Prospective randomized endoscopic study	Erosions, ulcers and mucosal inflammation at 7 and 28 days	Degree of gastroduodenal injury similar in HP$^+$ and HP$^-$ individuals Diffuse histological damage seen only in HP$^+$ subjects
Taha *et al.* (1995)	52 long-term NSAID users	None	Prospective observations study	Incidence of peptic ulcer at 0, 12 and 24 weeks	Incidence of ulceration with NSAIDs higher in HP$^+$ than HP$^-$ patients

Etod, etodolac; Pirox, piroxicam; Melox, meloxicam; Nap, naproxen; UGIB, upper gastrointestinal bleeding; HP$^+$, HP$^-$, *H. pylori* positive or negative.

436

free at inception, and it would be helpful if there were approximately equal distribution of other risk factors for peptic ulcer between the groups. This sort of major undertaking is unlikely to be completed in the near future, so the true nature of this relationship will remain obscure for some time yet. As has been pointed out, there is presently insufficient evidence for screening patients for HP before commencing NSAIDs.

9.3.2   Endoscopic studies of gastrointestinal toxicity with NSAIDs

This literature is widely disseminated and difficult to pull together. Since the advent of the modern fibre-optic endoscope, repeated studies have been conducted to document the acute and medium-term damage that occurs in individuals ingesting nonsteroidal NSAIDs (Lanza *et al.*, 1975, 1979, 1981, 1986, 1990; Caruso and Bianchi-Porro, 1980; Aabakken *et al.*, 1990; Friedman *et al.*, 1990; Bergmann *et al.*, 1992; Roth *et al.*, 1993; Laine *et al.*, 1995). The early studies were simply concerned to document an effect, and later there was interest in the extent to which the degree of damage varied between individual members of this class of drugs. More recently, most of the studies have been concerned with the efficacy of preventive measures or, as mentioned above, the importance of HP as a co-factor (Elliot *et al.*, 1994; Lipscombe *et al.*, 1995; Coch *et al.*, 1996; Hawkey, 1996; Laine, 1996; Porrow *et al.*, 1995).

The difficulty in interpreting endoscopic evidence of mucosal damage with these drugs is that it represents a 'surrogate' outcome. Surrogate outcomes are widely used in clinical research because they may allow quantification of benefit or harm in a shorter time period, and with smaller numbers of subjects, than would be necessary to measure the clinically significant outcome. In relation to NSAIDs, the outcome of interest is significant ulceration and its complications, bleeding, perforation and stenosis. The surrogate outcome that is measured in endoscopic studies is usually a scoring system for acute mucosal damage. Several rating scales have been proposed but the inter-rater reliability is not very good (Sonnenberg *et al.*, 1979; Cales *et al.*, 1990; Hudson *et al.*, 1994). The other problem in interpreting such data is that the study subjects are often healthy volunteers, rather than the elderly and sick, who are the main recipients of NSAIDs. In addition, acute ulceration is shown typically in up to 20% of subjects, whereas major gastrointestinal events occur in only 0.3–0.8% of subjects who ingest NSAIDs. The additional weakness of this approach is that it does not reflect the morbidity of individuals with upper gastrointestinal damage. There is no correlation between the amount of mucosal injury and the symptoms experienced by the individual (Graham *et al.*, 1994).

Despite these reservations, there is some parallel between the degree of mucosal damage and the level of risk of major and clinically significant outcomes. This was best shown in the studies of misoprostol protection against NSAID damage (Graham *et al.*, 1988; Raskin *et al.*, 1995; Silverstein *et al.*, 1995). A number of studies showed that acute endoscopic features were improved by co-prescription of misoprostol, and in the large

TABLE 9.2

Endoscopic studies of comparative damage from ibuprofen and other NSAIDs

Study	Subjects	n	Randomized	Blinded assessment	Duration	Drugs/doses	Findings in the stomach	Findings in the duodenum
Lanza et al. (1975)	Normal volunteers	20	Yes (crossover)	Yes	7 days	Ib 1200 mg, Phenyl 400 mg, Indo 100 mg, ASA 3600 mg, Placebo	ASA > Indo > Phenyl > Ibup	
Lanza et al. (1979)	Normal volunteers 21–45 years	40	Yes	Yes	7 days	Ib 1600 mg, Ib 2400 mg, Indo 100 mg, Indo 150 mg, Nap 500 mg, Nap 750 mg, ASA 3600 mg	ASA > Indo 750 > Indo 100 > Indo 150 > Ibup 2400 > Ibup 1600 > Placebo	
Caruso and Bianchi-Porro (1980)	Chronic RA or OA observational study	249 all ages	No	Yes	> 3 weeks	Various	ASA > Indo > Keto > Nap > Diclof > Ibup > Oxyphen > Diflun	
Lanza et al. (1981)	Normal volunteers aged 21–45 years	24	Yes	Yes	7 days	Ib 2400 mg, Tolm 2000, Indo 150 mg, Nap 750 mg, Placebo	Tolm > Nap > Ibup > Undo > Placebo	Tolm > Nap > Ibup > Indo > Ibup > Placebo
Lanza et al. (1986)	Normal volunteers (aged 18–50 years) Male	73	Yes	Yes	7 days	Ib 2400 mg, Nap 1000 mg, Indo 200 mg, Etod 600 mg Etod 1000 mg	Indo > Nap > Ibup > Placebo = Etod 1000 = Etod 600	Indo > Nap > Ibup > Etod 600 > Etod 1000 = Placebo
Friedman et al. (1990)	Normal volunteers	35	Yes	Yes	7 days	Ib 2400 mg, Ibup (Disp/W) 2400 mg, Ibup (Disp/O) 2400 mg, ASA 2825 mg	ASA > Ib/W > Ibup/O > Ibup	ASA > Ibup/W > Ib/O = Ib
Bergmann et al. (1992)	Normal volunteers (aged 23–34 years)	12	Yes (crossover)	Yes	Single dose	Keto 25 mg, Ib 200 mg, ASA 500 mg	ASA > Keto = Ibup	
Roth et al. (1993)	Patients with OA aged 60 years +	71	Yes	Yes	12 weeks	Ib 2400 mg Ib 2400 mg[+] Miso 800 µg, Nabum 1000 mg	Ibup > Ibup + Miso = Nabum	

ASA, acetylsalicylic acid; Diclo, diclofenac; Diflun, diflunisal; Etod, etodolac; Ib, ibuprofen; In, indomethacin; Keto, ketoprofen; Miso, misoprostol; Nabum, nabumetone; Nap, naproxen; Oxy, oxyphenbutazone; Phenyl, phenylbutazone; Tolm, tolmetin.

OA, osteoarthritis; RA, rheumatoid arthritis.

> indicates that the degree of mucosal damage was greater with this agent.

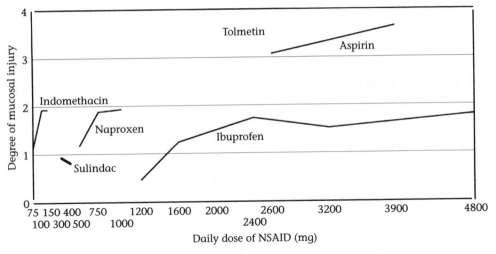

Figure 9.1: Summary of studies of endoscopic injury (from Lanza *et al.*, 1984).

MUCOSA study there was a reduction in major clinical endpoints that was similar in degree to the protection afforded in the endoscopic studies (Graham *et al.*, 1993; Raskin *et al*, 1995; Silverstein *et al.*, 1995).

In view of this, it is reasonable to consider endoscopic studies as providing pointers to the relative toxicity of individual NSAIDs. Of particular interest in this chapter is whether ibubrofen causes less damage than other NSAIDs.

The studies that we were able to uncover by the literature search mentioned earlier are summarized in Table 9.2. There were 8 studies that compared endoscopic damage observed with ibubrofen to that seen with a range of other nonsteroidal anti-inflammatory drugs (Lanza *et al.*, 1975, 1981, 1986; Lanza, 1984; Caruso and Bianchi-Porro, 1980; Friedman *et al.*, 1990; Bergmann *et al.*, 1992; Roth *et al.*, 1993). The design of these studies varied greatly, both in terms of the study participants (being either normal volunteers or older patients with arthritis), and in the duration of therapy, which ranged from a single dose to 12 weeks. The dose of ibuprofen most often used was 2400 mg daily. It can be seen that in this dose the drug was associated with a lesser degree of damage than aspirin, indomethacin or naproxen. These findings are consistent with a review published by Lanza in 1984 that summarized his experience with a series of endoscopic studies published between 1975 and 1983 (Lanza, 1984).

A feature of this series is the consistent methodology used. The studies always involved normal volunteers, usually required them to take a NSAID for 7 days, used a randomization process, and used standard endoscopic scoring by someone who was blind to the treatment assignment. The results reported by Lanza are summarized graphically in Figure 9.1. It can be seen that ibuprofen in doses up to 1600 mg/day was associated with a lesser degree of upper gastric mucosal damage than therapeutic doses of indomethacin

CHAPTER 9

or naproxen. The dose–response relationship with ibuprofen seems shallower than with these other NSAIDs. It is also apparent that the doses of aspirin used in these studies were associated with a substantial degree of mucosal damage. These results suggest that ibuprofen, in doses up to 1600 mg/day, is associated with a relatively low degree of gastric and duodenal mucosal damage. However, in doses of 2400 mg/day or above, the damage is similar to that seen with therapeutic doses of other commonly used NSAIDs. As will be seen later, these results parallel quite closely the findings of the large epidemiological studies that looked at major gastrointestinal complications. Another feature of the results is the relatively high risk seen with tolmetin, and the low level of endoscopic damage seen with sulindac. In the case of the latter, this apparent advantage was not confirmed in the epidemiological studies (see below). It should be noted that the dose of aspirin investigated in these studies was much higher than is used in typical practice today. Most epidemiological studies of the major gastrointestinal complications from aspirin have recorded low average doses, which reflects the widespread prophylactic use of aspirin, or its occasional use in low doses as an analgesic. It is seldom used in full anti-inflammatory doses.

The commonly used NSAIDs studied by Lanza (ibuprofan, naproxen and indo-methacin)l displayed fairly flat dose–response relationships, with the highest doses studied producing no more mucosal damage than the next highest dose (Figure 9.1). While this may be true for mucosal damage it is unclear whether it applies to major gastrointestinal complications, and the studies reported to date have not documented the upper end of the dose–response relationship. As much of the serious toxicity of NSAIDs is presumed to be systemic rather than local, it is best to assume that the level of risk increases in a linear fashion with increasing doses of NSAIDs or combinations of them.

9.3.3 Voluntary adverse reaction reports of gastrointestinal damage with NSAIDs

Voluntary adverse reaction reports are an important source of information on serious drug toxicity. Reports generally come from prescribing doctors or pharmacists, and less often from patients themselves. Usually the reports are collated by government-run reporting agencies or pharmaceutical manufacturers. ADR reports are a valuable signalling system, and the numbers of reports may give some idea of the incidence of a reaction in a community.

However, there are serious limitations to the interpretation of ADR reports. The main difficulty is that substantial under-reporting leads to a very uncertain numerator when attempts are made to calculate the incidence of ADRs. For instance, in the case of serious gastrointestinal reaction to NSAIDs, we have calculated from epidemiological and drug use data that less than 5% of cases of gastrointestinal bleeding or ulcer perforation occurring in Australian subjects on NSAIDs are reported to the Australian Adverse Drug Reactions Advisory Committee (unpublished observations). With this degree of under-reporting, a

TABLE 9.3

Studies of voluntary reports of serious gastrointestinal adverse reactions to NSAIDs

Drug	United Kingdom			United States		
	Reporting rate	Corrected reporting rate	Rank	Reporting rate	Corrected reporting rate	Rank
Ibuprofen	6.0	16.0	1	2.0	1.8	1
Fenoprofen	11.0	31.0	2	4.0	3.0	3
Diflunisal	13.0	32.0	3	8.5	2.8	2
Sulindac	13.0	34.0	4	4.98	3.6	5
Naproxen	18.0	46.0	5	4.2	3.1	4
Diclofenac	18.0	49.0	6	–	–	–
Indomethacin	18.0	50.0	7	–	–	–
Ketoprofen	30.0	80.0	8	–	–	–
Piroxicam	46.0	129.0	9	20.0	6.5	7
Tolmetin	77.0	213.0	10	7.9	5.9	6
Azapropazone	85.0	225.0	11	–	–	–

small increase in reporting rate with any particular compound, e.g. a new drug, will make this drug look much worse than other members of the class. However, it is hard to resist the temptation to carry out analyses of large collections of ADR reports, and this has been done in the United Kingdom using the 'yellow card system', and in the United States using the system for spontaneous reporting run by the Food and Drug Administration (FDA). In each country, series of gastrointestinal reactions to NSAIDs have been compiled and published (Bateman, 1996; Rossi *et al.*, 1987). In making their analyses, the investigators were well aware of the particular problems of comparing different drugs within the class of NSAIDs. The particular concerns in the interpretation include the following. (1) The marketing life-cycle. This should be controlled to avoid comparing drugs well into their life cycle with those that are in the first few years of marketing. This is because the reporting rates tend to be higher for recently marked compounds. (2) General trends in reporting rates have to be adjusted for. In many countries the rate of reporting of adverse reactions has risen through the 1980s and 1990s, and a drug marketed towards the end of this period will appear worse than one marketed at the beginning; the difference may simply be due to a rise in the 'background' reporting rate for all adverse reactions. Taking account of these possible sources of bias, both Rossi *et al.* (in relation to US data) and Bateman (for UK data) have published 'corrected' frequencies for individual NSAIDs (Bateman, 1996; Rossi *et al.*, 1987).

These data are summarized in Table 9.3. The crude reporting rates for serious gastro-intestinal reactions per million prescriptions written are generally higher in the United Kingdom than in the United States. This represents a true difference in the reporting rates for adverse drug reactions in general between the two countries. The corrected reporting rates for each country are very different, but this reflects the types of adjustments made by

CHAPTER 9

441

the authors. However, when the correct reporting rates are ranked, there is a similarity between the studies, with ibuprofen, diflunisal and fenoprofen tending to rank low for risk, while piroxican and tolmetin rank high. Ketoprofen and azapropazone ranked high for risk in the UK data, but the US data were not published in the paper by Rossi *et al.* The relationship of these rankings for risk of gastrointestinal toxicity to those obtained from epidemiological studies is considered later in this chapter.

9.3.4 Major controlled epidemiological studies of the risk of gastrointestinal complications with NSAIDs

From the results of the literature search, we identified controlled epidemiological studies that found a relationship between the use of NSAIDs in the community and the development of peptic ulcer complications necessitating admission to hospital (Somerville *et al.*, 1986; Carson *et al.*, 1987; Griffin *et al.*, 1991; Laporte *et al.*, 1991; Garcia-Rodriguez *et al.*, 1992; Nobili *et al.*, 1992; Abenhaim and Moride, 1993; Henry *et al.*, 1993; Kaufman *et al.*, 1993; Savage *et al.*, 1993; Garcia-Rodriguez and Jick, 1994; Langman *et al.*, 1994; Perez-Gutthann *et al.*, 1994). Some studies did not provide data on use of individual NSAIDs, failed to demonstrate the accepted association between NSAIDs and gastrointestinal damage, or did not meet current standards for epidemiological design or methods. These studies were excluded from further consideration. A list of these studies and reasons for their exclusion are available from the authors. The remaining studies were assessed by the following criteria: ascertainment and validation of study outcomes, selection and comparability of controls, ascertainment of exposure to NSAIDs, and control or adjustment for potential confounders. The results of this assessment are given in Tables 9.4 and 9.5.

From each paper we extracted the overall relative risk estimates for gastrointestinal bleeding, ulcer perforation or hospitalization with peptic ulceration for the group of NSAIDs that had been studied, and where given, how the estimated relative risks varied across different age groups, by sex, with different doses or durations of treatment, and according to the past history of peptic ulcer or its complications. Where both crude and multivariate relative risk estimates were provided, we used the adjusted data. Where data pooling seemed appropriate, studies were weighted according to the standard error of the natural logarithm of the adjusted odds ratio calculated from the confidence interval width, and were pooled using the random effects model of Der Simonian and Laird (1986). We then extracted the raw data relating to the use of *individual* NSAIDs by cases and controls. For the analysis of risk associated with use of individual drugs, we calculated for each study the odds ratio for each comparator drug, using exposure to ibuprofen (*rather than non-use of a NSAID*) as the reference category. Our other approach to the analysis was to attempt to find an order that best summarized the sequence of relative risks with all of the individual drugs that had been included in two or more studies, based on the rankings that were observed within the studies.

TABLE 9.4

Characteristics of the *ad hoc* epidemiological studies reviewed in this chapter

	Somerville et al. (1986)	Laporte et al. (1991)	Nobili et al. (1992)	Kaufman et al. (1993)	Savage et al. (1993)	Henry et al. (1993)	Langman et al. (1994)	Abenhaim and Moride (1993)
Study design	Matched case-control	Matched case-control	Matched case-control	Matched case-control	Matched case-control	Matched case-control	Matched case-control	Matched case-control
Study setting	Hospital-based, England	Multicentre hospital-based, Spain	Multicentre hospital-based, Italy	Multicentre hospital-based, International study	Hospital-based, New Zealand	Hospital-based, Australia	Multicentre hospital-based, UK	Hospital-based, Canada
Number of cases/controls	230/437 Aged ≥ 60 y	875/2682 All ages	441/1323 All ages	574/1159 Aged 18–79 y	494/972 All ages	644/1268 Aged ≥ 50 y	1144/2115 Aged ≥ 60 y	486/861 Aged ≥ 68 y
Outcome studied	Hospitalization with bleeding ulcers	Hospitalization with UGIB[a] due to ulcers or erosions	Hospitalization with UGIB	Hospitalization with major UGIB from stomach or duodenum	Hospitalization with UGIB or perforation	Hospitalization with UGIB or perforation	Hospitalization with bleeding ulcers	Hospitalization with UGIB or perforation
Ascertainment and validation of outcomes	Confirmed by endoscopy or surgery	Confirmed by endoscopy or surgery	Confirmed by endoscopy	Confirmed by endoscopy or radiology	Confirmed by endoscopy, surgery or autopsy	Confirmed by endoscopy or surgery	Confirmed by endoscopy or surgery	Outcomes verified by chart review
Selection and comparability of controls	Community and hospital controls. Matched for age and sex	Hospital controls. Matched for centre, age and sex	Hospital controls. Matched for hospital age and sex	Community and hospital controls. Matched for centre, age and sex	Hospital controls. Matched for age and sex	Hospital and community controls. Matched for age and sex	Community and hospital controls. Matched for centre, age and sex	Hospital controls. Matched for age and sex
Ascertainment of drug use and definition of exposure	Structured interview. Use within previous 7 days	Structured interview. Use within previous week	Structured interview. Use within previous week[b]	Structured interview. Use within previous week	Structured interview. Use within previous week	Structured interview. Use within previous week	Structured interview. Use within previous 3 months	Automated hospital prescription record. Exposure = record of supply that included index date

a UGIB, upper gastrointestinal bleeding.
b Used in analyses presented here.

TABLE 9.5

Characteristics of the epidemiological studies that used electronic record linkage or computerized medical records

	Carson et al. (1987)	Griffin et al. (1991)	Perez-Gutthann et al. (1994)	Garcia-Rodriguez et al. (1994)
Study design	Retrospective cohort study	Case-control study	Case-control study	Case-control study
Study setting	Record linkage, community-based, USA (Medicaid)	Record linkage, community-based, USA (Medicaid)	Record-linkage, community-based, Canada (Saskatchewan)	Computerized medical records, community-based, UK
Number of cases/controls	110 outcomes. All ages	1415/7063. Aged ≥ 65 y	1377/10 000. All ages	1457/10 000. Aged 25–79 y
Outcome studied	Hospitalization with ICD-9 codes compatible with UGIB[a]	Hospitalization with peptic ulcer or UGIB	Hospitalization with UGIB or perforation at gastric or duodenal sites	Hospitalization or referral with UGIB or perforation of stomach or duodenum
Ascertainment and validation of outcomes	ICD-9 codes only no validation of outcomes	Confirmed by endoscopy, radiology or surgery. Outcomes verified by chart review	Confirmed by endoscopy, radiology, surgery or autopsy. Outcomes verified by chart review	Outcomes verified by record review in a subsample
Selection and comparability of controls	Control group were a cohort of ibuprofen users. Analyses adjusted for age, sex and state	Stratified random community sample. Strata defined by age, sex, race and nursing home status	Random community sample. Analyses adjusted for age, sex and past history of ulcer	Random community sample. Analyses adjusted for age, sex, ulcer history and smoking
Ascertainment of drug use and definition of exposure	Automated prescription database. Exposure time window 1 month	Automated prescription database. 'Current use' = record of supply that included index date	Automated prescription database. 'Current use' = prescription filled in the month before the index date	Computerized medical record. Exposure = record of supply that included the index date.

[a] UGIB, upper gastrointestinal bleeding.

9.3.5   Design features

Twelve studies that reported relative risks of gastrointestinal complications with a total of 14 NSAIDs, and satisfied our criteria for inclusion, were identified through our literature search (Tables 9.4, 9.5). Twelve NSAIDs had been included in two or more studies and 11 studies provided comparative data on ibuprofen and other NSAIDs (Somerville *et al.*, 1986; Carson *et al.*, 1987; Griffin *et al.*, 1991; Laporte *et al.*, 1991; Garcia-Rodriguez *et al.*, 1992; Nobili *et al.*, 1992; Abenhaim and Moride, 1993; Henry *et al.*, 1993; Kaufman *et al.*, 1993; Savage *et al.*, 1993; Langman *et al.*, 1994; Garcia-Rodriguez and Jick, 1994; Perez-Gutthann *et al.*, 1994). Two reports were unpublished at the time of writing; one was an update and re-analysis of a previously published paper, the other has been published only as an abstract. Another two studies were updated by the authors at the investigators' workshop or in subsequent correspondence. All but one paper described case-control studies; 3 of the 12 employed linkage of administrative records, and one used computerized medical records. These designs have the advantage that the prescription record is created prior to the outcome, minimizing measurement biases. Comprehensive databases can provide estimates of incidence, and reduce selection biases, because all cases in the population are included. Such databases also act as a source of community controls, who can be selected randomly, thus avoiding some of the problems associated with finding an appropriate control group. However, the definition of exposure is based on a record of prescription, rather than consumption of the drugs of interest, and use of non-prescription drugs, cigarettes and alcohol is usually not recorded. Another potential weakness of these designs is reliance on recorded diagnoses. The inaccuracy of ICD coding of Medicaid patients in the United States has been a concern with all epidemiological studies that have relied on this data source.

All of the '*ad hoc*' studies employed classical case-finding techniques with diagnostic confirmation of case status, and ascertainment of prior drug use by structured interview. Controls in these studies were recruited from the community or from the same hospitals as the cases. Time windows for exposure also varied across the studies, from 1 week up to 3 months. The most common exposure period was 1 week.

9.3.6   Investigation of class effects

Despite quite marked variations in design and conduct, the overall results of these studies were very similar. Where they had been calculated, estimated overall relative risks (RR) of complications with use of NSAIDs lay mainly in the range 3–5. These results are consistent with the findings of meta-analyses published previously (Gabriel *et al.*, 1991; Bollini *et al.*, 1992).

There appeared to be no important difference between the results of the studies that used record linkage, or computerized medical records, and those that used traditional methods for case-finding and ascertainment of exposure (Tables 9.6 and 9.7).

CHAPTER 9

TABLE 9.6

Overall results of 'ad hoc' case-control studies

	Somerville et al. (1986)	Laporte et al. (1991)	Nobili et al. (1992)	Kaufman et al. (1993)	Savage et al. (1993)	Henry et al. (1993)	Langman et al. (1994)	Abenhaim and Moride (1993)
Overall relative risk (95% CI) NANSAID only[a]	2.7[b] (1.7–4.4) 3.8[b] (2.2–6.4)	NA	NA	NA	4.1 (2.8–5.9)	3.0 (2.3–3.8)	4.5 (3.6–5.6)	3.0 (2.2–4.1)
Effect of age on relative risk (95% CI)	NA	≤60 y 17.4 (9.3–32.6) >60 y 7.6 (4.8–12.2)[c]	<65 y 3.6 (2.2–5.9) ≥65 y 8.3 (4.9–14.0)	NA	<65 y 3.2 (1.9–5.4) 65+ y 6.2 (4.3–8.9)	<59 y 2.0 (1.2–3.4) 60–79 y 3.0 (2.2–4.0) 80+ y 4.2 (2.3–7.6)	60–69 y 4.2 (2.7–6.4) 70–79 y 4.4 (3.1–6.2) 80+ y 4.8 (3.2–7.3)	NA
Effect of duration of therapy on relative risk (95% CI)	NA	NA	NA	NA	NA	≤28 days 6.3 (3.5–11.3) >28 days 2.5 (2.0–3.3)	≤1 month 9.6 (5.5–16.8) ≥3 month 3.8 (2.9–5.1)	NA
Importance of dose on relative risk (95% CI)	NA	NA	NA	NA	NA	Lowest 2.1 (1.2–3.6) Highest 4.0 (2.6–6.1)	Lowest 2.5 (1.7–3.8) Medium 4.5 (3.3–6.0) Highest 8.6 (5.8–12.6)	NA
Previous ulcer history	NA	Yes 7.4 (2.4–23.0) No 8.0 (2.9–7.3)	Excluded subjects with previous history of ulcer	Excluded subjects with previous history of ulcer or UGIB	Yes 2.2 (1.4–3.6) No 6.7 (4.6–9.6)[c]	Yes 2.0 (1.5–2.8) No 3.3 (2.4–4.6)	NA	NA

[a] NANSAID, non-aspirin nonsteroidal anti-inflammatory drugs.
[b] Calculated from community and hospital controls, respectively.
[c] Estimated from authors' data.
NA, not available.

TABLE 9.7

Overall results of studies that used record-linkage or computerized medical records

	Carson et al. (1987)	Griffin et al. (1991)	Perez-Gutthann et al. (1994)	Garcia-Rodriguez et al. (1994)
Overall relative risk (95% CI)	NA	4.1 (3.5–4.7)	4.3 (3.7–5.0)	4.7 (3.8–5.7)
Effect of age on relative risk (95% CI)	NA	65–74 y 3.8 (3.0–5.0) 75–84 y 4.2 (3.4–5.2) 85+ y 4.3 (3.3–5.7)	15–59 y M 4.9 F 5.3 60–79 y M 4.1 F 5.0 80+ y M 2.9 F 6.5	<60 y 4.7 >60 y 4.7
Effect of duration of therapy on relative risk (95% CI)	NA	≤30 days 7.2 (4.9–10.5) 31–90 days 3.7 (2.7–5.2) 90+ days 3.9 (3.3–4.6)	1 pres 4.5 (3.5–5.7) 2–3 pres 4.4 (3.2–6.0) 4–6 pres 5.2 (3.7–7.3) 7–12 pres 3.7 (2.6–5.3) 12+ pres 2.9 (2.1–3.9)	1 pres 4.0 (2.7–6.1) 2–3 pres 3.2 (1.7–6.1) 4–6 pres 2.8 (1.3–6.0) 7–12 pres 6.7 (3.9–11.4) 13+ pres 6.4 (4.0–10.2)
Importance of dose	NA	Lowest 2.8 (1.8–4.3) Highest 8.0 (4.4–14.8)	Low 2.9 (2.2–3.8) Medium 4.2 (3.4–5.2) High 5.8 (4.0–8.6)	*Low dose* 1–6 pres 2.3 (1.4–3.7) ≥7 pres 3.8 (2.2–6.8) *High dose* 1–6 pres 5.4 (3.5–8.4) ≥7 pres 9.3 (5.9–14.8)
Previous ulcer history	NA	NA	No 4.6 (3.9–5.4) Yes 2.6 (1.7–4.0)	No 5.1 (4.1–6.3) Yes 2.8 (1.9–4.2)

F, female; M, male; pres, prescriptions.

All of the studies controlled or adjusted for age, eliminating the effect of this variable as a potential confounder. However, stratified analyses were conducted in several studies to determine whether age modified the effects of NSAIDs. Age was not found to be consistently associated with an increase in the estimated relative risk of upper gastrointestinal complications with NSAIDs. Three studies found that RR increased with age, while four found no effect of age, and one study found the RR to be lower in the older age group. Comparable data-sets could not be extracted from the studies and it was felt that pooling of the data on age would not be informative. Similarly, no consistent relationship was found between sex and RR with any NSAID (data not shown).

There was no evidence of confounding by ingestion of non-prescription aspirin, or use of cigarettes or alcohol in the '*ad hoc*' studies that collected this information.

Information on the relationship between a history of previous ulceration and the magnitude of the relative risk associated with use of any NSAID was obtained from five studies (Tables 9.6 and 9.7). The pooled relative risk in subjects with a previous history of ulcer or complications was 2.5 (1.9–3.2), compared with 4.9 (4.0–6.1) in subjects with no prior history.

The importance of duration of therapy was obtained from five studies (Tables 9.6 and 9.7). Consumption of NSAIDs for 1 month or less was associated with a pooled relative risk of 5.7 (4.3–7.7), compared with a pooled RR of 3.9 (3.3–4.5) with use for more than 1 month.

A positive relationship between the dose of NSAID taken and the relative risk of upper gastrointestinal complications was seen in all six studies that provided relevant data (Tables 9.6 and 9.7). Comparative and extractable data were available from five of the studies. Categorization of dosage was arbitrary. The pooled relative risk for the lowest category of dose used in each study was 2.7 (2.3–3.2), significantly lower than the relative risk with the highest dose category, 6.5 (5.0–8.5).

9.3.7 Relative risk of upper gastrointestinal complications with use of individual NSAIDs

The point estimates for the relative risks of serious gastrointestinal complications with the individual NSAIDs are given in Figure 9.2. There was a wide distribution of results, and the graphical display suggests that real differences exist between the drugs.

The pooled odds ratios for individual NSAIDs, calculated with exposure to ibuprofen as the reference, are given in Figure 9.3. The different numbers of studies that contributed to the analyses reflect their variable coverage of individual drugs. In each case the pooled odds ratio for exposure to the comparator, compared with exposure to ibuprofen, was significantly greater than 1. The data reviewed here indicate that the comparator drugs are associated with a 1.6-fold to 9.2-fold increase in the odds of serious upper gastrointestinal complications, compared with ibuprofen. These analyses include no adjustments for potential confounding factors as they were based on the authors' raw data.

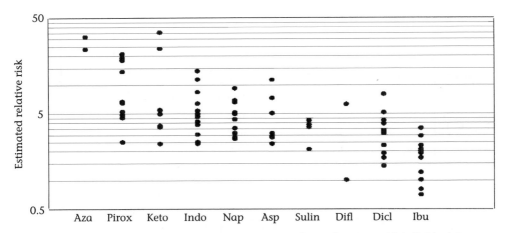

Figure 9.2: Estimated relative risks of major gastrointestinal complications with individual drugs (calculated with non-use of NSAIDs as the reference). Aza, azapropazone; Pirox, piroxicam; Keto, ketoprofen; Indo, indomethacin; Nap, naproxen; Asp, aspirin; Sulin, sulindac; Difl, diflunisal; Dicl, diclofenac; Ibu, ibuprofen.

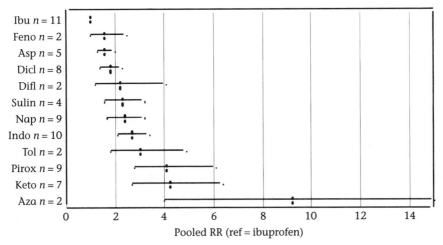

Figure 9.3: Estimated relative risks of major gastrointestinal complications with individual drugs. Abbreviations as in Figure 9.2; Feno, fenoprofen; Tol, tolmetin.

Figure 9.4 provides the summary statistics obtained using the ranking method. Drugs that appeared in two or more studies were included in the analysis to obtain a weighted summary order of the NSAIDs, according to relative risk. Twelve orderings achieved equal highest score. Ibuprofen ranked lowest on RR, diclofenac was next, and the data for the other drugs are summarized in Figure 9.4. An idea of the stability of each drug's position in the 12 top-scoring orderings can be obtained from a comparison of its highest and lowest values given in the figure. The values for fenoprofen seem unstable, probably owing to the fact that it was included in only two studies. The positions of the remaining NSAIDs

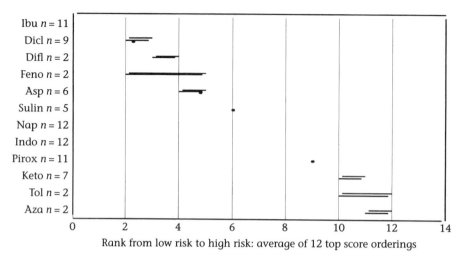

Figure 9.4: Estimated relative risks of major gastrointestinal complications with individual drugs: summary ranking method. Abbreviations as in Figures 9.2 and 9.3.

seem fairly stable, although the data from diflunisal, tolmetin and azapropazone must be treated with caution in view of the small numbers of contributing studies.

9.3.8 Relationship between drug half-life and relative risk of gastrointestinal complications

The results of these analyses are summarized in Table 9.8. In the first analysis (base case) we used the published half-life $(t_{1/2})$ for aspirin (around 30 min), and the quoted $t_{1/2}$ for the conventional formulation of ketoprofen. The correlation coefficient under these assumptions was 0.3692. This improved to 0.5038 when we used the published $t_{1/2}$ value for salicylic acid instead of aspirin, and the published $t_{1/2}$ value for sustained release ketoprofen rather than that for the conventional formulation. In the second sensitivity analysis we substituted the $t_{1/2}$ value of the sulfide metabolite of sulindac for that of the parent drug, but this made little further difference. Generally, the correlation coefficients were some-what unstable, indicating the sensitivity of these analyses to the underlying assumptions about which half-life estimates should be used. However the coefficients were significantly different from zero at the 10% significance level in all three studies.

9.3.9 Analysis by dosage of individual NSAIDs

Data on the distribution of relative risks according to the dose of the individual NSAIDs were available from five studies. Sample sizes were rather small, effectively limiting com-parisons to the commonly used NSAIDs. Extractable comparative data were available from five studies relating to three NSAIDs, ibuprofen, naproxen and indomethacin. Using the

TABLE 9.8

Comparison of ranking of individual NSAIDs by relative risk and by plasma half-life

Comparator	Rank by relative risk[a] (from lowest to highest RR)	Plasma half-lives (h)[b]		
		Main analysis	Sensitivity analysis 1	Sensitivity analysis 2
Ibuprofen	1	2.0	2.0	2.0
Diclofenac	2	1.5	1.5	1.5
Diflunisal	3	10.8	10.8	10.8
Fenoprofen	4	2.2	2.2	2.2
Aspirin	5	0.5	4.5	4.5
Sulindac	6	7.8	7.8	16.4
Naproxen	7	14.0	14.0	14.0
Indomethacin	8	3.8	3.8	3.8
Piroxicam	9	48.0	48.0	48.0
Ketoprofen	10	2.0	8.5	8.5
Tolmetin	11	6.8	6.8	6.8
Azapropazone	12	22.0	22.0	22.0
	Rank correlation Kendall's Tau	0.3692	0.5038	0.4733
	(p-value)	(0.0947)	(0.0226)	(0.0322)

[a] The ranking by relative risk was obtained from the results of the summary ranking procedure and the plasma half-life values were those published in reference texts.
[b] In the main analysis we used the $t_{1/2}$ for aspirin (rather than salicylic acid) and for ketoprofen in its conventional formulation. In sensitivity analysis 1 we used the $t_{1/2}$ for salicylic acid and the $t_{1/2}$ for ketoprofen in its sustained release formulation. Sensitivity analysis 2 was as for sensitivity analysis 1 except that we substituted the $t_{1/2}$ for the sulfide metabolite of sulindac for that of the parent drug.

arbitrary dose stratifications chosen by the authors (see Methods), the following pooled relative risks were obtained: 'Low dose': ibuprofen 1.6 (0.8–3.2), naproxen 3.7 (1.7–7.7) and indomethacin 3.0 (2.2–4.2). 'High dose': ibuprofen 4.2 (1.8–9.8), naproxen 6.0 (3.0–12.2) and indomethacin 7.0 (4.4–11.2). These data are presented graphically in Figure 9.5.

9.3.10 Other epidemiological studies

In addition to the classical epidemiological studies reviewed above, a major contribution has come from Jim Fries and his colleagues at Stanford University Medical Center. For many years they have been conducting analyses on data held in the Arthritis, Rheumatism and Ageing Medical Information System (ARAMIS). This database has been used over the last 20 years to measure the outcomes of treatment in patients with a range of rheumatic diseases. The data held relate to 17 000 subjects from 17 centres in the United States and Canada, with osteoarthritis, rheumatoid arthritis and other rheumatic disorders. Fries and colleagues have used the data to define the risk factors for development of serious toxicity from NSAIDs. Their main toxicity index includes measures of damage to different body systems, including the gastrointestinal tract, the skin, bone

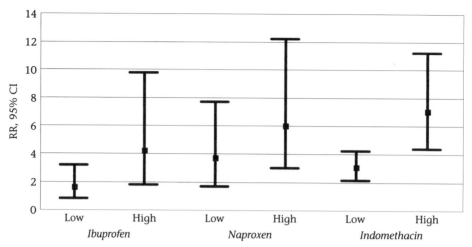

Figure 9.5: Effects of dose on relative risk of gastrointestinal complications with individual NSAIDs (calculated with non-use of NSAIDs as the reference).

marrow, kidneys and liver. However, they have also provided a separate report of gastrointestinal toxicity based on the number of hospitalizations with gastrointestinal disorders. These data are included in Table 9.8, which summarizes the rank order of risk for a different set of 10 NSAIDs derived from the various data sets reviewed earlier in this chapter.

As can be seen from Table 9.8, there is similarity in the rank order of gastrointestinal toxicity assessed by a variety of different methods. In constructing Table 9.8 we have used the rank order of risk from the major controlled epidemiological studies as the 'benchmark', and compared the ranks derived by Fries *et al.* from the endoscopic studies, and from the analysis of voluntary reports of adverse reactions in the United Kingdom and the United States. There is considerable similarity in these ranks. Ibuprofen is always at the lower end of the toxicity rating, whereas piroxicam and ketoprofen tend to appear at the higher end of the toxicity range. Diflunisal also tends to rank low for risk, although the position of diclofenac is somewhat variable. Sulindac ranks well in the studies of Fries *et al.*, and in the endoscopic studies but tends to hold the middle order in the epidemiological studies and voluntary adverse reaction reports. Naproxen and indomethacin tend to rank close together, with indomethacin appearing to have a somewhat higher risk rating. Tolmetin and azapropozone tend to rank poorly, with the latter having the worst rating.

It should be noted that aspirin does not appear in this summary table. In the early endoscopic ratings it invariably rates poorly, but the doses used were much higher than in modern clinical practice. In the lower doses used in modern epidemiological studies it has a middle order rank. However, there is no doubting the level of gastrointestinal toxicity that it induces when used in high doses.

9.4 CONCLUSIONS

There is a surprising degree of consistency in the findings of different studies regarding the relative gastrointestinal toxicity of ibuprofen. In doses of 1600 mg or less it has been associated with a lower degree of toxicity than other NSAIDs, and this has been consistent across the endoscopic studies, the analyses of voluntary adverse reaction reports, and the major controlled epidemiological studies. However, there is also evidence that, when used in doses of 2400 mg or more, it has a similar toxicity to other commonly used drugs, such as naproxen and indomethacin. The data reviewed here support the use of ibuprofen in a dose of 1600 mg/day as the preferred first-line therapy for patients who need moderate potency analgesic and anti-inflammatory drug therapy.

REFERENCES

AABAKKEN, L., LARSEN, S. and OSNES, M. (1990) Visual analogue skills for endoscopic evaluation of non-steroidal anti-inflammatory drug-induced mucosal damage in the stomach and duodenum. *Scandinavian Journal of Gastroenterology* 25, 443–448.

ABENHAIM, L. and MORIDE, Y. (1993) The effect of baseline susceptibility on the relative gastrotoxicity of individual NSAIDs in the elderly: a study with the Quebec database. Paper presented at the IXth International Conference on Pharmacoepidemiology, Washington DC, 1993.

BATEMAN, D.N. (1996) Re-evaluation of gut toxicity of NSAIDs. In: VANE, J. and BOTTING, R. (eds), *Improved Non-steroidal Anti-inflammatory Drugs. COX-2 Enzyme Inhibitors.* London, William Harvey Press/Dordrecht, Kluwer Academic Publishers, 189–201.

BERGMANN, J.S., CHASSANY, O., GENEVE, J., AVITEBOUL, M., CAULIN, C. and SEGRESTAA, J.M. (1992) Endoscopic evaluation of the effects of ketoprofen, ibuprofen, and aspirin on the gastroduodenal mucosa. *European Journal of Clinical Pharmacology* 42, 685–688.

BOLLINI, P., GARCIA-RODRIGUEZ, L.A., PEREZ-GUTTHANN, S. and WALKER, A.M. (1992) The impact of research quality and study design on epidemiological estimates of the effect of nonsteroidal anti-inflammatory drugs on upper gastrointestinal tract disease. *Archives of Internal Medicine* 152(6), 1289–1292.

CALES, P., ZABOTTO, B. and MESKENS, C. *et al.* (1990) Gastroesophageal endoscopical features in psoriasis, observer variability, interassociations in relationship to hepatic dysfunction. *Gastroenterology* 98, 156–162.

CARSON, J.L., STORM, B.L. and MORSE, M.L. *et al.* (1987) The relative gastrointestinal toxicity of the non-steroidal anti-inflammatory drugs. *Archives of Internal Medicine* 147, 1054–1059.

CARUSO, I. and BIANCHI PORRO, G. (1980) Gastroscopic evaluation of anti-inflammatory agents. *British Medical Journal* 280(6207), 75–78.

CLIVE, D.M. and STOFF, J.S. (1984) Renal syndromes associated with nonsteroidal anti-inflammatory drugs. *New England Journal of Medicine* **310**, 563–572.

COCH, N., DEZI, A., FERRARIO, S. and CAPURSO, I. (1996) Prevention of non-steroidal anti-inflammatory drug-induced gastrointestinal mucosal injury. A meta-analysis of randomised control clinical trials. *Archives of Internal Medicine* **56**(20), 2321–2322.

DER SIMONIAN, R. and LAIRD, N. (1986) Meta-analysis and clinical trials. *Controlled Clinical Trials* **7**, 177–188.

DOUTHWAITE, A.H. and LINTOTT, G.A.M. (1938) Gastroscopic observation of the effect of aspirin and certain other substances on the stomach. *Lancet* **2**, 1222–1225.

EL-ASSI, M.T., GENTA, R.M., KARTTUNEN, T.J. and GRAHAM, E.Y. (1996) Ulcer site and complications: relation to *Helicobacter pylori* infection and NSAID use. *Endoscopy* **28**(2), 229–233.

ELLIOT, S.L., YEOMANS, N.D., BUCHANAN, R.R. and SMALLWOOD, R.A. (1994) Efficacy of twelve months misoprostol as prophylaxis against NSAID-induced gastric ulcers. A placebo controlled trial. *Scandinavian Journal of Rheumatology* **23**(4), 171–176.

FRIEDMAN, H., SECKMAN, C.E., LANZA, F., ROYER, G., PERRY, K. and FRANCOM, S. (1990) Clinical pharmacology of pre-disintegrated ibuprofen 800 mg tablets: an endoscopic and pharmacokinetic study. *Journal of Clinical Pharmacology* **30**, 57–63.

FRIES, J. (1996) Toward an understanding of NSAID-related adverse events: The contribution of longitudinal data. *Scandinavian Journal of Rheumatology* **25**(Suppl. 102), 3–8.

FRIES, J.F., WILLIAMS, C.A. and BLOCH, D.A. (1991a) The relative toxicity of non-steroidal anti-inflammatory drug. *Arthritis and Rheumatism* **34**(11), 1353–1360.

FRIES, J.F., WILLIAMS, C.A., BLOCH, D.A. MICHEL, B.A. (1991b) Non-steroidal anti-inflammatory drug associated gastropathy: incidence and risk factor models. *American Journal of Medicine* **91**, 213–222.

GABRIEL, S.E., JAAKKIMAINEN, L. and BOMBARDIER, C. (1991) Risk for serious gastrointestinal complications related to use of nonsteroidal anti-inflammatory drugs. A meta-analysis. *Annals of Internal Medicine* **115**(10), 787–796.

GARCIA-RODRIGUEZ, L.A., WALKER, L.A.M. and PEREZ-GUTTHANN, S. (1992) Nonsteroidal anti-inflammatory drugs and gastrointestinal hospitalizations in Saskatchewan: a cohort study. *Epidemiology* **3**(4), 337–342.

GARCIA-RODRIGUEZ, L.A. and JICK, H. (1994) Risk of upper gastrointestinal bleeding and perforation associated with individual non-steroidal anti-inflammatory drugs. *Lancet* **343**, 769–772.

GRAHAM, D.Y. (1996) Non-steroidal anti-inflammatory drugs, *Helicobacter pylori*, and ulcers: where we stand. *American Journal of Gastroenterology* **92**(10), 2080–2086.

GRAHAM, D.Y., AGRAWAL, N.M. and ROTH, S.H. (1988) Prevention of NSAID-induced gastric ulcer with misoprostol: multicentre, double-blind, placebo-controlled trial. *Lancet* **2**(8623), 1277–1280.

GRAHAM, D.Y., WHITE, R.H. and MOERLAND, L.W. *et al.* (1993) Duodenal and gastric ulcer prevention with misoprostol in arthritis patients taking NSAIDs. Misoprostol study group. *Annals of Internal Medicine* **119**(4), 157–262.

GRIFFIN, M.R., PIPER, J.M., DAUGHERTY, J.R., SNOWDEN, M. and RAY, W.A. (1991) Non-steroidal anti-inflammatory drug use and increased risk for peptic ulcer disease in elderly persons. *Annals of Internal Medicine* **114**(4), 257–263.

GYÖMBER, E., VATTAY, P., SZABO, S. and RAINSFORD, K.D. (1996) Role of early vascular damage in the pathogenesis of gastric haemorrhagic mucosal lesions induced by indomethacin in rats. *International Journal of Experimental Pathology* **77**(1), 1–6.

HAWKEY, C.J. (1996) Non-steroidal anti-inflammatory drug gastropathy: causes and treatment. *Scandinavian Journal of Gastroenterology* **220**(Suppl.), 124–127.

HENRY, D.A. and LANGMAN, M.J.S. (1981) Drugs as gastric irritants. In: DYKES, P.W. and KEIGHLEY, M.R.V. (eds), *Drugs as Gastric Irritants*. Bristol, John Wright and Sons, 49–59.

HENRY, D., DOBSON, A. and TURNER, C. (1993) Variability in the risk of major gastrointestinal complications from non-aspirin nonsteroidal anti-inflammatory drugs. *Gastroenterology* **105**(4), 1078–1088.

HENRY, D., LIM, L. and GARCIA RODRIGUEZ, L.A. *et al.* (1996) Variability in risk of major upper gastrointestinal complications with individual NSAIDs: results of a collaborative meta-analysis. *British Medical Journal* **312**, 1563–1566.

HUDSON, M., EVERITT, S. and HAWKEY, C.J. (1994) Interobserver variation in assessment of gastroduodenal lesions association with non-steroidal anti-inflammatory drugs. *Gut* **35**, 1030–1032.

JANSSEN, M., DUJKMANS, B.A., LAMERS, C.B., ZWINDERMAN, A.H. and VAN DEN BROUCKE, J.P. (1994) A gastroscopic study of the predictive value of risk factors for non-steroidal anti-inflammatory drugs and associated ulcer disease in rheumatoid arthritis. *British Journal of Rheumatology* **35**(5), 449–454.

KAUFMAN, W., KELLY, J.P. and SHEEHAN, J.E. (1993) Nonsteroidal anti-inflammatory drug use in relation to major upper gastrointestinal bleeding. *Clinical Pharmacology and Therapeutics* **53**(4), 485–494.

LAINE, L. (1996) Non-steroidal anti-inflammatory drug gastropathy. *Gastrointestinal Endoscopy Clinics of North America* **6**(3), 489–504.

LAINE, L., COMINELLI, F., SLOANE, R., CASINI-RIGGI, V., MARIN-SORENSEN, M. and WEINSTEIN, W.M. (1995a) Interaction of NSAIDs and *Helicobacter pylori* on gastrointestinal injury and prostaglandin production: a controlled double-blind trial. *Alimentary Pharmacology and Therapeutics* **9**(2), 127–135.

CHAPTER 9

LAINE, L., SLOANE, R., FERRETI, M. and COMINELLI, F. (1995b) A randomised double-blind comparison of placebo, etodolac, and naproxen on gastrointestinal injury and prostaglandin production. *Gastrointestinal Endoscopy* **42**, 429–433.

LANGMAN, M.J.S. (1970) Epidemiological evidence for the association of aspirin and cute gastrointestinal bleeding. *Gut* **11**, 627–634.

LANGMAN, M.J.S., SPIRO, H.M. and INGELFINGER, S.J. (1974) Aspirin and the stomach. In: INGELFINGER, F.J., EBERT, R.V. and FINLAND, M. (eds), *Controversy and Internal Medicine 11*. Philadelphia: WE Saunders, 491–510.

LANGMAN, M.J.S., WEIL, J. and WAINRIGHT, P. (1994) Risks of bleeding peptic ulcer associated with individual non-steroidal anti-inflammatory drugs. *Lancet* **343**, 1075–1078.

LANZA, F.L. (1984) Endoscopic studies of gastric and duodenal injury after the use of ibuprofen, aspirin and other non-steroidal anti-inflammatory agents. *American Journal of Medicine* **77**(1A), 19–24.

LANZA, F., RACK, M.F., LYNN, M., WOLF, J. and SANDA, M. (1986) An endoscopic comparison of the effects of otodolac, indomethacin, ibuprofen, naproxen, and placebo on the gastrointestinal mucosa. *Journal of Rheumatology* **14**, 338–341.

LANZA, F.L., GRAHAM, D.Y., DAVIS, R.E. and RACK, M.F. (1990) Endoscopic comparison of cimetidine and sucralfate for the prevention of naproxen-induced acute gastroduodenal injury. *Digestive Diseases and Sciences* **35**(12), 494–999.

LANZA, F., ROYER, G. and NELSON, R. (1975) An endoscopic evaluation of the effects of non-steroidal anti-inflammatory drugs on the gastric mucosa. *Journal of Gastrointestinal Endoscopy* **21**(3), 103–105.

LANZA, F.L., ROYER, G.L., NELSON, R.S., CHEG, T.T., SECKMAN, C.E. and RACK, M.F. (1979) The effects of ibuprofen indomethacin aspirin naproxen and placebo on the gastric mucosa of normal volunteers. *Digestive Diseases and Sciences* **24**(11), 823–828.

LANZA, F.L., ROYER, G.L., NELSON, R.S., CHEG, T.T., SECKMAN, C.E. and RACK, M.F. (1981) A comparative endoscopic evaluation of the damaging effects of non-steroidal anti-inflammatory agents on the gastric and duodenal mucosa. *American Journal of Gastroenterology* **75**(1), 17–21.

LAPORTE, J.R., CARNE, X., VIDAL, X., MORENO, V. and JUAN, J. (1991) Upper gastrointestinal bleeding in relation to previous use of analgesics and non-steroidal anti-inflammatory drugs. Catalan countries study on upper gastrointestinal bleeding. *Lancet* **337**(8733), 85–89.

LIPSCOMBE, G.R., WALLIS, N., ARMSTRONG, G., GOODMAN, M.J. and REECE, W.D. (1995) Gastric mucosal adaptation to etodolac and naproxen. *Alimentary Pharmacology and Therapeutics* **9**(4), 379–385.

LIPSCOMBE, G.R., WALLIS, M., ARMSTRONG, G., GOODMAN, M.J. and REES, W.D. (1996) Influence of *Helicobacter pylori* on gastric mucosal adaptations to naproxen in man. *Digestive Diseases and Sciences* **41**(8), 1583–1588.

META, S., DASARATHY, S., TANDON, R.K., MATHUR, M. and MALAVIYA, A.N. (1992) A prospective randomised study of the injurious effects of aspirin and naproxen on the gastroduodenal mucosa in patients with rheumatoid arthritis. *American Journal of Gastroenterology* **87**(8), 996–1000.

MUIR, A. and COSSAR, I.A. (1955) Aspirin and ulcer. *British Medical Journal* 2, 7–12.

NOBILI, A., MOSCONI, P., FRANZOSI, M.G. and TOGNONI, G. (1992) Non-steroidal anti-inflammatory drugs and upper gastrointestinal bleeding, a post-marketing surveillance case-control study. *Pharmacoepidemiology and Drug Safety* 1, 65–72.

PEREZ-GUTTHANN, S., GARCIA-RODRIGUEZ, L.A. and RAIFORD, D.S. (1994) Individual non-steroidal anti-inflammatory drugs and the risk of hospitalization for upper gastrointestinal bleeding and perforation in Saskatchewan: a nested case-control study. I. *Pharmacoepidemiology and Drug Safety* 3(Suppl. 1), S63.

PORROW, G.B., MONTRONE, F., PETRILLO, M., CARUSO, I. and IMBESSI, V. (1995) Gastro-duodenal tolerability of nabumetone versus naproxen in the treatment of rheumatic patients. *American Journal of Gastroenterology* **90**(9), 1485–1488.

RASKIN, J.B., WHITE, R.H. and JACKSON, J.E. *et al.* (1995) Misoprostol dosage in the prevention of nonsteroidal anti-inflammatory drug-induced and duodenal ulcers: a comparison of three regimens. *Annals of Internal Medicine* **123**(5), 344–350.

ROSSI, A.C., HSU, J.P. and FAICH, G.A. (1987) Ulcerogenicity of piroxicam: an analysis of spontaneously reported data. *British Medical Journal* **294**(6565), 147–150.

ROTH, S.H., TINDALL, E.A. and JAIN, A.K. (1993) A controlled study comparing the effects of nabumetone ibuprofen plus misoprostol on the upper gastrointestinal tract mucosa. *Archives of Internal Medicine* **153**, 2565–2571.

SANTUCCI, L., FIORUCCI, S., PATOIA, L., DI MATTEO, F.M., BRUNORI, P.M. and MORELLI, A. (1995) Severe gastric mucosal damage induced by NSAIDs in healthy subjects associated with *Helicobacter pylori* infection and high levels of serum pepsinogens. *Digestive Diseases and Sciences* **40**(9), 2074–2080.

SAVAGE, R.L., MOLLER, P.W., BALLANTYNE, C.L. and WELLS, J. (1993) Variation in the risk of peptic ulcer complications with nonsteroidal anti-inflammatory drug therapy. *Arthritis and Rheumatism* **36**(1), 84–90.

SILVERSTEIN, F.E., GRAHAM, D.Y. and SENIOR, J.R. *et al.* (1995) Misoprostol reduces serious gastrointestinal complications in patients with rheumatoid arthritis receiving non-steroidal anti-inflammatory drugs. A randomised double-blind placebo controlled trial. *Annals of Internal Medicine* **123**(4), 241–249.

CHAPTER 9

SOMERVILLE, K., FAULKNER, G. and LANGMAN, M. (1986) Non-steroidal anti-inflammatory drugs in bleeding peptic ulcer. *Lancet* **1**, 462–464.

SONNENBERG, A., GIGER, M. and KERN, L. *et al.* (1979) How reliable is determination of ulcer size by endoscopy? *British Medical Journal* **2**, 1322–1324.

SVANES, C., OVREBOK, K. and SOREIDE, O. (1996) Ulcer bleeding and perforation: non-steroidal anti-inflammatory drugs or *Helicobacter pylori*. *Scandinavian Journal of Gastroenterology* **220**(Suppl.), 128–131.

TAHA, A.S., DAHILL, S., STURROCK, R.D., LEE, F.D. and RUSSELL, R.I. (1994) Predicting NSAID-related ulcers — assessment of clinical and pathological factors and importance of differences in NSAID. *Gut* **35**(7), 891–895.

TAHA, A.S., STURROCK, R.D. and RUSSELL, R.I. (1995) Mucosal erosions in long-term non-steroidal anti-inflammatory drug users: predisposition to ulceration and relation to *Helicobacter pylori*. *Gut* **36**(3), 334–336.

VANE, J.R. and BOTTING, R.M. (1997) Mechanism of action of aspirin-like drugs. *Seminars in Arthritis and Rheumatism* **26**(6 Suppl. 1), 2–10.

Renal Effects of Ibuprofen

M D MURRAY[1]* AND D CRAIG BRATER[2]

[1]Regenstrief Institute, Regenstrief Health Center, Indianapolis, Indiana,
USA and Purdue Pharmacy Programs, Purdue University School of
Pharmacy, Indianapolis, Indiana, USA
[2]Clinical Pharmacology Division, Department of Medicine,
Indiana University School of Medicine, Indianapolis, Indiana, USA

Contents

10.1 INTRODUCTION

NSAIDs can produce either acute, reversible or permanent renal toxicity and a variety of effects on electrolyte and water homeostasis (Clive and Stoff, 1984; Murray and Brater, 1993). Ibuprofen has been implicated in practically every type of renal disorder known to be caused by NSAIDs (Kleinknecht, 1993; Marasco *et al.*, 1987), but severe or irreversible toxicities are rare. These renal syndromes include acute ischemic renal insufficiency, alterations in sodium and water homeostasis, oedema and increased blood pressure, hyporeninemic-hypoaldosteronism, interstitial nephritis, papillary necrosis as well as other miscellaneous drug interactions from its renal effects. This chapter describes ibuprofen's role in these disorders and risk factors for their development.

In the United States, ibuprofen is the most commonly prescribed NSAID. It has accounted for 29% of all prescriptions for NSAIDs between 1991 and 1995 (IMS America, 1996). Each year during this period there were more than 20 million prescriptions written for the drug, with retail sales exceeding US$220 million. Moreover, since 1984, ibuprofen has been the leading nonsalicylate over-the-counter (OTC) NSAID. One popular ibuprofen product alone (Advil ®) held 13% of the $2.7 billion OTC analgesic market (*The Northern New Jersey Record*, 1995).

Given the widespread use of ibuprofen and the likelihood that it causes a variety of renal syndromes, the impact of these renal effects may be enormous. Notwithstanding, it is interesting to note that warnings to consumers of the effects of ibuprofen on the kidney cannot be found in the consumer literature accompanying the product (Bennett *et al.*, 1996) despite a number of attempts to implement a consumer warning in the accompanying OTC product labelling. (Ad Hoc Committee for the National Kidney Foundation, 1985; Bennett *et al.*, 1996)

Upon its introduction in the United Kingdom in 1967 and in the United States in 1974, there was little mention of the renal effects of ibuprofen (Kantor, 1979). Attention was mostly directed to the lower incidence of gastrointestinal toxicity of ibuprofen compared to aspirin and other available alternatives (Dornan and Regnolds, 1974; Blechman *et al.*, 1975; Lewis, 1976) and its central nervous system and ocular effects (Davies and Avery, 1971). Much attention was also paid to the lack of hepatic toxicity of ibuprofen. (Adams *et al.*, 1970). The focus upon the liver derived from the experience with the ibuprofen congener ibufenac, which had been removed from the market owing to its propensity to cause hepatotoxicity (Adams *et al.*, 1970).

There was little early evidence from animal studies to suggest that ibuprofen was nephrotoxic. Experiments performed on rats revealed that single lethal doses of 540 mg/kg/day produced slight renal tubular dilation and repeated doses of 180 mg/kg/day produced enlargement of the kidney (Adams *et al.*, 1969). The lack of early awareness of the renal effects of ibuprofen in humans might have been due to the low doses initially used. Indeed, the adult dosage upon marketing in the United Kingdom was a single

CHAPTER 10

200 mg tablet thrice daily with an additional tablet given at bedtime when needed. A dosage of six tablets per day (1200 mg) was recommended for a rapid response followed by reduction to the optimal daily dosage in 2–4 weeks (Davies and Avery, 1971). However, it soon became apparent that the dosage for anti-inflammatory effects needed to be higher than that initially recommended. As such, a new maximum of 2400 mg per day was soon set (The Upjohn Company, 1975). Thereafter, the renal effects of ibuprofen became manifest (Schooley *et al.*, 1977; Kimberly *et al.*, 1978), presumably reflecting its increased dosage and increased prevalence of use to treat patients with one of a variety of clinical conditions that make them susceptible to the renal effects of ibuprofen or other NSAIDs.

10.2   ROLE OF RENAL PROSTAGLANDINS IN IBUPROFEN'S RENAL EFFECTS

It has long been known that ibuprofen reduces the synthesis of renal prostaglandins (PGs) by the kidney (Fitzpatrick and Wynalda, 1976) and thereby influences renal function (Bowden *et al.*, 1977). The renal effects and toxicity of ibuprofen are best understood by examining the nephron's sites of autacoid synthesis and the physiology of these local hormones. Figure 10.1 shows the nephron and its many sites of prostanoid production. There are two fundamental compartments of autacoid production that explain most of the effects (Dunn and Zambraski, 1980; Änggård and Oliw, 1981). The *vascular compartment* includes the afferent arteriole, the glomerulus, the efferent arteriole, and the vasa recta. Effects of ibuprofen upon PGs in the vascular compartment explain its hemodynamic effects. The *tubular compartment* contains the proximal tubule, the loop of Henle, the distal tubule, and the collecting duct. Effects of ibuprofen upon the tubular compartment explain its effects on electrolyte homeostasis and water metabolism.

10.2.1   Nephron structure and function

Structure

As can be seen from Figure 10.1, the nephron contains numerous sites of eicosanoid synthesis (Änggård and Oliw, 1981; Schlondorff, 1986). Eicosanoids are precursors of prostaglandins (PGs) and thromboxane. Cyclooxygenase is present throughout the vasculature and tubules. Cytochrome P450 monooxygenase is also found in the proximal tubule and the medullary thick ascending loop of Henle (McGiff, 1991). Thus, products of cytochrome P450 monooxygenase may be formed *de novo* or vascular-derived PGs may become substrates at sites distal to the glomerulus such as within the medullary tubules and interstitium. Epoxides of arachidonic acid such as epoxyeicosatrienoic acids (EETs), and hydroxyeicosatetraenoic acids (HETEs) and omega-oxidation products are produced as metabolites of this system (McGiff, 1991).

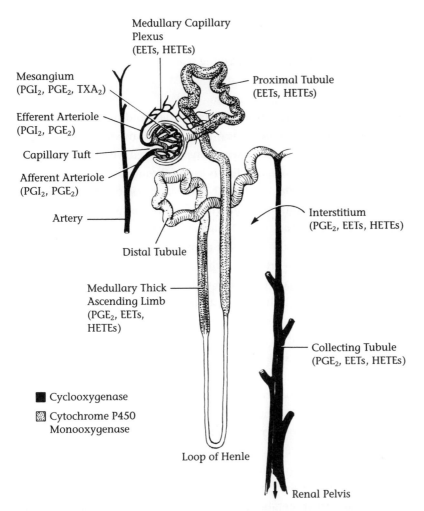

Medullary Capillary
Plexus
(EETs, HETEs)

Mesangium
(PGI$_2$, PGE$_2$, TXA$_2$)

Proximal Tubule
(EETs, HETEs)

Efferent Arteriole
(PGI$_2$, PGE$_2$)

Capillary Tuft

Afferent Arteriole
(PGI$_2$, PGE$_2$)

Artery

Interstitium
(PGE$_2$, EETs, HETEs)

Distal Tubule

Medullary Thick
Ascending Limb
(PGE$_2$, EETs,
HETEs)

Collecting Tubule
(PGE$_2$, EETs, HETEs)

■ Cyclooxygenase

▨ Cytochrome P450
Monooxygenase

Loop of Henle

Renal Pelvis

Figure 10.1: Distribution of renal autacoids within the nephron vasculature and tubular structures. EETs, epoxyeicosatrienoic acids; HETEs, hydroxyeicosatetraenoic acids; PG, prostaglandin; TX, thromboxane. (Reprinted from Murray and Brater (1993) with permission from Annual Reviews, Inc.)

The renal vasculature endothelium contains a variety of autacoids (Figure 10.1). Acute tubular ischemia and necrosis from ibuprofen occurs in some patients administered ibuprofen from a hemodynamic effect upon this vasculature. After entering the glomerulus, the afferent arteriole divides into four to six capillary tufts that are supported by an active network of mesangium and matrix (Klahr *et al.*, 1988; Latta, 1992). The matrix is exposed to many of the constituents found in blood and absorbs proteins and macromolecules (Latta, 1992). This is the site where interstitial nephritis from NSAIDs may begin. The efferent arteriole, the vessel that leaves the glomerulus, contains the effluent. It descends deep into the interstitium forming the medullary capillary plexus and vasa recta.

These latter vessels exchange water and electrolytes and provide oxygen and nutrients to the medulla. Studies of dogs demonstrate differential changes in renal blood among the cortex and medulla flow produced by ibuprofen (Young *et al.*, 1990).

Function

Renal autacoids produce many physiological effects. Understanding their effects is necessary for understanding the consequences of their depletion when ibuprofen is administered. PGs maintain renal perfusion in situations associated with reduced actual or effective circulating volume. PGI_2 (prostacyclin) is found throughout the vasculature and produces systemic and renovascular dilation (Nadler *et al.*, 1986). PGI_2 is also the predominant prostaglandin in the human glomerulus and the primary PG affecting glomerular hemodynamics (Patrono *et al.*, 1985; Nadler *et al.*, 1986). PGE_2 and PGI_2 affect afferent arteriolar tone by attenuating the effects of norepinephrine and angiotensin II, but only PGI_2 affects tone at the efferent arteriole (Palmer and Henrich, 1995). In patients with chronic glomerular disease, urinary excretion of PGI_2 correlates with glomerular filtration rate (Patrono *et al.*, 1985). With the administration of ibuprofen, removal of this mitigating effect of PGs can cause precipitous declines in renal blood flow and glomerular filtration in susceptible persons (Whelton *et al.*, 1990; Murray *et al.*, 1995). Hence, renal blood flow is controlled by the effects of a variety of autacoids upon the glomerular vasculature and mesangium. In addition to their vasodilatory effects throughout the vasculature, PGI_2 and PGE_2 affect the production of renin by the juxtaglomerular apparatus (Whorton *et al.*, 1977; Gerber *et al.*, 1978). Ibuprofen administration can thereby cause the syndrome of hyporeninemic-hypoaldosteronism and resultant hyperkalemia, but this is rare (DeFronzo, 1980; Marasco *et al.*, 1987).

Renal PGs within the tubular compartment and other autacoids affect sodium and potassium homeostasis, and water metabolism. The anatomical sites of autacoid production predict the activity of PGs and their metabolites at the site (Dunn, 1984a; Schlondorff, 1986). PGE_2 is the predominant PG produced by the medullary cells around the thick ascending loop of Henle and the cortical collecting duct. It has a profound effect on sodium and water metabolism. PGs have natriuretic effects (Ichikawa *et al.*, 1980). Natriuresis is the result of two effects of PGs. First, PGs cause vasodilation, which increases renal blood flow and thereby reduces proximal reabsorption of sodium. Second, PGs directly inhibit sodium reabsorption at the thick ascending limb of the loop of Henle and cortical collecting duct (Kaojarern *et al.*, 1983; Hébert *et al.*, 1991; Ling *et al.*, 1992).

Owing largely to these effects, administration of ibuprofen can cause sodium retention or blunting of the response to diuretics and antihypertensive drugs. In most persons, the sodium-retentive effects of NSAIDs are not clinically discernible. However, in patients sensitive to salt loads, such as those with chronic renal insufficiency or heart failure, sodium retention from ibuprofen can result in weight gain and oedema and interfere with the effects of antihypertensive drugs. At the collecting duct, PGE_2 inhibits antidiuretic hormone (arginine vasopressin). Ibuprofen can therefore promote water retention and lead to hyponatremia in some patients (Kimberly *et al.*, 1978; Blum and Aviram, 1980).

Some endothelial-derived autacoids such as nitric oxide and endothelin-1 also play a role in renal hemodynamics. Nitric oxide and endothelin-1 are ubiquitous throughout the vasculature. Nitric oxide is a renal vasodilator, whereas endothelin-1 is a potent vasoconstrictor (Henrich, 1991). It is becoming increasingly apparent that nitric oxide and endothelin-1 interact with prostaglandins in numerous ways in the kidney (Romero *et al.*, 1992). Unlike endothelin-1, endothelin-3 is a renal vasodilator producing its effect by increasing both nitric oxide and PG production, an effect that is partially blocked by the administration of ibuprofen, thereby resulting in a reduction in renal blood flow and glomerular filtration (Yamashita *et al.*, 1991).

The mesangium is richly endowed with vasoactive substances such as PGI_2, PGE_2 and intrinsic thromboxane A_2 (Klahr *et al.*, 1988). The effects of these eicosanoids, and macrophage and monocyte metabolites such as cytokines, interleukins and cell growth factors may predict glomerular morphology and pathology. But sometimes the effects are not so predictable. Co-administration of epidermal growth factor, a potent vasoconstrictor deriving from the mesangium, with ibuprofen results in renal vasodilation. Presumably, this effect is due to products formed via P450 metabolism, because the vasodilation is blocked by ketoconazole (Harris *et al.*, 1990).

Cytochrome P450 metabolites of PGs affect renal blood flow and glomerular filtration in the rat (Takahashi *et al.*, 1990) and dog (Feigen, 1984) and also produce natriuresis. HETEs are found in the proximal tubule and the medullary thick ascending limb of the loop of Henle. Their primary effect is inhibition of Na^+,K^+-ATPase at the S1 segment of the proximal tubule and medullary thick ascending limb. They may also produce vasodilation of the medullary capillary plexus (Takahashi *et al.*, 1990; McGiff, 1991). Hartupee *et al.* (1993) used inhibition of cyclooxygenase (with ibuprofen) and lipoxygenase in dogs to show that leukotrienes reduce urine osmolality and increase urine flow. Zeidel *et al.* (1991) have shown that interleukin-1 produces a natriuretic effect partly by stimulation of PGE_2 production by the collecting duct.

Cyclooxygenases 1 and 2

Until recently, there were large gaps in our understanding of the relationship between the effects of PGs in maintaining normal renal function and those that increase with disorders of inflammation. It is now known that there are at least two isoforms of cyclooxygenase. Cyclooxygenase-1 is a constitutive form that is responsible for normal physiological functions. Cyclooxygenase-2 is induced by nuclear factor- kappa B that occurs with inflammation (Yamamoto *et al.*, 1995). This discovery helps explain the effects of NSAIDs in the relief of pain and inflammation as well as their adverse renal effects.

Most existing NSAIDs inhibit both isoforms of cyclooxygenase (COX). As such, the therapeutic effects of these drugs come with a price in susceptible patients. Inhibition of

CHAPTER 10

COX-2 results in the relief of pain and inflammation, whereas inhibition COX-1, in clinical situations where certain physiological functions are dependent upon prostaglandins, results in dysfunction. For example, in the setting of prostaglandin-dependent renal function, administration of a NSAID that inhibits both isoforms would result in abrogation of the beneficial effects of the PG, resulting in an acute ischemic insult.

A measure of the relative activities of NSAIDs is the ratio of inhibition of COX-2 to COX-1. Vane and Botting (1996) have profiled the NSAIDs in terms of their selectivity in inhibiting COX-2. That of ibuprofen was intermediate between those of piroxicam and diclofenac. The intermediate ranking of ibuprofen in this profile could explain the intermediate effects of ibuprofen on renal function. New NSAIDs are being developed with selective COX-2 inhibition; this feature may impart favourable risk–benefit profiles.

The inhibition of cyclooxygenase by ibuprofen is a stereochemical process. This ability seems to reside almost entirely in the (S)-(+) enantiomer (Adams et al., 1976). Few data are available on the disposition of this enantiomer in relationship to its renal effects, particularly in its unbound form (Murray and Brater, 1990a; Williams, 1990). It is also now known that the (R)-(–) enantiomer also has clinically important effects (Villanueva et al., 1993). Because of the ability of the (R)-(–) enantiomer to be converted to the (S)-(+) enantiomer in vivo, it would seem to be important to consider the disposition of the separate enantiomers of ibuprofen as well as their effects on renal function concurrently. However, we have little insight into the integrative renal effects of the (S)-(+) and (R)-(–) enantiomers in humans.

10.3   IMPORTANCE OF IBUPROFEN'S PHARMACOKINETICS TO ITS RENAL EFFECTS

As described in previous chapters, the pharmacokinetic characteristics of ibuprofen include: (1) small volume of distribution, (2) extensive protein binding, (3) low intrinsic clearance, (4) low urinary excretion, and (5) short (2-hour) half-life. Because the kidney is the major organ for both concentrating and eliminating xenobiotics, its susceptibility to the toxic effects of many drugs is conceivable. It is somewhat surprising, however, that despite ibuprofen's extensive metabolism to inactive metabolites and little active drug being recovered from the urine, ibuprofen none the less can have a profound effect on renal function.

There are three dispositional aspects of ibuprofen relevant to a discussion of its renal effects, including (1) in vivo metabolic inversion of the (R)-(–) enantiomer into the (S)-(+) enantiomer; (2) altered protein binding of the enantiomers; and (3) altered clearance in certain clinical conditions. Arylpropionic acids such as ibuprofen are characterized by formation of acyl glucuronide conjugates, which are unstable and can be transformed back to the parent drug (Day et al., 1987). Even though ibuprofen itself is not eliminated by the kidney, it has been proposed that retention of the glucuronide conjugate could occur with cleavage back to active ibuprofen in patients with diminished renal function. Concentrations of ibuprofen would then increase (Verbeeck *et al.*, 1983) with intensified renal effects.

Accumulation of glucuronide conjugates of both *R* and *S* enantiomers could provide more (*R*)-(–) substrate for conversion to the active (*S*)-(+) enantiomer and allow a disproportionate increase in cyclooxygenase inhibition. Such accumulation has been demonstrated in uremic rabbits with 2-phenylpropionic acid, a compound structurally similar to the arylpropionic acid NSAIDs such as ibuprofen (Meffin, 1986). Until recently, clinical evidence of the relevance of this intriguing process to the renal effects of ibuprofen is lacking.

Rudy *et al.* (1995) determined the stereoselective disposition of ibuprofen administered to elderly persons with renal insufficiency and to elderly and young persons without renal insufficiency. Subjects received 800 mg thrice daily. They found that both groups of elderly had significantly decreased binding of (*S*)-(+)-ibuprofen compared to the young group. The half-life of elimination of the (*S*)-(+) enantiomer was greater for the elderly subjects with renal insufficiency compared to the young, and the unbound clearance of (*S*)-(+) was less. The fraction of the (*R*)-(–) enantiomer inverted to the (*S*)-(+) was the same in all groups, but the unbound clearances of glucuronidation and hydroxylation were reduced in the elderly with renal insufficiency. The results of this study highlight the importance of the relationship between the stereoselective pharmacokinetics of ibuprofen in patients at risk for renal effects.

Animal experiments provide other evidence, but it is uncertain whether it extrapolates to humans. In the isolated perfused rat kidney, there were no discernible differences noted in the pharmacokinetics of (*S*)-(+)- and (*R*)-(–)-ibuprofen (Cox *et al.*, 1991). (*S*)-(+) and to a lesser extent (*R*)-(–) decreased glomerular filtration and excretion of sodium, potassium, calcium and chloride. Accumulation in the kidney, of both enantiomers, was concentration-dependent. In their studies of rabbits, Chen *et al.* (1994) suggested that decreased clearance of (*S*)-(+)-ibuprofen, but not (*R*)-(–), contributed to the development of interstitial nephritis and tubular necrosis. However, similar evidence in man has not been forthcoming.

10.4   TYPES OF RENAL EFFECTS OF IBUPROFEN

Ibuprofen can cause practically all of the distinct renal syndromes produced by NSAIDs. There are four primary types of renal impairment from NSAIDs, namely acute ischemic renal insufficiency, effects on sodium, potassium, and water homeostasis with interference of the effects of diuretics and antihypertensive therapy, acute interstitial nephritis, and papillary necrosis. Ibuprofen's association with these adverse renal effects owes more to its widespread use than to any particular intrinsic characteristic of the drug per se. Severe, irreversible syndromes are rare. The experience of a patient treated with ibuprofen

CHAPTER 10

reported by Kimberly *et al.* (1978) exemplifies many of the features of ibuprofen-associated renal effects.

In their case series, Kimberly *et al.* (1978) found that ibuprofen, fenoprofen and naproxen produced a variety of renal effects in patients with systemic lupus erythematosus receiving diets controlled for sodium, potassium and fluid intake. It is of interest that within 3 days of ibuprofen administration (2400 mg/day) a 58-year-old woman manifested a variety of the renal effects of NSAIDs including:

(1) increase in serum creatinine from 80 to 265 µmol/l (0.9–3.0 mg/dl);
(2) increase in blood urea nitrogen from 5.5 to 15.5 mmol/l (16–43 mg/dl);
(3) increase in serum potassium from 4.7 to 6.1 mmol/l;
(4) decrease in serum sodium from 142 to 130 mmol/l;
(5) decrease in sodium excretion from 84 to 28 mmol/day;
(6) decrease in the urinary excretion of PGE from 48 to 20 ng/h;
(7) decrease in plasma renin activity from 2.34 to 0.12 ng/ml/h;
(8) decrease in urinary aldosterone excretion from 4.7 to 1.1 µg/day;
(9) increase in body weight of 2 kg.

When ibuprofen administration was stopped, the patient's renal functional parameters returned to baseline values. It is helpful to remember this patient's experience while discussing the renal effects of ibuprofen.

The literature abounds with similar reports of renal syndromes from ibuprofen, which underline their variety. Marasco *et al.* (1987) reported one 45-year-old patient with acute tubulointerstitial nephritis and summarized 20 previously reported cases found in the literature. Five of the 20 cases reported tubular necrosis, 5 hyperkalemia, 8 oliguria, 12 proteinuria, and 12 reported urinary sediment comprising red and white blood cells, and casts.

Since Marasco's report, additional case reports have been published of ibuprofen-associated renal syndromes including acute tubular necrosis (Wen *et al.*, 1992; Sanders, 1995), tubulointerstitial nephritis (McIntire *et al.*, 1993; DuBose, 1994; Wattad *et al.*, 1994), membranous nephropathy (Radford *et al.*, 1996), and lipoid nephrosis (Morgenstern *et al.*, 1989). The frequency of these renal syndromes has not been precisely estimated, but they appear to be uncommon.

10.4.1 Acute renal insufficiency

The most common form of ibuprofen-associated renal impairment is acute ischemic renal insufficiency. Usually it occurs as a transient acute hemodynamic effect within hours of the first dose in susceptible persons and is readily reversible after ibuprofen administration is stopped. If the drug continues to be administered, acute tubular necrosis with irreversible damage to the kidney can result (Carmichael and Shankel, 1985; Chan, 1987).

Healthy, euvolemic persons are not at risk for an acute hemodynamic effect from ibuprofen (Brater *et al.*, 1985; Passmore *et al.*, 1989, 1990). However, disorders, diseases or drugs that reduce actual or effective circulating volume set the stage for the development of acute renal insufficiency. Generally, they cause a homeostatic increase in the production of catecholamines such as norepinephrine and activation of the renin–angiotensin system (Clive and Stoff, 1984). Angiotensin II and catecholamines produce vasoconstriction within the renal vasculature that is countered by PGs so that renal blood flow and glomerular filtration are sufficiently maintained (Dunn and Zambraski, 1980; Dunn, 1984b). Clinical states in which decreased actual or effective circulating volume occur include dehydration, hemorrhage, congestive heart failure, cirrhosis with ascites, and excessive diuresis (Zipser *et al.*, 1979; Clive and Stoff, 1984; Brater, 1988). In these settings, renal impairment can occur upon ibuprofen administration and is manifest by increments in serum creatinine and blood urea nitrogen. Studies in the rat indicate that thromboxane synthesis may also be intimately involved (Kaufman, 1987a; Klausner *et al.*, 1989). Indeed, administration of thromboxane inhibitors has proved efficacious in preventing renal impairment in susceptible humans (Remuzzi *et al.*, 1992). Administration of PGE_1 has also been shown to prevent acute tubular necrosis in rats administered ibuprofen (Kaufman, 1987b). In patients with diabetes, the administration of PGE_1 as misoprostol has been shown to blunt the effects of ibuprofen on glomerular filtration (Bakris *et al.*, 1995).

Acute renal insufficiency from ibuprofen can also occur in the face of pre-existing chronic renal insufficiency (Ciabattoni *et al.*, 1984; Whelton *et al.*, 1990; Murray *et al.*, 1995). Renal function is rendered prostaglandin-dependent in patients with pre-existing renal insufficiency. Administration of NSAIDs removes the mitigating effect of PGs, thereby reducing renal blood flow and glomerular filtration. This is an area that we have probed with a variety of NSAIDs, including ibuprofen as a prototypic short-acting NSAID.

Acute renal toxicity of ibuprofen has been assessed using two distinct methodologies: acute interventional clinical studies and epidemiological studies. The advantage of the former is that specific clinical entities and mechanisms of renal insufficiency can be studied under controlled conditions. Using acute interventional methods, we have assessed the acute hemodynamic effects of ibuprofen in patients under dietary and fluid control. These studies tell us that the effect can occur and to what magnitude. Epidemiological studies, on the other hand, tell us how often these effects occur in the real world and provide more precise prevalence and incidence estimates and risk estimates for specific factors. For example, researchers who can follow a cohort of patients prescribed NSAIDs can ascertain the numbers of patients who develop renal insufficiency and determine whether patient risk is greater in selected populations such as elderly persons or those with heart failure. Hence, both acute interventional and epidemiological methodologies provide unique perspectives to our understanding of the effects of ibuprofen.

CHAPTER 10

10.4.2   Acute Interventional Studies

Acute interventional studies of small groups of preselected subjects demonstrate abrupt reductions in glomerular filtration rate of 9% to 69% following the administration of NSAIDs (Murray and Brater, 1990b). Zambraski and Dunn (1993) estimate that renal prostaglandin synthesis is reduced to about 50–60% of baseline with a maximum decrease of about 80% from NSAIDs. We have performed acute interventional studies of ibuprofen in patients with a variety of risk factors for renal impairment using clearance techniques (Murray *et al.*, 1995). We have studied the effects of ibuprofen and other NSAIDs on renal function in young persons and elderly persons with preserved renal function and those with mild to moderate renal insufficiency.

Patients are admitted to the clinical research centre where they ingest a controlled diet with fixed sodium and potassium intake. Within a week and after attaining sodium balance, a clearance study is performed with administration of the first dose of the NSAID. During this clearance study, control collections are obtained to determine baseline renal function using inulin as a marker of glomerular filtration rate. The first dose of ibuprofen or other NSAID is then administered, followed by a series of experimental collections to monitor the effect of the drug on renal function. Subjects are then maintained on the NSAID with daily monitoring of electrolyte excretion, serum electrolytes and creatinine clearance. This constitutes the balance portion of the study. With the last dose of NSAID another clearance study is performed. During this clearance study, control collections are again obtained; these values represent renal function on the background of chronic dosing with the NSAID. Experimental collections during this phase represent the effect of a single dose of NSAID superimposed on the background of chronic dosing.

Our studies have shown consistent effects from ibuprofen. In both normal controls and patients with renal insufficiency, glomerular filtration (as measured using inulin or creatinine clearance) and electrolyte excretion decrease with both the first dose (acute study) and the last dose (chronic study). Decrements from the short-acting NSAIDs such as ibuprofen and flurbiprofen were generally transient and soon returned to baseline.

Figures 10.2 and 10.3 reveal the effects on inulin and creatinine clearance following a single dose of ibuprofen 800 mg to elderly persons (73 ± 6 years of age) with preserved renal function (glomerular filtration rate > 1.17 ml/s) and those with moderate renal impairment (glomerular filtration rate 0.5–1.17 ml/s). Patients had not taken NSAIDs for 1 month prior to the study. Seven elderly patients had hypertension, but blood pressure was well controlled.

There are three important points about these time-response profiles of the effect of ibuprofen on inulin and creatinine clearance. First, there are no differences in the time profiles between patients with renal impairment and those with preserved renal function. Second, the effect occurred within 1 h and was fully reversible within several hours of the administered dose. Third, there was no chronic effect following repetitive decrements of

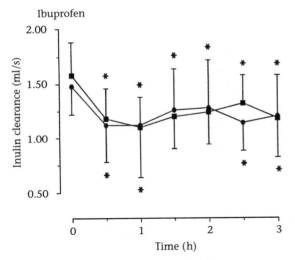

Figure 10.2: Inulin clearance after the first dose (squares) and last dose after 1 month of continuous dosing (circles) in 14 elderly persons *without* renal insufficiency (glomerular filtration rate > 1.15 ml/s (70 ml/min)). Baseline is time 0. Squares represent inulin clearance and circles represent creatinine clearance. Asterisks mark values that are significant at $p < 0.05$ after correcting for multiple testing. (Reprinted from Murray *et al.* (1995) with permission from Lippincott Raven Publisher.)

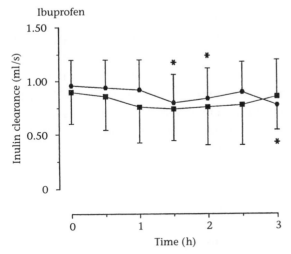

Figure 10.3: Inulin clearance after the first dose (squares) and last dose after 1 month of continuous dosing (circles) in 14 elderly persons *with* renal insufficiency (glomerular filtration rate 0.50–1.15 ml/s (30–70 ml/min)). Figure descriptions are the same as in Figure 10.2. (Reprinted from Murray *et al.* (1995) with permission from Lippincott Raven Publisher.)

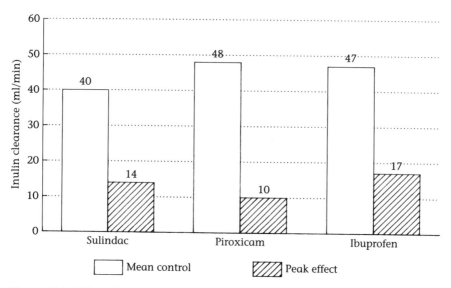

Figure 10.4: Effect of single doses of sulindac 200 mg, piroxicam 20 mg and ibuprofen 800 mg on inulin clearance in a patient susceptible to the renal effects of NSAIDs (see text). Each administration of NSAID was separated by at least 1 month. Mean control represents the patient's baseline measurements, immediately prior to NSAID administration. Peak effect is the nadir response within 3 h of dosing. (Reprinted from Murray and Brater (1993) with permission from Annual Reviews, Inc.)

multiple doses of ibuprofen. Glomerular filtration was fully reversible within the dosing interval after a single dose, and after multiple continuous dosing indicating no cumulative decrease in renal function. Of interest is the comparison of the clearance studies of baseline renal function (acute study, time zero) to renal function under the influence of several days to 1 month of NSAID administration (chronic study, time zero). For ibuprofen and other short-acting NSAIDs we have studied thus far, we have found no evidence to indicate an overall decline in renal function at 1 month (Murray *et al.*, 1992, 1995). Lack of cumulative effects of ibuprofen was also demonstrated by comparison of the baseline glomerular filtration rates from the clearance studies performed with administration of the first and last dose of NSAID.

Overall, we interpret these data to indicate that each dose of ibuprofen caused decrements in renal function, but that the effects were transient so that full recovery to baseline renal function occurred with repeated dosing. In contrast to the lack of effect of ibuprofen, the longer-acting NSAIDs sulindac and piroxicam produced small, but statistically significant, chronic decrements in glomerular filtration in these patients of 0.12 ml/s (7 ml/min) in these same patients.

Acute interventional studies of NSAIDs often unmask patients who are extremely susceptible to their renal effects. We and others have seen rapid, dramatic responses to ibuprofen and other NSAIDs. Figure 10.4 reveals the effect on inulin clearance in an elderly gentleman who was susceptible to the effects of ibuprofen, piroxicam and sulindac.

This 73-year-old man with osteoarthritis, hypertension, chronic renal insufficiency and atherosclerosis had excellent joint pain relief with ibuprofen. However, his serum creatinine rose from 177 µmol/l to 265 µmol/l (2.0 to 3.0 mg/dl) within 3 days and he had to have ibuprofen stopped. Our attempt to find a NSAID that he could tolerate failed. As can be seen from the figure, his inulin clearance decreased by 65%, 79% and 64% with sulindac, piroxicam and ibuprofen respectively. This patient's response to all three NSAIDs underlines the admonition that such patients who are susceptible to the acute hemodynamic effects of NSAIDs must have their renal function carefully monitored soon after the beginning of any NSAID.

In a randomized crossover study, Whelton et al. (1990) described the renal effects of ibuprofen, piroxicam and sulindac in 12 women with mild, stable renal insufficiency. Three women had their regimen of ibuprofen 800 mg three times daily stopped within 8 days owing to increased serum creatinine concentrations. Two of these three patients with exaggerated responses experienced similar effects with a dose of 400 mg three times daily. It is of interest that these three patients did not have similar renal responses to piroxicam 20 mg daily or sulindac 200 mg twice daily. However, the length of observation of patients may have been too short to accurately assess patient response to these longer-acting NSAIDs. As described above, our studies of elderly patients with mild to moderate renal insufficiency indicate that both sulindac and piroxicam cause decrements in renal function within a month of chronic dosing (Murray et al., 1995).

Ciabattoni et al. (1984) studied the renal effects of ibuprofen and sulindac in 20 patients with chronic glomerular disease. Ibuprofen 1200 mg or sulindac 400 mg per day were administered to 20 hospitalized women. In 10 patients, ibuprofen reduced by 80% urinary excretion of 6-ketoprostaglandin $F_{1\alpha}$ (the stable metabolite of PGI_2); serum creatinine concentrations increased by 40%, glomerular filtration (as measured by creatinine clearance) was reduced by 28%, and renal blood flow (as measured by p-aminohippurate clearance) was reduced by 35%. In the 10 patients who received sulindac, these renal effects were not observed.

Patrono et al. (1985) found that ibuprofen 1200 mg/day administered for 7 days to 11 patients with chronic glomerular disease was associated with decrements in 6-ketoprostaglandin $F_{1\alpha}$ and thromboxane B_2 (stable product of thromboxane A_2) and in reductions in creatinine and p-aminohippurate clearances of 25% and 35%, respectively. The correlation of creatinine clearance with urinary 6-ketoprostaglandin $F_{1\alpha}$ ($r = 0.87, p < 0.01$) highlights the importance of PGI_2 to the maintenance of renal function in these patients.

Finally, investigators found that ibuprofen administered to kidney transplant patients, instead of corticosteroids, increased the rejection rate of cadaveric kidneys (Kreis et al., 1984). The ibuprofen dosing protocol in this study was 50 mg/kg/day followed by a reduction to 25 mg/kg/day. Compared to corticosteroids, the rate of acute tubular necrosis was 51% higher in the ibuprofen recipients. Renal biopsy revealed evidence of glomerular ischemia in 11 of 12 ibuprofen recipients.

CHAPTER 10

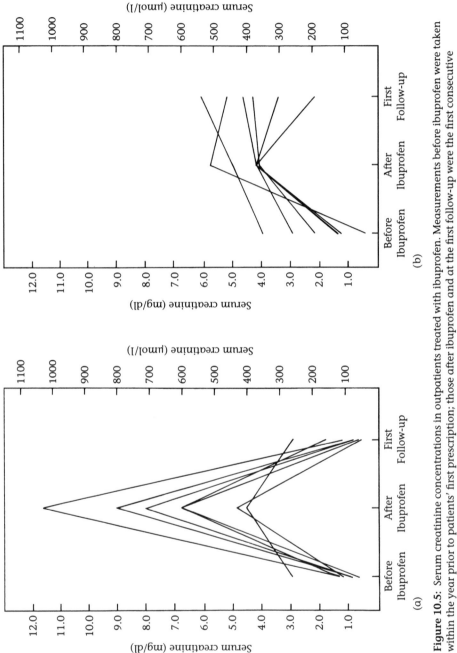

Figure 10.5: Serum creatinine concentrations in outpatients treated with ibuprofen. Measurements before ibuprofen were taken within the year prior to patients' first prescription; those after ibuprofen and at the first follow-up were the first consecutive measurements taken within the year after ibuprofen. Responses depicted in (a) are for patients in whom serum creatinine concentrations returned to baseline values. Responses depicted in (b) are for those in whom serum creatinine concentrations remained elevated at their first follow-up. Other factors besides ibuprofen could have contributed to these responses (see Figure 10.6).

10.4.3   Epidemiological studies

Epidemiological studies either use routine laboratory tests such as serum creatinine or blood urea nitrogen to measure changes in renal function with ibuprofen or they use hospital admission or discharge diagnoses for renal disorders. We studied ibuprofen-associated renal impairment in an unselected, adult general medical clinic population from Indianapolis, Indiana, USA, using a large clinical computing system called the Regenstrief Medical Record System (RMRS). We found that within a year of their first ibuprofen prescription, 18% of 1908 patients (who had sufficient laboratory tests) had clinically significant increments of serum creatinine, blood urea nitrogen, or both (Murray *et al.*, 1990). In this population, we determined a number of risk factors for renal insufficiency including age, gender, systolic blood pressure, pre-existing renal insufficiency, coronary artery disease, and diuretic use. Relative to patients prescribed acetaminophen, two factors were associated with renal insufficiency from ibuprofen, namely age ≥ 65 years and coronary artery disease.

In a broader general medicine clinic population we used the RMRS to identify 3909 adult patients from Indianapolis prescribed ibuprofen who had serum creatinine measurements the year before and after their first ibuprofen prescription. We found that 61 patients (1.6%) had increases in their serum creatinine values ≥ 88.4 µmol/l (1 mg/dl) within the year after their first prescription for ibuprofen. Figure 10.5 shows the serum creatinine values for 7 patients whose renal function returned to baseline values within the year following their first ibuprofen prescription (A) and 6 patients whose serum creatinine values remained elevated at least 88.4 µmol/l (1 mg/dl) above their baseline. As can be seen in Figure 10.6, the increase in the incidence is doubled with each additional risk factor.

We have also analyzed longitudinal data from these patients prescribed ibuprofen who had multiple serum creatinine measurements, using linear models. We analyzed 17 839 measurements on 1482 patients who had at least two serum creatinine measurements before and after their first prescription for ibuprofen. We found that the linear model that best described the data was one in which there was an abrupt increase in the serum creatinine after the prescription for ibuprofen followed by a decline. This model fits well with our other studies and suggests that when an acute hemodynamic insult occurs, discontinuation of ibuprofen results in a return to baseline values.

Other investigators have used epidemiological approaches to study these renal effects. Several of these epidemiological studies used renal diagnoses as the outcome of interest. The results of these studies indicate that ibuprofen use does not result in hospitalizations or other clinical encounters for important renal disorders. However, such studies are unable to detect lesser, though clinically important, changes in renal function that might not result in hospitalization, but could have been serious none the less (Fox and Jick, 1984; Johnson *et al.*, 1985; Beard *et al.*, 1988). Sandler *et al.* (1991) performed a multicentre case-control study of the risk of chronic renal disease, which was defined as hospitalization for chronic renal disease and an increase in serum creatinine > 133 µmol/l (1.5 mg/dl), and concluded that

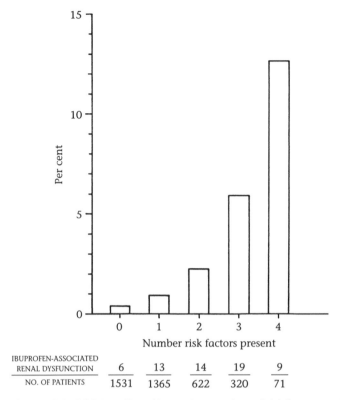

IBUPROFEN-ASSOCIATED RENAL DYSFUNCTION	6	13	14	19	9
NO. OF PATIENTS	1531	1365	622	320	71

Figure 10.6: Additive effect of increasing numbers of risk factors on the prevalence of ibuprofen-associated renal dysfunction in 3909 patients after their first prescription for ibuprofen. Risk factors from a multivariate model included a diagnosis of renal disease, prior blood urea nitrogen value, systolic blood pressure and prior hospitalization. Ibuprofen-associated renal dysfunction was defined as a change in serum creatinine from baseline of ≥ 88.4 µmol/l (1 mg/dl).

NSAIDs increase the risk of chronic renal disease in men > 65 years of age. There were too few patients using ibuprofen (9 cases but no controls) to accurately estimate its risk per se.

Other epidemiological studies excluded patients who may have been at risk for the renal effects of NSAIDs, such as frail elderly patients and patients with renal disease or insufficiency, with liver disease, or with advanced forms of other diseases (Bonney *et al.*, 1986). From these studies it can be concluded that ibuprofen administration rarely leads to a hospitalization for renal diagnoses and that young, healthy persons tolerate ibuprofen well. This latter point is consistent with the results of acute interventional studies.

Elderly persons are of particular concern. Because of the high prevalence of arthritis among them, they have the greatest need for continuous NSAID therapy. Their use of NSAIDs is more than 3.5 times greater than that of their younger counterparts (Baum *et al.*, 1985). Our own survey of elderly persons living in urban public housing complexes revealed that NSAIDs were the most frequently used over-the-counter and prescription drugs (Darnell, 1986). These subjects may also have multiple risk factors that make them susceptible to the renal effects of ibuprofen. (Murray and Brater, 1990b). Foremost is the likelihood of antecedent renal impairment in this population (Frocht and Fillit, 1984; Guralnik, 1989). Despite these overriding concerns, there have been few studies to determine the renal risk of NSAIDs in the elderly.

Our studies of elderly persons (Murray *et al.*, 1995) with preserved renal function demonstrate that they can safely receive ibuprofen and other NSAIDs unless there is another risk factor for ibuprofen-associated renal impairment. This is also the case for young patients. In contrast, elderly patients with renal insufficiency are at some risk. Our findings are supported by those of Cummings *et al.* (1988), who randomly assigned elderly patients (63–87 years of age) with osteoarthritis to either ibuprofen 400 mg (as the suspension) or aspirin 650 mg four times daily for 6 weeks. Serum creatinine and blood urea nitrogen were monitored weekly for 6 weeks. They found that neither regimen adversely affected renal function.

Similarly, Gurwitz *et al.* (1990) performed a prospective study of 114 elderly patients (87 ± 7 years of age) prescribed NSAIDs compared to a comparison group of 45 patients who were not receiving NSAIDs. Of the NSAID recipients, 101 (89%) were prescribed ibuprofen at a mean daily dosage of 1600 mg. Serum urea nitrogen values increased significantly with the first 5–7 days of treatment in those prescribed NSAIDs. Serum urea nitrogen increased > 50% in 13% of the patients compared to baseline; risk factors for this effect included concomitant treatment with a loop diuretic and a high NSAID dosage (> 2400 mg/day of ibuprofen).

10.4.4   Alterations in sodium and water homeostasis

Independent of its ability to cause acute and chronic renal impairment, ibuprofen may affect sodium and potassium homeostasis and water metabolism. Like the acute hemodynamic effect of ibuprofen, these renal syndromes are transient. Clinically, reduced excretion of sodium may result in formation of oedema, exacerbation of heart failure, or increased blood pressure. Finally, reduced excretion of water has rarely caused hyponatremia.

Although clinically detectable sodium retention occurs only infrequently in healthy subjects, occasionally sufficient sodium is retained to increase body weight or cause peripheral oedema. Abrogation of the effectiveness of diuretics and blunting of the effects of antihypertensive drugs may occur in patients prescribed these medications (Radack *et al.*, 1987).

All of these electrolyte and blood pressure effects could be more pronounced in elderly persons (Murray and Brater, 1990a; Johnson and Day, 1991; Gurwitz *et al.*, 1996; Murray *et al.*, 1997). Compared to young persons, the elderly have less capacity to conserve sodium (Epstein and Hollenberg, 1976; Luft *et al.*, 1987; Levi and Rowe, 1992), are more likely to have hyporeninemic-hypoaldosteronism (DeFronzo, 1980), often have mild to moderate renal impairment (Levi and Rowe, 1992), take other drugs and supplements that affect

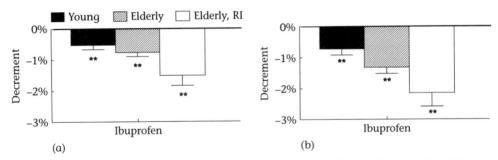

Figure 10.7: Maximum decrease in fractional excretion of sodium after the first dose (a) and last dose after 1 month of continuous administration (b) of ibuprofen 800 mg three times daily to young (*n* = 8) and elderly persons without renal insufficiency (*n* = 14) and elderly persons with renal insufficiency (RI) (*n* = 14). * $p < 0.05$; ** $p < 0.01$. (Reprinted from Murray *et al.* (1997) with permission from Lippincott Raven Publisher.)

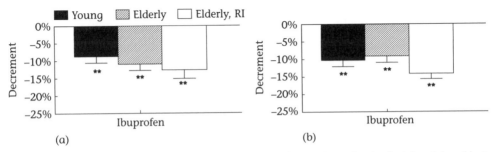

Figure 10.8: Maximum decrease in fractional excretion of potassium after the first dose (a) and last dose after 1 month of continuous administration (b) of ibuprofen. Legends and markings are the same as in Figure 10.7. (Reprinted from Murray *et al.* (1997) with permission from Lippincott Raven Publisher.)

sodium and potassium homeostasis (Adelman *et al.*, 1990), and often have poor diets (Roe, 1990).

We have recently examined the effects of ibuprofen on sodium and potassium homeostasis in elderly persons with renal insufficiency and in young and elderly persons without renal insufficiency (Murray *et al.*, 1997). The techniques used for these studies are the same as the acute interventional studies described above. Fractional clearance of the electrolytes was used to control for the effects of glomerular filtration on electrolyte excretion. Figure 10.7 shows the effect of ibuprofen on the fractional excretion of sodium for the first dose (a) and last dose after 1 month of continuous administration, (b) of ibuprofen administered to the three groups. As can be seen, the decrease in the fractional clearance of sodium from baseline after the first dose is most pronounced in elderly patients with renal insufficiency. This effect is more apparent after the last dose. Fractional excretion of potassium is also decreased relative to baseline in all groups, but with little difference among the groups (Figure 10.8a and b).

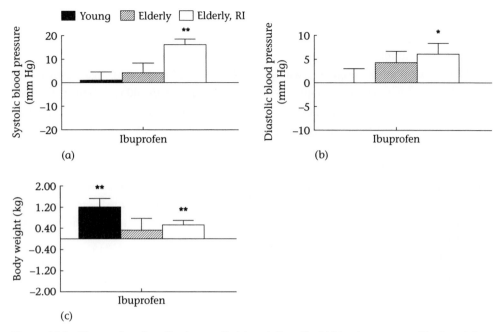

Figure 10.9: Change from baseline in systolic (a) and diastolic (b) blood pressure and body weight (c) after 1 month of continuous dosing of ibuprofen. Legends and markings are the same as in Figure 10.7. (Reprinted from Murray *et al.* (1997) with permission from Lippincott Raven Publisher.)

10.4.5   Effects of NSAIDs on blood pressure

Increased blood pressure and interference with antihypertensive therapy may occur in hypertensive patients prescribed ibuprofen. The mechanism is thought to be multi-factorial involving (1) removal of a systemic vasodilating effect of prostaglandins; (2) reduction of renal tubular PGE_2 causing sodium retention (Kaojarern *et al.*, 1983; Hébert *et al.*, 1991; Ling *et al.*, 1992). Administration of ibuprofen and other NSAIDs can cause sodium and water retention, heightened activity of vasopressors, and reduced effectiveness of diuretics and antihypertensive medications (Murray and Brater, 1993; Murray *et al.*, 1997).

Clinical effects deriving from the reduction in sodium excretion could include increases in patient body weight, oedema and blood pressure. As can be seen from Figure 10.9a and b, both systolic and diastolic blood pressures were increased after 1 month of chronic admin-istration of ibuprofen to elderly patients with renal insufficiency. Body weight was increased for young persons and elderly persons with renal impairment (c). These effects on blood pressure and weight are similar to that observed for flurbiprofen, particularly while patients are ingesting their usual sodium-containing diets (Murray *et al.*, 1992). Gurwitz *et al.* (1996) found that ibuprofen 1800 mg/day caused significant increases in systolic blood pressure in 22 elderly patients (> 60 years of age) in their placebo-controlled randomized trial. Patients' systolic blood pressures were 4 mm Hg higher 1 month after treatment with ibuprofen.

Using a case-control design, Gurwitz and colleagues (1994) also investigated the risk of beginning antihypertensive therapy in elderly New Jersey Medicaid recipients prescribed NSAIDs. They identified 9411 patients and 9629 controls over almost 9 years. They adjusted their risk estimates using age, gender, race and various health care system variables. The adjusted odds ratio (and 95% confidence interval) for use of NSAIDs within 60 days prior to the index date was 1.66 (1.54–1.80). Using standardized NSAID doses, they found a dose–response relationship in which the odds ratio was 1.55 for low dosages, 1.64 for medium and 1.82 for high dosages. Their sample was of sufficient size to permit risk estimates for individual NSAIDs. The odds of beginning antihypertensive therapy were 1.76, 2.12, 2.34 for ibuprofen, sulindac and piroxicam, respectively.

Radack and colleagues (1987) assessed the effects on blood pressure after 3 weeks of treatment with ibuprofen 400 mg every 8 h compared to acetaminophen 1 g every 8 h or placebo in 41 patients with essential hypertension. Blood pressure increases from baseline in the ibuprofen group were 6.3 mm Hg for supine diastolic blood pressure; 6.6 mm Hg for supine mean arterial pressure, and 5.8 mm Hg for sitting mean arterial pressure. Differences were significant compared to acetaminophen and placebo groups. In contrast, a crossover study by Wright and colleagues (1989) failed to reveal differences in blood pressure response to ibuprofen 800 mg four times daily in 12 hypertensive patients receiving hydrochlorothiazide compared to when these same patients were treated with hydrochlorothiazide alone. However, for 3 h after the morning dose, both systolic and diastolic blood pressures were at least 10 mm Hg greater while patients received ibuprofen, suggesting a transient effect and/or a lack of adequate statistical power.

Meta-analyzes of randomized controlled trials have been performed to estimate the effects of NSAIDs on blood pressure. Pope et al. (1993) analyzed data from 54 interventional studies of predominantly hypertensive patients (92%) and concluded that the effects of ibuprofen on blood pressure were negligible. Johnson et al. (1994a) used the results of 50 randomized controlled trials. The effect size of ibuprofen was not significant, but only 5 of the 50 trials included ibuprofen, which limited the power to detect an effect on blood pressure.

Houston et al. (1995) found no effect of adding ibuprofen 1200 mg/day to the regimen of 53 (otherwise healthy) hypertensive patients treated with verapamil. The study duration was 3 weeks. Minuz et al. (1990) found that compared to placebo, ibuprofen increased systolic blood pressure of 46 mildly hypertensive patients. Trimarco et al. (1985) found that such increases could be related to the ability of ibuprofen to interfere with sodium excretion in hypertensive patients.

Heerdink *et al.* (1996) studied a 10 519 patient cohort from the Netherlands using the PHARMO database and found that NSAIDs increased the risk of hospitalization for heart failure 2-fold. This estimate was stable after adjusting for patient age, gender, history of hospitalization and concurrent drug use. Incidence densities revealed that patients were 5 times more likely to be hospitalized for their heart failure within days of receiving a NSAID prescription compared to the rate 3 months later. This again indicates that the sodium-retentive effects of ibuprofen occur quickly and are capable of significant exacerbation of heart failure. Discontinuation of NSAID or increasing the dose of the patient's diuretic presumably diminished the likelihood of later exacerbations.

10.4.6 Effects of NSAIDs on serum potassium concentration

As previously described, inhibition of PGI_2 and PGE_2 synthesis at the juxtaglomerular apparatus by NSAIDs can produce hyporeninemic-hypoaldosteronism and result in hyperkalemia. Disorders prevalent in patients with this syndrome include age > 65 years, chronic renal insufficiency and diabetes mellitus (DeFronzo, 1980). The increase of serum potassium concentrations by NSAIDs has been used therapeutically in the treatment of Bartter's syndrome (Bartter *et al.*, 1976; Gill *et al.*, 1976). Because of ibuprofen's weak inhibition of PG synthesis at the juxtaglomerular apparatus, indomethacin is favoured over ibuprofen for the treatment of Bartter's syndrome (Bowden *et al.*, 1978).

Ordinarily, NSAID administration does not cause hyperkalemia in healthy subjects. Most case reports involve elderly patients with chronic renal insufficiency (Kimberly *et al.*, 1978; Tan *et al.*, 1979; Zimran *et al.*, 1985). Most cases involve indomethacin (Ponce *et al.*, 1985). Examples of hyperkalemia in patients prescribed ibuprofen are rare (Kimberly *et al.*, 1978; Tan and Burton, 1981; Lee *et al.*, 1986; Marasco *et al.*, 1987).

We also found in our acute interventional and epidemiological studies that ibuprofen administration rarely results in hyperkalemia. In our interventional studies of ibuprofen, any increases in serum potassium were transient and returned to normal within a month of ibuprofen administration. We also searched for the occurrence of ibuprofen-associated hyperkalemia in adult general medicine patients in Indianapolis using the RMRS. We defined as clinically significant a 20% increase in serum potassium from the last measurement within the 1 year prior to patients' first ibuprofen prescription date to the first serum potassium measurement following this date. Of 1163 ibuprofen recipients, 94 patients (8.1%) had clinically significant increases in their serum potassium; only 8 patients had values > 5.5 mmol/l. A review of the charts for these 8 patients revealed that ibuprofen-associated hyperkalemia was possible in only 3 patients. Relative to 2737 patients prescribed acetaminophen (instead of ibuprofen) we found a risk of ibuprofen-associated hyperkalemia of 1.1; 95% confidence interval, 0.84–1.48. Thus, the risk of developing hyperkalemia with ibuprofen use is extremely small.

10.4.7 Acute interstitial nephritis

Interstitial nephritis is a rare but severe form of ibuprofen nephrotoxicity. Incidence estimates indicate that it occurs in one of every 5000 to 10 000 patients using NSAIDs. Interstitial nephritis differs from the syndrome of acute ischemic renal insufficiency in its slower onset, greater severity and longer duration (Brater, 1988). Onset is usually within several months to 1 year from the start of NSAID administration (Porile *et al.*, 1990). Clinical characteristics include greatly elevated serum creatinine that may exceed 6 mg/dl, oedema, and proteinuria > 3.5 g/24 h in two-thirds of patients.

Renal biopsy demonstrates diffuse interstitial oedema and mild to moderate inflammation. Cellular infiltration of predominantly cytotoxic T cells is seen with smaller numbers of B cells and eosinophils (Bender *et al.*, 1984; Abt and Gordon, 1985). In contrast to acute interstitial nephritis caused by β-lactam antibiotics, eosinophiluria, eosinophilia, fever, and skin rash are infrequent. Most patients respond to discontinuation of the offending NSAID within 1–3 months (Brezin *et al.*, 1979; Porile *et al.*, 1990). Dialysis is sometimes necessary.

Arylpropionic NSAIDs, particularly fenoprofen, are frequently cited causes of acute interstitial nephritis. (Garella and Matarese, 1984; Pirani *et al.*, 1987; Porile *et al.*, 1990) Ibuprofen has also been reported (Regester 1980; Bender *et al.*, 1984; Kleinknecht *et al.*, 1986; Moss *et al.*, 1986; Marasco *et al.*, 1987; Pirani *et al.*, 1987; Tolins and Seel, 1987). There has been one report of a 20-year-old healthy female athlete whose disease progressively deteriorated after taking up to 1200 mg/day of OTC ibuprofen for 6 months to the extent that renal transplantation was required (Griffiths, 1992). Fortunately, such a tragic clinical course is not the rule.

A history of fenoprofen use is present in more cases than one might predict given its limited use. It was implicated in 20 of 43 cases (46%) of NSAID-associated interstitial nephritis in a recent case series review (Porile *et al.*, 1990). Although drugs from all of the other chemical classes of NSAIDs have been implicated, the high prevalence of fenoprofen-associated cases is much greater considering its limited use. It is possible that fenoprofen acyl glucuronide is capable of forming reactive metabolites by acyl glucuronide migration with irreversible binding to albumin or other haptens in a stereoselective fashion (Volland *et al.*, 1991). These complexes conceivably could be transported into the mesangium, causing release of cytokines, interleukins and other substances. Similarly, the fenoprofen–protein adduct could possess adverse immunological properties by increasing interleukin production of resident macrophages or cytotoxic T lymphocytes that may then be responsible for fenoprofen-associated interstitial nephritis (Ten *et al.*, 1988).

10.4.8 Membranous nephropathy

Radford *et al.* (1996) retrospectively reviewed charts using the Mayo Clinic indexing system to study the association of membranous nephropathy with the use of NSAIDs.

Using 20 years' of renal biopsy data, they identified 125 patients with membranous nephropathy of whom 29 were using NSAIDs at the time of its onset. Of these 29 patients, 13 patients met their criteria for being NSAID-related. Ibuprofen was implicated in 3 of the cases (23%). These were the first reports of ibuprofen causing this disorder. Patients were all males, aged 45, 49 and 50 years. Ibuprofen dosage ranged from 800 mg every other day to 1200 mg/day and duration of use ranged from 1 to 9 months. All patients had mild disease; one patient had associated interstitial nephritis. Two patients were treated with corticosteroids. Twenty-four-hour urinary protein declined to < 1 g/24 h within 8 months. The authors estimated that at least 10% of early-onset membranous nephropathy could be attributed to NSAID use.

10.4.9 Papillary necrosis

The most severe and often irreversible form of renal toxicity caused by NSAIDs is analgesic-associated nephropathy. There is little evidence to suggest that prolonged ibuprofen use results in papillary necrosis or analgesic nephropathy. Permanent damage to the kidney has occurred in persons who have abused analgesic mixtures for many years, particularly those containing phenacetin. The mechanism of this analgesic-associated nephropathy is poorly understood. Although several reports have appeared implicating the newer NSAIDs, including ibuprofen, as a cause of analgesic-associated nephropathy, there is little existing evidence to lead one to conclude that papillary necrosis from ibuprofen occurs.

There has been only one well-documented case implicating ibuprofen as a cause of papillary necrosis (Shah *et al.*, 1981; Rossi *et al.*, 1988). Several additional cases have been reported in which patients who were taking ibuprofen developed papillary necrosis, but these patients had other pathology such as necrotizing arthritis (Heaton and Bourke, 1976) and sickle-cell anemia (Lourie *et al.*, 1977) that also could be implicated. Seagasothy *et al.* (1994) questioned more than 2000 patients admitted to the medical wards about their analgesic consumption. Of these, 308 patients were considered to have abused analgesics. The analgesics for 38 patients who consumed excessive amounts of analgesics were profiled. Ibuprofen was not mentioned among these medications.

10.4.10 Renal interactions associated with ibuprofen

There are a number of interactions produced by ibuprofen that could result in important pharmacokinetic and pharmacodynamic changes to other drugs that are administered concurrently (Brater, 1986; Murray and Brater, 1990a; Johnson *et al.*, 1994b). Some of these interactions are real and others will require further documentation. Co-administration of ibuprofen with methotrexate could result in important decreases in the renal clearance of methotrexate (Tracy *et al.*, 1992) However, patients receiving lower doses (7.5 mg/week) of methotrexate in the treatment of rheumatoid arthritis may safely receive ibuprofen (Kremer and Hamilton, 1995).

Ibuprofen administered with angiotensin-converting enzyme inhibitors reduces natriuresis and can have a hemodynamic effect (Allon *et al.*, 1990). Ibuprofen may antagonize the effects of frusemide (furosemide) (Laiwah and Mactier, 1981), but this effect is more frequent with the more potent cyclooxygenase inhibitor indomethacin (Passmore *et al.*, 1989). Ibuprofen has also been reported to produce baclofen toxicity (Dahlin and George, 1984) and to decrease lithium clearance (Ragheb, 1987).

10.5 SUMMARY

Short-term use (1 month) of ibuprofen poses little threat of renal insult in normal, healthy persons at therapeutic dosages. However, NSAID administration to susceptible persons may cause decrements in renal plasma flow and glomerular filtration rate within hours. These acute renal effects are the most common effect of NSAIDs on the kidney and are caused by inhibition of products of arachidonic acid metabolism and other autacoids. Precipitous decrements in glomerular filtration and renal ischemia manifested by increased serum creatinine and urea nitrogen are possible. Patients susceptible to the sodium-retentive effects of ibuprofen may experience oedema, weight gain or increased blood pressure. However, these effects are usually fully reversible with prompt discontinuation of ibuprofen. Risk factors for the development of these acute renal effects are known, allowing clinicians to prospectively identify patients who are at risk and monitor them appropriately.

Acute interstitial nephritis is a rare form of renal toxicity that typically occurs over months of use. Renal impairment may be so severe as to require temporary hemodialysis or require kidney transplantation. As with the acute ischemic effects that occur with ibuprofen, however, renal function usually returns to normal upon discontinuation of NSAID. In contrast to the acute effects of NSAIDs, irreversible, analgesic-associated nephropathy manifested by papillary necrosis and chronic interstitial nephritis is extremely rare with ibuprofen (if it occurs). Clinically relevant drug interactions with ibuprofen are few.

In conclusion, although ibuprofen produces a variety of renal syndromes, with reasonable precautions, including improving consumer awareness and early renal monitoring by physicians of patients at risk for acute effects, it has an excellent safety profile.

REFERENCES

ABT, A.B. and GORDON, J.A. (1985) Drug-induced interstitial nephritis: coexistence with glomerular disease. *Archives of Internal Medicine* 145, 1063–1067.

ADAMS, S.S., BOUGH, R.G., CLIFFE, E.E., LESSEL, B. and MILLS, R.F.N. (1969) Absorption, distribution, and toxicity of ibuprofen. *Toxicology and Applied Pharmacology* 15, 310–330.

ADAMS, S.S., BOUGH, R.G., CLIFFE, E.E., DICKINSON, W., LESSEL, B., McCULLOUGH, K.F., MILLS, R.F.N., NICHOLSON, J.S. and WILLIAMS, G.A.H. (1970) Some aspects of the pharmacology, metabolism, and toxicity of ibuprofen. *Rheumatology and Physical Medicine* (Suppl. 9), 9–26.

ADAMS, S.S., BRESLOFF, P. and MASON, C.G. (1976) Pharmacological differences between the optical isomers of ibuprofen: evidence for metabolic inversion of the (–) isomer. *Journal of Pharmacy and Pharmacology* 28, 256–265.

ADELMAN, A.M., DALY, M.P. and MICHOCK, R.J. (1990) Alternate drugs. *Clinics in Geriatric Medicine* 6, 423–444.

AD HOC COMMITTEE FOR THE NATIONAL KIDNEY FOUNDATION (1985) Statement on the release of ibuprofen as an over-the-counter medicine [Editorial]. *American Journal of Kidney Diseases* 6, 4–5.

ALLON, M., PASQUE, C.B. and RODRIGUEZ, M. (1990) Interaction of captopril and ibuprofen on glomerular and tubular function in humans. *American Journal of Physiology* 259(2 Pt 2), F233–238.

ÄNGGÅRD, E. and OLIW, E. (1981) Formation and metabolism of prostaglandins in the kidney. *Kidney International* 19, 771–780.

BAKRIS, G.L., STARKE, U., HEIFETS, M., POLACK, D., SMITH, M. and LEURGANS, S. (1995) Renal effects of oral prostaglandin supplementation after ibuprofen in diabetic subjects: a double-blind, placebo-controlled, multicenter trial. *Journal of the American Society of Nephrology* 5, 1684–1688.

BARTTER, F.C., GILL, J.R. Jr., FROLICH, J.C., BOWDEN, R.E., HOLLIFIELD, J.W., RADFAR, N., KEISER, H.R., OATES, J.A., SEYBERTH, H. and TAYLOR, A.A. (1976) Prostaglandins are overproduced by the kidneys and mediate hyperreninemia in Bartter's syndrome. *Transactions of the Association of American Physicians* 89, 77–91.

BAUM, C., KENNEDY, D.L. and FORBES, M.B. (1985) Utilization of nonsteroidal anti-inflammatory drugs. *Arthritis and Rheumatism* 28, 686–692.

BEARD, K., PERERA, D.R. and JICK, H. (1988) Drug-induced parenchymal renal disease in outpatients. *Journal of Clinical Pharmacology* 28, 431–435.

BENDER, W.L., WHELTON, A., BESCHORNER, W.E., DARWISH, M.O., HALL-CRAGGS, M. and SOLEZ, K. (1984) Interstitial nephritis, proteinuria and renal failure caused by non-steroidal anti-inflammatory drugs. Immunologic characterization of the inflammatory infiltrate. *American Journal of Medicine* 76, 1006–1012.

BENNETT, W.M., HENRICH, W.L. and STOFF, J.S. (1996) The renal effects of nonsteroidal anti-inflammatory drugs: summary and recommendations. [Review]. *American Journal of Kidney Diseases* 28, S56–62.

BLECHMAN, W.J., SCHMID, F.R., APRIL, P.A., WILSON, C.H. and BROOKS, C.D. (1975) Ibuprofen or aspirin in rheumatoid arthritis therapy. *Journal of the American Medical Association* 233, 336–339.

CHAPTER 10

BLUM, M. and AVIRAM, A. (1980) Ibuprofen-induced hyponatremia. *Rheumatology and Rehabilitation* **19**, 258–259.

BONNEY, S.L., NORTHINGTON, R.S., HEDRICH, D.A. and WALKER, B.R. (1986) Renal safety of two analgesics used over the counter: ibuprofen and aspirin. *Clinical Pharmacology and Therapeutics* **40**, 373–377.

BOWDEN, R.E., KIMBERLY, R.P. and GILL, J.R. *et al.* (1977) Urinary prostaglandin E and renal function. *Clinical Research* **24**, 427A.

BOWDEN, R.E., GILL, J.R., JR., RADFAR, N., TAYLOR, A.A. and Keiser, H.R. (1978) Prostaglandin synthetase inhibitors in Bartter's syndrome. Effect on immunoreactive prostaglandin E excretion. *Journal of the American Medical Association* **239**, 117–121.

BRATER, D.C. (1986) Drug–drug and drug–disease interactions with nonsteroidal anti-inflammatory drugs. *American Journal of Medicine* **80**(Suppl. 1A), 62–77.

BRATER, D.C. (1988) Clinical aspects of renal prostaglandins and NSAID therapy. [Review]. *Seminars in Arthritis and Rheumatism* **17**, 17–22.

BRATER, D.C., ANDERSON, S., BAIRD, B. and CAMPBELL, W.B. (1985) Effects of ibuprofen, naproxen, and sulindac on prostaglandins in men. *Kidney International* **27**, 66–73.

BREZIN, J.H., MORIBER, KATZ, S., SCHWARTZ, A.B. and CHINITZ, J.L. (1979) Reversible renal failure and nephrotic syndrome associated with nonsteroidal anti-inflammatory drugs. *New England Journal of Medicine* **301**, 1271–1273.

CARMICHAEL, J. and SHANKEL, S.W. (1985) Effects of nonsteroidal anti-inflammatory drugs on prostaglandins and renal function. *American Journal of Medicine* **78**, 992–1000.

CHAN, X. (1987) Fatal renal failure due to indomethacin. *Lancet* **ii**, 340.

CHEN, C.Y., PANG, V.F. and CHEN, C.S. (1994) Assessment of ibuprofen-associated nephrotoxicity in renal dysfunction. *Journal of Pharmacology and Experimental Therapeutics* **270**, 1307–1312.

CIABATTONI, G., CINOTTI, G.A., PIERUCCI, A., SIMONETTI, B.M., MANZI, M., PUGLIESE, F., BARSOTTI, P., PECCI, G., TAGGI, F. and PATRONO, C. (1984) Effects of sulindac and ibuprofen in patients with chronic glomerular disease. Evidence for the dependence of renal function on prostacyclin. *New England Journal of Medicine* **310**, 279–283.

CLIVE, D.M. and STOFF, J.S. (1984) Renal syndromes associated with nonsteroidal anti-inflammatory drugs. *New England Journal of Medicine* **310**, 563–573.

COX, P.G., MOONS, W.M., RUSSEL, F.G. and VAN GINNEKEN, C.A. (1991) Renal handling and effects of (S)-(+)-ibuprofen and (R)-(−)-ibuprofen in the rat isolated perfused kidney. *British Journal of Pharmacology* **103**, 1542–1546.

CUMMINGS, D.M., AMADIO, P., JR., NETTLER, S. and FREEDMAN, M. (1988) Office-based evaluation of renal function in elderly patients receiving nonsteroidal anti-inflammatory drugs. *Journal of the American Board of Family Practice* **1**, 77–80.

DAHLIN, P.A. and GEORGE, J. (1984) Baclofen toxicity associated with declining renal clearance after ibuprofen. *Drug Intelligence and Clinical Pharmacy* **18**, 805–808.

DARNELL, J.D., MURRAY, M.D., MARTZ, B.L. and WEINBERGER, M. (1986) Medication use by ambulatory elderly. *Journal of the American Geriatrics Society* **34**, 1–4.

DAVIES, E.F. and AVERY, G.S. (1971) Ibuprofen: a review of its pharmacological properties and therapeutic efficacy in rheumatic disorders. *Drugs* **2**, 416–446.

DAY, R.O., GRAHAM, G.G., WILLIAMS, K.M., CHAMPION, G.D. and DE JAGER, J. (1987) Clinical pharmacology of non-steroidal anti-inflammatory drugs. *Pharmacology and Therapy* **3**, 383–433.

DE FRONZO, R.A. (1980) Hyperkalemia and hyporeninemic hypoaldosteronism. *Kidney International* **17**, 118–134.

DORNAN, J. and REYNOLDS, W.J. (1974) Comparison of ibuprofen and acetylsalicylic acid in the treatment of rheumatoid arthritis. *Canadian Medical Association Journal* **110**, 1370–1372.

DUBOSE, T.D. JR. (1994) Nephrotoxicity of nonsteroidal anti-inflammatory drugs. *Lancet* **344**, 515–518.

DUNN, M.J. (1984a) Nonsteroidal anti-inflammatory drugs and renal function. *Annual Review of Medicine* **35**, 411–428.

DUNN, M.J. (1984b) Role of eicosanoids in the control of renal function in severe hepatic disease. *Gastroenterology* **87**, 1392–1395.

DUNN, M.J. and ZAMBRASKI, E.J. (1980) Renal effects of drugs that inhibit prostaglandin synthesis. *Kidney International* **18**, 609–622.

EPSTEIN, M. and HOLLENBERG, N.K. (1976) Age as a determinant of renal sodium conservation in normal man. *Journal of Laboratory and Clinical Medicine* **87**, 411–417.

FEIGEN, L.P. (1984) Influence of renal lipoxygenase activity on the renal vascular response to arachidonic acid. *Journal of Pharmacology and Experimental Therapeutics* **228**, 140–146.

FITZPATRICK, F.A. and WYNALDA, M.A. (1976) *In vivo* suppression of prostaglandin biosynthesis by non-steroidal anti-inflammatory agents. *Prostaglandins* **12**, 1037–1051.

FOX, D.A. and JICK, H. (1984) Nonsteroidal anti-inflammatory drugs and renal disease. *Journal of the American Medical Association* **251**, 1299–1302.

FROCHT, A. and FILLIT, H. (1984) Renal disease in the geriatric patient. *Journal of the American Geriatric Society* **32**, 28–43.

GARELLA, S. and MATARESE, R.A. (1984) Renal effects of prostaglandins and clinical adverse effects of nonsteroidal anti-inflammatory agents. *Medicine* **63**, 165–181.

CHAPTER 10

GERBER, J.G., BRANCH, R.A., NIES, A.S., GERKENS, J.F., SHAND, D.G., HOLLIFIELD, J. and OATES, J.A. (1978) Prostaglandins and renin release: II. Assessment of renin secretion following infusion of PGI_2, E_2, D_2 into the renal artery of anesthetized dogs. *Prostaglandins* **15**, 81–88.

GILL, J.R. JR., FROLICH, J.C., BOWDEN, R.E., TAYLOR, A.A., KEISER, H.R., SEYBERTH, H.W., OATES, J.A. and BARTTER, F.C. (1976) Bartter's syndrome: a disorder characterized by high urinary prostaglandins and a dependence of hyperreninemia on prostaglandin synthesis. *American Journal of Medicine* **61**, 43–51.

GRIFFITHS, M.L. (1992) End-stage renal failure caused by regular use of anti-inflammatory analgesic medication for minor sports injuries: a case report. *South African Medical Journal* **81**, 377–378.

GURALNIK, J.M., LACROIX, A.Z., EVERETT, D.F. and KOVAR, M.G. (1989) Aging in the eighties: the prevalence of comorbidity and its association with disability. *Vital and Health Statistics of the National Center for Health Center for Statistics. Advance Data Report, no. 170.*

GURWITZ, J.H., AVORN, J., ROSS-DEGNAN, D. and LIPSITZ, L.A. (1990) Nonsteroidal anti-inflammatory drug-associated azotemia in the very old. *Journal of the American Medical Association* **264**, 471–475.

GURWITZ, J.H., AVORN, J., BOHN, R.L., GLYNN, R.J., MONANE, M. and MOGUN, H. (1994) Initiation of antihypertensive treatment during nonsteroidal anti-inflammatory drug therapy. *Journal of the American Medical Association* **272**, 781–786.

GURWITZ, J.H., EVERITT, D.E., MONANE, M., GLYNN, R.J., CHOODNOVSKIY, I., BEAUDET, M.P. and AVORN, J. (1996) The impact of ibuprofen on the efficacy of antihypertensive treatment with hydrochlorothiazide in elderly persons. *Journal of Gerontology, Series A, Biological*, M74–79.

HARRIS, R.C., MUNGER, K.A., BADR, K.F. and TAKAHASHI, K. (1990) Mediation of renal vascular effects of epidermal growth factor by arachidonate metabolites. *FASEB Journal* **4**, 1654–1660.

HARTUPEE, D.A., PASSMORE, J.C. and JIMENEZ, A. (1993) Effect of leukotrienes of renal water excretion. *Prostaglandins Leukotrienes and Essential Fatty Acids* **48**, 297–303.

HEATON, J.M. and BOURKE, E. (1976) Papillary necrosis associated with calyceal arthritis. *Nephron* **16**, 57–63.

HÉBERT, R.L., JACOBSON, H.R. and BREYER, M.D. (1991) Prostaglandin E_2 inhibits sodium transport in rabbit collecting duct by increasing intracellular calcium. *Journal of Clinical Investigation* **87**, 1992–1998.

HEERDINK, E.R., LEUFKENS, H.G., HERINGS, R.M.C., OTTERVANGER, J.P., STRICKER, B.H.C. and BAKKER, A. (1996) NSAIDs increase the risk of congestive heart failure in elderly patients on diuretics. *Archives of Internal Medicine* **158**.

HENRICH, W.L. (1991) Southwestern Internal Medicine Conference. The endothelium — a key regulator of vascular tone. *American Journal of the Medical Sciences* **302**, 319–328.

HENRICH, W.L. (1992) Functional and organic ischemic renal disease. In: SELDIN, D.W. and GIEBISCH, G. (eds), *The Kidney: Physiology and Pathophysiology*, vol. 3. New York, Raven Press, 3289–3292.

HOUSTON, M.C., WEIR, M., GRAY, J., GINSBERG, D., SZETO, C., KAIHLENEN, P.M., SUGIMOTO, D., RUNDE, M. and LEFKOWITZ, M. (1995). The effects of nonsteroidal anti-inflammatory drugs on blood pressures of patients with hypertension controlled by verapamil. *Archives of Internal Medicine* **155**, 1049–1054.

ICHIKAWA, I. and BRENNER, B.M. (1980) Importance of efferent arteriole vascular tone in regulation of proximal tubular fluid reabsorption and glomerulotubular balance in the rat. *Journal of Clinical Investigation* **65**, 1192–1201.

IMS AMERICA (1996) Totowa, New Jersey, 07512.

JOHNSON, A.G. and DAY, R.O. (1991) The problems of NSAID therapy in the elderly (Part I). *Drugs and Aging* **1**, 130–143.

JOHNSON, A.G., NGUYEN, T.V. and DAY, R.O. (1994a) Do nonsteroidal anti-inflammatory drugs affect blood pressure? A meta-analysis. *Annals of Internal Medicine* **121**, 289–300.

JOHNSON, A.G., SEIDEMANN, P. and DAY, R.O. (1994b) NSAID-related adverse drug interactions with clinical relevance: an update. *International Journal of Clinical Pharmacology and Therapeutics* **32**, 509–532.

JOHNSON, J.H., JICK, H., HUNTER, J.R. and DICKSON, J.F. (1985) A followup study of ibuprofen users. *Journal of Rheumatology* **12**, 549–552.

KANTOR, T.G. (1979) Ibuprofen: drugs five years later. *Annals of Internal Medicine* **91**, 877–882.

KAOJARERN, S., CHENNAVASIN, P., ANDERSON, S. and BRATER, D.C. (1983) Nephron site of effect of nonsteroidal anti-inflammatory drugs on solute, excretion in humans. *American Journal of Physiology* **244**, F134–F139.

KAUFMAN, R.P. JR., ANNER, H., KOBZIK, L., VALERI, C.R., SHEPRO, D. and HECHTMAN, H.B. (1987a) Vasodilator prostaglandins (PG) prevent renal damage after ischemia. *Annals of Surgery* **205**, 195–198.

KAUFMAN, R.P. JR., ANNER, H., KOBZIK, L., VALERI, C.R., SHEPRO, D. and HECHTMAN, H.B. (1987b) A high plasma prostaglandin to thromboxane ratio protects against renal ischemia. *Surgery, Gynecology and Obstetrics* **165**, 404–409.

KIMBERLY, R.P., BOWDEN, R.E., KEISER, H.R. and PLOTZ, P.H. (1978) Reduction of renal function by newer nonsteroidal anti-inflammatory drugs. *American Journal of Medicine* **64**, 804–807.

KLAHR, S., SCHREINER, G. and ICHIKAWA, I. (1988) The progression of renal disease. *New England Journal of Medicine* **318**, 1657–1666.

CHAPTER 10

KLAUSNER, J.M., PATERSON, I.S., KOBZIK, L., RODZEN, C., VALERI, C.R., SHEPRO, D. and HECHTMAN, H.B. (1989) Vasodilating prostaglandins attenuate ischemic renal injury only if thromboxane is inhibited. *Annals of Surgery* **209**, 219–224.

KLEINKNECHT, D. (1993) Diseases of the kidney caused by non-steroidal anti-inflammatory drugs. In: STEWARD, J.H. (ed.), *Analgesic and NSAID-induced Kidney Disease*. Oxford, Oxford University Press, 160–173.

KLEINKNECHT, D., LANDAIS, P. and GOLDFARB, B. (1986) Analgesic and nonsteroidal anti-inflammatory drug-associated acute renal failure: a prospective collaborative study. *Clinical Nephrology* **25**, 275–281.

KREIS, H., Chkoff, N., DROZ, D., NOEL, L.H., TOLANI, M., DESCAMPS, J.M., CHATENOUD, L., LACOMBE, M. and CROSNIER, J. (1984) Nonsteroid anti-inflammatory agents as a substitute treatment for steroids in ATGAM-treated cadaver kidney recipients. *Transplantation* **37**, 139–145.

KREMER, J.M. and HAMILTON, R.A. (1995) The effects of nonsteroidal anti-inflammatory drugs on methotrexate pharmacokinetics: impairment of renal clearance of methotrexate at weekly maintenance doses but not at 7.5 mg. *Journal of Rheumatology* **22**, 2072–2077.

LAIWAH, A.C.Y. and MACTIER, R.A. (1981) Antagonistic effect of non-steroidal anti-inflammatory drugs on frusemide-induced diuresis in cardiac failure. *British Medical Journal Clinical Research Edition* **283**(6293), 714.

LATTA, H. (1992) An approach to the structure and function of the glomerular mesangium. *Journal of the American Society of Nephrology* **2**(Suppl.), S65–S73.

LEE, T.H., SALOMON, D.R., RAYMENT, C.M. and ANTMAN, E.M. (1986) Hypotension and sinus arrest with exercise-induced hyperkalemia and combined verapamil/propranolol therapy. *American Journal of Medicine* **80**, 1203–1204.

LEVI, M. and ROWE, J.W. (1992) Renal function and dysfunction in aging. In: SELDIN, D.W. and GIEBISCH, G. (eds), *The Kidney: Physiology and Pathophysiology*. New York, Raven Press, 3433–3455.

LEWIS, J.R. (1976) Evaluation of ibuprofen (Motrin): A new antirheumatic agent. *Journal of the American Medical Association* **233**, 364–365.

LING, B.N., KOKKO, K.E. and EATON, D.C. (1992) Inhibition of apical Na^+ channels in rabbit cortical collecting tubules by basolateral prostaglandin E_2 is modulated by protein kinase. *Journal of Clinical Investigation* **90**, 1328–1334.

LOURIE, S.H., DENMAN, S.J. and SCHROEDER, E.T. (1977) Association of renal papillary necrosis and ankylosing spondylitis. *Arthritis and Rheumatism* **20**, 917–921.

LUFT, F.C., WEINBERGER, M.H., FINEBERG, N.S., MILLER, J.Z. and GRIM, C.E. (1987) Effects of age on renal sodium homeostasis and its relevance to sodium sensitivity. *American Journal of Medicine* **82**(Suppl. 1B), 9–15.

MARASCO, W.A., GIKAS, P.W., AZZIZ-BAUMGARTNER, R., HYZY, R., ELREDGE, C.J. and STROSS, J. (1987) Ibuprofen-associated renal dysfunction. Pathophysiologic mechanisms of acute renal failure, hyperkalemia, tubular necrosis, and proteinuria. *Archives of Internal Medicine* **147**, 210–216.

McGIFF, J.C. (1991) Cytochrome P450 metabolism of arachidonic acid. *Annual Review of Pharmacology and Toxicology* **31**, 339–369.

McINTIRE, S.C., RUBENSTEIN, R.C., GARTNER, J.C., GILBOA, N. and ELLIS, D. (1993) Acute flank pain and reversible renal dysfunction associated with nonsteroidal anti-inflammatory drug use. *Pediatrics* **92**, 459–460.

MEFFIN, P.J., SALLUSTIO, B.C., PURDIE, Y.J. and JONES, M.E. (1986) Enantioselective disposition of 2-arylpropionic acid nonsteroidal anti-inflammatory drugs. I. 2-Phenylpropionic acid disposition. *Journal of Pharmacology and Experimental Therapeutics* **238**, 280–287.

MINUZ, P., BARROW, S.E., COCKROFT, J.R. and RITTER, J.M. (1990) Effects of non-steroidal anti-inflammatory drugs on prostacyclin and thromboxane biosynthesis in patients with mild essential hypertension. *British Journal of Clinical Pharmacology* **30**, 519–526.

MORGENSTERN, S.J., BRUNS, F.J., FRALEY, D.S., KIRSCH, M. and BOROCHOVITZ, D. (1989) Ibuprofen-associated lipoid nephrosis without interstitial nephritis. *American Journal of Kidney Diseases* **14**, 50–52.

MOSS, A.H., RILEY, R., MURGO, A. and SKAFF, L.A. (1986) Over-the-counter ibuprofen and acute renal failure. *Annals of Internal Medicine* **105**, 303.

MURRAY, M.D. and BRATER, D.C. (1990a) Nonsteroidal anti-inflammatory drugs. *Clinics in Geriatric Medicine* **6**, 365–397.

MURRAY, M.D. and BRATER, D.C. (1990b) Adverse effects of nonsteroidal anti-inflammatory drugs on renal function [editorial]. *Annals of Internal Medicine* **112**, 559–560.

MURRAY, M.D. and BRATER, D.C. (1993) Renal toxicity of the nonsteroidal anti-inflammatory drugs. *Annual Review of Pharmacology and Toxicology* **32**, 435–465.

MURRAY, M.D., BRATER, D.C., TIERNEY, W.M., HUI, S.L. and McDONALD, C.J. (1990) Ibuprofen-associated renal impairment in a large general internal medicine practice. *Amercian Journal of Medical Sciences* **299**, 222–229.

MURRAY, M.D., GREENE, P.K., BRATER, D.C., MANATUNGA, A.K. and HALL, S.D. (1992) Effects of flurbiprofen on renal function in patients with moderate renal insufficiency. *British Journal of Clinical Pharmacology* **33**, 385–393.

MURRAY, M.D., BLACK, P.K., KUZMIK, D.D., HAAG, K.M., MANATUNGA, A.K., MULLIN, M.A., HALL, S.D. and BRATER, D.C. (1995) Acute and chronic effects of nonsteroidal anti-inflammatory drugs on glomerular filtration rate in elderly patients. *American Journal of the Medical Sciences* **310**, 188–197.

CHAPTER 10

MURRAY, M.D., LAZARIDIS, E.N., BRIZENDINE, E., HAAG, K., BECKER, P.K. and BRATER, D.C., (1997) Effect of NSAIDs on electrolyte homeostasis and blood pressure in young and elderly persons with and without renal insufficiency. *American Journal of Medical Sciences* **314**, 80–88.

NADLER, J.L., MCKAY, M., CAMPESE, V., VRBANAC, J. and HORTON, R. (1986) Evidence that prostacyclin modulates the vascular actions of calcium in man. *Journal of Clinical Investigation* **77**, 1278–1284.

PALMER, B.F. and HENRICH, W.L. (1995) Clinical acute renal failure with nonsteroidal anti-inflammatory drugs. [Review]. *Seminars in Nephrology* **15**, 214–227.

PASSMORE, A.P., COPELAND, S. and JOHNSTON, G.D. (1989) A comparison of the effects of ibuprofen and indomethacin upon renal hemodynamics and electrolyte excretion in the presence and absence of frusemide. *British Journal of Clinical Pharmacology* **27**, 483–490.

PASSMORE, A.P., COPELAND, S. and JOHNSTON, G.D. (1990) The effects of ibuprofen and indomethacin on renal function in the presence and absence of frusemide in healthy volunteers on a restricted sodium diet. *British Journal of Clinical Pharmacology* **29**, 311–319.

PATRONO, C., CIABATTONI, G., REMUZZI, G., GOTTI, E., BOMBARDIERI, S., DI MUNN, O., TARTARELLI, G., CINOTTI, G.A., SIMONETTI, B.M. and PIERUCCI, A. (1985) Functional significance of renal prostacyclin and thromboxane A2 production in patients with systemic lupus erythematosus. *Journal of Clinical Investigation* **76**, 1011–1018.

PIRANI, C.L., VALERI, A., D'AGATI, V. and APPEL, G.B. (1987) Renal toxicity of nonsteroidal anti-inflammatory drugs. *Contributions to Nephrology* **55**, 159–175.

PONCE, S.P., JENNINGS, A.E., MADIAS, N.E. and HARRINGTON, J.T. (1985) Drug-induced hyper-kalemia. *Medicine* **64**, 357–370.

POPE, J.E., ANDERSON, J.J. and FELSON, D.T. (1993) A meta-analysis of the effects of the non-steroidal anti-inflammatory drugs on blood pressure. *Archives of Internal Medicine* **153**, 477–484.

PORILE, J.L., BAKRIS, G.L. and GARELLA, S. (1990) Acute interstitial nephritis with glomeru-lopathy due to nonsteroidal anti-inflammatory agents: a review of its clinical spectrum and effects of steroid therapy. *Journal of Clinical Pharmacology* **30**, 468–475.

RADACK, K.L., DECK, C.C. and BLOOMFIELD, S.S. (1987) Ibuprofen interferes with the efficacy of antihypertensive drugs: a randomized, double-blind, placebo-controlled trial of ibuprofen compared with acetaminophen. *Annals of Internal Medicine* **107**, 628–635.

RADFORD, M.G., HOLLEY, K.E., GRANDE, J.P., LARSON, T.S., WAGONER, R.D., DONADIO, J.V. and MCCARTHY, J.T. (1996) Reversible membranous nephropathy associated with the use of nonsteroidal anti-inflammatory drugs. *Journal of the American Medical Association* **276**, 466–469.

RAGHEB, M. (1987) Ibuprofen can increase serum lithium level in lithium-treated patients. *Journal of Clinical Psychiatry* **48**, 161–163.

REGESTER, R.F. (1980) Nephrotic syndrome and renal failure associated with use of non-steroidal anti-inflammatory drugs. *Journal of the Tennessee Medical Association* **73**, 709–711.

REMUZZI, G., FITZGERALD, G.A. and PATRONO, C. (1992) Thromboxane synthesis and action within the kidney. *Kidney International* **41**, 1483–1493.

ROE, D.A. (1990) Geriatric nutrition. *Clinics in Geriatrics Medicine* **6**, 319–334.

ROMERO, J.C., LAHERA, V., SALOM, M.G. and BIONDI, M.L. (1992) Role of the endothelium-dependent relaxing factor nitric oxide on renal function. *Journal of the American Society of Nephrology* **2**, 1371–1387.

ROSSI, E., MENTA, R. and CAMBI, V. (1988) Partially reversible chronic renal failure due to long-term use of non-steroidal anti-inflammatory drugs. *Nephrology, Dialysis and Transplantation* **3**, 469–470.

RUDY, A.C., KNIGHT, P.M., BRATER, D.C. and HALL, S.D. (1995) Enantioselective disposition of ibuprofen in elderly persons with and without renal impairment. *Journal of Pharmacology and Experimental Therapeutics* **273**, 88–93.

SANDERS, L.R. (1995) Exercise-induced acute renal failure associated with ibuprofen, hydrochlorothiazide, and triamterene. *Journal of the American Society of Nephrology* **5**, 2020–2023.

SANDLER, D.P., BURR, F.R. and WEINBERG, C.R. (1991) Nonsteroidal anti-inflammatory drugs and the risk for chronic renal disease. *Annals of Internal Medicine* **115**, 165–172.

SCHLONDORFF, D. (1986) Renal prostaglandin synthesis: sites of production and specific actions of prostaglandins. *American Journal of Medicine* **81**(Suppl. 2B), 1–11.

SCHOOLEY, R.T., WAGLEY, P.F. and LIETMAN, P.S. (1977) Edema associated with ibuprofen therapy. *Journal of the American Medical Association* **237**, 1716–1717.

SEGASOTHY, M., SAMAD, S.A., ZULFIGAR, A. and BENNETT, W.M. (1994) Chronic renal disease and papillary necrosis associated with the long-term use of nonsteroidal anti-inflammatory drugs as the sole or predominant analgesic. *American Journal of Kidney Diseases* **24**, 17–24.

SHAH, G.M., MUHALWAS, K.K. and WINER, R.L. (1981) Renal papillary necrosis due to ibuprofen. *Arthritis and Rheumatism* **24**, 1208–1210.

TAKAHASHI, K., CAPDEVILA, J., KARARA, A., FALCK, J.R., JACOBSON, H.R. and BADR, K.F. (1990) Cytochrome P-450 arachidonate metabolites in rat kidney: characterization and hemodynamic responses. *American Journal of Physiology* **258**, F781–789.

TAN, S.Y. and BURTON, M. (1981) Hyporeninemic hypoaldosteronism. An overlooked cause of hyperkalemia. *Archives of Internal Medicine* **141**, 30–33.

CHAPTER 10

TAN, S.Y., SHAPIRO, R., FRANCO, R., STOCKARD, H. and MULROW, P.J. (1979) Indomethacin-induced prostaglandin inhibition with hyperkalemia: a reversible cause of hyporeninemic-hypoaldosteronism. *Annals of Internal Medicine* **90**, 783–785.

TEN, R.M., MILLINER, D.S., SCHWAB, T.R., HOLLEY, K.E., GLEICH, G.J. and TORRES, V.E. (1988) Acute interstitial nephritis: immunologic and clinical aspects. *Mayo Clinic Proceedings* **63**, 921–930.

THE NORTHERN NEW JERSEY RECORD (newspaper), 18 Oct. 1995.

THE UPJOHN COMPANY (1975) Motrin Product Literature.

TOLINS, J.P. and SEEL, P. (1987) Ibuprofen-induced interstitial nephritis and the nephrotic syndrome. *Minnesota Medicine* **70**, 509–511.

TRACY, T.S., KROHN, K., JONES, D.R., BRADLEY, J.D., HALL, S.D. and BRATER, D.C. (1992) The effects of salicylate, ibuprofen, and naproxen on the disposition of methotrexate in patients with rheumatoid arthritis. *European Journal of Clinical Pharmacology* **42**, 121–125.

TRIMARCO, B., DE SIMONE, A., CUOCOLO, A., RICCIARDELLI, B., VOLPE, M., PATRIGNANI, P., SACCA, L. and CONDORELLI, M. (1985) Role of prostaglandins in the renal handling of a salt load in essential hypertension. *American Journal of Cardiology* **55**, 116–121.

VANE, J.R. and BOTTING, R.M. (1996) Mechanism of action of anti-inflammatory drugs. [Review]. *Scandinavian Journal of Rheumatology — Supplement* **102**, 9–21.

VERBEECK, R.K., BLACKBURN, J.L. and LOEWEN, G.R. (1983) Clinical pharmacokinetics of nonsteroidal anti-inflammatory drugs. *Clinical Pharmacokinetics* **8**, 297–331.

VILLANUEVA, M., HECKENⱼERGER, R., STROBACH, H., PALMER, M. and SCHROR, K. (1993) Equipotent inhibition by (R)-(−), (S)-(+)- and racemic ibuprofen of human polymorphonuclear cell function *in vitro*. *British Journal of Clinical Pharmacology* **35**, 235–242.

VOLLAND, C., SUN, H., DAMMEYER, J. and BENET, L.Z. (1991) Stereoselective degradation of the fenoprofen acyl glucuronide enantiomers and irreversible binding to plasma protein. *Drug Metabolism and Disposition* **19**, 1080–1086.

WATTAD, A., FEEHAN, T., SHEPARD, F.M. and YOUNGBERG, G. (1994) A unique complication of nonsteroidal anti-inflammatory drug use. *Pediatrics* **93**, 693.

WEN, S.F., PARTHASARATHY, R., ILIOPOULOS, O. and OBERLEY, T.D. (1992) Acute renal failure following binge drinking and nonsteroidal antiinflammatory drugs. *American Journal of Kidney Diseases* **20**, 281–285.

WHELTON, A., STOUT, R.L., SPILMAN, P.S. and KLASSEN, D.K. (1990) Renal effects of ibuprofen, piroxicam, and sulindac in patients with asymptomatic renal failure. A prospective, randomized, crossover comparison [see comments]. *Annals of Internal Medicine*, **112**, 568–576.

WHORTON, A.R., MISONO, K., HOLLIFIELD, J., FROLICH, J.C., INGAMI, T., OATES, J.A. (1977) Prostaglandins and renin release: I. Stimulation of renin release from rabbit renal cortical slices. *Prostaglandins* **14**, 1095–1104.

WILLIAMS, K.M. (1990) Enantiomers in arthritic disorders. *Pharmacology and Therapy* **46**, 273–295.

WRIGHT, J.T., MCKENNEY, J.M., LEHANY, A.M., BRYAN, D.L., COOPOER, L.W. and LAMBERT, C.M. (1989) The effect of high-dose short-term ibuprofen on antihypertensive control with hydrochlorothiazide. *Clinical Pharmacology and Therapeutics* **46**, 440–444.

YAMAMOTO, K., ARAKAWA, T., UEDA, N. and YAMAMOTOT, S. (1995) Transcriptional roles of nuclear factor kappa B and nuclear factor interleukin-6 in the tumor necrosis factor alpha-dependent induction of cyclooxygenase-2 in MC3T3-E1 cells. *Journal of Biological Chemistry* **270**, 31315–31350.

YAMASHITA, Y., YUKIMURA, T., MIURA, K., OKUMURA, M. and YAMAMOTO, K. (1991) Effects of endothelin-3 on renal functions. *Journal of Pharmacology and Experimental Therapeutics* **259**, 1256–1260.

YOUNG, J.S., PASSMORE, J.C., HARTUPEE, D.A. and BAKER, C.H. (1990) Nutrient and non-nutrient renal blood flow. *Journal of Laboratory and Clinical Medicine* **115**, 680–687.

ZAMBRASKI, E. and DUNN, M.J. (1993) Effects of non-steroidal anti-inflammatory drugs on renal function. In: STEWARD, J.H. (ed.), *Analgesic and NSAID-induced Kidney Disease*. Oxford, Oxford University Press, 145–159.

ZEIDEL, M.L., BRADY, H.R. and KOHAN, D.E. (1991) Interleukin-1 inhibition of Na(+)-K(+)-ATPase in inner medullary collecting duct cells: role of PGE2. *American Journal of Physiology* **261**, F1013–1016.

ZIMRAN, A., KRAMER, M., PLASKIN, M. and HERSHKO, C. (1985) Incidence of hyperkalemia induced by indomethacin in a hospital population. *British Medical Journal* **291**, 107–108.

ZIPSER, R.D., HOEFS, J.C., SPECKART, P.F., ZIA, P.K. and HORTON, R. (1979) Prostaglandins: modulators of renal function and pressor resistance in chronic liver disease. *Journal of Clinical Endocrinology and Metabolism* **48**, 895–900.

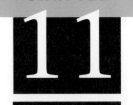

Adverse Drug Reactions Attributed to Ibuprofen: Effects Other Than Gastrointestinal

L J MIWA AND J K JONES

The Degge Group, Drug Safety Research and Information,
1616 North Fort Myer Drive, Suite 1430, Arlington,
VA 22209–3109, USA

Contents

11.1 INTRODUCTION

Nonsteroidal anti-inflammatory drugs (NSAIDs) are among the most widely used products in the world, with estimates that 1–2% of the populations of Europe and the United States take them daily (McGoldrick and Baile, 1997). Given their wide level of use, it would appear that this class of drugs is fairly safe, by and large. Nevertheless, NSAIDs do cause their share of adverse effects, the most common and best-known being gastrointestinal toxicity. This chapter focuses on the non-gastrointestinal adverse effects, which occur with less frequency than gastrointestinal toxicity but which are no less distressing to the patient and often confounding to the physician. Some of these reactions are mediated by the prostaglandin-inhibiting effect of NSAIDs; others cannot be so readily explained.

Although NSAID-associated gastrointestinal adverse effects have been examined in epidemiological studies in several countries that have provided a relatively consistent estimate of risk, quantitative risk estimates from such studies are lacking for the other NSAID-associated adverse effects. However, as the number of NSAIDs marketed has multiplied, the occurrence of these events has revealed a relatively consistent safety profile of NSAIDs as a class.

Much of what is known about these non-gastrointestinal adverse effects is based upon spontaneous reports of suspected associations, along with case series of these events. Although case reports are often used to make inferences as to the actual incidence of these events, it should be emphasized that only clinical trial and epidemiological study data can provide a basis for estimating population risk. Further, depending upon how the events are detected, and the populations in which such studies are done, even these quantitative estimates will vary. In the sections that follow, we describe the qualitative data based on case reports, including evidence from the pharmacological literature. When available, we describe clinical trials and epidemiological studies that provide a basis for a quantitative risk estimate for the particular adverse effect.

11.2 ALLERGY

Allergic or hypersensitivity reactions have always been a part of the profile of events associated with the use of NSAIDs. Some NSAID hypersensitivity reactions have been associated with aspirin sensitivity, in particular events associated with anaphylactoid and upper-airway allergic reactions; thus, presence of this condition is a contraindication for NSAID use. The experience with the NSAID zomepirac in the United States in the early 1980s heightened awareness of the potential for hypersensitivity reactions with this class of drugs. Zomepirac, developed and marketed for analgesic use, was associated with a number of episodes of anaphylaxis and was ultimately withdrawn from the market (Sandler, 1985; Corre and Spielberg, 1988).

CHAPTER 11

■ 499

Although serious hypersensitivity reactions with NSAIDs are rare (Henry, 1988), with movement of ibuprofen and other NSAIDs to non-prescription marketing status, the potential for these reactions remains a concern. Severe asthma and systemic reactions characterized by profound hypotension, fever, myalgias and rash have been reported with ibuprofen (Finch and Strottman, 1979; Lee *et al.*, 1983; Butterfield *et al.*, 1986; Ayres *et al.*, 1987). Reactions such as these represent, along with gastrointestinal effects, one of the two main categories of significant clinical NSAID-associated events that may occur in this setting.

11.2.1 Points to consider when evaluating allergy-type reactions to NSAIDs

Assessment of population risk for 'allergic' or 'hypersensitivity' events associated with NSAIDs is a complex undertaking for several reasons.

Variety of manifestations

From a clinical perspective, a number of clinical events may be labelled as 'hypersensitivity' reactions. These range from a variety of skin eruptions, to urticaria, to angio-oedema, to bronchospasm, and full-blown anaphylaxis. Depending upon how these events are classified, the rates of these reactions may vary considerably. These events have been covered extensively in reviews by many authors, including Bochner and Lichtenstein (1991), Hoigné *et al.* (1993) and Yocum and Khan (1994). Furthermore, the array of pathophysiological events associated with anaphylaxis includes a variety of alterations in the pulmonary, cardiovascular, cutaneous and gastrointestinal systems. Some symptom combinations may not be recognized or may be labelled as hypersensitivity reactions, and others are simply labelled as exacerbated asthma attacks (Picado *et al.*, 1989).

Study designs determine rates

Because of the wide range of possible events that may be classified as allergic reactions, literature estimates of the rate of hypersensitivity events may vary considerably, depending upon the methods used for detection and attribution of the multisystem events.

Multiple mechanisms

Understanding of rates of hypersensitivity reactions is further complicated by the fact that for NSAIDs there are two likely mechanisms associated with producing these events:

(1) *Pharmacological effects*. The pharmacology of the NSAIDs includes the ability to inhibit prostaglandin synthetase. Thus, in some persons, they may act to directly cause bronchospasm and possibly other related 'hypersensitivity' events;

(2) *IGE mediation*. The NSAIDs, being relatively small molecules, are also associated with the IGE-mediated mechanism of sensitization followed by subsequent true allergic reactions, including urticaria and anaphylaxis.

Data from spontaneous reports (Rossi and Knapp, 1982) and epidemiological studies (Strom *et al.*, 1987, 1988) suggest that the ability to cause events by both types of mechanisms may vary with the NSAID.

Variable effect of dose and dosing intervals

If most reactions are associated with the true allergic, or hypersensitivity, mechanism, one would not expect to see much of a dose relationship with hypersensitivity reactions, although some relationship to dose (e.g. with penicillin skin testing) may relate in part to route of exposure. If the pharmacological mechanism prevails, this may not be the case.

In general, it is proposed that for NSAID-associated hypersensitivity reactions there is less likely to be a difference in prescription and non-prescription use in relation to dose. On the other hand, dosing in the non-prescription setting may be *intermittent*, which in turn may predispose to greater risk of hypersensitivity reactions, as was the case for zomepirac (Strom *et al.*, 1987).

11.2.2   Epidemiology of allergy or hypersensitivity with NSAIDS

As noted by Bochner and Lichtenstein (1991), epidemiological data on anaphylaxis and other related hypersensitivity reactions is sparse. Our search for further data that could be used to understand the incidence of NSAID-associated anaphylaxis revealed a paucity of published quantitative data, though descriptive data and case series are common. In part this is due to the fact that serious hypersensitivity reactions are still quite uncommon as a whole, with rough estimates of rates of 1 event in 5000–10 000 persons for exposure to penicillins. Thus, the determination of the actual incidence in a population exposed to a single drug poses significant methodological challenges. We are aware that a case-control study of anaphylactic reactions is being conducted in the United States but have not obtained further details; this type of study will not provide incidence, though it has the potential to determine the relative risk for various prior exposures.

The studies described in the following section provide some insights into the population-based occurrence of hypersensitivity and anaphylactoid reactions associated with NSAIDs. This discussion assumes that dose is not a major factor; rather, any exposure to the drug at any dose (prescription or non-prescription) may convey roughly equal risk.

Epidemiology of allergic reactions in the hospital setting

The hospital setting is ideal for tabulating acute risks to drugs, such as acute allergy, since the potential for capturing serious events is high and the denominator is known. However, there are few recent data from this setting. A much earlier effort is cited for completeness as described below.

In the 1970s the Boston Collaborative Drug Surveillance Program set up a classical in-hospital monitoring programme in medical patients in 19 hospitals distributed in the

United States, New Zealand, Israel, Glasgow, Scotland and Canada (Miller and Greenblatt, 1976). Exposures and events were tabulated and a number of publications have provided baseline data on rates of events in this well-surveyed setting, despite the fact that the effort was discontinued in the late 1970s. With respect to NSAIDs, at the time the data were published, only aspirin, phenylbutazone and indomethacin were widely used and tabulated in the study.

Aspirin: Of 1615 aspirin-exposed patients, 77 had reactions and 2 (0.1% of total recipients) had hypersensitivity reactions. One patient had stomatitis and pharyngeal swelling that interfered with breathing.

Indomethacin: Of 205 patients exposed to indomethacin, 21 (10.2%) had associated events, of which only two (1%) were dermatological events (itching, rash); no other events that suggested clear hypersensitivity were listed.

Phenylbutazone: None of the 128 recipients of phenylbutazone was noted to have hypersensitivity reactions; however, this was commented upon by the authors, who noted that this type of reaction might be expected, citing a contemporaneous reference (Selwyn, 1967).

Although to some extent both the medications and methodology are outdated in that cautions with respect to ascertainment bias and causality assessment have evolved, the advantage of the close scrutiny after exposure provided in this study is likely to provide a reasonable estimate of rates occurring shortly after commencement of dosing. However, the small numbers of exposed patients also means that any estimate probably has a moderate to wide confidence interval.

Epidemiology studies in Medicaid databases

The experience with Zomax[R] (zomepirac, a NSAID marketed in the United States as an analgesic in 1980 and withdrawn in 1983) coincided with the development of Medicaid claims data as a source for postmarketing surveillance in the United States by the federal Food and Drug Administration, and the recognition of a need to determine whether known reactions could be detected. Strom *et al.* (1987, 1988) evaluated these hypersensitivity events using Medicaid data from several states. Incidence rates for each of the NSAIDs studied are provided in Table 11.1.

In an effort to place the very high spontaneous reporting rates for zomepirac relative to other NSAIDs into a population-based context, the authors first examined the relative risk (RR) for hypersensitivity reactions associated with zomepirac as compared with several other NSAIDs in the Florida Medicaid database. Important findings included the fact that the NSAIDs as a group were associated with an adjusted RR of 2.0 (95% confidence interval (CI), 1.3–2.9), which was higher for zomepirac than with all other NSAIDs. Risk was increased in those patients with a diagnosis of acute pain (RR = 3.6; 95% CI, 2.2–5.9) but not other indications, suggesting an association with intermittent use. Risk was higher in younger females, in patients with prior use of penicillin, and after the first NSAID prescription. The most common hypersensitivity ICD-9-CM code was 'urticaria, not otherwise specified'.

TABLE 11.1

NSAIDs and hypersensitivity reactions (Strom *et al.*, 1987)

NSAID	Incidence per 10 000 subjects (95% CI)
Fenoprofen	0 (0–8.5)
Ibuprofen	4.2 (1.8–8.3)
Indomethacin	5.1 (1.1–15.0)
Naproxen	0 (0–22.8)
Phenylbutazone	0 (0–45.3)
Sulindac	4.6 (1.5–10.6)
Tolmetin	0 (0–18.1)
Zomepirac	9.5 (5.3–15.6)

Hypersensitivity reactions included laryngeal spasm, upper respiratory tract hypersensitivity reactions (site unspecified), dermatitis due to drugs, urticaria, allergic urticaria, urticaria (unspecified), shock without mention of trauma, shock (unspecified), anaphylactic shock, angioneurotic oedema, unspecified adverse effect of a drug, medicinal and biological substances.

A follow-on study using Medicaid data in other states (Michigan, Minnesota, Missouri) focused on rates of hypersensitivity of tolmetin (an NSAID structurally related to zomepirac) versus other NSAIDs. A higher risk with tolmetin use was not found in this study (Strom *et al.*, 1988). Ibuprofen was not included in this study.

Epidemiology studies in the Netherlands

A case-cohort study was conducted in the Netherlands by Van der Klauw *et al.* (1993), first to determine the population-based rate of glafenine-associated anaphylactic reactions and further to determine the relative rates associated with other drugs causing admission for anaphylactoid and anaphylactic reactions. This study demonstrated a far higher risk for insects and food as a cause for anaphylaxis than for all drugs combined. For drugs, the relative risk (with 95% CI) was far highest for glafenine anaphylaxis (RR = 167.7 (63.0–446.4) in 1987; 128.6 (50.4–328.5) in 1988) compared with amoxycillin (15.2 (5.0–46.0) in 1987; 4.4 (1.0–18.9) in 1988) and diclofenac (6.1 (1.4–26.1) in 1988). Other NSAIDs grouped showed a RR of 3.19 to 3.67 for probable anaphylaxis, lower than the RR for the above drugs and penicillins.

Although the study design did not allow for precise incidence rate estimates, the authors stated that these findings were consistent with a rate of 1 event in 1000–2000 prescriptions for glafenine and 1 event in 10 000–20 000 prescriptions for diclofenac. Thus, using similar risk estimates for anaphylaxis with other NSAIDs, e.g. naproxen, it might be estimated in the range of 1 event in 20 000–40 000 prescriptions (0.005%). This latter estimate is lower than in the Medicaid study (Strom *et al.*, 1987); however, that study included hypersensitivity reactions other than anaphylaxis, such as urticaria.

NSAID hypersensitivity may manifest in different organ systems, such as the skin and liver. These events will be discussed under the sections specific to those organ systems.

CHAPTER 11

11.3 ADVERSE DERMATOLOGICAL EFFECTS

It has been said that the skin is the organ most commonly affected by adverse drug reactions (Felix and Smith, 1991). Spontaneous reports of NSAID-associated cutaneous adverse reactions are common (Alhava, 1994; Figueras *et al.*, 1994; Halpern, 1994), often being second only to gastrointestinal adverse reactions. A wide variety of cutaneous reactions has been associated with NSAIDs, and the association of a specific reaction may vary widely with individual NSAIDs. Albers (1992) compiled an exhaustive summary of NSAID-associated cutaneous reactions by drug and by reaction type. Epidemiological data are generally lacking for NSAID-associated adverse effects of the skin, except for the most serious and life-threatening types of reactions.

Cutaneous reactions to ibuprofen appear to be common complaints and range from nonspecific rashes to urticaria and pruritus, often as a component of a generalized hypersensitivity reaction (Halpern *et al.*, 1993; Halpern, 1994). Cutaneous reactions accounted for 25.5% of all suspected reactions to ibuprofen reported in the United Kingdom, second only to reports of gastrointestinal adverse effects (Halpern *et al.*, 1993). The frequencies of spontaneously reported cutaneous reactions were morbilliform (42%), angio-oedema (21.4%), urticaria (12.7%), photosensitivity reactions (5.3%), hair and nail disorders (3.7%), pruritus (3.1%), erythema multiforme/Stevens–Johnson syndrome/toxic epidermal necrolysis (3%), bullous eruptions (2.5%), erythema nodosum (0.1%), vasculitis (0.1%), and others (4.4%) (Halpern, 1994). Because skin reactions are quite noticeable and also occur soon after dosing, there is a greater likelihood of detection, attribution and reporting of these reactions than those less clinically noticeable or latent. Accordingly, although the relative frequency of skin reaction types among spontaneous reports may reflect their frequency of occurrence, only clinical trials and epidemiological studies can provide actual incidence rates for comparison.

In clinical trials, the overall incidence of cutaneous reactions was 1.1% (210 of 18 577 subjects) for which 40 patients (0.2% of total) required withdrawal of the drug (Halpern *et al.*, 1993; Halpern, 1994). The incidence in placebo controls in these clinical trials was not reported. The incidence of rash in single-dose, placebo-controlled trials of non-prescription ibuprofen (200 mg and 400 mg doses) was very low, 0.04% (one in 2579 patients) (Furey *et al.*, 1992). This low rate may have been due to the patient selection process, whereby patients with a history of salicylate or NSAID allergy were excluded, and to the short course of treatment.

Data from the Arthritis, Rheumatism and Aging Medical Information System (ARAMIS) that monitors events in patients with osteoarthritis and rheumatoid arthritis in the United States and Canada gives the incidence of nonspecific rash with ibuprofen as 10 events per 1000 patient-years. Similar rates were seen with other propionic acid derivatives. Indomethacin had the lowest rate, 5 events per 1000; piroxicam and meclofenamate had the highest rates, 31 and 39 per 1000 patient-years, respectively (Singh *et al.*, 1994). A similar ranking of NSAIDs was seen in reporting rates (the frequency of reported reactions to number of prescriptions in a defined time period) derived from the US Adverse Drug Reaction Reporting System of the American Academy of Dermatology (Stern and Bigby, 1984), which collected reports from dermatologists. These results are in concurrence with those from the epidemiological studies in terms of specific NSAIDs that appear to present the highest risk.

The few epidemiology studies of NSAID-associated adverse skin events have studied cases hospitalized for the target event. Results from an international collaborative case-control study of persons hospitalized for Stevens–Johnson syndrome (SJS) and toxic epidermal necrolysis (TEN) have been published (Naldi *et al.*, 1990; Roujeau *et al.*, 1990, 1995; Schopf *et al.*, 1991). Combined data from France, Germany, Italy and Portugal found that, among NSAIDs, only oxicam derivatives (e.g. piroxicam) were significantly associated with these diseases (Roujeau *et al.*, 1995). The multivariate relative risk for this class of NSAIDs was 22 (95% CI, 6.2–74). The risks associated with propionic acid NSAIDs (e.g. naproxen) and diclofenac were not significantly increased. A similar study done in Group Health Cooperative of Puget Sound found no NSAID-associated cases of erythema multiforme, SJS or TEN over a 14-year period representing approximately 3.8 million person-years of observation (Chan *et al.*, 1990). NSAIDs were not implicated in this study. A French study of all identified cases of TEN that occurred in France over a 5-year period (1981 to 1985) found NSAIDs to be the class of drugs most often associated (Roujeau *et al.*, 1990). When the number of cases of TEN associated with a specific drug were related to the defined daily doses (DDD) of that drug sold over the 5-year period (cases/sales), the highest ratio occurred with isoxicam. These studies are summarized in Table 11.2.

Thus, of all the NSAIDs, ibuprofen is one less frequently associated with cutaneous reactions. In addition to those reactions reported by Halpern (1994) listed above, fixed eruptions, purpura, lupus erythematosus-like events, Gougerot's syndrome, mucosal lesions, and alopecia were included by Albers in his review (1992).

11.4 HEPATOTOXICITY

Nearly all of the NSAIDs have been implicated in causing liver injury. Several have been withdrawn from clinical use because of associated hepatic injury (Koff, 1992; Boelsterli *et al.*, 1995). These have been summarized in recent reviews (Koff, 1992; Rabinovitz and Van Thiel, 1992; Boelsterli *et al.*, 1995; Manoukian and Carson, 1996).

In his review of NSAID-associated hepatotoxicity, Zimmerman (1990) noted that reports of serious liver toxicity with ibuprofen are rare. Halpern and colleagues (1993) reported that 56 reports of ibuprofen-associated liver disorders had been reported to the Committee on Safety of Medicines in 2644 total ibuprofen reports in the United Kingdom. Cases of ibuprofen hepatic injury have been primarily hepatocellular in nature. The

CHAPTER 11

TABLE 11.2

Summary of epidemiological studies of NSAID-associated severe cutaneous reactions

Study	Study design	Country	Overall incidence	Drug specific estimates of risk
Roujeau et al. (1990)	Retrospective survey of TEN cases over 5-year period	France	1.2–1.3 cases per million per year	Cases per million defined daily doses (DDD): isoxicam 0.41; oxyphenbutazone 0.18; fenbufen 0.13; piroxicam 0.04; diclofenac 0.02; indomethacin 0.01
Chan et al. (1990)	Retrospective survey of EM, SJS, TEN cases over 14-year period in HMO population	USA	7.4 cases per million person-years	NSAIDs not implicated
Naldi et al. (1990)	Retrospective survey of SJS, TEN over 5-year period. Prospective case-control surveillance of SJS, TEN over one year period	Italy	Retrospective: 0.6 case per million per year. Prospective: 1.2 cases per million per year	Not available
Schopf et al. (1991)	Retrospective survey of TEN, SJS over 5-year period	Germany	TEN: 0.93 case per million. SJS: 1.1 cases per million	Cases per million DDD: benoxaprofen 0.25; oxyphenbutazone 0.07; isoxicam 0.04; piroxicam 0.03; diclofenac 0.03; indomethacin 0.02
Roujeau et al. (1995)	Retrospective case-control study of TEN and SJS	France Germany Italy Portugal		Multivariate relative risk (95% CI): oxicam NSAIDs 22 (6.2–74); piroxicam 12 (3.1–45); propionic acid NSAIDs 1.7 (0.6–5.3); diclofenac 2.8 (0.7–10); pyrazolone derivatives 2 (0.6–6.8)

EM, erythema multiforme; TEN, toxic epidermal necrolysis; SJS, Stevens–Johnson syndrome.

mechanism is likely one of immunological idiosyncrasy (Zimmerman, 1990). Ibuprofen-mediated liver injury has also been reported in conjunction with Stevens–Johnson syndrome (Sternlieb and Robinson, 1978).

From a quantitative perspective, no hepatotoxicity was observed among 15 577 patients involved in ibuprofen clinical trials (Halpern et al., 1993). Freeland and co-workers (1988) evaluated aspartase aminotransferase (AST, SGOT) elevations in 1468 patients treated with aspirin, ibuprofen or oxaprozin in controlled, double-blind clinical trials. They found no elevations in ibuprofen-treated patients, concluding that ibuprofen was the safest of the three drugs studied. Elevated AST and ALT (alanine aminotransferase, SGPT) levels have been reported by other authors (Rabinovitz and Van Thiel, 1992).

Clinical trials that employ routine monitoring of liver function have the highest likelihood of ascertainment of any liver function abnormalities and have the considerable advantage of standard measures in defined time periods. Significant but asymptomatic liver toxicity will not be detected except in situations where other medical tests are done or toxicity is being specifically monitored. Thus, the only quantitative measure of effects on liver enzymes is within the clinical trial setting, since detection elsewhere is variable. However, the usefulness of these studies is often restricted owing to small numbers of patients and limited exposure times. Most problematic is the fact that few trials utilize uniform criteria or thresholds for assessing hepatic effects. The incidence rate of adverse liver events is greatly dependent upon the threshold of detection, whether it is an asymptomatic doubling or tripling of the transaminase level or hospitalization with jaundice. This variability confounds attempts to compare data between trials on different NSAIDs.

However, when utilizing clinically significant hepatic events in epidemiological studies, the incidence of serious, NSAID-associated liver disease is extremely low (Manoukian and Carson, 1996). A few cohort and case-control studies have attempted to quantify the risk of serious NSAID-associated liver disease. These are summarized in Table 11.3.

In a study of hospitalizations for acute liver injury in Saskatchewan, 16 cases were identified among 228 392 users of NSAIDs in the 5-year period (January 1982 to December 1986). One case was associated with diclofenac; this patient was also taking piroxicam. There was one case associated with ibuprofen. NSAIDs implicated in other cases included diclofenac, indomethacin, naproxen, sulindac and piroxicam (Garcia-Rodriguez et al., 1992). A case-control study of this same population found no significant difference in risk between these NSAIDs (Pérez-Gutthann and Rodriguez, 1993).

Two studies in the United Kingdom using computer-based medical records in the offices of general practitioners have been published (Jick et al., 1992; Garcia Rodriguez et al., 1994). The study by Garcia-Rodriguez and colleagues (1994) provided a comprehensive and rigorous examination of the data. Detection of a hepatic event was based upon notation by the general practitioner in the computer-based medical record and cases were validated. The incidence of acute liver injury per 100 000 users was 1.6 for ibuprofen. In this study, sulindac had the highest incidence rate at 148.1 per 100 000 users.

An earlier study in the United States used Medicaid claims data for inpatient and outpatient diagnoses in two states (Florida and Michigan) to identify potential cases of liver injury. Only patients whose records were retrieved and who were established to have acute non-viral liver injury were included as cases. There were no significant differences in risk for hepatic injury between types of NSAIDs, possibly because of the small number of cases of hepatic injury (Carson et al., 1993).

A study by Lanza et al. (1995) used automated insurance claims and medical records for 68 028 persons in a health maintenance organization population in the United States to determine the incidence of symptomatic liver function abnormalities, including subjects treated on an outpatient basis (Lanza et al., 1995). Only patients with at least one sign or

CHAPTER 11

TABLE 11.3

Summary of epidemiological studies of NSAID-associated hepatotoxicity

Study	Type of study	Outcome measured	Description of population			Results	Comments
			Geographic location	Study population size	Overall incidence rate (95% CI)	Drug-specific	
Lanza et al. (1995)	Retrospective cohort	Symptomatic liver dysfunction treated in the outpatient or inpatient setting	USA	68 028	0.3 (0.0–0.6) per 1000 NSAID users	Relative risk compared to naproxen 1.0: diclofenac 0.32 (0.2–1.9); piroxicam 0.00 (0.0–0.9); sulindac 2.9 (0.91–7.9); other NSAIDs 1.3 (0.30–4.2). Incidence per 1000 person-years: diclofenac 0.18; naproxen 0.56; piroxicam 0.00; sulindac 1.84; other NSAIDs 0.64	Case definition: at least one abnormal liver function text plus at one sign or symptom of liver dysfunction. Other NSAIDs: flurbiprofen, indomethacin, ketoprofen
Garcia-Rodriguez et al. (1994)	Retrospective cohort, nested case-control	Acute liver injury treated in the outpatient or inpatient setting	UK	625 307	0.04 (0.03–0.06) per 1000 NSAID users	Incidence per 1000 users: ibuprofen 0.02 (0.01–0.04); diclofenac 0.04 (0.01–0.09); naproxen 0.04 (0.02–0.1); mefenamic acid 0.03 (0.01–0.09); ketoprofen 0.09 (0.03–0.26); piroxicam 0.06 (0.02–0.22); fenbufen 0.12 (0.03–0.43); sulindac 1.48 (0.50–4.35)	Relative risk in rheumatoid arthritis patients: 10.9 (2.4–50.2) compared to osteoarthritis patients
Carson et al. (1993)	Case-control	(1) Idiopathic acute symptomatic liver disease resulting in hospitalization; (2) acute non-infectious hepatitis	FL, MI (USA)	107 cases 428 controls matched for sex and age by decade	(1) 0.022 (0.020–0.024) per 1000 persons annually; (2) 0.084 (0.078–0.090) per 1000 persons annually	Unadjusted odds ratio (95% CI): NSAID use: 1.4 (0.6–3.1); ibuprofen 1.3 (0.2–5.5); naproxen 0.6 (0.01–4.5); piroxicam 2.0 (0.03–38.9); sulindac 4.1 (0.8–22.4)	
Perez-Gutthann and Rodriguez (1993)	Nested case-control	Hospitalization for acute liver injury	Saskatchewan, Canada	228 392		Adjusted odds ratio (95% CI): NSAID use: 1.8 (0.8–3.7); ibuprofen 1.2 (0.1–12.0); indomethacin 2.6 (0.8–8.6); diclofenac 2.0 (0.2–17.4); naproxen 1.7 (0.5–6.4); piroxicam 2.0 (0.6–6.8); sulindac 5.0 (1.3–18.5)	Subset of 1992 Garcia-Rodriguez study
Garcia-Rodriguez et al. (1992)	Retrospective cohort	Acute liver injury resulting in hospitalization	Saskatchewan, Canada	228 392	For NSAID use: 0.09 (0.06–0.15) per 1000 person-years		Excess risk with current NSAID use = 0.05 per 1000 person-years. Adjusted RR = 1.7 (0.8–3.7)

CI, confidence interval; RR, relative risk.

symptom of liver disease and at least one abnormal liver function test were considered cases. No significant difference in risk was found between NSAIDs.

NSAID-associated hepatotoxicity occurs rarely and, with the possible exception of sulindac, no one NSAID appears to present more risk than the others.

11.5 HEMATOLOGICAL ADVERSE EFFECTS

NSAIDs have been implicated in a wide range of hematological adverse effects. Incidence estimates are lacking for most disorders. Hematological side-effects have been rarely associated with ibuprofen but they are potentially fatal. Halpern and colleagues (1993) reported that only 7% of ibuprofen adverse reaction reports to the Committee on Safety of Medicines (CSM) in the United Kingdom were hematological in nature, however they accounted for 28% of all ibuprofen fatalities. Platelet-related abnormalities were more frequent in the CSM reports than red or white cell disorders.

11.5.1 Neutropenia, agranulocytosis, and aplastic anemia

Ibuprofen has been implicated in case reports of neutropenia (Argen, 1975), agranulo-cytosis (Gryfe and Rubenzahl, 1976; Mamus *et al.*, 1986) and pancytopenia (Lindblad and Rodjer, 1991).

The International Agranulocytosis and Aplastic Anemia Study (IAAAS) was a population-based case-control study conducted in six European countries and Israel covering a total population of 22.3 million (IAAAS, 1986). The results are summarized in Table 11.4.

This study did not provide a specific estimate for ibuprofen, which fell into the category of 'other non-narcotic analgesics' and for which risk did not appear to be increased. Butazones (phenylbutazone, oxyphenbutazone) were well known to have adverse hematological effects (Inman, 1977). This study was the first to quantify a significant association of agranulocytosis and aplastic anemia with indomethacin use, though such an association had been noted

TABLE 11.4

Results from IAAAS: Multivariate rate ratio estimate (95% CI)

NSAID	Agranulocytosis[a]	Aplastic anemia[b]
Butazones	3.8 (1.3–10.7)	8.7 (3.4–22.3)
Indomethacin	8.9 (2.9–27.8)	12.7 (4.2–38.3)
Diclofenac	Not calculated	8.8 (2.8–27.3)
Other NSAIDs[c]	0.9 (0.3–3.1)	2.1 (0.8–5.9)

[a] Related to use 1 week prior to clinical onset of illness.
[b] Related to use 29 to 180 days prior to clinical onset of illness.
[c] Agranulocytosis cases includes exposures to ibuprofen, diclofenac, naproxen, piroxicam, flurbiprofen, ketoprofen, proquazone, niflumic acid, and glafenine. Aplastic anemia cases includes exposures to piroxicam, naproxen, indoprofen, ketoprofen, ibuprofen, etofenamate, sulindac, flurbiprofen, fluflenamic acid, glafenine, and niflumic acid.

earlier by other authors (Fowler, 1987). The strong association of diclofenac and aplastic anemia was also new. However, the width of the confidence intervals of the drug-specific risk estimates makes premature any conclusion of real differences between NSAIDs. More importantly, the excess risks for agranulocytosis and aplastic anemia presented by the drugs studied were 0.2–1.1 per million and 6.6–10.1 per million, respectively. Thus, the absolute risk for these blood dyscrasias is small.

Strom and colleagues conducted a population-based case-control study of NSAID-associated neutropenia using Medicaid claims data from six states (Strom *et al.*, 1993). The multivariate adjusted odds ratio for any NSAID use was 4.2 (90% CI, 2.0–8.7). Only the NSAID class of propionic acid derivatives reached statistical significance; however, the other classes had similar odds ratios and confidence intervals that overlapped, suggesting no real difference between classes.

11.5.2   Other blood disorders

Cases of ibuprofen-induced autoimmune hemolytic anemia (Guidry *et al.*, 1979) and immune thrombocytopenia (Meyer and Girma, 1993; Jain, 1994) have been reported, as for many NSAIDs. These have been summarized by Miescher (1986) and Rybak (1992).

NSAIDs other than aspirin cause reversible platelet inhibition that may minimally prolong the bleeding time. This effect generally is not clinically significant, even in patients with hemophilia (George and Shattil, 1991).

11.6   RENAL ADVERSE EFFECTS

Ibuprofen and all NSAIDs are known to exert effects on the kidney that are manifested in several ways, primarily disorders of sodium and water, direct renal toxicity (e.g. interstitial nephritis) and effects relating to the renal excretion of uric acid. The disorders of sodium and water handling are discussed in subsequent sections on Cardiovascular Adverse Effects and Drug Interactions (with antihypertensive agents).

Several extensive reviews of renal effects of NSAIDs have been published (Baisac and Henrich, 1994; DuBose, 1994; Delmas, 1995; Kleinknecht, 1995; Palmer, 1995; Palmer and Henrich, 1995; Bennett *et al.*, 1996). Through inhibition of prostaglandin synthesis, virtually all NSAIDs have been associated with reversible renal insufficiency (Delmas, 1995). Renal syndromes associated with NSAID use include oliguric or non-oliguric acute renal failure, interstitial nephritis, nephrotic syndrome, chronic renal failure, hyperkalemia, sodium, and water retention (Baisac and Henrich, 1994; Kleinknecht, 1995; Bennett *et al.*, 1996). Mechanisms of injury include inhibition of counterregulatory prostaglandins with loss of compensatory renal vasodilation under conditions of either systemic or renal hemodynamic instability, loss of natriuretic prostaglandins, hyporeninemic-hypoaldosteronism, enhanced antidiuretic hormone action, delayed hypersensitivity mediated through reactive arachidonic acid metabolites, and a combination of factors (Kleinknecht, 1995; Bennett *et al.*, 1996).

The most common NSAID-induced renal adverse effects are those mediated by NSAID inhibition of prostaglandin synthesis and include hemodynamically induced acute renal failure and disorders of salt and water retention. Risk factors for these adverse effects include those conditions that decrease effective arterial blood volume (Palmer, 1995; Palmer and Henrich, 1995). These include congestive heart failure, cirrhosis, nephrotic syndrome, sepsis, hemorrhage, diuretic therapy, third-spacing, volume depletion or hypotension. Conditions in which prostaglandins are important in maintaining intrarenal hemodynamics in the presence of normal or increased arterial blood volume are also risk factors. These include chronic renal failure, glomerulonephritis, advanced age, contrast-induced nephropathy, obstructive uropathy, and cyclosporin use (Baisac and Henrich, 1994; Palmer, 1995; Palmer and Henrich, 1995). NSAID-induced effects on sodium, potassium and water balance result in attenuation of the therapeutic effects of diuretics and antihypertensives, and increased risk for hyperkalemia in patients with altered potassium homeostasis. The latter include patients taking potassium-sparing diuretics, diabetic patients, and the elderly (Palmer, 1995).

Halpern and colleagues reported that 36 cases of renal impairment, including four deaths from renal failure, associated with ibuprofen had been reported in a 20-year period (Halpern *et al.*, 1993). These cases represented 1% of all adverse reactions associated with ibuprofen reported to the Committee on Safety of Medicines in the United Kingdom. Ibuprofen at 800 mg three times daily was found to worsen renal function in 3 of 12 patients with asymptomatic renal failure (Whelton *et al.*, 1990). Poirier, in an extensive review of the literature, identified 63 cases of reversible renal failure with ibuprofen (Poirier, 1984). Major but not uniform features of these cases included rapid reversibility within days of discontinuation of ibuprofen, variable duration of use, and variable doses within the therapeutic range. More recently, cases of acute reversible renal dysfunction with use of non-prescription ibuprofen in adult and paediatric patients have been reported (Moss *et al.*, 1986; Biljon, 1989; Spierto *et al.*, 1992; McIntire *et al.*, 1993).

In clinical trials, which tend to be of short duration, the frequency of NSAID-associated changes in renal function parameters appears to be low. Bonney and co-workers (1986) evaluated blood urea nitrogen and serum creatinine elevations in 1468 patients treated with aspirin, ibuprofen or oxaprozin in controlled, double-blind clinical trials. Patients took daily therapeutic doses of one of the three drugs for rheumatoid arthritis or osteoarthritis for up to 12 months' duration. All three drugs were associated with a low incidence of potentially significant elevations in renal laboratory tests. Three patients had serious elevations, one on oxaprozin, two on ibuprofen. All three patients were receiving concomitant diuretic therapy. The authors concluded that renal toxicity with NSAIDs is rare.

Understanding of the frequency of NSAID-associated adverse renal effects on a population level is complicated by the fact that results of epidemiological studies may vary

TABLE 11.5
Summary of selected epidemiological studies of NSAID-associated renal disease

Study	Study design	Results
Fox and Jick (1984)	(a) Intensive monitoring of 41 418 hospitalized patients (b) Retrospective cohort analysis of outpatients who received Rxs for NSAIDs	(a) 1.1% of NSAID users vs 1.3% of non-users had clinically diagnosed, elevations of BUN attributed to NSAID therapy (b) No hospitalizations for parenchymal renal disease
Johnson et al. (1985)	Retrospective cohort of 13 320 outpatients ≤ 65 years of age with ≥ 1 Rx for ibuprofen	No hospitalizations for acute kidney disease within 3 months after ibuprofen exposure
Beard et al. (1988)	Retrospective review of all persons hospitalized for new renal disease in 300 000 health maintenance organization population	No cases of NSAID-associated renal disease
Murray et al. (1990)	Retrospective cohort of outpatients who received ibuprofen Rx (1908) vs acetaminophen (3933)	18% of ibuprofen users developed renal impairment; 0.9% developed serious impairment. Adjusted OR for ibuprofen vs acetaminophen 1.1 (95% CI, 0.9–1.3). Increased risk in the elderly: 1.3 (1.1–1.7), and patients with coronary artery disease: 2.5 (1.4–4.7)
Derby and Jick (1991)	Retrospective cohort of outpatients who filled ≥ 1 Rx for ibuprofen (171 005), acetaminophen (309 961) or aspirin (125 244)	No cases of acute parenchymal renal disease attributed to these analgesics
Sandler et al. (1991)	Case-control study. Cases were patients hospitalized for newly diagnosed chronic renal dysfunction	Risk of chronic renal disease with previous daily use of NSAIDs: adjusted OR = 2.1 (95% CI, 1.1–4.1). Risk mainly in men older than 65 years: OR = 10.0 (1.2–82.7)
Beard et al. (1992)	Case-control study. Cases were patients undergoing renal biopsy	Risk of acute renal disease due to structural causes associated with NSAID exposure is nonsignificant: OR = 1.6 (95% CI, 0.9–3.0)
Perneger et al. (1994)	Case-control study. Cases were drawn from a population-based registry of patients with end-stage renal disease (ESRD)	Risk of ESRD associated with average annual intake ≥ 366 pills significant only for acetaminophen: adjusted OR = 2.1 (95% CI, 1.1–3.7). Risk of ESRD associated with cumulative lifetime intake of ≥ 5000 pills significant for acetaminophen (adjusted OR = 2.4 (1.2–4.8) and NSAIDs (adjusted OR = 8.8 (1.1–71.8)
Evans et al. (1995)	Case-control study. Cases were persons hospitalized for acute renal failure	Risk of hospitalization for acute renal failure significantly associated with recent NSAID use: OR = 2.2 (95% CI, 1.5–3.3) with community controls, 1.8 (1.1–2.9) with hospital controls
Perez-Gutthann et al. (1996)	Case-control study. Cases were persons hospitalized for acute renal failure	Current NSAID users had an adjusted OR for acute renal failure of 4.1 (95% CI, 1.5–10.8). Risk highest in the first month of use: OR = 8.5 (2.5–28.6), and with high doses OR = 9.8 (3.2–30.5)

Rx, prescription; OR, odds ratio; CI, confidence interval.

depending on the characteristics of the population studied (e.g. patients at risk may have been excluded), and whether renal dysfunction was defined by a recorded clinical diagnosis or abnormalities in renal laboratory parameters (e.g. serum creatinine).

When laboratory renal parameters (e.g. blood urea nitrogen or serum creatinine) were used to define renal dysfunction, 18% of ibuprofen users developed renal dysfunction; however the incidence of clinically serious renal dysfunction was much less, 0.9% (Murray *et al.*, 1990). As might be expected, elderly patients and patients with coronary artery disease were at higher risk. Two case-control studies of hospitalizations for acute renal failure found significantly increased risk associated with current or recent NSAID use (Evans *et al.*, 1995; Perez-Gutthann *et al.*, 1996). Another case-control study that looked at hospitalizations for newly diagnosed chronic renal failure found a significant doubling of risk associated with previous daily use of NSAIDs (Sandler *et al.*, 1991). Two case-control studies have found increased risk associated with high NSAID doses (Perneger *et al.*, 1994; Perez-Gutthann *et al.*, 1996). One case-control study found a low and non-significant association of NSAIDs and acute renal disease (Beard *et al.*, 1992). However, these cases were narrowly defined and the generalizability of these results to the broader NSAID-exposed population is not clear. These studies are summarized in Table 11.5.

NSAID-associated renal dysfunction serious enough to result in hospitalization appears to be uncommon (Murray *et al.*, 1990; Perez-Gutthann *et al.*, 1996). However, there are subpopulations of NSAID users who are at greater risk from NSAID-induced adverse renal effects. These include patients who are hemodynamically compromised or who have pre-existing renal dysfunction.

Suprofen, a NSAID with uricosuric properties, was apparently responsible for an acute flank pain syndrome associated with hematuria and acute renal failure (Strom *et al.*, 1989). The proposed pathogenic mechanism was acute, diffuse crystallization of uric acid in the renal tubules.

11.7 CARDIOVASCULAR ADVERSE EFFECTS

It is believed that NSAIDs may affect cardiovascular homeostasis by virtue of their effects on prostaglandins, which are thought to play important roles in normal cardiovascular functioning of the heart and coronary vessels (Beamish *et al.*, 1985). In addition to their known effects on sodium and water excretion, NSAIDs may have effects on coronary and other vasculature or direct effects on ischemic tissue.

The effects of NSAIDs in heart disease remain controversial owing to differential effects of different NSAIDs and their effect on the delicate balance between prostaglandin and thromboxane inhibition that governs cardiac pathophysiology (Beamish *et al.*, 1985). Animal models of cardiac ischemia indicate that some NSAIDs may have a detrimental effect on ischemic tissue. Other animal studies indicate that NSAIDs may either limit infarct size or contribute to its expansion (Wilson and Carruthers, 1992). One mechanism

CHAPTER 11

for this may relate to the finding of Serneri *et al.* (1990) that patients with angina experienced increased coronary vascular resistance after ketoprofen and aspirin in response to cold pressor (sympathetic) stimulation. In contrast, the NSAID sulfinpyrazone has been shown to prevent re-infarction and sudden death post myocardial infarction, an effect that may be due to the antiarrhythmic properties possessed by this particular agent (Beamish *et al.*, 1985).

Although NSAID-induced precipitation of cardiac decompensation is a concern because of the known effects of NSAIDs on water and sodium balance, it appears to have been little studied (Wilson and Carruthers, 1992). We are unaware of any epidemiological studies of NSAIDs and congestive heart failure.

One report from the Netherlands examined this association through a survey of physicians and a review of medical records at one hospital (Van Den Ouweland *et al.*, 1988). The survey went to 243 physicians, of whom 35% responded. It was not stated what proportion of the physician population was covered by this survey. Twenty respondents reported a total of 22 patients in whom congestive heart failure was observed after initiation of NSAIDs. Of the 22 patients, only 13 could be sufficiently documented. Of the 13 patients, 9 had suffered heart failure previously, and 4 were on diuretic therapy. The review of medical records encompassed 600 elderly patients hospitalized for congestive heart failure. The authors screened for patients with concomitant locomotor disease, as these patients were most likely to be receiving NSAID therapy. They identified 58 such patients, of whom 22 had been treated with an NSAID at the time of failure. Of the 22 cases, 17 had a probable cause of failure not related to the NSAID. Of the remaining five patients, one had moderate cardiac compromise and had been on diuretic therapy. The other four had no apparent heart disease and ranged in age from 74 to 82 years. Mean creatinine clearance was 76 ± 15 ml/min. The authors concluded that NSAID-induced congestive heart failure may occur in the elderly without a history of cardiac disease.

11.8 ADVERSE EFFECTS ON REPRODUCTION

11.8.1 Animal studies of teratogenic and reproductive effects

Most NSAIDs have had no teratogenic effects in animal studies, though some have been associated with other reproductive effects, often at maternally toxic doses.

Reproductive toxicity studies in rabbits and rats have found no teratogenic effects with fenoprofen, ibuprofen, nabumetone, phenylbutazone, piroxicam and suprofen (Shepard, 1992). In these studies, piroxicam was associated with decreased fetal growth and growth retardation at maternally toxic doses. Suprofen suppressed fetal weight in rats, and delayed fetal ossification in rabbits. Nabumetone at high doses reduced postnatal weight gain in rats; fetal mortality increased in rabbits (Shepard, 1992).

Ibuprofen, but not naproxen, significantly inhibited fetal implantation in rats in one study (Gupta *et al.*, 1984). In a study that looked at the potency of various NSAIDs in blocking parturition in rats, ibuprofen, tolmetin and phenylbutazone were the least effective, and piroxicam, sudoxicam and flurbiprofen showed the greatest potency (Powell and Cochrane, 1982).

In rats, meclofenamate sodium and pirprofen had no teratogenic effects (Shepard, 1992). Increased postimplantation loss, prolonged gestation, decreased weanling weights, and increased weanling loss were seen at maternally toxic doses of meclofenamate (Petrere *et al.*, 1985).

Ketoprofen has been tested in rats, mice and monkeys without adverse effect on the fetus (Shepard, 1992). No teratogenic effects were seen in rats or mice with sulindac (Brooks and Needs, 1989). Tenoxicam produced no malformations in mice, rats or rabbits. Embryolethality occurred at the highest doses in rabbits, and increased neonatal deaths in rats (Shepard, 1992). Tolmetin in rabbits had no teratogenic effect. At high doses, dam weight gain was decreased and fetal mortality was increased (Shepard, 1992).

Indomethacin produced skeletal defects in mouse fetuses (Shepard, 1992). Positive and negative animal studies for diclofenac-associated teratogenicity exist. Brooks and Needs (1989) concluded that there is no clear evidence of mutagenic effects with diclofenac in doses used in humans.

Reproductive toxicity studies in animals are a required part of the drug development process. Such studies are generally done in at least two species (the rat and the rabbit) and should 'allow exposure of mature adults and all stages of development from conception to sexual maturity' (Mathieu, 1994). In general, drug effects are examined in mature animals from pre-mating through pregnancy and lactation, and in their offspring from conception through postnatal growth and development. Although the lack of reproductive toxicity in animals provides some reassurance regarding the reproductive safety of a drug, the possibility exists that a particular animal model may not appropriately reflect human pharmacological response. For this reason, clinical experience with a drug in pregnant women is required to more fully assess the reproductive safety of a specific drug.

11.8.2   Reports of teratogenic effects in humans

There have been scattered spontaneous reports of suspected NSAID-associated birth defects. Brooks and Needs (1989) noted two reports of possible malformations associated with indomethacin. One of these was a case of phocomelia and agenesis of the penis (Briggs *et al.*, 1990). Aselton reported one congenital defect among 50 infants exposed to indomethacin (Aselton *et al.*, 1985). No further information was provided.

One report of women taking phenylbutazone in the first trimester reported six minor and one major malforfamations (Kullander and Kallen, 1976). Briggs cites one other report, stating that the causal relationship was not established (Briggs *et al.*, 1990).

Phenylbutazone has been shown to produce chromosomal abnormalities in treated patients, which in males presents a theoretical risk of chromosomally imbalanced sperm (Fowler, 1987).

One retrospective study found one child with a congenital defect associated with ibuprofen among 51 exposed during the first trimester (Aselton *et al.*, 1985). A report of postmarketing surveillance of ibuprofen exposures indicated five exposed infants with various defects and an unclear relationship to the ibuprofen exposure (Briggs *et al.*, 1990).

A prospective study of 45 women with rheumatic disease who took NSAIDs during their pregnancies reported no difference in pregnancy outcome, duration of labour, complications at delivery, neonatal health, or health and development in the offspring (Østensen and Østensen, 1996). NSAIDs used during pregnancy were naproxen (23 women), ibuprofen (8 women), indomethacin (4 women), ketoprofen (3 women) and piroxicam (6 women). Five women took aspirin. Generally, epidemiological studies are required to determine the association between a drug exposure and a congenital malformation. An exception exists in the situation when a drug is a potent teratogen that commonly causes a congenital malformation that is otherwise rare in the population. Thalidomide and phocomelia are the classic example of this circumstance. Often in case reports, precise information on dose and time of drug exposure relative to the critical period of embryonic development are lacking. Generally, the aetiology of the defect is unknown and some may be fairly common in the general population. For these reasons, a conclusion of causality is generally not possible from individual case reports. However, these may serve as a signal of possible teratogenic effects of a drug. Based on animal data, the paucity of case reports in the literature, and their high prevalence of use, most of the NSAIDs appear to be free of teratogenic effects.

11.8.3 Perinatal adverse effects associated with therapeutic use

NSAIDs, primarily indomethacin, have been used in the treatment of premature labour (Repke and Niebyl, 1985; Varvarigou *et al.*, 1996; Moise *et al.*, 1988). Indomethacin has also been used to treat polyhydramnios (Cabrol *et al.*, 1987). The adverse effects associated with the use of indomethacin for premature labour are well documented and include premature closure of the ductus arteriosus, primary pulmonary hypertension of the newborn, oligohydramnios, and renal complications in the neonatal period including oliguria, azotemia, non-oliguric renal failure, and chronic renal failure accompanied by renal histological changes (Repke and Niebyl, 1985; Heymann, 1986; Kaplan *et al.*, 1994; van der Heijden and Gubler, 1995). NSAIDs may also displace bilirubin from albumin binding sites increasing the risk for kernicterus (Repke and Niebyl, 1985).

Many factors may influence the individual risk to a fetus or neonate, including gestational age, dose, timing, duration of exposure, differences in NSAID potency, differences in sensitivity of the ductal tissue and pulmonary vasculature, presence of other risk factors (e.g. hypoxemia), and time from last exposure to delivery (Rudolph, 1981; Heymann, 1986; Ferner and Smith, 1991). Twin pregnancies may be particularly at risk for renal complications (Kaplan *et al.*, 1994; van der Heijden and Gubler, 1995). Animal studies support differential effects of NSAIDs on cerebral blood flow and other regional hemodynamics (Malcolm *et al.*, 1993; Chemtob *et al.*, 1991).

A strong association of indomethacin with oligohydramnios has been demonstrated by several studies and case reports (Itskovitz *et al.*, 1980; de Wit *et al.*, 1988; Goldenberg *et al.*, 1989; Hickok *et al.*, 1989; Hendricks *et al.*, 1990; Kirshon *et al.*, 1991; Kaplan *et al.*, 1994). Ibuprofen has been implicated as well (Cantor *et al.*, 1980; Hickok *et al.*, 1989; Hendricks *et al.*, 1990; Wiggins and Elliott, 1990; Kaplan *et al.*, 1994).

Ketoprofen, indomethacin and ibuprofen have been implicated in case reports of neonatal renal dysfunction, including acute and chronic renal failure (Simeoni *et al.*, 1989; Cantor *et al.*, 1980; Kaplan *et al.*, 1994; van der Heijden and Gubler, 1995).

Premature closure of the ductus with persistent pulmonary hypertension and severe hypoxemia has been reported with naproxen (Wilkinson *et al.*, 1979) and indomethacin (Manchester *et al.*, 1976; Truter *et al.*, 1986; Demandt *et al.*, 1990). Indomethacin also has been implicated in neonatal ischemic brain injury demonstrated on cerebral ultrasonography (Haddad *et al.*, 1990).

11.8.4 Other reproductive effects

NSAIDs have been implicated in reversible ovulatory failure in women receiving chronic NSAID therapy for inflammatory arthritis. Smith and colleagues (1996) reported the investigation for infertility of three women with ankylosing spondylitis, rheumatoid arthritis and seronegative inflammatory polyarthritis. Diclofenac, naproxen and piroxicam were the NSAIDs in use. NSAID therapy was associated with recurrent development of luteinized unruptured ovarian follicles. Normal ovulation followed discontinuation of NSAID therapy (Smith *et al.*, 1996).

Impotence or loss of libido have been reported with nearly all of the NSAIDs. Since prostaglandins have been shown to influence penile erection, the association of NSAIDs with sexual dysfunction is a plausible one (Beeley, 1991).

11.9 ENDOCRINE AND METABOLIC ADVERSE EFFECTS

Halpern and colleagues (1993) reported rare cases of altered glucose metabolism associated with ibuprofen submitted to the Committee on Safety of Medicines in the United Kingdom. Increased serum levels of uric acid (Vrhovac, 1984) and decreased plasma albumin (Swaminathan, 1991) have been reported with ibuprofen, but the clinical significance of these reports is unknown. Metabolic acidosis has been reported with ibuprofen overdose (Linden and Townsend, 1987).

CHAPTER 11

NSAIDs potentiate the antidiuretic response to vasopressin through inhibition of prostaglandin synthesis (Jackson, 1996). Symptomatic hyponatremia has been reported with several NSAIDs, including ibuprofen (Swaminathan, 1991). The effects of ibuprofen on water, sodium and potassium balance are discussed in the section on Renal Adverse Effects.

Goitre and hypothyroidism have been reported with phenylbutazone (Fowler, 1987). Butazones inhibit thyroid hormone synthesis by blocking the organic binding of iodine (Yeung and Cockram, 1991). Fenclofenac and phenylbutazone interfere with thyroid function tests, potentially leading to misdiagnosis (Fowler, 1987; Yeung and Cockram, 1991). Phenylbutazone, azapropazone and mefenamic acid may lower serum uric acid levels owing to their mild uricosuric properties (Harth, 1992).

11.10   CENTRAL NERVOUS SYSTEM EFFECTS

11.10.1   General CNS effects

Reports of central nervous system (CNS) effects of ibuprofen appear to be common at therapeutic dosages. In a review of ibuprofen adverse effects reported to the Committee on Safety of Medicines in the United Kingdom from 1969 to 1991, CNS toxicity ranked third overall, accounting for 341 (13%) of adverse drug reaction reports (Halpern *et al.*, 1993). Fifty-six per cent of CNS reports dealt with problems such as headache, dizziness, ataxia, and paraesthesia; 46% were psychiatric in nature, including depression, somnolence, confusion, nightmares and hallucinations.

Headache is a common side-effect of NSAIDs (Coles *et al.*, 1983; Singh *et al.*, 1994; Inman and Rawson, 1987), especially with indomethacin. Headaches due to indomethacin have been attributed to its chemical similarity to serotonin, a major neurotransmitter and vasoactive substance (Henry, 1988). Vertigo and tinnitus also appear to be common complaints with NSAID therapy (Coles *et al.*, 1983; Singh *et al.*, 1994).

In a clinical trials analysis of 3029 adverse drug reactions reported among 18 577 patients, 635 (20.9%) complained of CNS symptoms such as dizziness, headache, depression, and somnolence; however, withdrawal occurred in only 1.3% of these cases (Halpern *et al.*, 1993).

In an investigation of the safety of over-the-counter ibuprofen in 15 double-blinded, single-dose, placebo-controlled trials (878 patients), CNS effects occurred in descending order of frequency as follows: drowsiness, tiredness, dizziness, light-headedness, nervousness, irritability and unsteadiness (Furey *et al.*, 1992). The overall incidence of CNS effects was 0.8%.

11.10.2   Aseptic meningitis

In 1991 Hoppmann and colleagues reviewed 23 cases of NSAID-associated aseptic meningitis (Hoppmann *et al.*, 1991). Additional cases continue to appear in the literature

(Durback *et al.*, 1988; Mifsud, 1988; Grimm and Wolf, 1989; Agus *et al.*, 1990; Chez *et al.*, 1990; Davis *et al.*, 1994; Hanson and Morgan, 1994; Kaplan *et al.*, 1994). Most reports have involved ibuprofen, but sulindac, naproxen and tolmetin have also been implicated (Durback *et al.*, 1988; Mifsud, 1988; Grimm and Wolf, 1989; Agus *et al.*, 1990; Chez *et al.* 1990; Hoppmann *et al.*, 1991; Davis *et al.*, 1994; Hanson and Morgan, 1994; Kaplan *et al.*, 1994). Many of these patients had systemic lupus erythematosus and these patients seem to be particularly at risk. Evidence from these cases indicates that aseptic meningitis is a hypersensitivity-mediated reaction (Hoppmann *et al.*, 1991).

11.10.3   Cognitive dysfunction

NSAID-associated cognitive dysfunction in the elderly has been suggested, but confirmation by prospective trials is lacking (Goodwin and Regan, 1982; Wysenbeek *et al.*, 1988). A recent epidemiological study lends further support to this association (Saag *et al.*, 1995). Saag and colleagues (1995) used the population of the Iowa 65+ Rural Health Study, one of the National Institute on Aging's Established Populations for Epidemiological Studies in the Elderly, to examine this issue. Memory decline was assessed by a change in immediate word recall in a 3-year interval. The three most commonly used NSAIDs in this population were piroxicam, ibuprofen and naproxen. High-dose NSAID use was second only to functional status as the strongest risk factor (odds ratio = 2.06 (95% CI, 1.1–3.9)) for significant decline in immediate word recall. Specific individual NSAIDs were no more likely than any other to be significantly associated with recall decline. However, when propionic acid derivatives (ibuprofen, naproxen, ketoprofen, fenoprofen) were analyzed together, the increased risk neared significance (odds ratio = 3.7 (95% CI, 0.92–10.0)).

11.10.4   Psychiatric adverse effects

NSAIDs have been reported to cause psychiatric adverse effects including paranoia, depression, anxiety, disorientation and hallucinations, though these effects have not been reported with all NSAIDs (Anonymous, 1993). Indomethacin has been most often associated with adverse psychiatric effects including depression, paranoia and hallucinations (Hoppmann *et al.*, 1991). Reports associated with fenbufen, ibuprofen and sulindac also exist (Griffith *et al.*, 1982; Davison and Hassanyeh, 1991; Hoppmann *et al.*, 1991). The single case report of ibuprofen-associated paranoid psychosis occurred in a 37-year-old male receiving 1600 mg ibuprofen daily for back pain. He reportedly displayed paranoid symptoms after the fourth dose of ibuprofen and after 10 more days of therapy he was arrested for shooting a gun at people (Griffith *et al.*, 1982). Although the initiation of ibuprofen appears to be temporally related to the man's symptoms, he had a history of psychiatric illness and his symptoms persisted for 2 months after discontinuation of the ibuprofen, making the causal relationship of the NSAID to his problems less clear.

CHAPTER 11

519

11.11 OCULAR ADVERSE EFFECTS

Ocular side-effects, relating either to effects on the optic nerve or to other eye functions, are infrequently associated with NSAIDs. The National Registry of Drug-Induced Ocular Side-Effects, a registry of reports from ophthalmologists in the United States, reported a total of 144 cases of optic nerve toxicity associated with NSAIDs. There were 120 reports of optic or retrobulbar neuritis associated with 14 NSAIDs. Sixty-two per cent ($n = 74$) of the cases were associated with propionic acid derivatives, with ibuprofen accounting for the largest number of these reports ($n = 43$). There were fewer reports of papilloedema ($n = 24$) associated with 8 of the 14 NSAIDs. Ibuprofen, indomethacin and naproxen accounted for 17 of these reports. The authors acknowledge that direct cause and effect cannot be definitively established from registry data. However, the data suggest that all NSAIDs have the potential to cause disc oedema, papilloedema, pseudotumor cerebri or optic neuritis (Fraunfelder and Samples, 1994). The mechanism by which drugs cause pseudotumor cerebri is unknown but is believed to involve salt and water retention, with intracranial fluid redistribution (Blain and Lane, 1991).

The literature contains several case reports of ibuprofen-associated visual disturbance, including decreased visual acuity and macular oedema (Nicastro, 1989), iridocyclitis (Kaplan *et al.*, 1994), vortex keratopathy (Fitt *et al.*, 1996), contrast sensitivity (Ridder and Tomlinson, 1992) and toxic amblyopia (Palmer, 1972). In 1993, Halpern *et al.* (1993) and colleagues reported that 68 cases of visual or other ocular disorders had been reported in the United Kingdom, where ibuprofen has been marketed since 1969. This compares with 731 cases of gastrointestinal adverse effects reported in the same period. Most of these 68 cases were reports of abnormal vision (Halpern *et al.*, 1993).

Data from the Arthritis, Rheumatism and Aging Medical Information System (ARAMIS,) which prospectively monitors approximately 3000 patients with rheumatic diseases, indicates complaints of blurred vision occur with nearly all NSAIDs. The incidence with ibuprofen was 6 events per 1000 patient-years. Indomethacin had the highest incidence with 11 events per 1000 patient-years (Singh *et al.*, 1994).

11.12 DRUG INTERACTIONS

The prevalence and incidence of adverse drug interactions involving NSAIDs are unknown (Johnson *et al.*, 1994). One drug utilization review conducted at a health maintenance organization of 42 000 members found, in a 1-month period, that 8% of prescriptions for NSAIDs were written to patients also receiving potentially interacting medications (Mead and McGhan, 1988). Most clinically significant NSAID drug interactions result from the ability of NSAIDs to inhibit cyclooxygenase, thereby reducing prostaglandin biosynthesis. Some NSAID drug interactions result from the fact that NSAIDs are highly bound to plasma proteins and thus may compete with other drugs for binding sites. Few

NSAID drug interactions result from NSAID inhibition of the hepatic metabolism of other drugs (Verbeeck, 1990; Hansten and Horn, 1993). An exhaustive review of drug interactions with NSAIDs was recently published (Johnson *et al.*, 1994). Some of the clinically significant drug interactions with NSAIDs are discussed below.

NSAID–antihypertensives interactions

The mechanism by which NSAIDs blunt the effect of antihypertensive therapy is not completely understood, however inhibition of prostaglandin-mediated effects in the kidney and vasculature are likely. Calcium channel blockers and centrally acting α-agonists seem less likely to interact with NSAIDs than other antihypertensive agents. This topic has been reviewed (Mene *et al.*, 1995).

A meta-analysis of randomized trials assessing the effect of NSAIDs on blood pressure found that NSAIDs elevated supine mean blood pressure by 5.0 mm Hg (95% CI, 1.2–8.7). Among trials involving treated hypertensive patients exposed to NSAIDs the pooled mean change was statistically significant (5.4 mm Hg (95% CI, 1.2–9.6)). Of three categories of antihypertensive therapy (β-blockers, vasodilators and diuretics), the increase in supine mean blood pressure was substantially greater for β-blockers and vasodilators than for diuretics. However, this reached statistical significance only for the β-blockers (6.2 mm Hg (95% CI, 1.0–11.4)). Of the nine NSAIDs studied, piroxicam, indomethacin and ibuprofen produced the largest increases in supine mean blood pressure. However, only piroxicam reached statistical significance. Aspirin, sulindac and flurbiprofen produced the smallest changes. Increases seen with tiaprofenic acid, diclofenac and naproxen were intermediate in magnitude. These results differ from an earlier meta-analysis in which naproxen and indomethacin had the most effect and sulindac, ibuprofen and aspirin had the least effect. Johnson and colleagues suggested that duration of NSAID use may not be an important factor, as the effect seen was similar whether patients received single-dose antihypertensive therapy or had been controlled for weeks to months (Johnson *et al.*, 1994).

A recent review of NSAIDs and hypertension concluded that we do not yet know what risk, if any, follows from NSAID-associated increases in blood pressure, nor whether these increases are sustained over time since the studies have all been relatively short-term. Certain patient subgroups may be at risk for this NSAID effect: the elderly, patients with salt-sensitive hypertension, and patients with pre-existing hypertension receiving antihypertensive medication (de Leeuw, 1996).

A case-control study of elderly Medicaid enrollees found a statistically significant, dose-related, increased risk for initiation of antihypertensive therapy among persons who were recent NSAID users compared to non-users. The overall adjusted odds ratio was 1.66 (95% CI, 1.54–1.80). The risk increased with NSAID dose: 1.55 (95% CI, 1.38–1.74) for low dose; 1.64 (95% CI, 1.44–1.87) for medium dose; 1.82 (95% CI, 1.62–2.05) for high dose (Gurwitz *et al.*, 1994).

These same investigators performed a randomized, double-blind, two-period crossover trial of ibuprofen (1800 mg/day) vs placebo, administered to 25 patients > 60 years of age with hypertension controlled with hydrochlorothiazide. Treatment (ibuprofen or placebo) was given for 4 weeks, followed by a 2-week washout period, followed by 4 weeks with the other treatment. Patients continued their usual thiazide dose during the study and 22 completed the study. Systolic blood pressures, supine and standing, were significantly increased by ibuprofen (Gurwitz *et al.*, 1996).

A three-phase, randomized, double-blind, placebo-controlled multicentre study of 162 patients aged 18–75 years with essential hypertension controlled with once-daily verapamil examined the effects on blood pressure of ibuprofen, naproxen or placebo. Each treatment was given for 3 weeks. No significant differences in sitting, standing or supine blood pressure occurred with ibuprofen or naproxen (Houston *et al.*, 1995).

It is clear that NSAID therapy may interfere with antihypertensive therapy, primarily to effect reversal of the hypotensive effects of diuretics, β-blockers and ACE-inhibitors. The interactions associated with specific antihypertensives are described below.

NSAID–diuretic interactions

Reduced diuretic and antihypertensive effects with loop diuretics (bumetanide, furosemide) have specifically been reported with indomethacin, ibuprofen, naproxen, flurbiprofen, sulindac and piroxicam.

Indomethacin, diclofenac and ibuprofen, when combined with the potassium-retaining diuretic triamterene, produced in significant decreases in creatinine clearance resulting in acute renal failure (Hansten and Horn, 1993a).

NSAID–β-adrenergic blocker interactions

Decreased antihypertensive effects of β-blockers have specifically been associated with propranolol, pindolol, labetalol, atenolol and oxprenolol given with indomethacin. Piroxicam and naproxen may have a similar effect. Sulindac may be least likely to have an effect (Hansten and Hornn, 1993; Tatro, 1997).

NSAID–angiotensin-converting enzyme inhibitor interactions

A decreased antihypertensive effect was reported specifically with indomethacin and captopril, particularly in low-renin hypertensives. Studies show a similar effect of indomethacin on enalapril and lisinopril. However, sulindac appeared to have no effect on captopril and enalapril. In some circumstances, the potential exists for additive effects of NSAIDs and ACE inhibitors to reduce renal blood flow. One retrospective study of patients receiving both NSAIDs and ACE inhibitors found three cases of reversible renal failure (Hansten and Horn, 1993i).

NSAID–oral anticoagulant interactions

All NSAIDs can prolong the bleeding time through inhibition of platelet function. Platelet effects, the ability of NSAIDs to potentiate the hypoprothrombinemic response to oral anticoagulants, and the known risk of gastrointestinal bleeding with NSAIDs makes the combination of NSAIDs and oral anticoagulants one to avoid if possible (Chan, 1995).

In studies, diclofenac, etodolac, fenbufen, ibuprofen, indomethacin, ketoprofen, ketorolac, nabumetone, naproxen, nimesulide, sulindac, tenoxicam and tolmetin had no effect on the hypoprothrombinemic response of the oral anticoagulants tested. Fenoprofen is capable of displacing warfarin from binding sites, but information is otherwise limited. Case reports of bleeding complications exist for ibuprofen, indomethacin, ketoprofen, sulindac and tolmetin. Additional cases in which loss of anticoagulant control occurred without bleeding have also been reported. Meclofenamate, mefenamic acid, piroxicam and lornoxicam increased the hypoprothrombinemic effect in studies. A study found excessive hypoprothrombinemic effect with flurbiprofen, with resulting bleeding in some patients. A case of increased warfarin response and bleeding has been reported with azapropazone, an NSAID chemically related to phenylbutazone. Phenylbutazone and oxyphenbutazone may interact with oral anticoagulants by two mechanisms, displacement of warfarin from protein-binding sites and inhibition of metabolism of the most potent S enantiomer of warfarin. The result is a dramatic increase in hypoprothrombinemic effect. These two NSAIDs should be considered contraindicated in patients receiving anticoagulant therapy (Hansten and Horn, 1993d; Mieszczak and Winther, 1993; Tatro, 1997; Chan, 1995; Gabb, 1996).

A retrospective cohort study of Tennessee Medicaid enrollees 65 years of age and older examined the risk of gastrointestinal bleeding in the elderly with concurrent use of NSAIDs and anticoagulants. The incidence of hospitalization for peptic ulcer disease was estimated to be 7 per 1000 person-years. The adjusted incidence of hospitalization for ulcer disease was 14.3 per 1000 person-years in current users of oral anticoagulants, 6.4 per 1000 person-years among non-users, and 26.3 per 1000 person-years in persons currently using both NSAIDs and oral anticoagulants. Compared to non-users of either drug, the relative risk was 12.7 (95% CI, 6.3–25.7). Among current oral anticoagulant users, 10% of hospitalizations for hemorrhagic ulcers were attributable to concomitant NSAID use. Data on individual NSAIDs, e.g. naproxen, were not presented (Shorr *et al.*, 1993).

In conclusion, although the interaction between NSAIDs and oral anticoagulants may not always produce significant adverse outcomes, the data are strongly suggestive that, because of their pharmacological characteristics alone, these agents should be used together only in very special circumstances where monitoring of coagulation and bleeding are assured. An extensive review of interactions between warfarin and NSAIDs has been published (Chan, 1995; Frazee and Reed, 1995).

CHAPTER 11

NSAID–aminoglycoside interactions

Aminoglycosides are eliminated through glomerular filtration. NSAIDs have the potential to decrease renal blood flow and glomerular filtration through effects on renal prostaglandins. Indomethacin significantly increased peak and trough concentrations of aminoglycosides in pre-term infants (Zarfin *et al.*, 1985). A study in rats found that prolonged administration (27 days) of diclofenac or ibuprofen potentiated gentamicin nephrotoxicity. This effect was not seen with short-term NSAID use (Farag *et al.*, 1996).

NSAID–oral hypoglycemic interactions

Phenylbutazone has been shown to prolong the half-life or increase the serum concentrations of several oral hypoglycemic drugs. This interaction may result from phenylbutazone inhibition of metabolism of the oral hypoglycemic, as well as protein binding displacement. There are limited data on other NSAIDs. Studies have shown no interaction between pirprofen and glyburide, between tolmetin or naproxen and tolbutamide, between tenoxicam and glybornuride, or between ibuprofen and glyburide (Kubacka *et al.*, 1996; Hansten and Horn, 1993f).

NSAID–cyclosporin interactions

Although the results are not well understood, patients receiving cyclosporin who then received an NSAID (diclofenac, sulindac and mefenamic acid have been specifically implicated) experienced elevated serum creatinine concentrations, sometimes accompanied by increased cyclosporin concentrations (Hansten and Horn, 1993e).

NSAID–lithium interactions

In studies, diclofenac, ibuprofen, indomethacin, ketorolac, naproxen and phenylbutazone increased plasm lithium concentrations, resulting in symptoms in some patients. Mefenamic acid and piroxicam have been implicated in case reports of lithium toxicity. Sulindac produces a temporary reduction of serum lithium concentrations. A change in lithium dose in unlikely to be necessary, but monitoring is recommended (Hansten and Horn, 1993).

NSAID–methotrexate interactions

Azapropazone, diclofenac and flurbiprofen were implicated in case reports of methotrexate toxicity following addition of the NSAID. NSAIDs reduce the renal clearance of methotrexate. Separate studies have shown ibuprofen to decrease the renal clearance of methotrexate and to have a lack of significant effect on methotrexate kinetics (Hansten and Horn, 1993).

TABLE 11.6

Summary of incidence estimates from epidemiological studies of selected NSAID-associated non-gastrointestinal adverse effects

Adverse effect	Rate per 1000 persons, unless otherwise specified	Comment
Hypersensitivity	0–0.95	Primarily urticaria (Strom *et al.*, 1987)
Anaphylaxis	0.025–1 per 1000 prescriptions	Primarily anaphylaxis (van der Klauw *et al.*, 1993)
Severe cutaneous reactions	0.0006–0.0074	Both SJS and TEN. Combined studies (see Table 11.2)
Hepatotoxicity	0.022–0.27	Includes symptomatic liver dysfunction treated in the outpatient or inpatient setting. Combined studies (see Table 11.3)
Hematological: agranulocytosis	0.0017–0.009	From IAAS: 8 geographical regions
Hematological: aplastic anemia	0.0006–0.0031	From IAAS: 8 geographical regions

SJS, Stevens–Johnson syndrome; TEN, toxic epidermal necrolysis; IAAS, International Agranulocytosis and Aplastic Anemia Study.

11.13 FUTURE NEEDS

A complete understanding of the overall population risk associated with NSAID use is still lacking owing to the paucity of incidence data on their non-gastrointestinal effects. Data are gradually accumulating, however, as evidenced by a number of population-based studies on hypersensitivity, serious skin disorders and hepatic events. To a lesser extent, renal effects, cardiovascular events and drug interactions with antihypertensives and anti-coagulants have also been studied. Table 11.6 provides a crude comparison of data from epidemiological studies. These data tend to support the original contention that, overall, serious NSAID-associated adverse events occur with relatively low frequency. Even NSAID-associated gastrointestinal bleeding, although the most common of NSAID adverse effects, has a fairly low rate of occurrence in the population. However, as discussed throughout this chapter, the risk for NSAID adverse events is often increased by various risk factors, the presence of compromised cardiovascular, hepatic or renal function in particular. In these circumstances, careful benefit-to-risk assessments of the NSAID therapy coupled with appropriate monitoring for these increasingly well-understood effects is required.

As yet, the differences in risk profiles between NSAIDs are generally not known, since the majority of studies have had insufficient power to determine differential effects. Further, the risk for any NSAID relative to another often varies between studies, probably owing to factors that include differential NSAID prescribing, study design and definition of outcomes.

In conclusion, the incidence rates of NSAID-associated, non-gastrointestinal adverse drug reactions need further study in population-based databases. Several population-based studies of NSAID-associated gastropathy exist that have helped to define the overall incidence rate, the lack of real differences between most NSAIDs, the strength of risk factors and those populations at greatest risk. Clinical trials are unable to provide this type of information. Insurance claims databases (e.g. Medicaid), or computer-based patient record databases (e.g. MediPlus[R]) are the only viable means of assessing population incidence for these rare adverse effects. Even these resources are limited in their ability to capture the non-prescription use of drugs, which is becoming an increasingly important issue as more of these products move to over-the-counter status.

REFERENCES

ANONYMOUS (1993) Drugs that cause psychiatric symptoms. *Medical Letter on Drugs and Therapeutics* **35**(901), 65–69.

AGUS, B., NELSON, J., KRAMER, N., MAHAL, S.S. and ROSENSTEIN, E.D. (1990) Acute central nervous system symptoms caused by ibuprofen in connective tissue disease *Journal of Rheumatology* **17**, 1094–1096.

ALBERS, H.J. (1992) Dermatological aspects of nonsteroidal anti-inflammatory drugs. In: BORDA, I.T. and KOFF, R.S. (eds), *NSAIDs: A Profile of Adverse Effects*. Philadelphia, Hanley and Belfus, 185–217.

ALHAVA, E. (1994) Reported adverse drug reactions and consumption of non-steroidal anti-inflammatory drugs. *Pharmacology and Toxicology* **75**(Suppl. 2), 37–43.

ARGEN, R.J. (1975) Ibuprofen therapy. *Arthritis and Rheumatism* **118**(4), 380–381.

ASELTON, P., JICK, H., MILUNSKY, A., HUNTER, J.R. and STERGACHIS, A. (1985) First-trimester drug use and congenital disorders. *Journal of the American College of Obstetricians and Gynecologists* **65**(4), 451–455.

AYRES, J.G., FLEMING, D.M. and WHITTINGTON, R.M. (1987) Asthma death due to ibuprofen. *Lancet* **2**, 1082.

BAISAC, J. and HENRICH, W.L. (1994) Nephrotoxicity of nonsteroidal anti-inflammatory drugs. *Mineral and Electrolyte Metabolism* **20**(4), 187–192.

BEAMISH, R.E., DAS, P.K., KARMAZYN, M. and DHALLA, N.S. (1985) Prostaglandins and heart disease. *Canadian Journal of Cardiology* **1**(1), 66–74.

BEARD, K., PERERA, D.R. and JICK, H. (1988) Drug-induced parenchymal renal disease in out-patients. *Journal of Clinical Pharmacology* **28**(5), 431–435.

BEARD, K., LAWSON, D.H. and MACFARLANE, G.J. (1992) Non-steroidal anti-inflammatory drugs and acute renal disease: a case control study. *Pharmacoepidemiology and Drug Safety* **1**, 3–9.

BEELEY, L. (1991) Drug-induced sexual dysfunction and infertility. In: DAVIES, D.M. (ed.), *Textbook of Adverse Drug Reactions*, 4th edn. New York, Oxford University Press, 771–787.

BENNETT, W.M., HENRICH, W.L. and STOFF, J.S. (1996) The renal effects of nonsteroidal anti-inflammatory drugs: summary and recommendations. *American Journal of Kidney Diseases* 28(Suppl. 1), S56–62.

BILJON, G. (1989) Reversible renal failure associated with ibuprofen in a child. A case report. *South African Medical Journal* 76, 34–35.

BLAIN, P.G. and LANE, R.J.M. (1991) Neurological disorders. In: DAVIES, D.M. (ed.), *Textbook of Adverse Drug Reactions*, 4th edn. New York, Oxford University Press, 534–566.

BOCHNER, B.S. and LICHTENSTEIN, L.M. (1991) Anaphylaxis. *New England Journal of Medicine* 324(25), 1785–1790.

BOELSTERLI, U.A., ZIMMERMAN, H.J. and KRETZ-ROMMEL, A. (1995) Idiosyncratic liver toxicity of nonsteroidal anti-inflammatory drugs: molecular mechanisms and pathology. *Critical Reviews in Toxicology* 25(3), 207–235.

BONNEY, S.L., NORTHINGTON, R.S., HEDRICH, D.A. and WALKER, B.R. (1986) Renal safety of two analgesics used over the counter: ibuprofen and aspirin. *Clinical Pharmacology and Therapeutics* 40(4), 373–377.

BRIGGS, G.G., FREEMAN, R.K. and YAFFE, S.J. (1990) *Drugs in Pregnancy and Lactation*, 3rd edn. Baltimore, Williams and Wilkins.

BROOKS, P.M. and NEEDS, C.J. (1989) The use of antirheumatic medication during pregnancy and in puerperium. *Rheumatic Diseases Clinics of North America* 15(4), 789–806.

BUTTERFIELD, J.H., SCHWENK, N.M., COLVILLE, D.S. and KUIPERS, B.J. (1986) Severe generalized reactions to ibuprofen: report of a case. *Journal of Rheumatology* 13(3), 649–650.

CABROL, D., LANDESMAN, R., MULLER, J., UZAN, M., SUREAU, C. and SAZENA, B.B. (1987) Treatment of polyhydraminos with prostaglandin synthetase inhibitor (indomethancin). *American Journal of Obstetrics and Gynecology* 157, 422–426.

CANTOR, B., TYLER, T. and NELSON, R.M. (1980) Oligohydramnios and transient neonatal anuria. A possible association with the maternal use of prostaglandin synthetase inhibitors. *Journal of Reproductive Medicine* 24(5), 220–223.

CARSON, J.L., STROM, B.L., DUFF, A., GUPTA, A. and DAS, K. (1993) Safety of nonsteroidal anti-inflammatory drugs with respect to acute liver disease. *Archives of Internal Medicine* 153(11), 1331–1336.

CHAN, H.L., STERN, R.S., ARNDT, K.A., LANGLOIS, J., JICK, S.S., JICK, H. and WALKER, A.M. (1990) The incidence of erythema multiforme, Stevens–Johnson syndrome, and toxic epidermal necrolysis. A population-based study with particular reference to reactions caused by drugs among outpatients. *Archives of Dermatology* 126(1), 43–47.

CHAPTER 11

CHAN, T.Y.K. (1995) Adverse interactions between warfarin and nonsteroidal anti-inflammatory drugs: mechanisms, clinical significance, and avoidance. *Annals of Pharmacotherapy* **29**(12), 1274–1283.

CHEMTOB, S., BEHARRY, K., BARNA, T., VARMA, D.R. and ARANDA, J.V. (1991) Differences in the effects in the new-born piglet of various nonsteroidal antiinflammatory drugs on cerebral blood flow but not on cerebrovascular prostaglandins. *Pediatric Research* **30**(1), 106–111.

CHEZ, M., SILA, C.A. and RANSOHOFF, R. (1990) Ibuprofen meningitis. *Neurology* **40**, 866–867.

COLES, L.S., FRIES, J.F., KRAINES, R.G. and ROTH, S.H. (1983) From experiment to experience: side-effects of nonsteroidal anti-inflammatory drugs. *American Journal of Medicine* **74**, 820–828.

CORRE, K.A. and SPIELBERG, T.E. (1988) Adverse drug reaction processing in the United States and its dependence on physician reporting: zomepirac (Zomax) as a case in point. *Annals of Emergency Medicine* **17**(2), 145–149.

DAVIS, B.J., THOMPSON, J., PEIMANN, A. and BENDIXEN, B.H. (1994) Drug-induced aseptic meningitis caused by two medications. *Neurology* **44**, 984–985.

DAVISON, K. and HASSANYEH, F. (1991) Psychiatric disorders. In: DAVIES, D.M. (ed.), *Textbook of Adverse Drug Reactions*, 4th edn. New York, Oxford University Press, 601–642.

DE LEEUW, P.W. (1996) Non-steroidal anti-inflammatory drugs and hypertension. The risks in perspective. *Drugs* **51**(2), 179–187.

DELMAS, P.D. (1995) Non-steroidal anti-inflammatory drugs and renal function. *British Journal of Rheumatology* **34**(Suppl. 1), 25–28.

DEMANDT, E., LEGIUS, E., DEVLIEGER, H., LEMMENS, F., PROESMANS, W. and EGGERMONT, E. (1990) Prenatal indomethacin toxicity in one member of monozygous twins; a case report. *European Journal of Obstetrics, Gynecology and Reproductive Biology* **35**(2–3), 267–269.

DERBY, L.E. and JICK, H. (1991) Renal parenchymal disease related to over-the-counter analgesic use. *Pharmacotherapy* **11**, 467–471.

DE WIT, W., VAN MOURIK, I. and WIESENHAAN, P.F. (1988) Prolonged maternal indomethacin therapy associated with oligohydramnios. Case reports. *British Journal of Obstetrics and Gynaecology* **95**, 303–305.

DUBOSE, T.D. (1994) Nephrotoxicity of non-steroidal anti-inflammatory drugs. *Lancet* **344**(8921), 515–518.

DURBACK, M.A., FREEMAN, J. and SCHUMACHER, H.R. JR. (1988) Recurrent ibuprofen-induced aseptic meningitis: third episode after only 200 mg of generic ibuprofen. *Arthritis and Rheumatism* **31**(6), 813–815.

EVANS, J.M., MCGREGOR, E., MCMAHON, A.D., MCGILCHRIST, M.M., JONES, M.C., WHITE, G., MCDEVITT, D.G. and MACDONALD, T.M. (1995) Non-steroidal anti-inflammatory drugs and hospitalization for acute renal failure. *Quarterly Journal of Medicine* **88**(8), 551–557.

FARAG, M.M., MIKHAIL, M., SHEHATA, R., ABDEL-MEGUID, E. and ABDEL-TAWAB, S. (1996) Assessment of gentamicin-induced nephrotoxicity in rats treated with low doses of ibuprofen and diclofenac sodium. *Clinical Science* **91**(2), 187–191.

FELIX, R.H. and SMITH, A.G. (1991) Skin disorders. In: DAVIES, D.M. (ed.), *Textbook of Adverse Drug Reactions*, 4th edn. New York, Oxford University Press, 514–534.

FIGUERAS, A., CAPELLA, D., CASTEL, J.M. and LAPORTE, J.R. (1994) Spontaneous reporting of adverse drug reactions to non-steroidal anti-inflammatory drugs: a report from the Spanish system of pharmacovigilance, including an early analysis of topical and enteric-coated formulations. *European Journal of Clinical Pharmacology* **47**, 297–303.

FINCH, W.R. and STROTTMAN, M.P. (1979) Acute adverse reactions to ibuprofen in systemic lupus erythematosus. *JAMA* **241**(24), 2616–2618.

FITT, A., DAYAN, M. and GILLIE, R.F. (1996) Vortex keratopathy associated with ibuprofen therapy. *Eye* **10**(Pt 1), 145–146.

FOWLER, P.D. (1987) Aspirin, paracetamol and non-steroidal anti-inflammatory drugs. A comparative review of side-effects. *Medical Toxicology Adverse Drug Experiences* **2**(5), 338–366.

FOX, D.A. and JICK, H. (1984) Nonsteroidal anti-inflammatory drugs and renal disease. *JAMA* **251**(10), 1299–1300.

FRAUNFELDER, F.T. and SAMPLES, J.R. (1994) Possible optic nerve side-effects associated with nonsteroidal anti-inflammatory drugs. *Journal of Toxicology, Cutaneous and Ocular Toxicology* **13**(4), 311–316.

FRAZEE, L.A. and REED, M.D. (1995) Warfarin and nonsteroidal antiinflammatory drugs: why not? *Annals of Pharmacotherapy* **29**, 1289–1291.

FREELAND, G.R., NORTHINGTON, R.S., HEDRICH, D.A. and WALKER, B.R. (1988) Hepatic safety of two analgesics used over the counter: ibuprofen and aspirin. *Clinical Pharmacology and Therapeutics* **43**(5), 473–479.

FUREY, S.A., WAKSMAN, J.A. and DASH, B.H. (1992) Nonprescription ibuprofen: side effect profile. *Pharmacotherapy* **12**(5), 403–407.

GABB, G.M. (1996) Fatal outcome of interaction between warfarin and a non-steroidal anti-inflammatory drug. *Medical Journal of Australia* **164**(11), 700–701.

GARCIA-RODRIGUEZ, L.A., PEREZ GUTTHANN, S., WALKER, A.M. and LUECK, L. (1992) The role of non-steroidal anti-inflammatory drugs in acute liver injury. *British Medical Journal* **305**(6858), 865–868.

CHAPTER 11

GARCIA-RODRIGUEZ, L.A., WILLIAMS, R., DERBY, L.E., DEAN, A.D. and JICK, H. (1994) Acute liver injury associated with nonsteroidal anti-inflammatory drugs and the role of risk factors. *Archives of Internal Medicine* **154**(3), 311–316.

GEORGE, J.N. and SHATTIL, S.J. (1991) The clinical importance of acquired abnormalities of platelet function. *New England Journal of Medicine* **324**(1), 27–39.

GOLDENBERG, R.L., DAVIS, R.O. and BAKER, R.C. (1989) Indomethacin-induced oligo-hydramnios. *American Journal of Obstetrics and Gynecology* **160**(5 Pt 1), 1196–1197.

GOODWIN, J.S. and REGAN, M. (1982) Cognitive dysfunction associated with naproxen and ibuprofen in the elderly. *Arthritis and Rheumatism* **25**, 1013–1015.

GRIFFITH, J.D., SMITH, C.H. and SMITH, R.C. (1982) Paranoid psychosis in a patient receiving ibuprofen, a prostaglandin synthesis inhibitor: case report. *Journal of Clinical Psychiatry* **43**(12), 499–500.

GRIMM, A.M. and WOLF, J.E. (1989) Aseptic meningitis associated with nonprescription ibuprofen use. *Annals of Pharmacotherapy* **23**, 712.

GRYFE, C.I. and RUBENZAHL, S. (1976) Agranulocytosis and aplastic anemia possibly due to ibuprofen. *CMA Journal* **114**, 877.

GUIDRY, J.B., OGBURN, C.L. JR. and GRIFFIN, F.M. JR. (1979) Fatal autoimmune hemolytic anemia associated with ibuprofen. *JAMA* **242**(1), 68–69.

GUPTA, U., THOMAS, K.J., DATTA, H. and MATHUR, V.S. (1984) Effect of ibuprofen and naproxen on implantation and pregnancy in rat. *Indian Journal of Experimental Biology* **22**, 282–283.

GURWITZ, J.H., AVORN, J., BOHN, R.L., GLYNN, R.J., MONANE, M. and MOGUN, H. (1994) Initiation of antihypertensive treatment during nonsteroidal anti-inflammatory drug therapy. *JAMA* **272**(10), 781–786.

GURWITZ, J.H., EVERITT, D.E., MONANE, M., GLYNN, R.J., CHOODNOVSKIY, I., BEAUDET, M.P. and AVORN, J. (1996) The impact of ibuprofen on the efficacy of antihypertensive treatment with hydrochlorothiazide in elderly persons. *Journal of Gerontology A: Biological Sciences and Medical Sciences* **51**(2), M74–M79.

HADDAD, J., MESSER, J., CASANOVA, R., SIMEONI, U. and WILLARD, D. (1990) Indomethacin and ischemic brain injury in neonates. *Journal of Pediatrics* **116**(5), 839–840.

HALPERN, S.M. (1994) Cutaneous toxicity of ibuprofen. *Archives of Dermatology* **130**, 259–260.

HALPERN, S.M., FITZPATRICK, R. and VOLANS, G.N. (1993) Ibuprofen toxicity: a review of adverse reactions and overdose. *Adverse Drug Reactions and Toxicological Reviews* **12**(2), 107–128.

HANSON, L. and MORGAN, H.J. (1994) Ibuprofen-induced aseptic meningitis. *Journal of the Tennessee Medical Association* **87**(2), 58.

HANSTEN, P.D. and HORN, J.R. (1993a) Diuretic drug interactions. In: *Drug Interactions and Updates*. Applied Therapeutics, 507–524.

HANSTEN, P.D. and HORN, J.R. (1993b) Nonsteroidal anti-inflammatory drug interactions. In: *Drug Interactions and Updates*. Applied Therapeutics, 605–623.

HANSTEN, P.D. and HORN, J.R. (1993c) Antineoplastic drug interactions. In: *Drug Interactions and Updates*. Applied Therapeutics, 401–421.

HANSTEN, P.D. and HORN, J.R. (1993d) Anticoagulant drug interactions. In: *Drug Interactions and Updates*. Applied Therapeutics, 285–329.

HANSTEN, P.D. and HORN, J.R. (1993e) Immunosuppressant drug interactions. In: *Drug Interactions and Updates*. Applied Therapeutics, 569–578.

HANSTEN, P.D. and HORN, J.R. (1993f) Antidiabetic drug interactions. In: *Drug Interactions and Updates*. Applied Therapeutics, 373–387.

HANSTEN, P.D. and HORN, J.R. (1993g) Differences in nonsteroidal anti-inflammatory drug interactions. In: *Drug Interactions and Updates*. Applied Therapeutics, 99–101.

HANSTEN, P.D. and HORN, J.R. (1993h) Beta-adrenergic blocker drug interactions. In: *Drug Interactions and Updates*. Applied Therapeutics, 435–457.

HANSTEN, P.D. and HORN, J.R. (1993i) Angiotensin-converting enzyme inhibitor drug interactions. In: *Drug Interactions and Updates*. Applied Therapeutics, 127–135.

HARTH, M. (1992) Rare miscellaneous adverse drug reactions and interactions of non-steroidal anti-inflammatory drugs. In: BORDA, I.T. and KOFF, R.S. (eds), *NSAIDs: A Profile of Adverse Effects*. Philadelphia, Hanley and Belfus, 219–231.

HENDRICKS, S.K., SMITH, J.R., MOORE, D.E. and BROWN, Z.A. (1990) Oligohydramnios associated with prostaglandin synthetase inhibitors in preterm labour. *British Journal of Obstetrics and Gynaecology* 97, 312–316.

HENRY, D.A. (1988) Side-effects of non-steroidal anti-inflammatory drugs. *Baillière's Clinical Rheumatology* 2(2), 425–454.

HEYMANN, M.A. (1986) Non-narcotic analgesics. Use in pregnancy and fetal and perinatal effects. *Drugs* 32(Suppl. 4), 164–176.

HICKOK, D.E., HOLLENBACH, K.A., REILLEY, S.F. and NYBERG, D.A. (1989) The association between decreased amniotic fluid volume and treatment with nonsteroidal anti-inflammatory agents for preterm labor. *American Journal of Obstetrics and Gynecology* 160(6), 1525–1531.

HOIGNÉ, R., SCHLUMBERGER, H.P., VERVLOET, D. and ZOPPI, M. (1993) Epidemiology of allergic drug reactions. In: DUKOR, P., HANSON, L.A., KALLOS, P., SHAKIB, F., TRNKA, Z., WAKSMAN, B.H. and BURR, M.L. (eds), *Monographs in Allergy*, 31st edn. Basel, S. KARGER, 147–170.

CHAPTER 11

HOPPMANN, R.A., PEDEN, J.G. and OBER, S.K. (1991) Central nervous system side effects of nonsteroidal anti-inflammatory drugs aseptic meningitis, psychosis, and cognitive dysfunction. *Archives of Internal Medicine* **151**, 1309–1313.

HOUSTON, M.C., WEIR, M., GRAY, J., GINSBERG, D., SZETO, C., KAIHLENEN, P.M., SUGIMOTO, D., RUNDE, M. and LEFKOWITZ, M. (1995) The effects of nonsteroidal anti-inflammatory drugs on blood pressures of patients with hypertension controlled by verapamil. *Archives of Internal Medicine* **155**(10), 1049–1054.

INMAN, W.H.W. (1977) Study of fatal bone marrow depression with special reference to phenylbutazone and oxyphenbutazone. *British Medical Journal* **1**, 1500–1505.

INMAN, W.H.W. and RAWSON, N.S.B. (1987) Prescription-event monitoring of five non-steroidal anti-inflammatory drugs. In: RAINSFORD, K.D. and VELO, G.P. (eds), *Side-effects of Anti-inflammatory Drugs Part One: Clinical and Epidemiological Aspects*. Lancaster, MTP Press, 111–124.

IAAS (International Agranulocytosis and Aplastic Anemia Study) (1986) Risks of agranulo-cytosis and aplastic anemia: a first report of their relation to drug use with special reference to analgesics. *JAMA* **256**(13), 1749–1757.

ITSKOVITZ, J., ABRAMOVICI, H. and BRANDES, J.M. (1980) Oliogohydramnion, meconium and perinatal death concurrent with indomethacin treatment in human pregnancy. *Journal of Reproductive Medicine* **24**, 137–140.

JACKSON, E.K. (1996) Vasopressin and other agents affecting the renal conservation of water. In: HARDMAN, J.G., LIMBIRD, L.E. and GILMAN, A.G. (eds), *Goodman and Gilman's The Pharmacological Basis of Therapeutics*, 9th edn. New York, McGraw-Hill, 715–731.

JAIN, S. (1994) Ibuprofen-induced thrombocytopenia. *British Journal of Clinical Practice* **48**(1), 51.

JICK, H., DERBY, L.E., GARCIA RODRIGUEZ, L.A., JICK, S.S. and DEAN, A.D. (1992) Liver disease associated with diclofenac, naproxen, and piroxicam. *Pharmacotherapy* **12**(3), 207–212.

JOHNSON, A.G., SEIDEMANN, P. and DAY, R.O. (1994) NSAID-related adverse drug interac-tions with clinical relevance. An update. *International Journal of Clinical Pharmacology and Therapeutics* **32**(10), 509–532.

JOHNSON, J.H., JICK, H., HUNTER, J.R. and DICKSON, J.F. (1985) A followup study of ibuprofen users. *Journal of Rheumatology* **12**(3), 549–552.

KAPLAN, B.H., NEVITT, M.P., PACH, J.M. and HERMAN, D.C. (1994) Aseptic meningitis and iridocyclitis related to ibuprofen. *American Journal of Ophthalmology* **117**(1), 119–120.

KAPLAN, B.S., RESTAINO, I., RAVAL, D.S., GOTTLIEB, R.P. and BERNSTEIN, J. (1994) Renal failure in the neonate associated with in utero exposure to non-steroidal anti-inflammatory agents. *Pediatric Nephrology* **8**(6), 700–704.

KIRSHON, B., MOISE, K.J. JR., MARI, G. and WILLIS, R. (1991) Long-term indomethacin therapy decreases fetal urine output and results in oligohydramnios. *American Journal of Perinatology* **8**(2), 86–88.

KLEINKNECHT, D. (1995) Interstitial nephritis, the nephrotic syndrome, and chronic renal failure secondary to nonsteroidal anti-inflammatory drugs. *Seminars in Nephrology* **15**(3), 228–235.

KOFF, R.S. (1992) Liver disease induced by nonsteroidal anti-inflammatory drugs. In: BORDA, I.T. and KOFF, R.S. (eds), *NSAIDs: A Profile of Adverse Effects*. Philadelphia, Hanley and Belfus, 133–145.

KUBACKA, R.T., ANTAL, E.J., JUHL, R.P. and WELSHMAN, I.R. (1996) Effects of aspirin and ibuprofen on the pharmacokinetics and pharmacodynamics of glyburide in healthy subjects. *Annals of Pharmacotherapy* **30**(1), 20–26.

KULLANDER, S. and KALLEN, B. (1976) A prospective study of drugs and pregnancy. 4. Miscellaneous drugs. *Acta Obstetrica et Gynecologica Scandinavica* **55**(4), 287–295.

LANZA, L.L., WALKER, A.M., BORTNICHAK, E.A., GAUSE, D.O. and DREYER, N.A. (1995) Incidence of symptomatic liver function abnormalities in a cohort of NSAID users. *Pharmacoepidemiology and Drug Safety* **4**, 231–237.

LEE, R.P., KING, E.G. and RUSSELL, A.S. (1983) Ibuprofen: a severe systemic reaction. *Canadian Medical Association Journal* **129**, 854–855.

LINDBLAD, R. and RODJER, S. (1991) Case report: a case of severe pancytopenia caused by ibuprofen. *Journal of Internal Medicine* **229**, 281–283.

LINDEN, C.H. and TOWNSEND, P.L. (1987) Clinical and laboratory observations: metabolic acidosis after acute ibuprofen overdosage. *Journal of Pediatrics* **111**(6 Pt 1), 922–925.

MALCOLM, D.D., SEGAR, J.L., ROBILLARD, E. and CHEMTOB, S. (1993) Indomethacin compromises hemodynamics during positive-pressure ventilation, independently of prostanoids. *Journal of Applied Physiology* **74**, 1672–1678.

MAMUS, S.W., BURTON, J.D., GROAT, J.D., SCHULTE, D.A., LOBELL, M. and ZANJANI, E.D. (1986) Ibuprofen-associated pure white-cell aplasia. *New England Journal of Medicine* **314**(10), 624–625.

MANCHESTER, D., MARGOLIS, H.S. and SHELDON, R.E. (1976) Possible association between maternal indomethacin therapy and primary pulmonary hypertension of the newborn. *American Journal of Obstetrics and Gynecology* **126**(4), 467–469.

MANOUKIAN, A.V. and CARSON, J.L. (1996) Nonsteroidal anti-inflammatory drug-induced hepatic disorders. Incidence and prevention. *Drug Safety* **15**(1), 64–71.

MATHIEU, M. (1994) *New Drug Development: A Regulatory Overview*, 3rd edn. Waltham, Parexel International Corporation.

CHAPTER 11

McGOLDRICK, M.D. and BAILIE, G.R. (1997) Nonnarcotic analgesics: prevalence and estimated economic impact of toxicities. *Annals of Pharmacotherapy* 31, 221–227.

McINTIRE, S.C., RUBENSTEIN, R.C., GARTNER, J.C. JR. and GILBOA, N. (1993) Acute flank pain and reversible renal dysfunction associated with nonsteroidal anti-inflammatory drug use. *Pediatrics* 92, 459–460.

MEAD, R.A. and McGHAN, W.F. (1988) Use of nonsteroidal anti-inflammatory drugs in a health maintenance organization. *American Pharmacist*, NS28, 29–31.

MENE, P., PUGLIESE, F. and PATRONO, C. (1995) The effects of nonsteroidal anti-inflammatory drugs on human hypertensive vascular disease. *Seminars in Nephrology* 15(3), 244–252.

MEYER, D. and GIRMA, J. (1993) von Willebrand factor: structure and function. *Thrombosis and Haemostasis* 70(1), 99–104.

MIESCHER, P.A. (1986) Blood dyscrasias secondary to non-steroidal anti-inflammatory drugs. *Medical Toxicology* 1(Suppl. 1), 57–70.

MIESZCZAK, C. and WINTHER, K. (1993) Lack of interaction of ketoprofen with warfarin. *European Journal of Clinical Pharmacology* 44(2), 205–269.

MIFSUD, A.J. (1988) Drug-related recurrent meningitis. *Journal of Infection* 17, 151–153.

MILLER, R.R. and GREENBLATT, D. (1976) *Drug Effects in Hospitalized Patients*. New York, Wiley.

MOISE, K.J. JR., HUHTA, J.C., SHARIF, D.S., OU, C.N., KIRSHON, B. and WASSERSTRUM, N. (1988) Indomethacin in the treatment of premature labor. Effects on the fetal ductus arteriosus. *New England Journal of Medicine* 319(6), 327–331.

MOSS, A.H., RILEY, R., MURGO, A. and SKAFF, L.A. (1986) Over-the-counter ibuprofen and acute renal failure. *Annals of Internal Medicine* 105(2), 303.

MURRAY, M.D., BRATER, D.C., TIERNEY, W.M., HUI, S.L. and McDONALD, C.J. (1990) Ibuprofen-associated renal impairment in a large general internal medicine practice. *American Journal of the Medical Sciences* 299(4), 222–229.

NALDI, L., LOCATI, F. and CAINELLI, T. (1990) Incidence of toxic epidermal necrolysis in Italy. *Archives of Dermatology* 126, 1103–1104.

NICASTRO, N.J. (1989) Visual disturbances associated with over-the-counter ibuprofen in three patients. *Annals of Ophthalmology* 21(12), 447–450.

ØSTENSEN, M. and ØSTENSEN, H. (1996) Safety of nonsteroidal anti-inflammatory drugs in pregnant patients with rheumatic disease. *Journal of Rheumatology* 23(6), 1045–1049.

PALMER, B.F. (1995) Renal complications associated with use of nonsteroidal anti-inflammatory agents. *Journal of Investigative Medicine* 43(6), 516–533.

PALMER, B.F. and HENRICH, W.L. (1995) Clinical acute renal failure with nonsteroidal anti-inflammatory drugs. *Seminars in Nephrology* 15(3), 214–227.

PALMER, C.A.L. (1972) Toxic amblyopia from ibuprofen. *British Medical Journal* 3, 705.

PEREZ-GUTTHANN, S. and RODRIGUEZ, L.A.G. (1993) The increased risk of hospitalizations for acute liver injury in a population with exposure to multiple drugs. *Epidemiology* **4**(6), 496–501.

PEREZ-GUTTHANN, S., GARCIA RODRIGUEZ, L.A., RAIFORD, D.S., DUQUE OLIART, A. and RIS ROMEU, J. (1996) Nonsteroidal anti-inflammatory drugs and the risk of hospitalization for acute renal failure. *Archives of Internal Medicine* **156**(21), 2433–2439.

PERNEGER, T.V., WHELTON, P.K. and KLAG, M.J. (1994) Risk of kidney failure associated with the use of acetaminophen, aspirin, and nonsteroidal antiinflammatory drugs. *New England Journal of Medicine* **331**(25), 1675–1679.

PETRERE, J.A., HUMPHREY, R.R., ANDERSON, J.A., FITZGERALD, J.E. and DE LA IGLESIA, F.A. (1985) Studies on reproduction in rats with meclofenamate sodium, a nonsteroidal anti-inflammatory agent. *Fundamental and Applied Toxicology* **5**, 665–671.

PICADO, C., CASTILLO, J.A., MONTSERRAT, J.M. and AGUSTI-VIDAL, A. (1989) Aspirin-intolerance as a precipitating factor of life-threatening attacks of asthma requiring mechanical ventilation. *European Respiratory Journal* **2**(2), 127–129.

POIRIER, T.I. (1984) Reversible renal failure associated with ibuprofen: case report and review of the literature. *Drug Intelligence Clinical Pharmacology* **18**, 27–32.

POWELL, J.G. and COCHRANE, R.L. (1982) The effects of a number of non-steroidal anti-inflammatory compounds on parturition in the rat. *Prostaglandins and Leukotrienes in Medicine* **23**(4), 469–488.

RABINOVITZ, M. and VAN THIEL, D.H. (1992) Hepatotoxicity of nonsteroidal anti-inflammatory drugs. *American Journal of Gastroenterology* **87**(12), 1696–1704.

REPKE, J.T. and NIEBYL, J.R. (1985) Role of prostaglandin synthetase inhibitors in the treatment of preterm labor. *Seminars in Reproductive Endocrinology* **3**(3), 259–272.

RIDDER, W.H. and TOMLINSON, A. (1992) Effect of ibuprofen on contrast sensitivity. *Optometry and Vision Science* **69**(8), 652–655.

ROSSI, A.C. and KNAPP, D. (1982) Tolmetin-induced anaphylactoid reactions. *New England Journal of Medicine* **307**(8), 499–500.

ROUJEAU, J.C., GUILLAUME, J.C., FABRE, J.P., PENSO, D., FLECHET, M.L. and GIRRE, J.P. (1990) Toxic epidermal necrolysis (Lyell syndrome) incidence and drug aetiology in France, 1981–1985. *Archives of Dermatology* **126**, 37–42.

ROUJEAU, J.C., KELLY, J.P., NALDI, L. *et al.* (1995) Medication use and the risk of Stevens–Johnson syndrome or toxic epidermal necrolysis. *New England Journal of Medicine* **333**(24), 1600–1607.

RYBAK, M.E.M. (1992) Hematologic effects of nonsteroidal anti-inflammatory drugs. In: BORDA, I.T. and KOFF, R.S. (eds), *NSAIDs: A Profile of Adverse Effects*. Philadelphia, Hanley and Belfus, 113–132.

CHAPTER 11

SAAG, K.G., RUBENSTEIN, L.M., CHRISCHILLES, E.A. and WALLACE, R.B. (1995) Nonsteroidal antiinflammatory drugs and cognitive decline in the elderly. *Journal of Rheumatology* 22(11), 2142–2147.

SANDLER, D.P., BURR, F.R. and WEINBERG, C.R. (1991) Nonsteroidal anti-inflammatory drugs and the risk for chronic renal disease. *Annals of Internal Medicine* 115, 165–172.

SANDLER, R.H. (1985) Anaphylactic reactions to zomepirac. *Annals of Emergency Medicine* 14(2), 171–174.

SCHOPF, E., STUHMER, A., RZANY, B., VICTOR, N., ZENTGRAF, R. and KAPP, J.F. (1991) Toxic epidermal necrolysis and Stevens–Johnson syndrome. *Archives of Dermatology* 127, 839–842.

SELWYN, J.G. (1967) Hypersensitivity reactions to phenylbutazone. *British Medical Journal* 4, 487–488.

SERNERI, G.G.N., GENSINI, G.F., ABBATE, R., CASTELLANI, S., BONECHI, F., CARNOVALI, M., ROSTAGNO, C., DABIZZI, R.P., DAGIANTI, A. and ARATA, L. (1990) Defective coronary prostaglandin modulation in anginal patients. *American Heart Journal* 120(1), 12–21.

SHEPARD, T.H. (1992) *Catalog of Teratogenic Agents*, 7th edn. Baltimore, Johns Hopkins University Press.

SHORR, R.I., RAY, W.A., DAUGHERTY, J.R. and GRIFFIN, M.R. (1993) Concurrent use of non-steroidal anti-inflammatory drugs and oral anticoagulants places elderly persons at high risk for hemorrhagic peptic ulcer disease. *Archives of Internal Medicine* 153(14), 1665–1670.

SIMEONI, U., MESSER, J., WEISBURD, P., HADDAD, J. and WILLARD, D. (1989) Neonatal renal dysfunction and intrauterine exposure to prostaglandin synthesis inhibitors. *European Journal of Pediatrics* 148, 371–373.

SINGH, G., RAMEY, D.R., MORFELD, D. and FRIES, J.F. (1994) Comparative toxicity of non-steroidal anti-inflammatory agents. *Pharmacology and Therapeutics* 62(1–2), 175–191.

SMITH, G., ROBERTS, R., HALL, C. and NUKI, G. (1996) Reversible ovulatory failure associated with the development of luteinized unruptured follicles in women with inflammatory arthritis taking non-steroidal anti-inflammatory drugs. *British Journal of Rheumatology* 35(5), 458–462.

SPIERTO, R.J., KAUFMAN, M.B. and STOUKIDES, C.A. (1992) Acute renal failure associated with use of over the counter ibuprofen. *Annals of Pharmacotherapy* 26, 714.

STERN, R.S. and BIGBY, M. (1984) An expanded profile of cutaneous reactions to non-steroidal anti-inflammatory drugs: reports to a specialty-based system for spontaneous reporting of adverse reactions to drugs. *JAMA* 252(11), 1433–1437.

STERNLIEB, P. and ROBINSON, R.M. (1978) Stevens–Johnson syndrome plus toxic hepatitis due to ibuprofen. *New York State Journal of Medicine* 78(8), 1239–1243.

STROM, B.L., CARSON, J.L., MORSE, M.L., WEST, S.L. and SOPER, K.A. (1987) The effect of indication on hypersensitivity reactions associated with zomepirac sodium and other nonsteroidal antiinflammatory drugs. *Arthritis and Rheumatism* **30**(10), 1142–1148.

STROM, B.L., CARSON, J.L., SCHINNAR, R., SIM, E. and MORSE, M.L. (1988) The effect of indication on the risk of hypersensitivity reactions associated with tolmetin sodium vs other nonsteroidal antiinflammatory drugs. *Journal of Rheumatology* **15**(4), 695–699.

STROM, B., WEST, S., SIM, E. and CARSON, J. (1989) The epidemiology of the acute flank pain syndrome from suprofen. *Clinical Pharmacology and Therapeutics* **46**(6), 693–699.

STROM, B.L., CARSON, J.L., SCHINNAR, R., SNYDER, E.S., SHAW, M. and LUNDIN, F.E. JR. (1993) Nonsteroidal anti-inflammatory drugs and neutropenia. *Archives of Internal Medicine* **153**, 2119–2124.

SWAMINATHAN, R. (1991) Disorders of metabolism 2. In: DAVIES, D.M. (ed.), *Textbook of Adverse Drug Reactions*, 4th edn. New York, Oxford University Press, 399–490.

TATRO, D.S. (1997) *Drug Interaction Facts*. St. Louis, Facts and Comparisons.

TRUTER, P.J., FRANSZEN, S., VAN DER MERWE, J.V. and COETZEE, M.J. (1986) Premature closure of the ductus arteriosus causing intra-uterine death. A case report. *South African Medical Journal* **70**(9), 557–558.

VAN DEN OUWELAND, F.A., GRIBNAU, F.W.J. and MEYBOOM, R.H.B. (1988) Congestive heart failure due to nonsteroidal anti-inflammatory drugs in the elderly. *Age and Ageing* **17**, 8–16.

VAN DER HEIJDEN, B. and GUBLER, M.C. (1995) Renal failure in the neonate associated with in utero exposure to non-steroidal anti-inflammatory agents. *Pediatric Nephrology* **9**(5), 675.

VAN DER KLAUW, M.M., STRICKER, B.H., HERINGS, R.M., COST, W.S., VALKENBURG, H.A. and WILSON, J.H. (1993) A population based case-cohort study of drug-induced anaphylaxis. *British Journal of Clinical Pharmacology* **35**(4), 400–408.

VARVARIGOU, A., BARDIN, C.L., BEHARRY, K., CHEMTOB, S., PAPAGEORGIOU, A. and ARANDA, J.V. (1996) Early ibuprofen administration to prevent patent ductus arteriosus in premature newborn infants. *JAMA* **275**(7), 539–544.

VERBEECK, R.K. (1990) Pharmacokinetic drug interactions with nonsteroidal anti-inflammatory drugs. *Clinical Pharmacokinetics* **19**(1), 44–66.

VRHOVAC, B. (1984) Anti-inflammatory analgesics and drugs used in gout. In: DUKES, M.N.G. (ed.), *Meyler's Side Effects of Drugs*, 10th edn. New York, Elsevier, 153–171.

WHELTON, A., STOUT, R.L., SPILMAN, P.S. and KLASSEN, D.K. (1990) Renal effects of ibuprofen, piroxicam, and sulindac in patients with asymptomatic renal failure. *Annals of Internal Medicine* **112**, 568–576.

CHAPTER 11

WIGGINS, D.A. and ELLIIOTT, J.P. (1990) Oligohydramnios in each sac of triplet gestation caused by Motrin — fulfilling Koch's postulates. *American Journal of Obstetrics and Gynecology* **162**(2), 460–461.

WILKINSON, A.R., AYNSLEY-GREEN, A. and MITCHELL, M.D. (1979) Persistent pulmonary hypertension and abnormal prostaglandin E levels in preterm infants after maternal treatment with naproxen. *Archives of Disease in Childhood* **54**, 942–945.

WILSON, T.W. and CARRUTHERS, S.G. (1992) Renal and cardiovascular adverse effects of nonsteroidal anti-inflammatory drugs. In: BORDA, I.T. and KOFF, R.S. (eds), *NSAIDs: A Profile of Adverse Effects*. Philadelphia, Hanley and Belfus, 81–112.

WYSENBEEK, A.J., KLEIN, Z., NAKAR, S. and MANE, R. (1988) Assessment of cognitive function in elderly patients treated with naproxen. *Clinical and Experimental Rheumatology* **6**, 399–400.

YEUNG, V.T.F. and COCKRAM, C.S. (1991) Endocrine disorders. In: DAVIES, D.M. (ed.), *Textbook of Adverse Drug Reactions*, 4th edn. New York, Oxford University Press, 344–369.

YOCUM, M.W. and KHAN, D.A. (1994) Assessment of patients who have experienced anaphylaxis: a 3-year survey. *Mayo Clinic Proceedings* **69**, 16–23.

ZARFIN, Y., KOREN, G., MARESKY, D., PERLMAN, M. and MACLEOD, S. (1985) Possible indomethacin-aminoglycoside interaction in preterm infants. *Journal of Pediatrics* **106**(3), 511–513.

ZIMMERMAN, H.J. (1990) Update of hepatotoxicity due to classes of drugs in common clinical use: non-steroidal drugs, anti-inflammatory drugs, antibiotics, antihypertensives, and cardiac and psychotropic agents. *Seminars in Liver Disease* **10**(4), 322–338.

Human Toxicity of Ibuprofen

GLYN VOLANS* AND RITA FITZPATRICK

Medical Toxicology Unit, Guy's and St Thomas' Hospital Trust, London, UK

*CONTACT NUMBER

Tel: +44 (0)171 771 5315 Fax: +44 (0)171 771 5306
Email: Volans@medtox.demon.co.uk

Contents

12.1 INTRODUCTION

In the experience of Poisons Information Centres, all drugs, whatever their formulation and intended use, have the potential to be misused in overdosage, either deliberately or accidentally. Although some drugs, such as anti-cancer drugs, are rarely taken in overdosage by healthy adults, others, such as CNS active drugs, including anxiolytics, antidepressants and analgesics, are commonly misused and overdosage represents an important health care problem. Against that background, the taking of ibuprofen in overdosage demonstrates the importance of toxicovigilance, i.e. the surveillance of incidents of human overdosage and the use of the data thus gained to improve drug safety.

For the first 14 years of its availability in the United Kingdom (10 years in the United States), as a prescription-only anti-inflammatory drug, ibuprofen was seldom reported to have been taken in overdosage. This finding was similar for all NSAIDs available at that time but was striking for ibuprofen. An average 12–13 million prescriptions for ibuprofen were issued per year between 1978 and 1980, but during 1980 and 1981 there were only 75 enquiries to the National Poisons Information Service, London (NPIS(London)) out of a total 58 000 reported overdoses (Court *et al.*, 1983). Nevertheless it was possible to demonstrate that ibuprofen toxicity in overdosage appeared to be low and these findings contributed to the evidence considered by the regulatory authorities in the United Kingdom and the United States when OTC licences were granted (Boots Company plc, 1982; American Home Products Corporation, 1983).

The reasons for this low incidence of overdosage with a group of widely prescribed drugs have not been fully explained, but are likely to include both patient- and product-related factors. Thus the incidence of overdosage and suicide attempts by patients with rheumatoid disease seems to be low, and such patients generally treat their drugs with care and store them safely.

Once ibuprofen became available OTC as an analgesic rather than as an anti-inflammatory drug, it was entirely predictable that it would figure more frequently in overdosage. Indeed, not only was there ample evidence from many countries that analgesics were the drugs most frequently encountered in overdosage, there was also epidemiological evidence from the United Kingdom that in 50–76% of adult self-poisonings with analgesics the drugs concerned were purchased OTC (National Poisons Information Service Monitoring Group, 1981).

Within two years of the OTC release of ibuprofen it was possible to demonstrate the predicted increased frequency of deliberate overdosage in adults and accidental ingestion by children (Perry *et al.*, 1987). These trends have continued with the increased sales of OTC products, and at the time of writing, 13–14 years after the first OTC licences were granted, ibuprofen has established itself as one of the top drugs in enquiries to Poisons Centres in the United Kingdom and the United States (see Tables 12.1, 12.2 and 12.3) (Litovitz *et al.*, 1997; National Poisons Information Service (London), unpublished).

TABLE 12.1

Ibuprofen enquiries to Poisons Information Centres (London and United States)

Year	Number of enquiries re ibuprofen to NPIS(London)	Total of all enquiries (all agents) to NPIS(London)	Percentage of total London enquiries	Number of enquiries re ibuprofen to US poison centres	Total of all enquiries to US poison centres (all agents)	Percentage of total
1991	2311	100 813	2.3	31 576	1 837 939	1.7
1992* Sample	430	115 220	2.6	33 465	1 864 188	1.8
Extrapolated total	3010					
1993* Sample	552	134 208	2.9	33 013	1 751 476	1.9
Extrapolated total	3864					
1994	3781	153 130	2.5	35 703	1 926 438	1.9
1995	2624	172 861	1.5	39 361	2 023 189	1.9

TABLE 12.2

Substances most frequently involved in human exposures reported to NPIS(London) 1996

Rank	Substance name	Number of enquiries 1996	Percentage of total enquiries
1	Paracetamol	41 834	21.8
2	Aspirin	13 777	7.2
3	Ibuprofen	10 220	5.3
4	Diazepam	9 570	5.0
5	Temazepam	8 982	4.7
6	Coproxamol	7 641	4.0
7	Caffeine	7 362	3.8
8	Dothiepin	6 804	3.5
9	Fluoxetine	5 950	3.1
10	Zopiclone	4 837	2.5

TABLE 12.3

Substances most frequently involved in human exposures reported to US Poison Centres 1996

Rank	Substance name	Number of enquiries 1996	Percentage of total enquiries
1	Cleaning substances	221 261	10.3
2	Analgesics*	208 305	9.7
3	Cosmetics	184 799	8.6
4	Plants	113 619	5.3
5	Cough and cold preparations	106 823	5.0
6	Bites/envenomations	95 283	4.4
7	Pesticides	86 912	4.0
8	Foreign bodies	84 392	3.9
9	Topicals	77 269	3.6
10	Food products/poisoning	73 947	3.4

* Includes 43 777 enquiries involving ibuprofen.

The management of cases of analgesic overdosage represents a major health care problem (Hawton and Fagg, 1992; Gunnell *et al.*, 1997) and consumes financial resources that could have been put to better use. A comprehensive review of experience with ibuprofen overdosage is thus important in order to propose measures to optimize management and, if possible, to reduce the size of the problem.

12.2 MECHANISM OF TOXICITY IN OVERDOSAGE

In contrast to aspirin and paracetamol, ibuprofen does not appear to manifest an additional pathophysiological mechanism in overdosage (Halpern *et al.*, 1993). Thus it would be expected that toxic effects would be related to its known pharmacological actions through inhibition of prostaglandin synthesis (Chapter 5) and that any new dose-related effects

CHAPTER 12

would be attributable to accumulation of its metabolites 2-hydroxyibuprofen and 2-carboxyibuprofen (Chapter 2). Any review of the clinical presentation and management of ibuprofen overdosage must therefore look for acute toxic effects that represent an extension of either intended therapeutic benefits or of unwanted adverse effects.

12.3   REVIEW OF THE EFFECTS OF IBUPROFEN IN OVERDOSAGE

The earliest surveys of ibuprofen overdosage all found a low incidence of toxic effects, but their authors also emphasized the need for continuing surveillance for new problems that might emerge only after some years, as had been the case with paracetamol (Clark *et al.*, 1973). Annual Reports from Poisons Centres in the United States and United Kingdom (Litovitz *et al.*, 1997; NPIS(London), unpublished) have, however, supported earlier observations and there is adequate evidence that toxicity is low even after large doses have been ingested.

Typical of such reports is the one from the NPIS(London) covering the three-year period 1985 to 1988 (Halpern *et al.*, 1993). During that time there were a total of 1515 ibuprofen enquiries concerning 1033 (68%) adults and 482 (32%) children under 12 years of age. When co-ingestion of other drugs was excluded there remained 1089 cases, 705 (65%) of which were asymptomatic, while 199 (18%) experienced mild symptoms and only 23 (2%) experienced moderate toxicity. There were no cases with severe or fatal effects in this series. For 162 (15%) patients, symptoms were not known at the time of enquiry. Vomiting was the most frequent effect reported: 70 (35%) of the 199 patients with mild effects and 6 out of 23 (26%) patients with moderate effects had vomiting. Drowsiness and abdominal pain were also reported.

Similar overall conclusions have been reached by other investigators, no series of cases producing a greater frequency of toxic effects or unexpected toxic effects. In that situation, it is more relevant to consider the evidence for dose–response and toxicokinetics and to review all cases reports where more serious toxicity has been demonstrated. This approach was taken in an earlier review of ibuprofen toxicity that covered ADRs and effects of overdosage, both those reported to the NPIS(London) and those in the published literature up to 1992 (Halpern *et al.*, 1993). The present review follows on from this, covering a further 5 years' surveillance (1991–1995 inclusive) of referrals to the NPIS(London), presented in Table 12.1, and a review of more recent published reports.

12.4   REPORTS OF DEATHS AFTER IBUPROFEN OVERDOSE

Extensive literature searches have, to date, identified only seven published reports of fatal overdosages associated with ibuprofen (Court and Volans, 1983; Hall *et al.*, 1986; Bernstein *et al.*, 1992; Kunsman and Rohig; 1993; Levine *et al.*, 1993). It is therefore important to review the details of each case in order to ensure that any risk factors are properly identified. This has been done in Table 12.4; however, it can be seen that in each case assessment of

TABLE 12.4

Published reports of deaths after ibuprofen overdosages

Reference	Age/sex	Dose of ibuprofen	Highest plama ibuprofen	Other drugs	Symptoms/signs	Comment
Court et al. (1983)	67 years F	N/K	N/A	Aspirin	Confused hyperventilating, deaf, cardiac arrest	Severe salicylate toxicity at modest levels
Hall et al. (1986)	16 months	469 mg/kg	N/A	None	Apnoea, aspiration, pneumonitis	Death from sepsis at 7 days
Steinmetz et al. (1987)	48 years M	N/K	80.8 mg/l post mortem	Paracetamol 200 mg/l post mortem	Found dead	Past history: multiple drug overdoses, peptic ulceration, renal failure, cachexic
Hall et al. (1988)	Adult	> 20 g	N/A	None recorded	Oliguric sepsis	Hemodialysis refused; might have survived if treated
Bernstein et al. (1992)	54 years F	N/K	N/A	Theophylline sustained release, 31.3 mg/l Formed bezoar	Lethargic tachycardia	Past history: obstructive airways disease, diabetes mellitus, peptic ulcer, atrial fibrillation, death cardiac arrest
Kunsman and Rohig (1993)	26 years M	N/K	340 mg/l post mortem	None	Found dead	Past history of drug abuse; cause of death 'ibuprofen toxicity'; manner of death 'not known'
Levine et al. (1993)	19 years M	N/K	130 mg/l	Cyclobenzaprine, phenylpropanolamine, chlorphenyramine. Phenytoin, lignocaine — therapeutic concentrations.	Tachycardia, metabolic acidosis	'Due to multiple drug ingestion'

ibuprofen toxicity is limited either by lack of information or by evidence for complicating factors, such as co-ingestion of other drugs (including aspirin, cyclobenzaprine, phenyl-propanolamine, chlorpheniramine and paracetamol) or secondary problems, e.g. sepsis following aspiration or hypotension following deliberate self-exsanguination.

A review of fatal cases recorded by Poisons Information Centres may duplicate published reports and often the cases will be less thoroughly documented by the centre. Nevertheless, this information can be useful in confirming the low frequency of fatal toxicity in cases where hospital treatment is attempted. It is, therefore, interesting to note that during the nine years 1985–1993 the US Poisons Information Centres recorded only three deaths due to ibuprofen (all deliberate ingestions by adults) compared with 147 deaths due to paracetamol and 167 due to aspirin over the same period (Jones, personal communication, 1994).

It is not possible from present evidence, therefore, to define a potentially fatal dose of ibuprofen in humans on a dose per kilogram basis. However, it is important to stress the possibility of increased toxicity in patients who take multiple overdoses or who are suffering from underlying diseases. Clearly, all cases of suspected fatal toxicity should be fully reported to regulatory agencies and manufacturers and, when appropriate, published in the literature.

12.5 DOSE–RESPONSE AND TOXICOKINETICS

Ingestion of more than 400 mg/kg carries a high risk of serious toxicity (Halpern *et al.*, 1993; Hall *et al.*, 1986). Survival has been reported in a small number of patients after allegedly very large overdoses. The largest ingestion to date is claimed by Wolfe (1995): 72 g taken by a 44-year-old man whose weight was not stated. Ibuprofen was not measured in the blood but nevertheless the circumstantial evidence and the severity of the clinical effects, including acidosis, renal insufficiency and rhabdomyolyisis, offer strong support for the alleged dose. In other cases very high plasma ibuprofen concentrations have been measured in patients with relatively few symptoms, for example, the adult patient reported by Court *et al.* (1983) with a plasma ibuprofen concentration of 704 mg/l (more than 20 times the peak plasma concentration seen after a single dose of 400 mg ibuprofen), who was asymptomatic.

When ibuprofen concentrations have been measured in fatal cases, they are difficult to interpret when the timing of the sample in relation to the time of ingestion is unknown, as is usually the case, or if the measurements have been made on post-mortem samples.

At the other end of the scale, there is plenty of evidence that doses of less than 100 mg/kg of ibuprofen do not cause toxic effects and that between 200 and 400 mg/kg is likely to be associated with only mild to moderate symptoms. These findings have been taken into account in a recent study where healthy adult human volunteers took ibuprofen 75 mg/kg in a single oral dose as a marker substance for a study of whole-bowel irrigation, used as a method to aid removal of poisons from the gastrointestinal tract. In fact, the volunteers in question were taking as a single dose approximately 8 g of ibuprofen, i.e. up to 10 times the normal maximum single therapeutic dose. They reported no adverse affects. One cannot imagine similar studies using 10 times the maximum therapeutic dose for either paracetamol or aspirin!

Any changes in the pharmacokinetics after ibuprofen overdosage appears to be small and of little or no clinical significance for the vast majority of patients. Thus, absorption is rapid and the first samples taken after ingestion (usually 2–6 h after ingestion) invariably produce the highest levels recorded in the individual patient even after the largest doses. Metabolism does not appear to be saturable and, in consequence, the largest overdoses result in high levels of acidic metabolites (see below). In absence of renal failure, excretion of unchanged ibuprofen and its metabolites is sufficient to avoid any clinically significant prolongation of the relevant half-lives. Patients with renal failure should be regarded differently.

Based on these observations and on the low incidence of severe toxicity, it is not surprising that the measurement of ibuprofen plasma concentrations has not proved useful in the management of ibuprofen overdosages, in contrast with the important role of drug measurement in management of overdosage with paracetamol or aspirin. Hall *et al.* (1986) produced a nomogram that they believed could be a useful prognostic indicator for those patients who are asymptomatic on presentation at hospital but develop symptoms later. However, the scatter of the data is wide and the correlations are weak, and when Jenkinson *et al.* (1988) applied a pharmacokinetic model they found the best fit for the relationship between symptoms and timed ibuprofen concentrations was an exponential equation. Ultimately, both groups accepted that this model has poor specificity and sensitivity and is of no use in clinical practice.

The role of measurement of blood concentrations of ibuprofen in clinical practice is thus largely limited to confirming diagnosis in cases with serious clinical effects (when they should preferably be supported by a full analytical screen for co-ingested drugs) or cases where there may be other diagnostic implications, for example, cases of suspected child abuse by drugs.

CHAPTER 12

12.6 GASTROINTESTINAL EFFECTS

In spite of the relatively low incidence of gastrointestinal intolerance to ibuprofen in therapeutic doses (Chapter 9), it might be predicted that this advantage would be lost in acute overdosage owing simply to dose–response effects and confounding variables such as co-ingestants or underlying disease. In practice, gastrointestinal symptoms are the most frequent symptoms recorded after acute ibuprofen overdosage, but they are seldom severe. The incidence of nausea, vomiting and abdominal discomfort varies from over 40% (McElwee *et al.*, 1990) to between 6% and 10% (Court *et al.*, 1983; Hall *et al.*, 1986).

The only two series that used blood concentrations and toxicokinetics as an index of dose rather than relying on the clinical history alone (Hall *et al.*, 1986; Jenkinson *et al.*, 1988) indicate that this variation is most likely to be dose related.

Other adverse gastrointestinal events described after therapeutic doses of ibuprofen include tablets lodging in the oesophagus, ulceration, bleeding and strictures in the small bowel, and colitis. None have been described after acute overdose. Surprisingly, there are no reports of gastrointestinal hemorrhage in the published literature up to 1997.

12.7   RENAL EFFECTS

Ibuprofen, in common with other NSAIDs, can be shown to cause renal toxicity through inhibition of cyclooxygenase, which in turn blocks production of the renal vasodilators PGE_2 and prostacyclin. Renal function then declines as a result of reduced renal blood flow and glomerular filtration, with consequent effects upon fluid and electrolyte balance followed by renal failure (Chapter 10). Rare cases of interstitial nephritis due to ibuprofen have been described but this has not been seen in overdose.

Patients with evidence of renal impairment related to long-term use of ibuprofen and other NSAIDs are a regular experience in nephrology clinics. There was thus an understandable concern that the wider OTC use of ibuprofen would be associated with potentially serious or even life-threatening renal failure from unsupervised therapeutic use or overdosage. For this reason, it has been important to monitor the incidence of renal problems in all reported series of ibuprofen overdosage and to publish case reports where severe renal toxicity has been encountered.

The earliest series of cases (Court *et al.*, 1983) identified only one report of possible renal toxicity in 168 cases. This involved an elderly male who ingested between 9.6 and 16 g of ibuprofen and experienced a transient rise in urea and creatinine that could have been related to an underlying impairment in renal function. Similarly, Hall *et al.* (1986) reported two adults who developed transient renal impairment in a series of 126 cases and, although they subsequently reported a death from renal failure (Hall *et al.*, 1988), they considered that recovery would have occurred if permission for hemodialysis had not been withheld. Jenkinson *et al.* (1988) reviewed the relationship between clinical effects and pharmocokinetics in their patients and other published cases. It was concluded that evidence of renal toxicity was more likely with plasma ibuprofen concentrations greater than 280 mg/l within 10 h after ingestion and it was acknowledged that pre-existing renal disease could seriously increase this risk. Overall, it was felt that minor changes in renal function probably go unnoticed in patients who remained well after the overdosage.

The case reports of serious renal toxicity published to date can be divided into those where there was massive overdosage and those where additional factors appear to have been operating.

12.7.1   Cases of massive overdose

A 52-year-old woman who ingested 54 g ibuprofen developed metabolic acidosis and oliguric renal failure. She required dialysis but recovered normal renal function over a period of 17 days (Bennett *et al.*, 1985). A 23-year-old male took 30 g of ibuprofen plus an unknown but probably insignificant amount of sublingual nitroglycerin. A qualitative toxicology screen was negative, but 18 h after ingestion the plasma ibuprofen concentration was 324 mg/l. He developed hypotension and metabolic acidosis and was treated by hemofiltration/hemodialysis. On day 3, he developed adult respiratory distress syndrome (ARDS) and required further intensive-care support before being discharged on day 20. Hemodialysis was continued on an outpatient basis for one further week, but by day 35 both the blood urea and creatinine were normal without renal support (Le *et al.*, 1994).

12.7.2   Cases affected by additional factors

There have been three reports of acute renal failure following the use of NSAIDs after binge drinking (Blau, 1987; Elsasser *et al.*, 1988; Wen *et al.*, 1992). In these, the patients all reported flank/low back pain for which they took ibuprofen in repeated high therapeutic/excessive doses. There was biopsy evidence of acute tubular necrosis and it seems likely that these findings could be transferable to all NSAIDs since similar observations were made in a patient who took aspirin (Wen *et al.*, 1992). All these patients recovered over several days with symptomatic management for acute renal failure and none required dialysis.

Acute renal failure was reported in a previously healthy 25-year-old soldier who developed a severe dental infection/abscess but could not report immediately for treatment. He took twice the normal maximum dose of ibuprofen for 5 days and was febrile and anuric on admission. He recovered without recourse to dialysis and returned to active duties one week after discharge from hospital (Shelley *et al.*, 1994).

The patient described above was previously fit and knew that he was taking an excessive dose of ibuprofen. In another case, however, a 73-year-old male with known chronic renal failure took the correct lower dose of ibuprofen (1.2 g daily) for one week and developed acute on chronic renal failure (Spierto *et al.*, 1992). He had previously been warned against the use of Motrin (a brand of ibuprofen in the United States) but had self-medicated with Advil, unaware that the two drugs were the same. He recovered his previous renal function after 3 days in hospital.

Most recently, Mattana *et al.* (1997) reported the case of a 41-year-old male who, after ingesting 36 g of ibuprofen over a 3–4 day period, developed renal failure. He had a long history of drug abuse and took the ibuprofen for symptomatic relief of painful leg ulcers caused by skin-popping. He presented with pulmonary oedema, bradycardia and severe renal failure that required emergency treatment by hemodialysis. He was subsequently found to be HIV-positive but he did not have AIDS and responded to treatment, although requiring regular dialysis. After several months there was a gradual improvement in renal function, sufficient to allow dialysis to be discontinued. Unfortunately, at that stage he was lost to follow-up.

Acute renal insufficiency has also been described in a 2-year-old child after a massive accidental ingestion of ibuprofen equivalent to 640 mg/kg and associated with a plasma ibuprofen concentration at 4 h, more than 6 times the maximum therapeutic level (Kim *et al.*, 1995). Normalization of renal function occurred after 12 h.

In summary, therefore, the expected nephrotoxicity has been demonstrated after both acute and chronic ibuprofen overdosage. Its frequency, however, is low and is related either to massive doses (greater than 400 mg/kg) or to complicating factors such as underlying chronic renal disease, serious infection or the metabolic consequences of binge drinking. Treatment is supportive and recovery of normal renal function is often rapid without hemodialysis. Nevertheless, there are well-described cases where dialysis has been life-saving and recovery of renal function has occurred after several months.

Attention must be given to the information provided to patients on the risks of ibuprofen toxicity, particularly nephrotoxicity, in order to prevent patients inadvertently taking chronic overdoses by consuming more than one brand of medication containing the same active ingredient.

12.8 METABOLIC EFFECTS

Metabolic acidosis is an uncommon but initially alarming clinical finding in both adults and children after acute ibuprofen overdosage. It appears to be mainly dose-related but may also be influenced by co-ingested drugs and other problems, notably renal failure (Halpern *et al.*, 1993).

The most severe case so far reported (Downie *et al.*, 1993) involved a 33-year-old male who ingested 60 g of ibuprofen, 250 mg of diclofenac and ethanol. He was admitted 9 h after ingestion, unconscious and hypotensive with small, reactive pupils and no spontaneous movements. Investigation demonstrated a severe metabolic acidosis (pH 7.0, P_{CO_2} 4.0 kPa, P_{O_2}, 17.8 kPa, HCO_3^- 9.3 mmol/l, base excess −22.6 mmol/l). There was mild renal impairment and the toxicology screen demonstrated ibuprofen 1000 mg/l, ethanol 1.1 g/l with no diclofenac or other drugs detected. Resuscitation with 7.5 litres of crystalloid and 3.5 litres of colloid over 12 h resulted in prompt recovery of blood pressure and renal output. Initially the acidosis worsened, but this responded to slow administration of 200 mmol of 8.4% high-strength sodium bicarbonate and the patient regained consciousness after 24 h. He made a complete recovery and was discharged after several days.

Similar cases have been reported in children by Linden and Townsend (1987), typically with a pH as low as 7.27 and ibuprofen concentrations over 600 mg/l. Recovery with prompt treatment was rapid and followed a similar pattern to that described in adults.

To date, no concentrations of ibuprofen metabolites have been measured in cases of metabolic acidosis following ibuprofen overdosage. One could surmise, however, that, although both the parent drug and the metabolites would contribute to the acidosis, they might not explain its severity. It might be predicted, therefore, that there would be a degree of inhibition of oxidative metabolism similar to that seen in salicylate poisoning. Whatever the mechanism, rapid treatment, combined with the effects of rapid metabolism and excretion of the ibuprofen/metabolites appears to account for the short critical period in most cases unless there is pre-existing renal failure.

12.9   CENTRAL NERVOUS SYSTEM (CNS) EFFECTS

CNS depression, from drowsiness to coma, may occur in ibuprofen overdosage in addition to nystagmus, blurred vision, tinnitus, dizziness and headache. In most patients, however, these effects are transient and are not severe, with recovery occurring over 12–24 h. McElwee *et al.* (1990) reported such symptoms in 99 (30%) of 329 patients but others, including Hall *et al.* (1986), found the incidence of these effects to be nearer 20% and even lower in children. These differences probably relate primarily to dosage and to the presence or absence of co-ingested drugs.

The few cases of severe coma related to overdosage of ibuprofen alone have all been associated with acidosis and renal impairment (see above).

The role of co-ingestants was reviewed by Halpern *et al.* (1993), who concluded that the contribution of the individual drugs to the CNS effects experienced was often difficult to determine. They noted that hypotension may have been a factor in some cases.

On balance, therefore, management of CNS effects is of concern only infrequently after ibuprofen overdosage. There is no antidote, but equally there is probably no risk of interaction if the commonly used antidotes naloxone or flumazenil are given in the belief that opioids or benzodiazapines have been ingested/co-ingested. Coma due to acidosis responds to treatment of that cause and otherwise the clinician needs to bear in mind the possibility that CNS depression in ibuprofen overdosage may be due to co-ingestants and thus to investigate and treat accordingly.

12.10   CARDIOVASCULAR EFFECTS

Hypotension and arrhythmias (both tachycardia and bradycardia) were recorded in only 14 (4.3%) of the series of ibuprofen overdose cases reported by McElwee *et al.* (1990), and Halpern *et al.* (1993) found that such effects were only generally seen in cases where there were known co-ingestants. More recently, McCune and O'Brien (1993) reported a 35-year-old male with a previous history of chest pain from oesophagitis and an identified mild mitral regurgitation who developed atrial fibrillation after an overdose of 12 g of ibuprofen. He was given treatment with amiodarone for 3 days before reverting to sinus rhythm. ECG investigations demonstrated a short PR interval, indicating that a possible hidden accessory pathway could have been a predisposing factor. On balance, cardiovascular effects in ibuprofen overdose are infrequent and require only supportive treatment.

12.11   RESPIRATORY EFFECTS

Drug-induced asthma from ibuprofen and aspirin is a well-recognized side-effect and there appears to be complete or near-complete cross-sensitivity. Deaths have been reported in such cases (Antonicelli and Tagliabracci, 1995) and it might be predicted, therefore, that asthma or bronchitis could be precipitated after an ibuprofen overdose. No such cases have been reported; on the contrary, beneficial anti-inflammatory effects have been claimed in patients with cystic fibrosis after long-term treatment with ibuprofen in 20–30 mg/kg doses (Konstan *et al.*, 1995).

Occasional symptoms of dyspnoea or painful breathing have been reported (McElwee *et al.*, 1990; Hall *et al.*, 1986). A 16-month-old child who was involved in an accidental overdose of ibuprofen developed an apnoeic episodes and seizures and suffered a fatal aspiration pneumonia (Hall *et al.*, 1986). Fortunately, this experience does not appear to have been repeated in other cases and, overall, it appears that specific attention to respiratory function is generally not required in ibuprofen overdosage.

12.12   HEMATOLOGICAL EFFECTS

Although hematological adverse effects (aplastic anemia, agranulocytosis, thrombocytopenia) from therapeutic doses of ibuprofen are rare, they have accounted for a disproportionate number of deaths (Halpern *et al.*, 1993). No serious hematological effects have been described after ibuprofen overdose, although thrombocytopenia occurred in one patient who also suffered hepatorenal and respiratory failure (Lee and Finkler, 1986). Full recovery was reported.

12.13   SKIN REACTIONS

Although skin reactions represent the second most frequent type of ADR from ibuprofen, none have been reported after overdosage.

12.14   IBUPROFEN TOXICITY IN CHILDREN

In the above review, observations on children have been included where they contribute to the overall assessment of toxicity. It is important, however, to recognize that the usage of ibuprofen in children differs from that in adults, principally in its role as an antipyretic syrup that is now available both on prescription and, for children over 1 year of age, over the counter.

The debate on the value and safety of antipyretic drugs in childhood fever continues and in the case of ibuprofen there have been calls for randomized controlled trials (Mitchell and Lesko, 1995) and somewhat alarmist debates on the severity of its adverse effects in this age group (Anonymous, 1991; Casteels-Van Daele, 1991; Choonara *et al.*, 1992; Debuse, 1992; Kluger, 1992; Pisacane, 1992). The resolution of that debate is outside the remit of this review, but it is probably worth noting that pharmacokinetic studies of ibuprofen in children did not reveal any unexpected findings (Kauffman and Nelson, 1992), while a practitioner-based randomized clinical trial of paediatric ibuprofen versus paracetamol involving nearly 84 000 children (Lesko and Mitchell, 1996) demonstrated that the incidence of gastrointestinal bleeding, acute renal failure and anaphylaxis was not increased.

In acute overdosage it appears that children can suffer the same range of problems as adults. There have been case reports of transient renal impairment (Kim *et al.*, 1995; Kovesi *et al.*, 1998), acidosis (Linden and Townsend, 1986; Zuckerman and Uy, 1995) and coma (Garrettson *et al.*, 1982; Perry *et al*; 1987; Court *et al.*, 1991). All of these cases recovered with conventional treatment. Serious cases are extremely rare and we have only found one published report of death (Hall *et al.*, 1986).

There are probably other, unpublished, cases of serious toxicity, but it seems likely that any truly new observations would have been reported in the literature or to the regulatory agencies. On balance, therefore, we could conclude that ibuprofen is no more toxic in children than in adults and that the high incidence of asymptomatic cases after childhood accidents with ibuprofen is related to the fact that in most cases the dosage is below that at which symptoms occur and to the absence of co-ingested drugs or underlying disease.

These conclusions do not remove the need for careful monitoring and reporting of all cases of serious childhood poisoning due to ibuprofen, particularly following the OTC licensing of ibuprofen syrup. A continuing vigilance for the unexpected is required.

12.15 IBUPROFEN IN PREGNANCY AND BREAST FEEDING

The use of ibuprofen in pregnancy is not contraindicated, although physicians are recommended to consider alternatives and users of the OTC product are cautioned to consult their doctor. Nevertheless, it seems likely that many patients will receive ibuprofen during pregnancy either as treatment started before conception was diagnosed or because the drug was considered necessary. It is reassuring, therefore, that a review of maternal and fetal considerations in NSAID therapy concluded that there was no evidence to link ibuprofen with congenital defects and that ibuprofen is compatible with breast feeding (Schoenfeld *et al.*, 1992).

12.16 CHRONIC ABUSE OF IBUPROFEN

Analgesic abuse with aspirin and phenacetin was unrecognized for many years, and led to an epidemic of analgesic nephropathy often leading to death from renal failure or a need

CHAPTER 12

for dialysis/transplantation (Dubach *et al.*, 1991). By the time ibuprofen became available for non-prescription use, doctors were well aware of the possible dangers from chronic analgesic abuse and the product was licensed with a clear indication that it was not to be used regularly for more than 72 h without consulting a doctor. In spite of this, it is inevitable that some patients will misuse this drug and suffer avoidable adverse effects, notably gastrointestinal bleeding and acute renal failure.

To date, however, there have been no reports of analgesic abuse with ibuprofen either for supposed psychological effect or for relief of chronic pain on a scale similar to the earlier experience with OTC analgesics. It might be hoped that such problems would not arise, since there is no evidence to suggest that ibuprofen has effects that would make it a likely candidate for abuse and there is extensive knowledge of the long-term use of ibuprofen in the management of patients with rheumatoid disease. In addition, the OTC products have been licensed with a very clear indication that they should not be used continuously for more than 72 h unless a doctor has been consulted.

12.17   CONCLUSIONS

12.17.1   Management of ibuprofen overdosage

The accumulated experience of ibuprofen overdosage is now such that it is possible to summarize the expected toxic effects and their duration according to estimated dose and time of ingestion. This is presented in Table 12.5, which is based on the experience of the National Poisons Information Service (London) and is compatible with information given on the computerized poisons information system *Toxbase* (Scottish Poisons Information Bureau, 1998) and *Poisindex* (Rumack *et al.*, 1998).

12.17.2   Continuing surveillance

After more than 14 years' experience of the wider OTC use of ibuprofen, it is tempting to suggest that we now know all that is necessary about its effect in overdose. Such a view may prove to be correct, but we would suggest that, given the relatively small numbers of reports of serious poisoning, continuing surveillance is necessary and all severely poisoned cases should be reported to Poisons Information Centres.

12.17.3   Comparative human toxicity — Ibuprofen versus other NSAIDs and non-opioid analgesics

Acute analgesic poisoning has been prominent among the problems referred to Poisons Information Centres since their origins more than forty years ago. Although it seems unlikely that anything could be done to completely prevent the problem without seriously

TABLE 12.5

Management of ibuprofen overdose

	Treatment at dose ingested		
	< 100 mg/kg	100–400 mg/kg	> 400 mg/kg
Children	Supportive care	Activated charcoal 1 g/kg within 1 h of ingestion Observation for 4 h minimum.	Activated charcoal 1 g/kg within 1 h of ingestion Observation for 4 h minimum with symptomatic care Maintain good urine output and monitor renal function as required
Adults (Ingested doses tend not to correlate well with clinical effects therefore all patients should be treated symptomatically)	Supportive care	Activated charcoal within 1 h of ingestion Observation for 4 h minimum	Gastric lavage within 1 h of ingestion followed by activated charcoal. Observation for 4 h minimum with symptomatic care. Maintain good urine output and monitor renal function as required

Cautions

Patients with any of the following conditions should be treated symptomatically after exposure to any dose of ibuprofen:
- history of peptic ulceration
- aspirin sensitivity
- asthma
- bleeding disorders
- renal, hepatic or cardiac impairment

restricting access to an essential form of treatment, this should not be used as an excuse for inaction.

We have reviewed both the history and current situation with respect to acute human toxicity from NSAIDs and non-opioid analgesics in both adults and children (Volans and Fitzpatrick, 1998), and were able to conclude that ibuprofen in overdosage is safer than paracetamol, aspirin and some other NSAIDs such as mefenamic acid. Thus, the wider OTC use of ibuprofen can be seen as a measure to improve drug safety.

We further suggested that a review of measures to improve safety, including restriction of OTC availability, and to improve product information was long overdue. It is note-worthy, therefore, that a review by the Medicines Control Agency in the United Kingdom has resulted in new legislation for OTC aspirin and paracetamol that will reduce the pack sizes and introduce additional, carefully worded statements about the risks associated with overdosage (Department of Health, 1997). OTC ibuprofen was not affected by these changes. In conclusion, we believe that these recent measures support our views on the safety of ibuprofen in overdosage. We consider, however, that the effectiveness of the new measures needs to be monitored and our surveillance programme will continue. We note also that, in some countries, the NSAIDs ketoprofen and piroxicam have now been given OTC licences, and no doubt other NSAIDs will also be given OTC licences in the future. In each case, it will be important to confirm that safety in overdosage is comparable to that now established for ibuprofen.

REFERENCES

AMERICAN HOME PRODUCTS CORPORATION (1983) *Summary of Safety and Efficacy Data for Advil (Ibuprofen) submitted to the Food and Drug Administration.*

ANONYMOUS (1991) Management of childhood fever. *Lancet* **338**, 1049–1050.

ANTONICELLI, L. and TAGLIABRACCI, A. (1995) Asthma death induced by ibuprofen. *Monaldi Archives for Chest Disease* 50, 76–78.

BENNETT, R.R., DUNKELBERG, J.C. and MARKS, E.S. (1985) Acute oliguric renal failure due to ibuprofen overdose. *Southern Medical Journal* 78, 490–491.

BERNSTEIN, G., JEHLE, D., BERNASKI, E. and BRAEN, G.R. (1992) Failure of gastric emptying and charcoal administration in fatal sustained release theophylline overdose: phar-macobezoar formation. *Annals of Emergency Medicine* 21, 1388–1390.

BLAU, E. B. (1987) Ibuprofen and ethanol overdose-induced acute tubular necrosis. *Wisconsin Medical Journal* 86, 23–24.

BOOTS COMPANY plc (1982) *Summary of Safety and Efficacy Data Submitted to the Committee on the Safety of Medicines for Nurofen (Ibuprofen).*

CASTEELS-VAN DAELE, M. (1991) Management of childhood fever. *Lancet* **338**, 1408.

CHOONARA, I., NUNN, A.J. and BARKER, C. (1992) Drugs for childhood fever. *Lancet* **339**, 69–70.

CLARK, R., THOMPSON, R.P.H., BORIRAKCHANYAVAT, V., WIDDOP, B., DAVIDSON, A.R., GOULDING, R. and WILLIAMS, R. (1973) Hepatic damage and death from overdose of paracetamol. *Lancet* **i**, 66.

COURT, H., STREETE, P.J. and VOLANS, G.N. (1981) Overdose with ibuprofen causing unconsciousness and hypotension. *British Medical Journal* **282**, 1073.

COURT, H., STREETE, P. and VOLANS, G.N. (1983) Acute poisoning with ibuprofen. *Human Toxicology* **2**, 381–384.

DEPARTMENT OF HEALTH (1997) New measures to improve safety of over-the-counter painkillers, Press Release, 97/204 (26 Aug.).

DEBUSE, P. (1992) Drugs for childhood fever. *Lancet* **339**, 70.

DOWNIE, A., ALI, A. and BELL, D. (1993) Severe metabolic acidosis complicating massive ibuprofen overdose. *Postgraduate Medical Journal* **69**, 575–577.

DUBACH, U.C., ROSNER, B. and STURMER, T. (1991) An epidemiological study of abuse of analgesic drugs: effects of phenacetin and salicylate on mortality and cardiovascular morbidity (1968–1987). *New England Journal of Medicine* **324**, 155–160.

ELSASSER, G.N., LOPEZ, L. and EVANS, E. (1988) Reversible acute renal failure associated with ibuprofen ingestion and binge drinking. *Journal of Family Practice* **27**, 221–222.

GARRETTSON, L.K., GOPLERUD, J.M. and SAADY, J.J. (1982) Ibuprofen overdose with sedation. *Veterinary and Human Toxicology* **23**(Suppl. 1), 48.

GUNNEL, D., HAWTON, K., MURRAY, V., GARNIER, R., BISMUTH, C., FAGG, J. and SIMKIN, S. (1997) Use of paracetamol for suicide and non-fatal poisoning in the UK and France: are restrictions on availability justified? *Journal of Epidemiology and Community Health* **51**, 175–179.

HALL, A.H. and RUMACK, B.H. (1988) Treatment of patients with ibuprofen overdose. *Annals of Emergency Medicine* **17**, 184–185.

HALL, A.H., SMOLINSKI, F.C. and CONRAD, F.L. (1986) Ibuprofen overdose: 126 cases. *Annals of Emergency Medicine* **15**, 1308–1313.

HALL, A.H., SMOLINSKI, F.C., KULIG, K. and RUMACK, B.H. (1988) Ibuprofen overdose — a prospective study. *Western Journal of Medicine* **148**, 653–656.

HALL, A.H., SMOLINSKI, F.C., STOVER, B., CONRAD, F.L. and RUMACK, B.H. (1992) Ibuprofen overdose in adults. *Clinical Toxicology* **30**, 23–37.

HALPERN, S.M., FITZPATRICK, R. and VOLANS, G.N. (1993) Ibuprofen toxicity. A review of adverse reactions and overdose. *Adverse Drug Reactions and Toxicological Reviews* **12**, 107–128.

CHAPTER 12

HAWTON, K. and FAGG, J. (1992) Trends in deliberate self poisoning and self injury in Oxford, 1976–90. *British Medical Journal* **304**, 1409–1410.

JENKINSON, M.L., FITZPATRICK, R., STREETE, P.J. and VOLANS, G.N. (1988) The relationship between plasma ibuprofen concentrations and toxicity in acute ibuprofen overdose. *Human Toxicology* **7**, 319–324.

KAUFFMAN, R.E. and NELSON, M.V. (1992) Effect of age on ibuprofen pharmacokinetics and antipyretic response. *Journal of Pediatrics* **121**, 969–973.

KIM, J., GAZARIAN, M., VERJEE, Z. and JOHNSON, D. (1995) Acute renal insufficiency in ibuprofen overdose. *Paediatric Emergency Care* **11**, 107–108.

KLUGER, M.J. (1992) Drugs for childhood fever. *Lancet* **339**, 70.

KONSTAN, M.W., BYARD, P.J., HOPPEL, C.L. and DAVIS, P.B. (1995) Effect of high-dose ibuprofen in patients with cystic fibrosis. *New England Journal of Medicine* **332**, 848–854.

KOVESI, T.A., SWARTZ, R. and MACDONALD, N. (1998) Transient renal failure due to simultaneous ibuprofen and aminoglycoside therapy in children with cystic fibrosis. *New England Journal of Medicine* **338**, 65.

KUNSMAN, G.W. and ROHIG, T.P. (1993) Tissue distribution of ibuprofen in a fatal overdose. *American Journal of Forensic Medicine and Pathology* **14**, 48–50.

LE, H.T., BOSSE, G.M. and TSAIM, Y. (1994) Ibuprofen overdose complicated by renal failure, adult respiratory distress syndrome, and metabolic acidosis. *Journal of Toxicology and Clinical Toxicology* **32**, 315–320.

LEE, C.Y. and FINKLER, A. (1986) Acute intoxication due to ibuprofen overdose. *Archives of Pathology and Laboratory Medicine* **110**, 747–749.

LESKO, S.M. and MITCHELL, A.A. (1995) An assessment of the safety of pediatric ibuprofen. A practitioner-based randomized clinical trial. *Journal of the American Medical Association* **273**, 929–933.

LEVINE, B., JONES, R., SMITH, M.L., GUDEWICZ, T.M. and PETERSON, B. (1993) A multiple drug intoxication involving cyclobenzaprine and ibuprofen. *American Journal of Forensic Medicine and Pathology* **14**, 246–248.

LINDEN, C.H. and TOWNSEND, P.L. (1987) Metabolic acidosis after acute ibuprofen overdosage. *Journal of Pediatrics* **11**, 922–925.

LITOVITZ, T.L., SMILKSTEIN, M., FELBERG, L., KLEIN-SCHWARTZ, W., BERLIN, R. and MORGAN, J.L. (1997) Annual Report of the American Association of Poison Control Centers Toxic Exposure Surveillance System. *American Journal of Emergency Medicine* **15**, 447–500.

MATTANA, J., PERINHASEKAR, S. and BROD-MILLER, C. (1997) Near-fatal but reversible acute renal failure after massive ibuprofen ingestion. *American Journal of the Medical Sciences* **313**, 117–119.

McELWEE, N.E., VELTRI, J.C., BRADFORD, D.C. and ROLLINS, D.E. (1990) A prospective, population based study of acute ibuprofen overdose: complications are rare and routine serum levels not warranted. *Annals of Emergency Medicine* **19**, 657–662.

McCUNE, K.H. and O'BRIEN, C.J. (1993) Atrial fibrillation induced ibuprofen overdose. *Postgraduate Medical Journal* **69**, 325–326.

MITCHELL, A.A. and LESKO, S.M. (1995) When a randomised controlled trial is needed to assess drug safety. The case of paediatric ibuprofen. *Drug Safety* **13**, 15–24.

NATIONAL POISONS INFORMATION SERVICE MONITORING GROUP (1981) Analgesic poisoning: A multi-centre prospective survey. *Human Toxicology* **1**(7), 23–25.

NATIONAL POISONS INFORMATION SERVICE (London), unpublished, *Annual Report 1996*.

PERRY, S.J., STREETE, P.J. and VOLANS, G.N. (1987) Ibuprofen overdose: the first two years of over-the-counter sales. *Human Toxicology* **6**, 173–178.

RUMACK, B.H., RIDER, P.K. and GELMAN, C.R. (eds) (1998) *Poisindex(R) System*. Englewood, CO, Micromedex Inc.

PISACANE, A. and SIMEONE, C. (1992) Drugs for childhood fever. *Lancet* **339**, 70.

SCOTTISH POISONS INFORMATION BUREAU (1998) *TOXBASE Clinical Toxicology Database*. Edinburgh, Scottish Poisons Information Bureau.

SCHOENFIELD, A., BAR, Y., MERLOB, P. and OVADIA, Y. (1992) NSAIDs: maternal and fetal considerations. *American Journal of Reproductive Immunology* **28**, 141–147.

SHELLEY, J.J., SHIPMAN, G.L. and HECHT, R.C. (1994) Adverse reaction to ibuprofen overdose. *General Dentistry* **42**, 414–416.

SPIERTO, R.J., KAUFMAN, M.B. and STOUKIDES, C.A. (1992) Acute renal failure associated with the use of over-the-counter ibuprofen. *Annals of Pharmacotherapy* **26**, 714.

STEINMETZ, J.C., LEE, C.Y. and WU, A.Y. (1987) Tissue levels of ibuprofen after fatal overdosage of ibuprofen and acetaminophen. *Veterinary and Human Toxicology* **29**, 381–383.

VOLANS, G.N. and FITZPATRICK, R. (1998) Acute human toxicity from NSAIDs and analgesics. In RAINSFORD, K.D. and POWANDA, M.C. (eds), *Safety and Efficacy of Non-prescription (OTC) Analgesics and NSAIDs*. Dordrecht, Kluwer Academic Publishers, 93–100.

WEN, S.F., PARTHASARATHY, R., ILIOPOULOS, O. and OBERLEY, T.D. (1992) Acute renal failure following binge drinking and nonsteroidal anti-inflammatory drugs. *American Journal of Kidney Diseases* **20**, 281–285.

WOLFE, T. (1995) Ibuprofen overdose. *American Journal of Emergency Medicine* **13**, 375.

ZUCKERMAN, G.B. and UY, C.C. (1995) Shock, metabolic acidosis and coma following ibuprofen overdose in a child. *Annals of Pharmacotherapy* **29**, 869.

CHAPTER 12

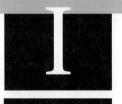

Some Brands of Ibuprofen in Various Countries

Brand name	Composition	Manufacturer
UNITED KINGDOM		
Nurofen	200 mg coated tablets 400 mg coated tablets Microgranules 400 mg powders Soluble 200 mg tablets 400 mg coated tablets Gel 5%	Crookes Healthcare, Nottingham
Cuprofen	400 mg coated tablets 200 mg coated tablets Soluble 200 mg effervescent tablets	Seton, Manchester
Advil	200 mg coated tablets 400 mg coated tablets	Whitehall Labs, Maidenhead
Nurofen Plus	200 mg coated tablets/codeine 12.5 mg	Crookes Healthcare, Nottingham
Ibuleve	Gel 5% Spray 5% Sports gel 5%	Dendron, Watford
Nurofen Cold & Flu	200 mg/pseudoephedrine 30 mg tablets	Crookes Healthcare, Nottingham
Ibugel	Gel 5%	Dermal, Hitchin
Hedex Ibuprofen	200 mg coated tablets	SB Consumer Healthcare, Brentford
Junifen	100 mg/5 ml suspension	Crookes Healthcare, Nottingham
Solpaflex	200 mg tablets/codeine 12.5 mg	SmithKline Beecham, Brentford
Proflex	Cream 5% 300 mg sustained release capsules 200 mg coated tablets	Novartis Consumer, Horsham
Deep Relief	Gel 5%	Mentholatum, Glasgow
Reclofen	400 mg tablets 200 mg tablets	Cox, Barnstaple
Fenbid	Gel 5%	Goldshield, Croydon
Lemsip Power+	Powders 400 mg/pseudoephedrine 60 mg	Reckitt and Colman, Hull
Vicks Action	Cold & Flu 200 mg/pseudoephedrine 30 mg coated tablets	Proctor and Gamble H/C, Weybridge
Ibuspray	Spray 5%	Dermal, Hitchin
Radian B Ibuprofen	Gel 5%	Roche Consumer HTH, Welwyn Garden City
Librofem	200 mg tablets	Novartis Consumer, Horsham
Inoven	200 mg coated tablets	J and J MSD Consumer, High Wycombe
Phor Pain	200 mg coated tablets 400 mg coated tablets	Goldshield, Croydon

Brand name	Composition	Manufacturer
Pacifene	400 mg coated tablets 200 mg coated tablets	Sussex Pharm., East Grinstead
Migrafen	200 mg coated tablets	Chatfield Labs, London
Anadin	Ibuprofen 200 mg tablets	Whitehall Labs, Maidenhead
Femafen	200 mg capsules	Roche Consumer Healthcare, Welwyn Garden City
Novaprin	200 mg tablets	Pharmexco
Seclodin	200 mg capsules	Whitehall Labs, Maidenhead
UNITED STATES Advil	200 mg tablets 200 mg film-coated tablets 200 mg gel caplet 200 mg gelatin-coated tablet	Whitehall-Robins
Motrin IB	200 mg tablets 200 mg gelatin-coated tablets	Upjohn
Children's Motrin	100 mg/5 ml suspension 100 mg film-coated tablets 400 mg/1 ml drops oral 50 mg chewable tablets	Upjohn
Advil Cold & Sinus	200 30 mg film-coated tablets 200 30 mg coated tablets	Whitehall-Robins
Nuprin	200 mg tablets 200 mg coated tablets	
Advil Children's	100 mg/5 ml suspension	Whitehall-Robins
Motrin IB Sinus	200 mg/pseudoephedrine 30 mg tablets	Upjohn
Dimetapp All/Sinus	Film-coated tablets	Whitehall-Robins
Midol IB	200 mg tablets	
Arthritis Foundation Ibuprofen	200 mg tablets	
Nuprin Backache	200 mg film-coated tablets	
Bayer Select Arthritis	200 mg film-coated tablets	Bayer
Haltran	200 mg tablets	
Exedrin 1B	200 mg caplets 200 mg film-coated tablets 200 mg tablets	
Dimetapp Sinus	200 mg coated tablets	Whitehall-Robins
Ibuprin	200 mg coated tablets	
Aches-N-Pain	200 mg tablets	
Medipren	200 mg film-coated tablets 200 mg tablets	

Brand name	Composition	Manufacturer
Midol 200	200 mg tablets	
Pamprin-Ib	200 mg coated tablets	
Trendar	200 mg tablets	
SPAIN		
Nurofen	400 mg coated tablets 200 mg coated tablets	Boots Healthcare
Dorival	200 mg tablets	Bayer, Barcelona
Doctril	200 mg coated tablets	Abello, Madrid
Nurogrip	200 mg/pseudoephedrine 300 mg coated tablets	
Salvarina	200 mg capsules	Salvat, Barcelona
Leonal	200 mg tablets	Byk, Leo
Altior	200 mg capsules	Penser
Isdol	200 mg tablets	Isdin, Barcelona
Aldospray Analges	Aero pres.aero.top 5% spray	Ado Union
Kalma	200 mg powders	Schering Plough, Madrid
Noalgil	200 mg coated tablets	Pharmacia Upjon, Barcelona
Narfen	200 mg tablets	Alter, Madrid
Sadefen	200 mg coated tablets	Roche Nicolas
Cusialgil	200 mg tablets	Cusi
Liderfeme	200 mg powders	Farmalider
FRANCE		
Advil	200 mg coated tablets	Whitehall, Paris
Nureflex	200 mg coated tablets	Boots Healthcare, Courbevoie
Rhinadvil	200 mg/pseudoephedrine 30 mg tablets	Whitehall, Paris
Nurofen	200 mg coated tablets	Boots Healthcare, Courbevoie
Intralgis	Gel 5%	Urgo, Chenove
Ibutop	Gel 5% gel	Chefaro Ardeval, Saint Denis
Rhinureflex	200 mg/pseudoephedrine 30 mg film-coated tablets	Boots Healthcare, Courbevoie
Gelufene	200 mg capsules, 5% gel	Cooper Melun, Melun
Tiburon	Gel 5% gel 200 mg capsules	Lipha Monot, Lyon
Vicks Rhume	200 mg/pseudoephedrine 30 mg tablets	Lachartre, Neuilly-Sur-Seine
Ergix	200 mg film-coated tablets	Lipha Monot, Lyon
Dogit	Cream 5%	Lipha Sante, Lyon

Brand name	Composition	Manufacturer
Oralfene	200 mg capsules	Pierre Fabre Santé, Boulogne
Algifene	200 mg layered tablets	Roche Nicholas, Gaillard
Analfene	200 mg film-coated tablets RPG 200 mg capsules	Bouchara, Levallois Perret
Antarene	200 mg tablets	Elerte, Aubervilliers
Analgyl	200 mg layered tablets	Rhôn-Poulenc Rorer, Antony
Solufen	200 mg capsules	Galephar, Erstein
ITALY Moment	200 mg coated tablets Drops oral 200 mg powders	Angelini Francesco
Antalgil	200 mg tablets	Johnson and Johnson, Pomezia
Nurofen	200 mg coated tablets	Boots Healthcare, Nottingham
Algofen	200 mg coated tablets	Restiva
Calmine	200 mg capsules	SIT, Mede
Dolocyl	200 mg enteric-CT tablets	Sandoz, Milano
Brufen Crema	10% cream	Rivizza
Neo Mindol	200 mg capsules	Bracco, Milano
Brufort	Ointment 10%	Lampugnani
Arfen Pronto	1.4 g vaginal liquid	Lisapharma
Arfen	Gel 10%	Lisapharma
Prontalgin	200 mg tablets	SPA
GERMANY Dolormin	200 mg film-coated tablets 200 mg effervescent tablets	Woelm Pharma, Eschwege
Aktren	200 mg coated tablets 200 mg powders	Bayer, Leverkusen
Ibutop	Cream 5% Gel 5%	Chefaro Deutsch, Waltrop
Optalidon 200	200 mg film-coated tablets 200 mg effervescent tablets	Novartis Consumer Healthcare
Pfeil Azhnschmerz	200 mg film-coated tablets	Stada, Bad Vibel
Dolgit	Cream 5%	Dolorgiet, Bonn
Dismenol N	200 mg film-coated tablets	Merz, Frankfurt
Ilvico Grippal	200 mg tablets	Merck, Darmstadt
Vivmed	200 mg film-coated tablets	Dr Mann Pharma, Berlin
Dolgit Mikrogel	Gel 5%	Dolorgiet, Bonn
Urem	200 mg coated tablets	Kade, Berlin

Brand name	Composition	Manufacturer
Mensoton 200	200 mg tablets	Berlin Chem/Menari, Berlin
Dolo-Sanol	200 mg film-coated tablets	Sanol, Monheim
Ibu 200	200 mg coated tablets	Bipharm
Togal N	200 mg film-coated tablets	Togal, Munich
Seclodin	200 mg coated tablets	Whitehall-Much, Haan
Imbun	200 mg effervescent tablets	Merckle, Ulm
Trauma Dolgit	Gel 5%	Dolorgiet, Bonn
Dimidon	200 mg film-coated tablets	Samedpharm
Denitigoa Forte	200 mg film-coated tablets	Scheurich, Appenweler
Contraneural	200 mg film-coated tablets	Pfleger, Bamberg
Gynofug	200 mg film-coated tablets	Wolff Bielefeld, Bielefeld
Tempil	200 mg soluble tablets	Temmler, Marburg
Ibumerck	200 mg film-coated tablets	Merck Generika, Darmstadt
Jenaprofen	200 mg film-coated tablets	Jenapharm, Jena
Fibraflex	200 mg film-coated tablets	Nycomed Arzneimittel, Munich
Medokal SL	200 mg tablets	Goldham, Zusmarshausen
Mobilat Schmerztab	200 mg film-coated tablets	Luitpold, Munich
Exneural	200 mg film-coated tablets	BASF Generics, Mannheim
Ibubest	200 mg film-coated tablets	CT Arzneimittel, Berlin
Logomed Schmerz	200 mg film-coated tablets	Merz, Frankfurt
Pyracophen Rapid	200 mg chewable tablets	Wero Medical
Dismenol N	200 mg film-coated tablets	Simons
Fibraflex	200 mg film-coated tablets	Nycomed Arzneimittel, Munich
Stadasan	200 mg film-coated tablets	Stada, Bad Vibel
AUSTRALIA		
Nurofen	200 mg tablet	Boots, Australia
Nurofen Junior	100 mg/5 ml suspension	Boots, Australia
ACT-3	200 mg liquid filled gel capsule 200 mg tablet	
Triprofen	200 mg tablet	
Actiprofen	200 mg tablet	
Brufen	400 mg tablet	Boots, Australia
Rafen	200 mg tablet	

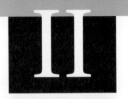

Methods for Analysis of Ibuprofen in Biological Systems

K D RAINSFORD

Division of Biomedical Sciences, Sheffield Hallam University, Pond Street,
Sheffield S1 1WB, UK

Some methods that have been developed for the analysis of ibuprofen and its metabolites in biological matrices are briefly described here. Most modern methods employed for the assay of ibuprofen in plasma or tissues employ high-performance liquid chromatography (HPLC) or gas chromatography (GC) with or without coupled mass spectrometry (GC-MS) (Davies, 1997). It is also often necessary to determine the proportion of the respective enantiomers, and for this chiral chromatographic columns are necessary. A recent review by Davies (1997) gives a detailed assessment of currently available methods and lists a comprehensive selection of stereospecific HPLC assay methods (Table A.1; reproduced with permission of the publishers of *Journal of Chromatography*, Elsevier Science).

Recently, methods have been developed for the analysis of ibuprofen by capillary electrophoresis (Shihabi and Hinsdale, 1996; Reijenga *et al.*, 1997). As applied for the analysis of *rac*-ibuprofen in serum, the method requires that the samples be first deproteinized by addition of acetonitrile; then the extract is applied directly to the capillary column, which is run in 0.15 mol/l borate buffer, pH 8.5 (Reijenga *et al.*, 1997). The method is suitable for analysis of samples containing > 10 µg/ml. A method has been reported for the chiral separation of ibuprofen enantiomers (Williams and Vigh, 1997) that could be applied to analyses in biological matrices.

A non-invasive method for detecting enantiomers and metabolites of ibuprofen *in vivo* has been developed that employs ^{13}C-nuclear magnetic resonance (NMR) spectrometry (Chen *et al.*, 1996). It has been applied for the detection of ibuprofen and metabolites in rats following oral administration of 50–200 mg/kg of (*R*)-(–)- or (*S*)-(+)-[2- ^{2}H,2-^{13}C]ibuprofen. No attempts were made at quantifying the amount of drug present.

REFERENCES

CHEN, C.-N., WANG, P.C., SONG, H.-F., LIU, Y.C. and CHEN, C.-S. (1996) Non-invasive detection of ibuprofen *in vivo* ^{13}C-NMR signals in rats. *Chemical and Pharmaceutical Bulletin* **44**, 204–207.

DAVIES, N.M. (1997) Methods for the analysis of chiral non-steroidal anti-inflammatory drugs. *Journal of Chromatography B* **691**, 229–261.

REIJENGA, J.C., INGELSE, B.A. and EVERAERTS, F.M. (1997) Training software for chiral separations in capillary electrophoresis. *Journal of Chromatography A* **772**, 195–202.

SHIHABI, Z.K. and HINSDALE, M.E. (1996) Analysis of ibuprofen in serum by capillary electrophoresis. *Journal of Chromatography B* **683**, 115–118.

WILLIAMS, B.A. and VIGH, B. (1997) Determination of effective mobilities and chiral separation selectivities from partially separated enantiomer peaks in a racemic mixture using pressure mediated capillary electrophoresis. *Analytical Chemistry* **69**, 4410–4418.

TABLE A.1

Stereospecific Chromatographic (GC, GC-MS or HPLC) assay methods

MQ (mg/l)	V (ml)	DR	MP	λ (nm)	Column	IS	Specimen	Reference
NR	NR	Thionyl chloride, (R)-(+)-α-methylbenzylamine	Nitrogen	NA	U-shaped (5 m × 3 mm I.D.) of 1% OV-17	NR	Urine	(1)
1.0	1.0	Thionyl chloride, 1,1'-carbonyldiimidazole, (S)-(−)-α-methylbenzylamine	Helium, hydrogen, oxygen	NA	U-shaped (1.5 m × 3 mm I.D.) of 3% OV-17	n-Tidecanoic acid	Plasma, urine	(2)
0.5	1	(S)-(+)-2-Octanol	0.05% Isopropyl alcohol in heptane	220	Two 5 μm silica (25 × 0.46 cm)	4-n-Pentyl, phenyl-acetic acid	Plasma, synovial fluid	(3)
10	9.0	Thionyl chloride, benzylamine	Hexane–isopropanol–acetonitrile (95:5:1)	254	DNPG 5 μm (4.6 mm × 25 cm) and MS	NR	Equine urine	(4)
0.05	1.0	(S)-(+)-2-Octanol	NR	NA	GCMS	D14 ibuprofen	Plasma	(5)
0.75	1.0	1,1'-Carbonyldiimidazole, (S)-(+)-amphetamine	Helium, hydrogen, air	NA	Fused-silica capillary (12 m × 0.2 mm I.D.)	p-Methoxy-, phenyl-acetic acid	Plasma, urine	(6)
0.1	NR	1,1'-Carbonyldiimidazole, (S)-(−)-phenylethylamine	NR	NA	DB-5 capillary column (30 m × 0.25 mm)	2-Chlorobiphenylpropionic acid	Plasma, urine	(7)
1.0	0.5	1-Hydroxybenzotriazole, 1-(3-dimethylaminopropyl)-3-ethyl carbodiimide hydrochloride (S)-(−)-1-(1-naphthyl)ethylamine (NEA)	Hexane–ethylacetate (4:1)	254	Hypersil 10 μm (250 × 4.5 mm I.D.)	p-Chlorophenoxyacetic acid	Plasma	(8)
0.1	0.5	Ethylchloroformate, (S)-(−)-1-(1-NEA)	Acetonitrile–water–acetic acid–triethylamine (55:45:0.1:0.02, v/v) pH 4.9	232	Partisil 5-ODS-3 (4.6 mm × 10 cm)	(±)-2-(4-Benzoylphenyl)butyric acid	Plasma	(9)
6.25	1.0	Methylene chloride, ECF, 4-methoxyaniline	Hexane–chloroform–2-propanol (18:2:1)	254	Pirkle covalent column (25 cm × 4.6 mm I.D.) with α-aminopropyl packing packing of 5 μm spherical particles with (R)-N-(3, 5-dinitrobenzoyl)phenylglycine	α-Phenylpropionic acid	Plasma, urine	(10)

0.1	0.5, 0.1, 0.1	NA	Acetonitrile–0.1% triethylammonium acetate buffer (30:70, v/v) pH = 7.5	220	Cyclobond I (250 mm × 4.5 mm I.D.)	NR	Plasma, urine, dog bile	(11)
0.1, 1.0	0.2	Thionyl chloride, (S)-(−)-1-phenylethylamine	Isopropanol–heptane (2.5:97.5)	216	Hibar Lichrosorb 5-Si60 (250 mm × 4 mm I.D.)	NR	Total plasma, unbound plasma	(12)
0.1	0.5	NA	0.5% 2-propanol 5 mmol/l DMOA in 20 mmol/l phosphate buffer (pH 6.7)	220	Enantiopac (100 mm × 4.0 mm I.D.)	(S)-Ketoprofen	Plasma	(13)
1	1.0	NA	1.2% v/v 2-propanol 1.2 mmol/l N,N-dimethyloctylamine (DMOA) in 0.02 mmol/l sodium dihydrogen phosphate	227	Chiral-AGP (100 mm × 4 mm I.D.)	4-Pentyl-phenyl-acetic acid	Plasma	(14)
NR	NR	Thionyl chloride (1R,2S,5R)-(−)-menthol	Hexane–diethyl ether (100:1)	354	2 Whatman Partisil columns 10 μm (2 × 4.6 mm I.D. × 25 cm)	NR	Plasma	(6)
0.25	0.25, 0.5	ECF, (R)-(+)-α-phenylethylamine	Acetonitrile–water–acetic acid–tetraethylamine (46.5: 53.5:0.1:0.03, v/v) pH 4.9	225	Phenomenex C_{18} 5-ODS (10 cm × 4.6 mm I.D.)	Fenoprofen	Rat/human plasma	(15)
0.1	0.5	ECF, (S)-(−)-1-(1-naphthyl)-ethylamine (NEA) acetonitrile	Water–acetic acid–triethylamine (60:40:0.1:0.02, v/v) pH 5.0	Ex 280 Em 320	Partisil 5-ODS-2 RAC II (4.6 mm I.D. × 10 cm)	Fenoprofen	Plasma	(16)
NR	0.5	EEDQ or ECF, (S)-NEA	Acetonitrile–water–acetic acid (55:45:0.1:0.02, v/v)	232	Ultrasphere 5-ODS (100 × 4.6 mm I.D.)	NR	Plasma	(17)
2.5	0.5	EEDQ, p-nitrobenzylamine hydrochloride (PNBA)	Hexane–isopropanol (35:5, v/v)	235	CSP (R)-(−)-(1-naphthyl)ethylurea (100 × 4.6 mm I.D. 3 μm, aminopropyl silanized silica)	Tidecanoid acid	Dog plasma	(17)

TABLE A.1 (continued)

MQ (mg/l)	V (ml)	DR	MP	λ (nm)	Column	IS	Specimen	Reference
0.4	NR	(−)-APMB, DPDS, TPP	NR	Ex 320 Em 380	Reversed-phase column	NR	Rat plasma	(18)
0.003	0.2	ECF, dexamphetamine	Helium	NA	25 m × 0.32 m I.D.	Naproxen	Plasma, synovial fluid	(19)
0.005	0.1	(R)-(−)-2,2,2-trifluoro-1-(9-anthryl)ethanol oxalyl chloride	Helium	BA	2.0 m × 2 mm I.D. glass column	4-methoxyphenyl acetic acid	Plasma	(20)

Abbreviations: MQ, minimum reported quantifiable concentration of each component; V, volume; DR, derivatizing reagent; MP, mobile phase (liquid for HPLC; gas for GC or GC-MS); λ, wavelength of detection (nm) for HPLC; IS, internal standard; NA, not applicable; NR, not reported; ECF, ethyl chlorformate; EEDQ, 2-ethoxy-1-(1-ethoxycarbonyl)-1,2-dihydroquinolone

References: (1) Brooks, C.J.W. and Gilbert, M.T. (1974) *Journal of Chromatography* **99**, 541. (2) Van Gessen, G.J. and Kaiser, D.G. (1975) *Journal of Pharmaceutical Science* **64**, 798. (3) Lee, E.J.D. et al. (1984) *Journal of Pharmaceutical Science* **73**, 1542.
(4) Crowther, J.B. et al. (1984) *Analytical Chemistry* **56**, 2921.
(5) Asami, M. and Nakamura, K.-I. (1995) *Chirality* **7**, 28.
(6) Chen, C.Y. et al. (1991) *Journal of the Formosan Medical Association* **90**, 437.
(7) Young, M.A. et al. (1986) *Journal of Pharmacy and Pharmacology* **38**, 60P.
(8) Averginos, A. and Hutt, A.J. (1987) *Journal of Chromatography* **415**, 75.
(9) Mehvar, R. et al. (1988) *Clinical Chemistry* **34**, 493.
(10) Nicoll-Griffith, D.A. et al. (1988) *Journal of Chromatography* **428**, 103. (11) Geisslinger, G. et al. (1989) *Journal of Chromatography* **491**, 139.
(12) Evans, A.M. et al. (1989) *European Journal of Clinical Pharmacology* **36**, 283.
(13) Mezel-Soglowek, S. et al. (1990) *Journal of Chromatography* **532**, 295.
(14) Petterson, K.J. and Olsson, A. (1991) *Journal of Chromatography* **563**, 414.
(15) Wright, M.A. et al. (1992) *Journal of Chromatography* **583**, 259. (16) Lemko, C.H. et al. (1993) *Journal of Chromatography* **619**, 330.
(17) Ahn, H.Y. et al. (1994) *Journal of Chromatography* A **653**, 163.
(18) Peterson, P. and Markides (1992) *Journal of Chromatography* **584**, 189.
(19) Jack, D.S. et al. (1992) *Journal of Chromatography* **584**, 189.
(20) Zhao, M.-J. et al. (1994) *Journal of Chromatography* A **656**, 441.

Index

Note: references are to *ibuprofen*, except where otherwise stated. Main chapter pages are shown in **bold**.